# Emerging Technologies in Dermatology

# Emerging Technologies in Dermatology

Editor: Adrien Cameron

AMERICAN
MEDICAL PUBLISHERS
www.americanmedicalpublishers.com

AMERICAN
MEDICAL PUBLISHERS
www.americanmedicalpublishers.com

Cataloging-in-Publication Data

Emerging technologies in dermatology / edited by Adrien Cameron.
p. cm.
Includes bibliographical references and index.
ISBN 979-8-88740-091-4
1. Dermatology--Technological innovations. 2. Dermatology.
3. Skin--Diseases--Diagnosis--Technological innovations.
4. Skin--Diseases--Treatment--Technological innovations.
I. Cameron, Adrien.
RL72 .E44 2023



American Medical Publishers,
41 Flatbush Avenue,
1st Floor, New York,
NY 11217, USA

ISBN 979-8-88740-091-4 (Hardback)

# Contents

# Preface

This book aims to highlight the current researches and provides a platform to further the scope of innovations in this area. This book is a product of the combined efforts of many researchers and scientists, after going through thorough studies and analysis from different parts of the world. The objective of this book is to provide the readers with the latest information of the field.

The branch of medicine that deals with the medical and surgical aspects of skin is called dermatology. There are various specialized fields in dermatology such as cosmetic dermatology, dermatopathology, trichology, immunodermatology, Mohs surgery, teledermatology, etc. Immunodermatology is a field that specializes in curing immune-mediated skin diseases such as lupus, bullous pemphigoid, pemphigus vulgaris, etc. Another speciality known as Mohs surgery targets the excision of skin cancers, employing the technique for intraoperative assessment of deep tumor margins. A type of dermatological practice which involves telecommunication technologies to exchange medical information and treatment through audio, visual, and data communication is called teledermatology. Therapies that are used frequently in dermatology include cryosurgery for the treatment of warts, skin cancers and other dermatoses; laser therapy for the treatment of birth marks, skin disorders, tattoo removal and cosmetic rejuvenation; and photodynamic therapy for the treatment of skin cancers and precancerous growth. This book unravels the recent studies in the field of dermatology. Its aim is to present the emerging technologies within this field. This book will serve as a reference to a broad spectrum of readers.

I would like to express my sincere thanks to the authors for their dedicated efforts in the completion of this book. I acknowledge the efforts of the publisher for providing constant support. Lastly, I would like to thank my family for their support in all academic endeavors.

**Editor**

# 1

# Toward Machine-Learning-Based Decision Support in Diabetes Care: A Risk Stratification Study on Diabetic Foot Ulcer and Amputation

*Zeinab Schäfer[1]*, Andreas Mathisen[1], Katrine Svendsen[2], Susanne Engberg[3], Trine Rolighed Thomsen[4,5] and Klaus Kirketerp-Møller[3,6]*

[1] Department of Computer Science, Aarhus University, Aarhus, Denmark, [2] Research Unit for Mental Public Health, Department of Public Health, Aarhus University, Aarhus, Denmark, [3] Steno Diabetes Center, Copenhagen, Denmark, [4] Department of Chemistry and Biosciences, Center for Microbial Communities, Aalborg University, Aalborg, Denmark, [5] Life Science, Danish Technological Institute, Taastrup, Denmark, [6] Department of Dermatology, Venereology and Wounds, Copenhagen Wound Healing Center, Bispebjerg Hospital, Copenhagen, Denmark

***Correspondence:**
*Zeinab Schäfer*
*zeinab.schaefer@cs.au.dk*

Diabetes mellitus is associated with serious complications, with foot ulcers and amputation of limbs among the most debilitating consequences of late diagnosis and treatment of foot ulcers. Thus, prediction and on-time treatment of diabetic foot ulcers (DFU) are of great importance for improving and maintaining patients' quality of life and avoiding the consequent socio-economical burden of amputation. In this study, we use Danish national registry data to understand the risk factors of developing diabetic foot ulcers and amputation among patients with diabetes. We analyze the data of 246,705 patients with diabetes to assess some of the main risk factors for developing DFU/amputation. We study the socioeconomic information and past medical history of the patients. Factors, such as low family disposable income, cardiovascular disorders, peripheral artery, neuropathy, and chronic renal complications are among the important risk factors. Mental disorders and depression, albeit not as pronounced, still pose higher risks in comparison to the group of people without these complications. We further use machine learning techniques to assess the practical usefulness of such risk factors for predicting foot ulcers and amputation. Finally, we outline the limitations of working with registry data sources and explain potentials for combining additional public and private data sources in future applications of artificial intelligence (AI) to improve the prediction of diabetic foot ulcers and amputation.

**Keywords: risk assessment, amputation, prediction models, cohort analyses, diabetic foot ulcer**

## 1. INTRODUCTION

Diabetes mellitus, a worldwide pandemic that is expected to rise to 700 million cases by 2045, is a serious challenge for both patients and healthcare professionals [1]. The alarming numbers in the prevalence of diabetes and the high social and financial costs associated with the disease indicate a pressing need for further improving effective control and prevention strategies [6]. Among the most disabling, complex, and costly complications of diabetes are diabetic foot ulceration (DFU) and amputation [2–5]. Various studies have investigated risk factors for developing DFU [7, 8].

Such studies have traditionally been conducted with controlled cohorts that allow for adjustment of the most likely confounding variables but often with study scale as the main trade-off. However, the abundance of digital medical data available today presents new opportunities to drastically increase the scale of future risk stratification studies and explore different risk factors. Moreover, through the combination of different data sources and incorporating risk analysis studies, it becomes more tractable to develop decision support based on machine learning, e.g., to support early detection or monitoring of certain conditions.

In order to model a decision system that is able to assess the risk of developing DFU/ amputation, it is required to understand the best set of underlying features and how their combination can improve the prediction. In numerous studies, the impact of different socio-economic status of patients in relation to diabetes has been studied [9]. As an example, it has been shown that the income level is inversely correlated with diabetes (type 2) [10, 11]. In Cosgrove [9] and Pouwer et al. [12], the effect of stress, stressful life events, such as changes in family status, salary income, and working condition in relation to diabetes have been assessed.

In a study conducted by Hangaard et al. [8], a cohort analysis of 5,588 patients with type 1 diabetes and 7,113 patients with type 2 diabetes has been applied where risk factors for first-time foot ulcers have been shown using general clinical information that is already obtained during routine follow-ups. Among the risk factors were long diabetes duration, history of cardiovascular disease, decreased visual acuity, diabetic retinopathy, and self-reported neuropathic symptoms. Engberg et al. [7] also show being male, having type 2 diabetes, and smoking increase the risk of getting a recurrent foot ulcer in their cohort study with 780 people. In addition, they present that patients with neuro-ischaemic or critically ischaemic ulcers have a higher risk of developing recurrent ulcers compared to patients with neuropathic ulcers.

Sen et al. [13] used a meta-analysis approach, coalescing findings from multiple risk stratification studies specifically about amputation for patients with a diabetic foot infection. Based on a set of inclusion criteria, they included 25 articles in their study totaling 6,132 patients. Among the predictors for amputation in patients with diabetic foot infection were a previous history of amputation, peripheral arterial disease, retinopathy, osteomyelitis, and gangrene/necrosis. While most risk stratification studies largely confirm and report on similar factors, we are still to see larger studies on nationwide diabetes populations, which also include more factors about general socio-economic well-being.

We therefore assess the risk level of developing DFU/amputation and the mortality using the available socio-economic registry data and available medical registrations of patients. The purpose of this study is 2-fold. The first aim is to investigate risk factors and features based on a large readily available medical dataset, which can be used for early detection of patients who are at high risk of developing DFU or amputation. Among the significant risk factors are the traditional major complications of diabetes, disposable income, mental disorders, such as depression and dementia. While there are limitations with the precision of the available data, we believe that the volume of our study strengthens the findings that both confirm existing risk factors and indicate new features promising to be scrutinized further in the field. Accordingly, this part also serves to assess how existing large data sources can be used to assess known risk factors, explore new risk factors, and to understand the weaknesses of such data analysis. The second aim is to utilize machine learning (ML) approaches to predict the occurrence of DFU and amputation in order to assess the practical usefulness of risk factors based on general socio-economic information of patients and their medical history. Thus, the long-term goal of our work is to unfold the potential of using different sporadic health-care data sources which may be combined for better machine-learning-based decision support in the future.

## 2. MATERIALS AND METHODS

### 2.1. Data Sources

Healthcare data is usually scattered throughout multiple systems maintained by different entities and each with a different level of detail and granularity. In Denmark, the data sources can generally be divided into three categories; the national registers, local care data, and personalized tracked data. This study relies on the national registers[1], which are population-wide databases that historically have been established for administrative purposes, but they also serve as sources to compute general statistics about the entire population, e.g., to support policymaking. All data in the national registers are connected through a personal identification number (CPR) from the Danish Civil Registration System [14], which allows unambiguous linkage of the registers. The Danish Civil Registration System contains information about all residents in Denmark, including citizenship, birth, and family status. Among the more prominent medical register, are the Danish National Patient Register (LPR) [15] and the Danish National Prescription Registry [16]. Using all these national registry systems, we have access to diagnoses, treatments, procedures, and prescribed medications, as well as general socioeconomic information, such as salary, public welfare benefits, employment status, and addresses. Other different data sources, such as personal tracked data and local care data will be used for our future studies (see **Figure 1**). For more details see section 4.1.

### 2.2. Population Data Statistics

We conduct a population cohort study on Danish national registers with citizens born between 1900 and 1968, which includes the data from 3,500,877 citizens. We only have the available medical and socio-economic data from the years 2000 to 2018. The focus of our study is on the time period since the first onset of diabetes from 2000 to DFU and amputation. In cases where none of these events occur, we consider the death year or the end of the study being 2018. As we do not have access to the entire life history of the patients (only the period between 2000 and 2018), it is challenging to obtain the exact year of a diabetes diagnosis. Therefore, we assume the earliest recorded

[1] The project was approved by Statistic Denmark as project number 707670.

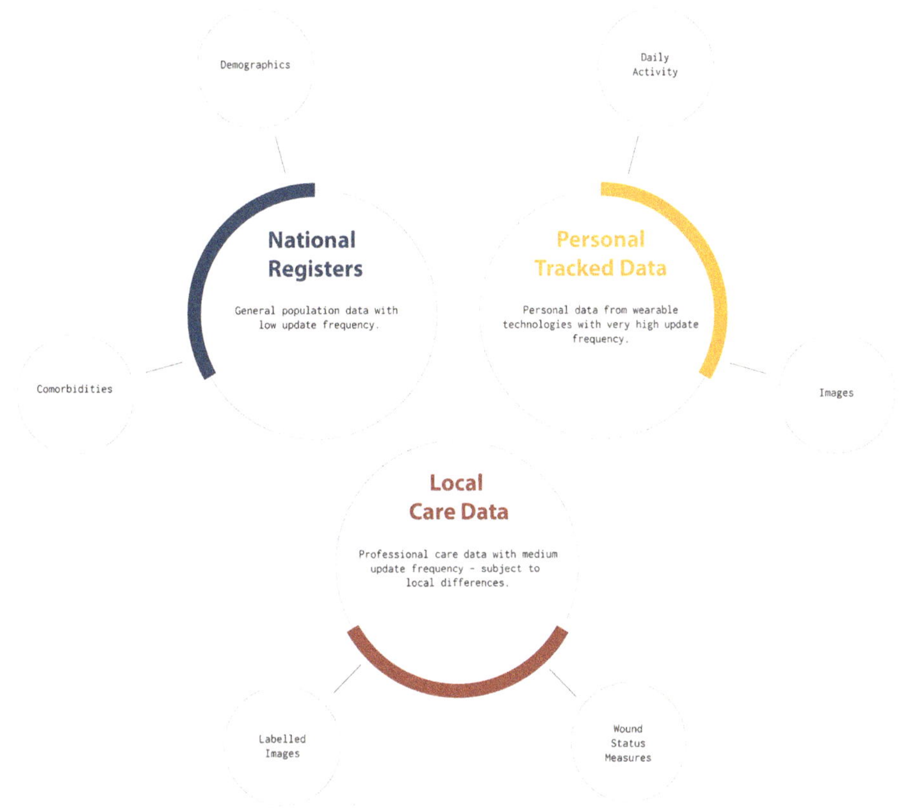


**FIGURE 1 |** A general overview of existing diabetes related data sources in Denmark. The current study is based on data from national registry. Potential future data sources include the local care and personal tracked data.

year of diabetes diagnosis in the period of 2000 to 2018 to be the onset of diabetes for the patients.

Among the full population, there are 247,208 citizens that have been diagnosed with any type of diabetes at some point. We exclude entries with incomplete data, as well as entries where general foot-ulcer, amputation, or death were registered before the diabetes diagnosis. Thus, in total, we consider a population of 246,705 patients with diabetes (among them, 531 patients are younger than 31 years old at the time of diabetes diagnosis, and we kept them in the dataset). Among the population of patients with diabetes, there are 13,695 registered cases of DFU and 7,540 cases of amputation. The median observation period for the patients with a registered DFU or amputation diagnosis (time period since diabetes year until DFU or amputation) based on our data is 8 years (mean of 7.74 ± 5.8) and 6 years (mean of 6.8 ± 5.29), respectively. The median follow-up duration for patients without DFU or amputation complication is 9 years (mean of 9.4 ± 5.8 years). It is important to state that because of a lack of access to the entire patient history described earlier, the reported duration is not accurate and subject to bias.

All codes for diagnosis of diseases are based on the *international classification of diseases ICD-10* [17]. Codes corresponding to different medications are based on the ATC/DDD index [18]. For example, to identify patients with diabetes, we use all diagnosis codes from the diabetes diagnoses tree as well as codes for relevant antidiabetic medicine. In Denmark, we further use a coding scheme named SKS, which incorporates ICD-10 but extends certain parts of the tree. SKS is governed by The Danish Health Data Authority and is used by all public healthcare institutions. This is in particular useful for identifying patients diagnosed with DFU. A recent paper has described how ICD-10 codes provide poor positive predictive values for DFU [19]. In their study, they use the diabetes codes E10.5–14.5, which cover both diabetic gangrene, peripheral angiopathy, and ulcer for different diabetes types—i.e., these codes do not only cover DFU and therefore they are subject to false positives. The SKS coding scheme further subdivides E10.5–14.5 into A-D, which means that the codes E10.5B–E14.5B that have been used for this study are specifically for DFU. All codes used in this study have been included in the section 1.1 in **Supplementary Material**. We discuss some of the limitations with regard to the coding system and the fixed time period in section 4.1.

Using the available population data, we extract the following features and information: the presence of any of the following medical conditions before the event of interest (i.e., foot ulcer or amputation); and cardiovascular-related disorders, neuropathy disorders, peripheral artery diseases, hypertension, hyperlipidemia, chronic renal disorder, urinary tract infection, retinopathy, mental disorder, depression, dementia with

Alzheimer, and nervous system disorder (see **Appendix** in **Supplementary Material** for the corresponding ICD-10 codes). The socio-economical features used are as follows:

- The past medical history of the patients
- The average number of Statins and diabetic-related medication prescribed annually
- The number of changes in the home address registry
- Household disposable income
- Age, gender, and Ethnic background (Danish and immigrant citizen)
- The number of changes in the family status
- Effect of different medical conditions on the risk of DFU/amputation.

We use the Cox proportional-hazard model [20] and Aalen Johansen model to analyze the risk effect of the listed covariates in the study. The event of interest considered is the occurrence of amputation and foot ulcers. It is important to state that in the available database, 30% of amputation registries have been recorded in the same year as the foot ulcer (42% of people who got amputations had no foot ulcer registration code). From 2,402 patients that have foot ulcers and amputation registered in the same year, in 75% of the cases, the events are registered with a difference of 2 months or less apart. We believe that this could be due to inaccurate recording of the diagnoses or significant delays in diagnosing foot ulcers. Despite an overlap in the coding registration, we analyze the two events of foot ulcer and amputation separately, as amputation occurs as a consequence of a delayed treated foot ulcer.

## 2.3. Statistical Models

The survival function $S(t)$ is defined as the probability of a person not experiencing the event of interest until a specified time $t$. It is denoted as $S(t) = Pr\{T \leq t\} = 1 - F(t)$ where $T$ is a continuous random variable for a person's survival time, $t$ is a specific value of interest for $T$ and $F(t) = Pr\{t < T\}$ is the cumulative distribution function of the random variable $T$ (see chapter 1 of [20]).

Given that an individual has survived up to time $t$, the hazard function (also known as the condition failure rate) $h(t)$ is the instantaneous potential that the event of interest occurs at time $t$. Mathematically the hazard function is defined as

$$h(t) := \lim_{\Delta t \to 0} \frac{P(T \leq t + \Delta t \mid T \geq t)}{\Delta t}, \tag{1}$$

This definition implies that $h(t) \geq 0$. Note that $h(t)$ is not a probability and in particular has no upper bound.

Using the same terminology as above, the Cox PH model is essentially a linear regression to the (log) hazard function. The Cox PH model parameterizes the hazard function as follows:

$$h(t, X) = h_0(t) \exp\left(\sum_i \beta_i X_i\right) \tag{2}$$

where $h_0(t)$ is the *baseline hazard function* and the $\beta_i$ correspond to the coefficients in a linear combination of explanatory variables $X_i$.

The Cox model expresses the hazard at time $t$ for a person with given specific explanatory variables (covariates). In this model, the baseline hazard function depends on the time $t$; however, the explanatory variables are not time-dependent. The coefficients $\beta_i$ are computed through maximum likelihood estimation. For more details regarding the model and estimation techniques, see chapter 3 of [20].

The *hazard ratio* is defined as the hazard rate of a person with a set of specific predictor variables divided by the hazard for a different individual. That this ratio is a constant is the basic assumption of the Cox model. The expression $\exp(\beta_i)$ hence corresponds to the hazard ratio of a patient with feature $X_i = 1$ vs. a patient with $X_i = 0$ and with exactly the same features apart from that.

### 2.3.1. Extended Time-Varying Cox (TVC) Model

Unlike the basic Cox PH model, the TVC model assumes that the indicator variables $X_i(t)$ depend on the time $t$. This leads to the following expression for the hazard function.

$$h(t, X) = h_0(t) \exp\left(\sum_i \beta_i X_i(t)\right) \tag{3}$$

The regression coefficients $\beta_i$ are computed in a similar way as for the basic Cox model using maximum likelihood estimation. For a complete description of the methodology, see chapter 6 of [20]. We used the lifelines package, an open-source python library to conduct our survival analysis studies.

In our application, the variables $X_i(t)$ track the onset time of a particular disorder. Before the onset of a disease we set $X_i(t) = 0$ and afterwards, until the end of the study we have $X_i(t) = 1$. We also stratify the population-based on sex and age where it is assumed that the baseline hazards are distinct (chapter 6, [20]). In addition, we apply the Mann-Whitney $U$-test to gauge which features are significant contributors to the risk of developing complications, such as foot ulcers or amputation.

### 2.3.2. The Aalen Johansen Model

The Cox PH model estimates the conditional probability of developing DFU or amputation, i.e., the probability assuming zero mortality. This model is mainly useful for a qualitative assessment of the increase in risk due to other complications. On the other hand, the model slightly overestimates the true probability of developing DFU or amputation. We, therefore, used the Aalen Johansen Model to estimate the probability of developing DFU or amputation, while accounting for mortality, that is to take into account *competing events* that may preclude the event of interest from occurring.

The Aalen Johansen model is a non-parametric approach for computing the cumulative hazard rate and is expressed as $F(t, j) = P(T \leq t, J = j)$ where $T$ is the time since origin to the event of interest or competing for an event and $J$ denotes the type of event (see [21] for more details). Due to the high average age of our population and high mortality during the study period, we compute the cumulative density for the following two cases:

1. The risk of getting DFU/amputation

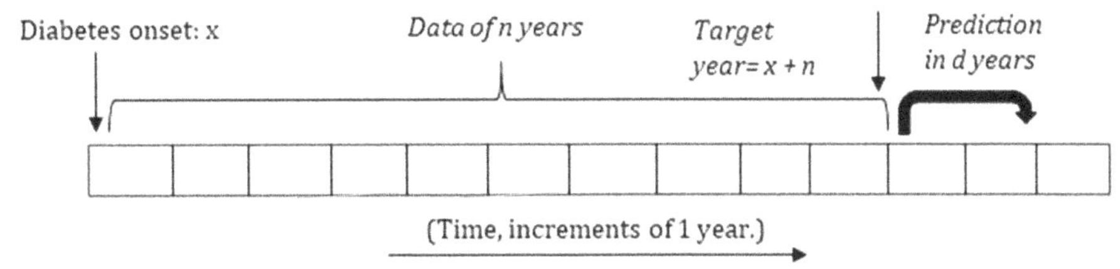


**FIGURE 2 |** Structure of using the past data for predicting the future occurrence of amputation or foot ulcer in the next *d* years (setup 2). The variable n is set between 3 and 11 years.

2. The mortality

We apply a separate model for female and male patients at different age groups. For comparison, we also produce a baseline model that considers the total population with any type of medical condition for the specific age group.

## 2.4. Applying Machine Learning Methods

After assessing the different risk factors, we apply machine learning to predict the occurrence of DFU/amputation at different time-intervals. As duration since diabetes to DFU/amputation is a key element in our study, we divide the data as follows: For a fixed number of years $n$, ranging from $n = 3$ to $n = 11$, we first get the data from diabetes onset until $n$ years after. This is referred to as the target year. We remove the patients that die within this period (where they have less than $n$ years of data available) unless they developed DFU/amputation within this time period. **Figure 2** presents a small illustration of the timeline and its structure.

We use two model setups. In setup 1, we divide the remaining patients into two classes. The first class consists of all patients who developed DFU/amputation within the target year. The second class consists of all patients who did not develop any DFU/amputation for at least the first $n$ years after the onset of diabetes. The goal is to classify between the two classes, which serves to demonstrate that the two classes can be distinguished at all based on the provided features. For each class, features are based on data from diabetes onset until either the occurrence of DFU/amputation or until the target year. Thus, this setup models whether patients get DFU/amputation at all given their medical history up until a maximum of $n$ years.

For setup 2, we take the information of patients for the first $n$ years since diabetes onset and predict whether they will develop DFU/amputation within the next $d$ years. Thus, in this setup patients with a similar history of no DFU/amputation in the first $n$ years of their diabetes history are compared and it is specified for which period prediction is done.

Setup 1 has less practical value compared to setup 2, as patients are compared based on ideal points in time of their diabetes lifespan, i.e., using all information right up until the occurrence of DFU/amputation or until the end of the fixed study period. Setup 2 more directly models predictive potential in real-life settings, but it is also much more restrictive in that it only compares patients with similar time periods of no DFU/amputation. Thus, in reality, the true predictive potential of the data in this study may lie somewhere in between the two model setups.

In both cases, for scalar features, such as the number of address changes, average family income, and medication intake,

**TABLE 1 |** Data characteristics of the patients included in the study.

| | **Patients with diabetes ($N = 246,705$)** | | |
|---|---|---|---|
| | **No complication ($n = 229,681$) *n* (%)** | **Foot ulcer ($n = 13,695$) *n* (%)** | **Amputation ($n = 7,540$) *n* (%)** |
| **Gender** | | | |
| Male | 131,852 (57.4) | 9,520 (69.5) | 5,439 (72.1) |
| Female | 97,829 (42.6) | 4,175 (30.5) | 2,101 (27.9) |
| **Age** | | | |
| <31 | 491 (0.2) | 37 (0.3) | 14 (0.2) |
| 31–54 | 62,728 (27.3) | 4,382 (32.0) | 1,979 (26.2) |
| 55–63 | 60,000 (26.1) | 3,682 (26.9) | 1,952 (25.9) |
| 64–71 | 52,007 (22.6) | 2,888 (21.1) | 1,753 (23.2) |
| 72–98 | 54,453 (23.7) | 2,706 (19.8) | 1,842 (24.4) |
| **Ethnic background** | | | |
| Danish | 204,765 (89.2) | 12,843 (93.8) | 7,185 (95.3) |
| Immigrant | 24,560 (10.7) | 829 (6.1) | 347 (4.6) |
| Descendant | 356 (0.2) | 23 (0.2) | 8 (0.1) |
| **Family disposable income** | | | |
| DKK <179,001 | 74,434 (32.4) | 5,343 (39.0) | 3,634 (48.2) |
| DKK 179,001–292,000 | 76,713 (33.4) | 4,639 (33.9) | 2,446 (32.4) |
| DKK >292,000 | 78,277 (34.1) | 3,691 (27.0) | 1,448 (19.2) |
| Bone fracture | 55,904 (24.3) | 3,565 (26.0) | 1,628 (21.6) |
| Cardiovascular disease | 53,410 (23.3) | 11,046 (80.7) | 5,502 (73.0) |
| Chronic kidney complication | 18,483 (8.0) | 1,894 (13.8) | 1,087 (14.4) |
| Dementia | 1,606 (0.7) | 40 (0.3) | 22 (0.3) |
| Depression | 606 (0.3) | 25 (0.2) | 7 (0.1) |
| Neuropathy | 11,119 (4.8) | 2,042 (14.9) | 1,093 (14.5) |
| Retinoathy | 9,707 (4.2) | 961 (7.0) | 467 (6.2) |
| Hyperlipidemia | 4,320 (1.9) | 207 (1.5) | 76 (1.0) |
| Hypertension | 27,465 (12.0) | 1,680 (12.3) | 756 (10.0) |
| Mental disorders | 17,364 (7.6) | 1,015 (7.4) | 432 (5.7) |
| Nervous system disorder | 57,805 (25.2) | 4,420 (32.3) | 1,984 (26.3) |
| Periphery artery disorder | 10,488 (4.6) | 2,023 (14.8) | 1,695 (22.5) |
| Urinary tract infection | 21,208 (9.2) | 1,302 (9.5) | 620 (8.2) |
| Multiple unspecified complications | 14,681 (6.4) | 2,967 (21.7) | 1,933 (25.6) |

the yearly average is used. In order to make the intake of medications comparable between different patients, the data is normalized based on the duration time since diabetes onset to the occurrence of DFU/amputation or end of the study for the patient (which is either death or end of the study in case of no event observation). Boolean features, such as the occurrence of any medical condition are only taken into account if they occur before and including the target year and before the development of DFU/amputation. In both setups, logistic regression (LR) and random forest (RF) classifiers are used and compared against the results of a baseline classifier.

## 3. RESULTS

In **Table 1**, we present an overview of data along with the statistics of different medical conditions. Results corresponding to some of the entries in the table are based on the quality of data which we discuss in the limitation section. In the following, we present the risk analysis of the medical conditions outlined previously and the socio-economic factors.

### 3.1. Risk Factors for Diabetic Foot Ulceration and Amputation

**Figure 3** shows the log hazard ratio for average household disposable income for patients with foot ulcers, amputation, and those with amputations who also had foot ulcers. We group the data into three groups, which are split at the 33rd and 66th percentiles, respectively. A Cox PH model is applied for every percentile if the subject falls within that group.

The survival probability of DFU/amputation for a population of Danes and immigrants is included in **Figure 4** where we apply a Kaplan Meier estimator at four distinct age groups for the Danish (blue line) and immigrant population (yellow line). The x-axis presents the number of years since diabetes onset, and the y-axis is the corresponding probability of surviving DFU (plot a) and amputation (plot b). The survival probability for the immigrants is slightly higher than the Danish population of patients. As we explain in the discussion, this can be related to a generally younger population of immigrants as well as a smaller sample size.

**Figure 5** shows the hazard ratio for different medical conditions. The predictors for every medical condition are age, gender and the event of interest is the observation of DFU/amputation. The duration from diabetes until the occurrence of DFU/amputation has been corrected for individuals deceased during the study period. The study period for these individuals has been set to the date of death. In other cases, the study period is the end of the study in 2018 or the year in which the event has occurred. The models are stratified based on age and gender in plots (a,c) and applied separately for female and male populations as in (b,d). Results indicate the level of increase in the hazard rate for developing DFU/amputation for each medical category. The risk of amputation stratified based on major or minor cases and those who have foot ulcer have been included in **Supplementary Figure 2** in **Supplementary Material**.

### 3.2. The Aalen Johansen Model on Medical Conditions and Mortality

In **Figure 6** we compare mortality against the risk of DFU and amputation (see **Supplementary Figures 3–5** in **Supplementary Material** for other medical conditions and the risk plots for DFU event). The risk of getting amputation and DFU for patients with cardiovascular complications is higher than the average risk of all patients with diabetes. A similar pattern is observed for neuropathy, chronic kidney, and nervous system disorder for both amputation and DFU events. In particular, the mortality risk for patients with diabetes and chronic kidney disorder is significantly above the average mortality risk of the population of all patients with diabetes. The risk values are observed to be slightly higher for men than female through all age groups.

### 3.3. Predictive Models

Based on the model setups described in section 2.4, we use the following features for LR and RF models:

1. Occurrence of any of the following medical conditions before and including the target year: neuropathy, retinopathy, hypertension, bone fracture, urinary tract infection, cardiovascular disease, chronic renal disease, hyperlipidemia, peripheral artery disorder, depression, dementia and Alzheimer, mental disorder, nervous system disorder, and DFU (for prediction of amputation)
2. Annual number of antidiabetic medicine, statin intake, and family disposable income up to and including the target year.
3. Annual average dose prescriptions of diabetes medication and statin up to and including the target year
4. Number of address changes up to and including the target year
5. Age (at the time of diagnosis of diabetes), Gender, family status, and background of patients.

We randomly split the data into train and test sets and apply an RF model and an LR for prediction (25% of samples are used for the testing and 75% for training). The plot in **Figure 7** shows the accuracy of the models vs. the baseline and the ROC curves. The baseline in (a) represents the accuracy of a baseline classifier, where the output is always no occurrence of amputation within $n$ years since this is the largest class. The baseline in (b) corresponds to the diagonal line that has an area under the curve of 0.5 (a random classifier). A high value of true positive and zero false positive rates is the ideal situation of a perfect classifier.

The plots in **Figures 8A–C** correspond to average ROC predictions of amputation occurrence at $d = 2, 3, 5$ years after the target year. We plot the mean and standard deviation of the ROC curves for different $n$. In addition the prediction results for DFU and amputation for those who have DFU have been included in **Supplementary Figure 1** in **Supplementary Material**.

## 4. DISCUSSION

**Figure 3C** clearly shows a higher hazard for patients with a lower household income. The finding have been confirmed and investigated before in several studies (see [22–25]). In this

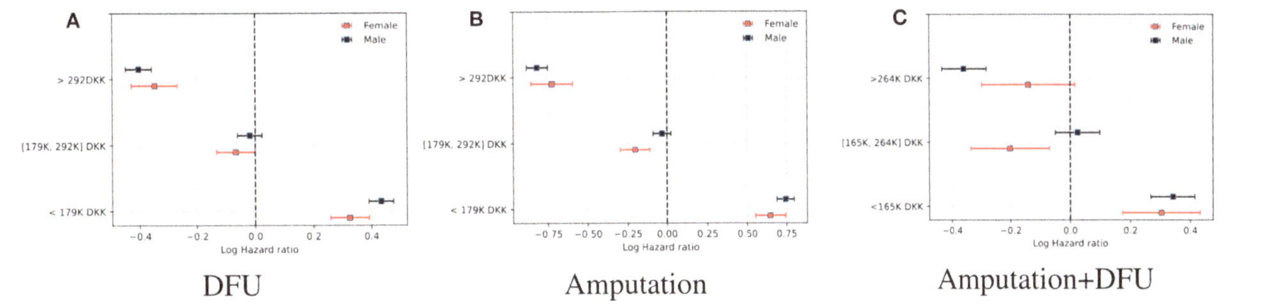


**FIGURE 3 |** The log hazard ratio for household disposable income for patients with diabetes and foot ulcer, amputation, and those who have foot ulcer and amputation. The risk of DFU/amputation event is higher for the 33rd percentile. **(A)** DFU. **(B)** Amputation. **(C)** Amputation + DFU.

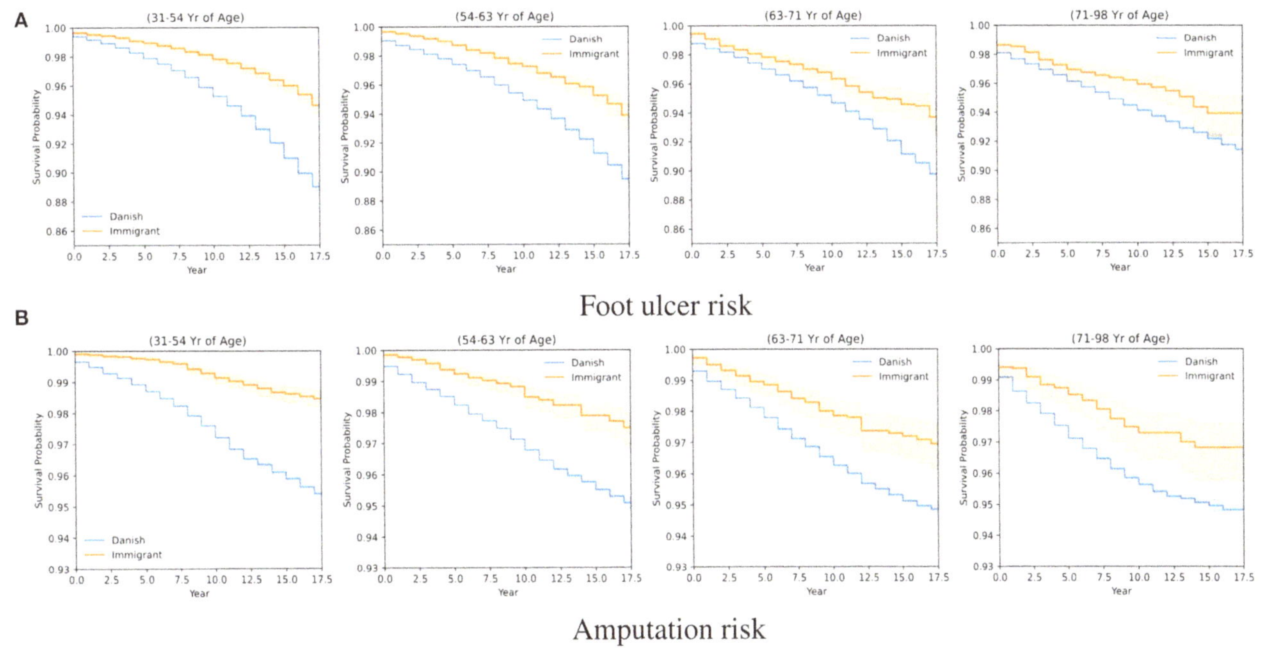


**FIGURE 4 |** Kaplan-Meier estimates for different age groups and backgrounds and the corresponding risk levels for foot ulcer and amputation. **(A)** Foot ulcer risk. **(B)** Amputation risk.

study, a similar outcome can be concluded with regard to the serious consequences of diabetes, namely DFU and amputation among lower-income families as well. The model is stratified on age for all three percentiles. By that, we mean that data is split into $m$ smaller datasets based on age. Every dataset has a different baseline hazard rate; however, they all share the same regression parameters. The covariates that have been used for each dataset are the same, therefore the age is not shown separately in the results.

The plots in **Figure 4** compare the survival probabilities between populations of Danes and immigrants over different years. Two factors that can explain the higher survival probability of the immigrant population over the Danish population can be explained in terms of the population size and the fact that the population of immigrants is younger than the Danish population in general (56.9±11.4 vs. 62.4±11.4 years old). As the population of immigrants is smaller as well, we split the data into four age groups and fit a separate model for each category. The number of Danes and immigrants for each age group is (56,277, 11,282), (57,447, 6,969), (51,463, 4,233), and (55,141, 2,986), respectively. We did not include the population of descendants in the study since the sample size is small and is subject to high variation. As the age increases, the standard deviation in the estimated survival probabilities increases, potentially narrowing the gap between the two different population backgrounds.

Beside the socioeconomic factors, the assessment of the risk of mortality and DFU/amputation for different medical conditions can be summarized as follows: diabetes patients with cardiovascular disorders, peripheral artery, neuropathy, and chronic renal complication are among populations with a high risk of developing DFU and amputation (see **Figure 5**). Similar results are obtained for major and minor amputations (see **Supplementary Figure 2** in **Supplementary Material**). The high standard deviation for some cases in **Supplementary Figure 2** in

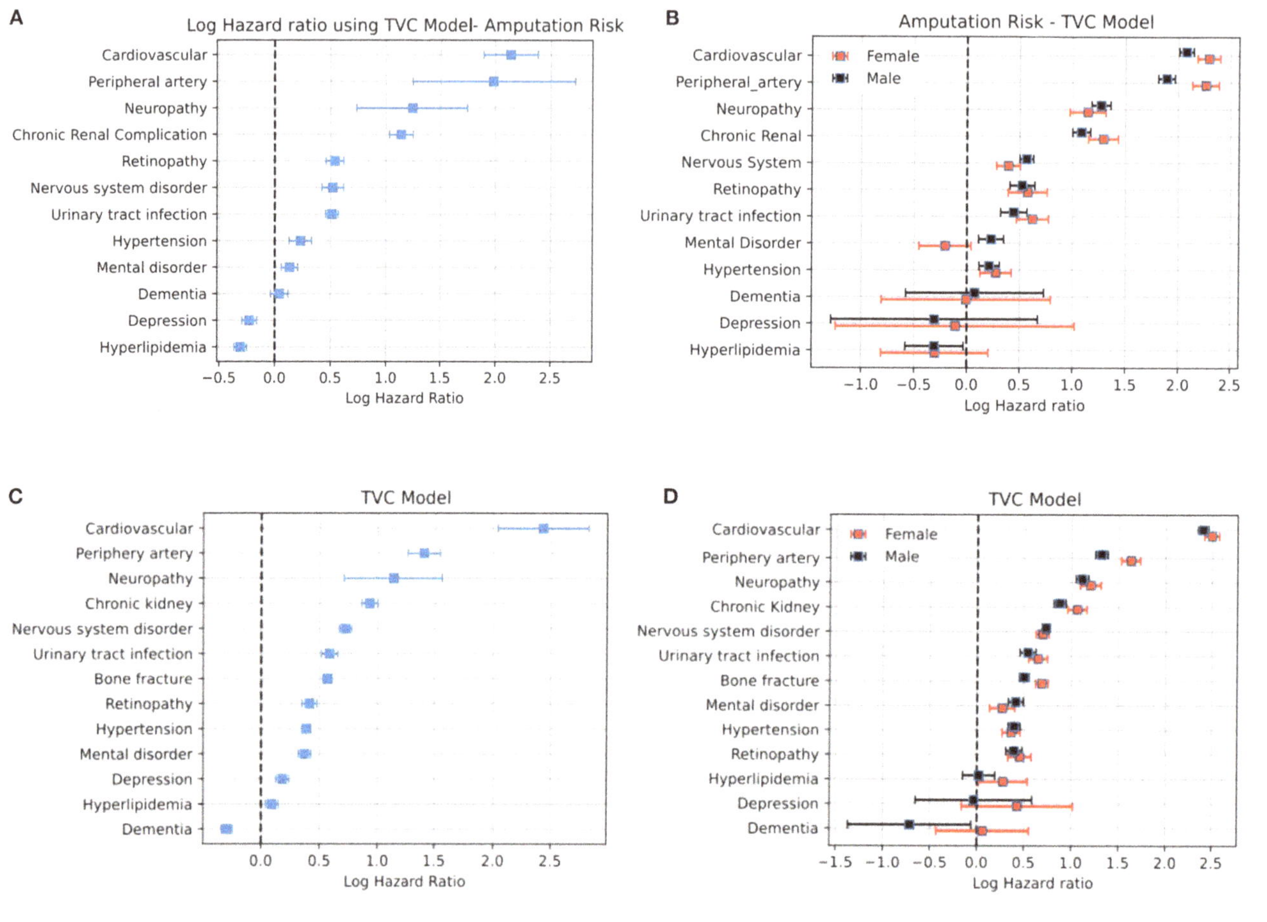


**FIGURE 5 |** Plots **(A–D)** correspond to the log-hazard ratio of patients who get amputation and foot ulcer, respectively.

**Supplementary Material** is due to the relatively small population sizes because of stratification. This is more pronounced for depression, mental disorder, and dementia where it becomes difficult to report significant results. We used a separate Cox model for each medical condition to avoid the issue of confounding variables. This means that we cannot account for interactions between different risk factors. We leave such a study for potential future work.

As the age group increases in **Figure 6** (**Supplementary Figures 3–5** in **Supplementary Material**) and the duration since diabetes onset, the mortality risk increases significantly above the amputation risk for most medical conditions. However, in the lower age group, for cardiovascular and neuropathy, the risk of amputation is higher than the mortality risk at the beginning, and above the baseline for the general population of diabetes. This is highly expected as peripheral neuropathy is one of the contributors to DFU occurrence. This consequently increases the risk of amputation.

After assessing different risk factors, we use ML in two setups to evaluate the predictive value of the features with regard to DFU/amputation. The first model is set up to distinguish between two classes of people w/o amputation, we show the accuracy results for different target years in **Figures 8A,B**. The plots show the following: in (a) we exclude the first 2 years and last 6 years since the number of classes is significantly unbalanced. The number of people who get amputation only a year or two after diabetes onset is very low, therefore the baseline classifier has a high prediction accuracy (slightly above 97% accuracy). This number reduces as the number of years increases and the classes become more balanced. The lowest accuracy corresponds to within 10 years after diabetes onset using the logistic regression model which is at 95%, about 4% above the baseline predictions. Plot b corresponds to the ROC curves, which is independent of the class sample size.

The ROC curves of predictive models in **Figure 8** for different *d* values (results have been averaged over *n*) illustrate the preliminary results of using the registry information. It is a more challenging task to predict the occurrence of DFU/amputation in the next coming years, based solely on the extracted socioeconomic features and past medical conditions. Therefore, we clearly observe a lower performance in the ROC curve in comparison to the classification task. Although the features that have been used in the study can be used for prediction models (based on the classifier results), they are not sufficient enough for accurate prediction of DFU/amputation. More detailed

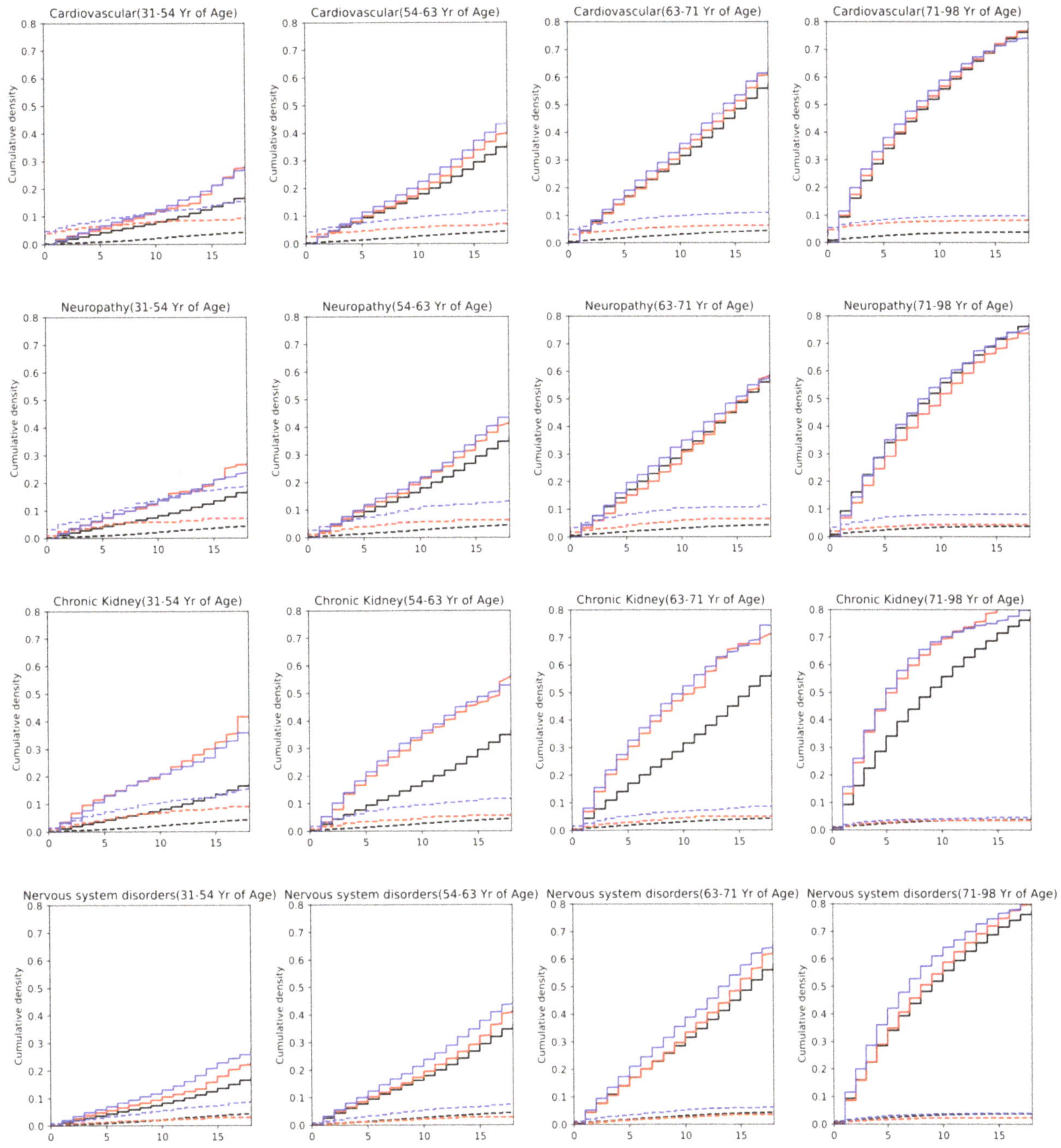


**FIGURE 6 |** Risk of developing amputation or death for males and females at different age groups. Plots correspond to having diabetes and one of the medical conditions. Red (Female)/Blue (Male)/Black (Baseline) dashed lines: risk of developing amputation. Red/Blue/Black solid: (Female/Male/Baseline) risk of mortality. The x-axis denotes the number of years since diabetes onset. The baseline corresponds to the population of all people with diabetes.

features and a higher time resolution are required for better predictive models.

## 4.1. Limitations and Strengths

Doing a study on existing medical data comes with added uncertainty as we have little control over the data collection process. In our study, we rely entirely on data from various national registers, thus the existing coding is used to identify all conditions. Although the coding is done by professionals, it may differ across regions, hospitals, and doctors subject to different coding preferences. While we do account for different ways of coding, e.g., diabetes and DFU, we may not have included all

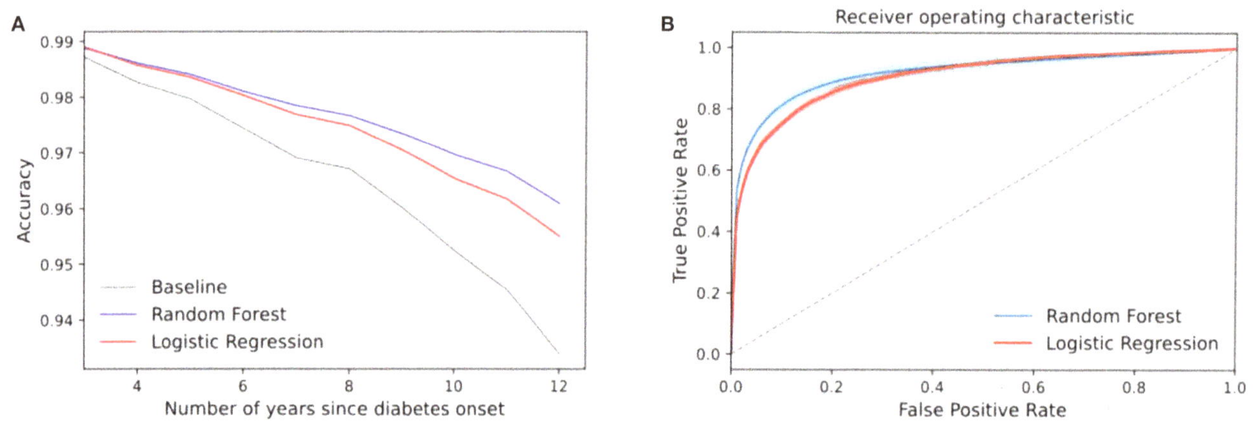


**FIGURE 7 | (A)** Accuracy of the amputation classifier for different *n* years using a random forest and logistic regression. Baseline corresponds to a classifier that outputs no amputation. **(B)** Averaged ROC curves for *n* years. The diagonal line corresponds to a random classifier. Plots correspond to setup 1.

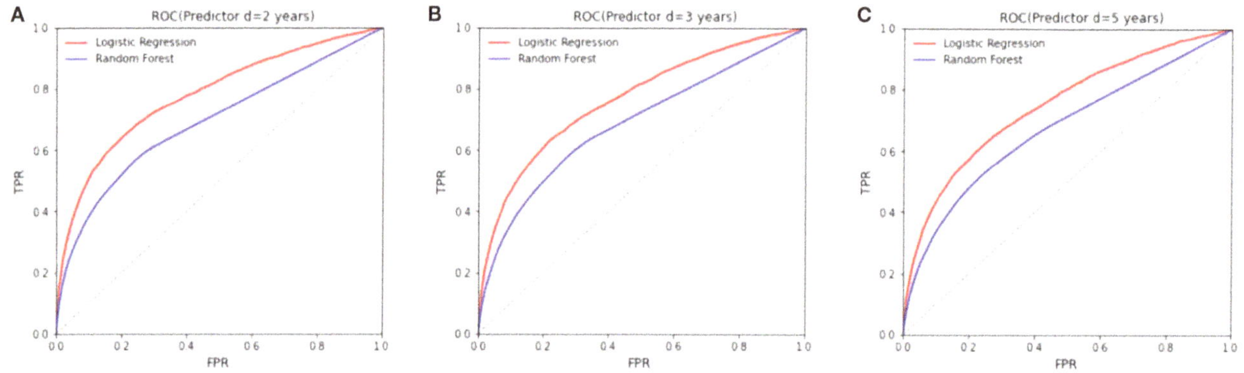


**FIGURE 8 |** The ROCs for the prediction models of amputation in the next 2, 3, and 5 years, respectively (setup 2). The diagonal line is the baseline where predictions are random. **(A)** ROC (Predictor $d = 2$ years). **(B)** ROC (Predictor $d = 3$ years). **(C)** ROC (Predictor $d = 5$ years).

ways. This is also true for other diabetes-related comorbidities. As a result of the existing coding practice, certain complications have a low representation in the data used for the analysis. For example, one would expect that most patients suffering from DFU also suffer from neuropathy or some form of lowered nerve functioning in their feet. However, in the data of this study, only 14.9% have been diagnosed with neuropathy prior to DFU. This is in part a result of poor coding practice and the fact that data is not available for the entire lifespan of the participants. Some doctors may even use a single code named “diabetes with multiple complications” for patients suffering from more than one diabetes complication, which means it is impossible to distinguish exactly which complications are present after the fact. Another reason for the low prevalence of some conditions is the fact that only complications identified prior to DFU or amputation are included since the goal was to assess the practical usefulness of the available data for prediction. In several cases, complications are diagnoses at the same time as DFU, thus omitted in our analysis.

In addition to missing cases, we also expect some false positives in the data. Christensen et al. [19] recently described how using ICD-10 codes to identify DFU will give several false positives, as the current codes cover more diagnoses than just DFU. However, in our study, we use the Danish SKS coding scheme that, besides the ICD-10 codes, for example have specific codes for DFU (see section 2.2). Consequently, our results should contain fewer false positives compared to the results presented by Christensen et al. [19].

Another limiting factor in our study is the fact that we do not have medical and socio-economic data for the entire lifespan of the patients, since we only have data from 2000 until 2018. Thus, there are certain features that cannot be reliably estimated. For example, we are unable to compute whether a DFU diagnosis is a first-time incident or a recurrent one. Therefore, our study focuses on DFU occurrence in general, which means that we do not consider factors that are specific to first time or recurrent incidents. For instance, prior foot ulceration would likely be a strong predictor for recurrent ones. If we focused only on the recurrent DFU, we would limit our dataset significantly. In the same way, earlier diabetes diagnosis before 2000 cannot be ascertained, and this introduces a bias in the estimation of the target year.

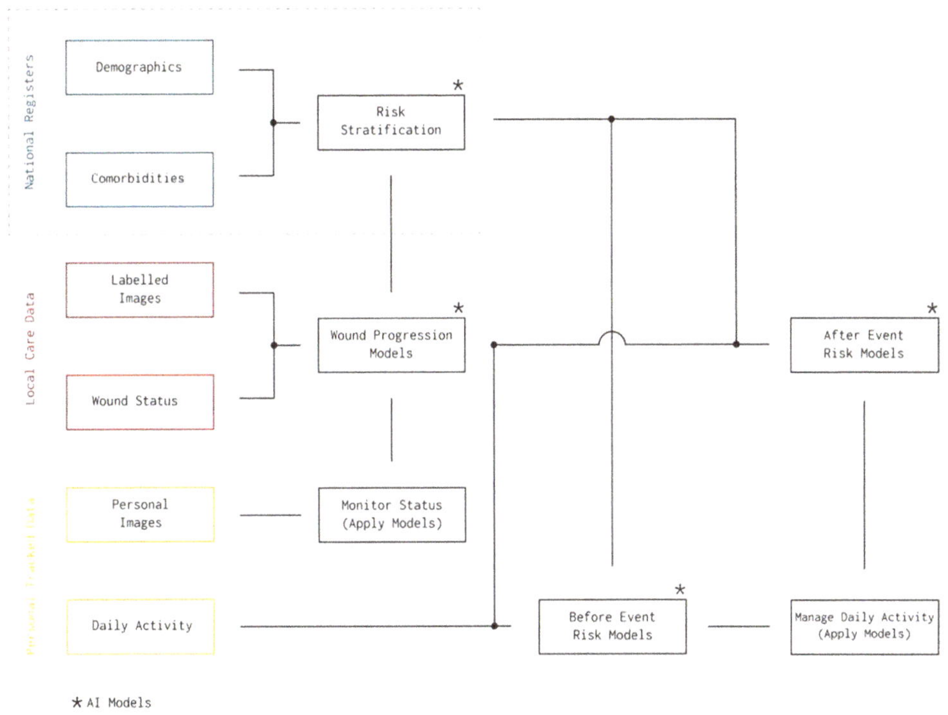


**FIGURE 9 |** The flowchart-like graph depicts a potential future interplay between different data sources for application of AI in the domain of diabetic foot care.

The overlap between the foot ulcer registration year with the amputation registration year is also a disadvantage of the study, which further reveals the shortcomings with registry data in general. As mentioned previously in section 2.3, for patients with both amputation and foot ulcers, more than half of the cases occur in the same year. The separate analysis of the two events did not yield significantly different results due to the high overlap. This in particular signals a general delayed diagnosis of a foot ulcer or delayed registration of codes, which makes it challenging to design sensible predictive models for such conditions with register data alone. Despite the limiting factors of the data, the size of the dataset is a major strength. In fact, several of the factors that we show to significantly increase the risk of DFU/amputation replicate findings from other smaller studies, implying that the volume of the data mitigates some of the limitations. Assessing the usefulness of the available medical data for prediction purposes is therefore still very relevant in order to inform future studies and eventually practical applications.

### 4.1.1. Future Work

**Figure 9** depicts a potential future interplay between different data sources and different applications of AI that we aim to pursue in the upcoming studies. It highlights how the promised value of AI may be unlocked by combining existing data repositories with detailed quantified self data (personal tracking data), and how the result of one analysis can support the development of new and more advanced analysis models. The upper part of **Figure 9** outlined by the dashed box represents the work on risk stratification presented in this paper. While risk stratification in itself is useful to learn about diabetes and its complications, the results from such an analysis can also directly be used in more precise and timely risk models that combine results from large cohort studies, with more detailed data about the everyday life of patients. This data could be provided by local care personnel and the patients themselves (see **Figure 1**).

One example is the opportunity to build machine learning models with existing wound image data and labels describing the current state of the wounds. Image recognition for diabetic feet is already an active field of research in which problems, such as wound segmentation [26, 27], ulcer detection [28], and recognition of ischemia and infection [26, 29] have been investigated. Thus, the next step may be to combine such methods with general risk factors to develop better models that are able to automatically label new images with information about the state of the wound progression. Such a wound progression model would be directly applicable in new tools both for patients and for doctors - patients would be able to self-monitor their wounds and doctors would be able to get detailed wound history that could support better medical advice.

Going even further, risk stratification and wound progression can serve as input to fine-grained risk models, both for predicting certain events and for predicting additional complications once an event has occurred. For instance, patients with slow healing progress may have a higher risk of getting an amputation, i.e., a wound progression model may be used to generate features for a model that tries to predict amputation. The presented flowchart is merely one suggestion of how we may combine detailed personal activity data with general risk factors and wound progression information to develop better prediction models in the area of diabetes. Still, there is much research needed to utilize the current data sources for accurate and reliable models that can be used for prediction of diabetes complications.

## 5. CONCLUSION

The risk assessment of different medical and socioeconomic features indicates that there is a high hazard of developing DFU or amputation for patients with diabetes and cardiovascular, peripheral artery disease, neuropathy, and chronic renal complications. It is also observed that mental disorders can slightly increase the risk; however, this is subject to more investigation as the category of mental disorders that have been used in this study covers a broad range of diagnoses. Family disposable income is inversely correlated with the risk of DFU and amputation. We did not find any significant correlation between DFU/amputation occurrence and the number of changes in the family-status or changes in the number of the home registry. However, the type of transitions in the family status, along with possible registered medical disorders are part of future investigation to single out different stressful events. Based on medical condition history and socioeconomic features, we were able to distinguish between patients with diabetes w/o DFU/amputation with an accuracy above the baseline over different years. This shows that in principle the two populations can be distinguished based on the available features. However, the results corresponding to the prediction of DFU/amputation in the next years require improvements. This has to be done by applying more feature engineering and obtaining more information on the medical and physiological history of the patients. Changing the timeline of the study is also one of the main factors for modeling future events. In addition, utilization of different data sources, such as images and user tracking data will allow for models that utilize data closer to the time of interest, thus allowing for more timely predictions that may better support current medical practices.

## AUTHOR CONTRIBUTIONS

ZS has contributed to the processing, analyzing the data, preparing the manuscript, discussion of results, revision of the manuscript, and the final approval. AM contributed to processing, design of the study, data visualization, preparing the manuscript, and discussion of results. SE, TR, and KK-M contributed to the idea and design of the study, discussions of the results, the revision of the manuscript, and final approval. KS contributed with data extraction and discussions regarding the results. All authors contributed to the article and approved the submitted version.

## REFERENCES


1. International Diabetes Federation (IDF) (2019). Available online at: https://www.idf.org/aboutdiabetes/what-is-diabetes/facts-figures.html (accessed February 05, 2021).
2. Pop-Busui R, Boulton AJ, Feldman EL, Bril V, Freeman R, Malik RA, et al. Diabetic neuropathy: a position statement by the American Diabetes Association. *Diabetes Care.* (2017) 40:136–54. doi: 10.2337/dc16-2042
3. Lavery LA, Armstrong DG, Wunderlich RP, Tredwell J, Boulton AJ. Diabetic foot syndrome: evaluating the prevalence and incidence of foot pathology in Mexican Americans and non-Hispanic whites from a diabetes disease management cohort. *Diabetes Care.* (2003) 26:1435–8. doi: 10.2337/diacare.26.5.1435
4. Bergman M, Buysschaert M, Schwarz PE, Albright A, Narayan KV, Yach D. Diabetes prevention: global health policy and perspectives from the ground. *Diabetes Manage.* (2012) 2:309. doi: 10.2217/dmt.12.34
5. Kirketerp-Møller K, Svendsen OL, Jansen RB. The management of diabetic foot ulcers in Danish hospitals is not optimal. *Danish Med J.* (2015) 62:1–4.
6. Sortsø C, Green A, Jensen P, Emneus M. Health economics societal costs of diabetes mellitus in Denmark. *Diabetic Med J.* (2015) 33:877–85. doi: 10.1111/dme.12965
7. Engberg S, Kirketerp-Møller K, Ullits Andersen H, Rasmussen A. Incidence and predictors of recurrent and other new diabetic foot ulcers: a retrospective cohort study. *Diabet Med.* (2019) 36:1417–23. doi: 10.1111/dme.13964
8. Hangaard S, Rasmussen A, Almdal T, Nielsen AA, Nielsen KE, Siersma V, et al. Standard complication screening information can be used for risk assessment for first time foot ulcer among patients with type 1 and type 2 diabetes. *Diabetes Res Clin Pract.* (2019) 151:177–86. doi: 10.1016/j.diabres.2019.04.021
9. Cosgrove M. Do stressful life events cause type 1 diabetes? *Occupat Med.* (2004) 54:250–4. doi: 10.1093/occmed/kqh047
10. Rabi DM, Edwards AL, Southern DA, Svenson LW, Sargious PM, Norton P, et al. Association of socio-economic status with diabetes prevalence and utilization of diabetes care services. *BMC Health Serv Res.* (2006) 6:124. doi: 10.1186/1472-6963-6-124
11. Hsu CC, Lee CH, Wahlqvist ML, Huang HL, Chang HY, Chen L, et al. Poverty increases type 2 diabetes incidence and inequality of care despite universal health coverage. *Diabetes Care.* (2012) 35:2286–92. doi: 10.2337/dc11-2052
12. Pouwer F, Kupper N, Adriaanse MC. Does emotional stress cause type 2 diabetes mellitus? A review from the European Depression in Diabetes (EDID) Research Consortium. *Discov Med.* (2010) 9:112–8.
13. Sen P, Demirdal T, Emir B. Meta-analysis of risk factors for amputation in diabetic foot infections. *Diabetes Metab Res Rev.* (2019) 35:e3165. doi: 10.1002/dmrr.3165
14. Pedersen CB. The Danish civil registration system. *Scand J Public Health.* (2011) 39:22–5. doi: 10.1177/1403494810387965
15. Lynge E, Sandegaard JL, Rebolj M. The Danish national patient register. *Scand J Public Health.* (2011) 39:30–3. doi: 10.1177/1403494811401482
16. Wallach Kildemoes H, Toft Sørensen H, Hallas J. The Danish national prescription registry. *Scand J Public Health.* (2011) 39:38–41. doi: 10.1177/1403494810394717
17. World Health Organization. *Classification of Diseases.* (2019). Available online at: https://icd.who.int/browse10/2019/en (accessed February 05, 2021).
18. WHO Collaborating Centre for Drug Statistics Methodology. *International Language for Drug Utilization Research.* (2019). Available online at: https://www.whocc.no/atc_ddd_index/?code=c10aa (accessed February 05, 2021).
19. Christensen DH, Knudsen ST, Nicolaisen SK, Andersen H, Callaghan BC, Finnerup NB, et al. (2019). Can diabetic polyneuropathy and foot ulcers in patients with type 2 diabetes be accurately identified based on icd-10 hospital diagnoses and drug prescriptions? *Clin. Epidemiol.* 11:311–21. doi: 10.2147/CLEP.S197474
20. Kleinbaum DG, Klein M. *Survival Analysis.* Vol. 3. Springer (2010).
21. Edwards JK, Hester LL, Gokhale M, Lesko CR. Methodologic issues when

estimating risks in pharmacoepidemiology. *Current Epidemiol Rep.* (2016) 3:285–96. doi: 10.1007/s40471-016-0089-1

22. Deladoëy J, Henderson M, Geoffroy L. Linear association between household income and metabolic control in children with insulin-dependent diabetes mellitus despite free access to health care. *J Clin Endocrinol Metab.* (2013) 98:E882–5. doi: 10.1210/jc.2013-1212
23. Bird Y, Lemstra M, Rogers M, Moraros J. The relationship between socioeconomic status/income and prevalence of diabetes and associated conditions: a cross-sectional population-based study in Saskatchewan, Canada. *Int J Equity Health.* (2015) 14:93. doi: 10.1186/s12939-015-0237-0
24. Dallongeville J, Cottel D, Ferrières J, Arveiler D, Bingham A, Ruidavets JB, et al. Household income is associated with the risk of metabolic syndrome in a sex-specific manner. *Diabetes Care.* (2005) 28:409–15. doi: 10.2337/diacare.28.2.409
25. Shin W, Kim H, Lee T, Jeon DH, Ha K, Kim D, et al. Combined effects of diabetes and low household income on mortality: a 12-year follow-up study of 505 677 Korean adults. *Diabet Med.* (2018) 35:1345–54. doi: 10.1111/dme.13695
26. Wang C, Yan X, Smith M, Kochhar K, Rubin M, Warren SM, et al. A unified framework for automatic wound segmentation and analysis with deep convolutional neural networks. In: *2015 37th Annual International Conference of the IEEE Engineering in Medicine and Biology Society (EMBC).* Milan: IEEE (2015). p. 2415–8.
27. Goyal M, Yap MH, Reeves ND, Rajbhandari S, Spragg J. Fully convolutional networks for diabetic foot ulcer segmentation. In: *2017 IEEE International Conference on Systems, Man, and Cybernetics (SMC).* IEEE (2017). p. 618–623. doi: 10.1109/SMC.2017.8122675
28. Goyal M, Reeves ND, Davison AK, Rajbhandari S, Spragg J, Yap MH. Dfunet: convolutional neural networks for diabetic foot ulcer classification. *IEEE Trans Emerg Top Comput Intell.* (2018). 4, 728–739. doi: 10.1109/TETCI.2018.2866254
29. Goyal M, Reeves ND, Rajbhandari S, Ahmad N, Wang C, Yap MH. Recognition of ischaemia and infection in diabetic foot ulcers: dataset and techniques. *Comput Biol Med.* (2020) 117:103616. doi: 10.1016/j.compbiomed.2020.103616

# 2

# Accuracy of Deep Neural Network in Triaging Common Skin Diseases of Primary Care Attention

*Mara Giavina-Bianchi*, Eduardo Cordioli and André P. dos Santos*

*Department of Telemedicine, Hospital Israelita Albert Einstein, São Paulo, Brazil*

***Correspondence:***
*Mara Giavina-Bianchi*
*marahgbianchi@gmail.com*

Access to dermatological care can be challenging in certain regions of the world. The triage process is usually conducted by primary care physicians; however, they may not be able to diagnose and assign the correct referral and level of priority for different dermatosis. The present research aimed to test different deep neural networks to obtain the highest level of accuracy for the following: (1) diagnosing groups of dermatoses; (2) correct referrals; and (3) the level of priority given to the referral compared to dermatologists. Using 140,446 images from a teledermatology project, previously labeled with the clinical diagnosis, and their respective referrals, namely biopsy, in-person dermatologist visits or monitoring the case via teledermatology along with the general physician, 27 different scenarios of neural networks were derived, and the algorithm accuracies in classifying different dermatosis, according to the group of the diagnosis they belong to, were calculated. The most accurate algorithm was then tested for accuracy in diagnosis, referral, and level of priority given to 6,945 cases. The GoogLeNet architecture, trained with 24,000 images and 1,000 epochs, using weight random initialization and learning rates of $10^{-3}$ was found to be the most accurate network, showing an accuracy of 89.72% for diagnosis, 96.03% for referrals and 92.54% for priority level in 6,975 image testing. Our study population, however, was confined to individuals with chronic skin conditions and, therefore, it has limited value as a triage tool because it has not been tested for acute conditions. Deep neural networks are accurate in triaging, correct referral and prioritizing common chronic skin diseases related to primary care attention. They can also help health-care systems optimize patients' access to dermatologists.

**Keywords: primary care attention, common skin lesions, dermatology, deep neural network, articial intelligence**

## INTRODUCTION

Health access is a serious challenge for most of the worldwide population. It becomes even more evident when the necessary assistance requires a specialized professional. In Brazil, the specialty of Dermatology was the second-most referred to by primary care physicians, amounting to 17.78% of all the referrals with the average waiting time being more than 100 days for an appointment (1, 2).

A large number of dermatologist referrals occur mainly due to the wide variety of dermatoses, which makes the diagnosis challenging for primary care physicians. A study conducted by the Brazilian Society of Dermatology indicated that, in 2018, only 9.1% Brazilian municipalities had specialists in dermatology (3). This heterogeneous distribution of the medical population,

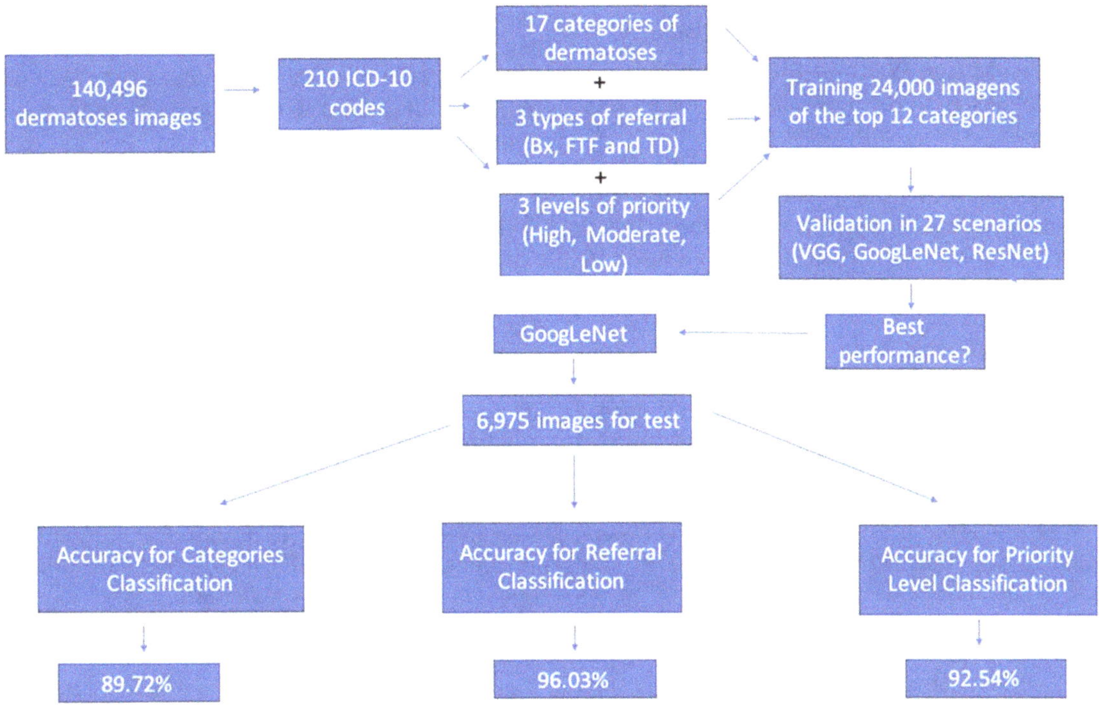


**GRAPHICAL ABSTRACT |** Graphical Abstract showing the research flow from the dataset base images, classification of the dermatoses according to categories, referral and level of priority; training and validation in different scenarios to the final test, using the algorithm with the best performance.

especially in remote areas, contributes to the increase in seeking means of care such as telemedicine. The effectiveness, accuracy, and reliability of dermatological diagnosis via telemedicine have been widely studied and are considered equivalent to those performed by dermatologists in face-to-face consultations (4–6).

The digital nature of these services, added to the recent developments in the field of image processing, provide an extremely fertile environment for research related to the application of artificial intelligence (AI) in the identification and diagnosis of skin lesions. In 2016, Shrivastava developed an algorithm based on support vector machine (SVM) capable of identifying psoriasis with 99.81% accuracy (7).

In 2018, in a research by Han et al., a classification algorithm built with deep neural networks showed 91% accuracy in the task of differentiating pigmented lesions between benign and malignant using a sample of 21,306 images (8). A large body of research in the literature points to a satisfactory accuracy of AI algorithms in identifying various types of skin diseases, ranging from simple onychomycosis (9) to melanomas (10–12).

However, previous studies generally focused on one disease or a limited group of diseases. To study the application of these technologies in the larger context of public health, a broader approach is needed to classify the dermatoses in established categories and suggest appropriate treatment approaches. In addition to focusing on the diagnosis of a single disease, it was observed that many studies have utilized image acquisition protocols and equipment designed specifically for AI in order to enhance the accuracy of classification algorithms. However, these image-acquisition protocols are too time consuming for health-care professionals to implement, and the equipment used are not available in most primary health-care units. This hinders the implementation of the algorithm in the public health system.

The authors identified an opportunity to evaluate the performance of these techniques in a broader context which does not classify lesions as belonging or not belonging to a specific diagnosis, rather in a more comprehensive classification, using simple protocols that can be applied by day-to-day primary health-care professionals.

The image acquisition equipment used in the present study are available among primary care networks. The purpose of the study was to optimize stages of the diagnostic process to provide health-care professionals with a diagnostic support tool that is capable of correctly and quickly screening and referring to cases to the specialist, according to their priority level.

The primary goal of the current work was to evaluate the accuracy of different algorithms of deep neural networks for triage and support diagnosis of skin lesions. The second aim was to test the accuracy of the algorithm for the best performance on the diagnosis, referral and level of priority, compared to those performed by dermatologists, using a test with clinical images *in silico*.

# MATERIALS AND METHODS

## Acquisition of Clinical Images for the Development of the Neural Network

The present study was approved by the Ethics Committee of the Hospital Israelita Albert Einstein (project number: 3541-18). 140,446 images were utilized corresponding to 57,568 skin lesions, obtained between July 2017 and August 2018 from a philanthropic assistance project between Albert Einstein Israel-Brazilian Benevolent Society and the São Paulo City Hall. The project and its results have been described in detail previously (1).

Briefly, patients requiring primary care attention and waiting for an appointment with a dermatologist in the public healthcare system of the city were directed to three municipal hospitals, where photos of their skin lesions were collected by health technicians using the default Samsung Galaxy S7 smartphone camera in conventional offices. These images, together with the demographic data and a brief clinical history, were uploaded to the Amazon Web Services platform and diagnosed by 13 dermatologists who had to choose among three possible referrals: (1) biopsy of the lesion; (2) a face-to-face visit to the dermatologist; or (3) suggesting the best conduct for the treatment and/or monitoring the cases via teledermatology along with the primary care physician. The 57,568 diagnosed lesions were classified into 210 International Classification of Diseases-10 (ICD-10) codes, which were grouped into 17 categories based on the nature of the dermatoses for better evaluation of the results. The categories are described in **Table 1** and are the targets for predicting the diagnosis in the present study. The total number of images in each category, their corresponding percentage, the number of images used to test the algorithm and referrals with their respective priorities, according to our dermatologists' standards of care are shown in **Table 1**. The ICD-10 codes and the main diseases that make up each category are listed in **Supplementary Table 1**.

## Development of Artificial Neural Networks

To mitigate the problem of lack of focus on injuries, all the images were cut individually using Microsoft Paint so that only the region of interest related to the lesion was preserved for analysis. Following this, in order to standardize the network input, images were resized to 224 × 224 pixels. The errors obtained in the classification of the training set and validation were calculated using the mean square error equation (MSE). It was chosen among the various loss functions used for the classification field because it was the most frequent supervisioned learning in medical literature at the time of the experiment. More technical information on algorithm pipeline is found in **Supplementary Material 2**.

The programming language used was Python; all neural network models were trained and tested on Keras API using Tensorflow as the backend in two Amazon instances: p 2.xlarge with a single Nvidia Tesla k80 GPU, g3.4xlarge with a single Nvidia Tesla M60 GPU.

## Experiments

Two initial exploratory experiments conducted previously to the following are presented in **Supplementary Material 3**.

**TABLE 1** | Categories of target classes dermatological diseases, their contribution in the dataset of images, referral and level of priority, according to our dermatologists' standard of care.

| | Category | Total images dataset (*n*) | Total images dataset (%) | Test images (*n*) | Referral | Priority |
|---|---|---|---|---|---|---|
| 1 | Benign tumor | 31,998 | 22.78 | 1,600 | TD | low |
| 2 | Eczema | 25,217 | 17.95 | 1,261 | TD | moderate |
| 3 | Pigmentation disorder | 19,825 | 14.12 | 992 | TD | low |
| 4 | Superficial infection/Infestation | 18,963 | 13.50 | 949 | TD | moderate |
| 5 | Inflammatory disorder | 15,228 | 10.84 | 762 | TD | moderate |
| 6 | Benign cyst | 7,776 | 5.54 | 389 | FTF | low |
| 7 | External cause | 5,916 | 4.21 | 296 | TD | low |
| 8 | Genetic cause | 5,077 | 3.61 | 254 | TD | low |
| 9 | Not grouped | 2,474 | 1.76 | 123 | TD | low |
| 10 | Metabolic cause | 2,438 | 1.74 | 121 | FTF | low |
| 11 | Malignant tumor | 2,375 | 1.69 | 118 | BIOPSY | high |
| 12 | Pre-malignant (actinic keratosis) | 2,200 | 1.57 | 110 | BIOPSY | high |
| 13 | Connective tissue disorder | 371 | 0.26 | 0 | FTF | high |
| 14 | Adverse drug reaction | 339 | 0.24 | 0 | TD | moderate |
| 15 | Deep/systemic infection | 128 | 0.09 | 0 | FTF | high |
| 16 | Bullous disease | 61 | 0.04 | 0 | TD | high |
| 17 | Factitial dermatitis | 60 | 0.04 | 0 | TD | low |
| 18 | Total | 140,446 | 100% | 6,975 | – | – |

*TD, teledermatology; FTF, face-to-face dermatologist.*

**TABLE 2** | Results of the first experiment to test the accuracy of different neural networks according to architecture, weights and learning rate.

| Scenario | Architecture | weight Initialization | Learning rate | Training accuracy | Validation accuracy | Training error | Validation error | Validation specificity | Validation sensitivity |
|---|---|---|---|---|---|---|---|---|---|
| **1** | **VGG** | **FFE** | $\mathbf{10^{-3}}$ | **99.97%** | **87%** | **0.0120** | **0.7359** | **96.76%** | **87.76%** |
| 2 | VGG | EMRW | $10^{-3}$ | 76.61% | 66.66% | 0.5899 | 0.8782 | 91.50% | 68.2% |
| 3 | VGG | RI | $10^{-3}$ | 97.72% | 86.45% | 0.0722 | 0.7367 | 96.51% | 86.6% |
| 4 | GoogLeNet | FFE | $10^{-3}$ | 100% | 88% | 0.0002 | 0.6811 | 88.59% | 97.01% |
| 5 | GoogLeNet | EMRW | $10^{-3}$ | 92.46% | 58.33% | 0.1943 | 2,027 | 89.75% | 62% |
| **6** | **GoogLeNet** | **RI** | $\mathbf{10^{-3}}$ | **98.09%** | **90.62%** | **0.0774** | **0.4928** | **97.73%** | **90.86%** |
| 7 | ResNet | FFE | $10^{-3}$ | 19.53% | 20% | 1.6094 | 1.6094 | 80% | 20% |
| 8 | ResNet | EMRW | $10^{-3}$ | 98.55% | 25% | 0.0288 | 8,040 | 80% | 20% |
| 9 | ResNet | RI | $10^{-3}$ | 15.27% | 14% | 1.6094 | 1.6094 | 79% | 16% |
| 10 | VGG | FFE | $10^{-6}$ | 51.92% | 60% | 1,2061 | 1,181 | 89.95% | 62.26% |
| 11 | VGG | EMRW | $10^{-6}$ | 56.85% | 51.04% | 1.1603 | 1.2 | 87.98% | 54.33% |
| 12 | VGG | RI | $10^{-6}$ | 20% | 26% | 1.6094 | 1,6093 | 80% | 20% |
| 13 | GoogLeNet | FFE | $10^{-6}$ | 88.16% | 84% | 0.3768 | 0.4937 | 95.94% | 85% |
| 14 | GoogLeNet | EMRW | $10^{-6}$ | 66.21% | 40.62% | 0.899 | 1,66716 | 85.13% | 43.3% |
| 15 | GoogLeNet | RI | $10^{-6}$ | 43.28% | 38.54% | 1.3286 | 1.6240 | 84.65% | 40.59% |
| 16 | ResNet | FFE | $10^{-6}$ | 17.37% | 26% | 1.6109 | 1,608 | 80.26% | 21% |
| 17 | ResNet | EMRW | $10^{-6}$ | 79.77% | 25% | 0.5516 | 1,99700 | 80% | 20% |
| 18 | ResNet | RI | $10^{-6}$ | 34.87% | 30% | 1,44680 | 1.6094 | 82.74% | 33.32% |
| 19 | VGG | FFE | $10^{-9}$ | 20% | 20% | 1,77511 | 1,66637 | 80% | 20% |
| 20 | VGG | EMRW | $10^{-9}$ | 20.24% | 20.83% | 1.6809 | 1,66434 | 80% | 20% |
| 21 | VGG | RI | $10^{-9}$ | 20.76% | 14.58% | 1,694 | 1.6094 | 80% | 20% |
| 22 | GoogLeNet | FFE | $10^{-9}$ | 19.81% | 25% | 1.7363 | 1.6406 | 81.12% | 25.2% |
| 23 | GoogLeNet | EMRW | $10^{-9}$ | 18.26% | 11.45% | 1,66825 | 1.7704 | 77.47% | 11.20% |
| 24 | GoogLeNet | RI | $10^{-9}$ | 20.22% | 16.66% | 1,685 | 2,22818 | 79.50% | 17.60% |
| 25 | ResNet | FFE | $10^{-9}$ | 22.7% | 19% | 1.6269 | 0.04 | 79.75% | 19% |
| 26 | ResNet | EMRW | $10^{-9}$ | 18.85% | 14% | 2.1515 | 1.8448 | 79.69% | 18.66% |
| 27 | ResNet | RI | $10^{-9}$ | 19.42% | 15% | 1,833 | 2,33286 | 79.35% | 16.79% |

*FFE, fixed feature extractors; EMRW, extension of the model and reinitialization of weights; RI, random initialization.*
*The bold in lines for scenarios 1 and 6 of the this table, they were the best results obtained in the first experiment.*

## First Experiment

To test the accuracy of different neural networks, 24,000 random images were utilized to train the 12 groups of most frequently identified dermatoses (**Table 1**), corresponding to 99.32% of the total volume of the diagnosed diseases. The 12 groups were composed of the classes: benign tumor, eczema, pigmentation disorder, superficial infection/infestation, inflammatory disorder, benign cyst, external cause, genetic cause, not grouped, metabolic cause, malignant tumor and pre-malignant. The category "Pre-malignant" had only 2,200 images and was the only one in which the same images were used both in the training and validation sets (**Table 1**).

Twenty seven scenarios were evaluated based on architectural variations, the initialization strategy, the weights, and the learning rates. The VGG, GoogLeNet and ResNet architectures were evaluated using weight initialization of fixed feature extractors (FFE), extension of the model and reinitialization of weights (EMRW), and random initialization (RI). We have chosen those architectures based on previous works (8, 9, 13), which showed interesting results with them. As the first experiment intended to be exploratory, we used different initialization techniques, including random initialization, which could be seen as not seen suitable for our dataset. IMAGEnet was the base assembly to apply for weight initialization. The learning rate value was adjusted between test scenarios. The parameter variations were 1e-03, 1e-06, and 1e-09, respectively.

The other parameters of the architectures followed the configuration presented in the literature (14). For training, momentum rate with a value of 0.9 and images of the dataset were processed in groups of 32 images simultaneously were used. The training was carried out over 1,000 epochs. To avoid data unbalance due to the disparity between the number of images in each group, the same number of images were used in each of the 12 groups for training and validation. For the validation, 200 random images, which were not present in the training set of each group, were used.

## Second Experiment

During the second experiment, in the final test with the algorithm yielding the best performance among the deep neural networks, 5% of images from each category of dermatoses were used with 7.022 images belonging to the 17 groups, as shown in **Table 1**. The five groups presented at the bottom of the table (connective tissue disorder, adverse drug reaction, deep/systemic infection, bullous disease and factitial dermatitis), however, were disregarded due to the small number of cases, resulting in a total of 6,975 cases tested.

# RESULTS

## First Experiment

**Table 2** presents the results of 27 different scenarios tested in the first experiment to determine which neural network achieves the best performance.

In the training phase, the best accuracy was observed in scenarios with a learning rate of $10^{-3}$. All three architectures showed an accuracy of 98–100%. However, when verifying the values of the validation phase, the GoogLeNet architecture

**TABLE 3** | Confusion matrix of this diagnostic accuracy for GoogLeNet architecture.

| | Genetic cause | Metabolic cause | Traumatic cause | Benign cyst | Pigmentation disorder | Eczema | Superficial infection | Inflammation of unknown cause | Not grouped | Benign tumor | Malignant tumor | Pre-malignant tumor |
|---|---|---|---|---|---|---|---|---|---|---|---|---|
| Genetic cause | 236 | 1 | | 9 | | 53 | 9 | | 3 | 38 | | |
| Metabolic cause | | 119 | 2 | | | 34 | 7 | 6 | 4 | | 4 | |
| External cause | 1 | | 272 | | | 3 | 5 | | 1 | 14 | | 2 |
| Benign cyst | 5 | | | 352 | 27 | 24 | 23 | 12 | 5 | | | |
| Pigmentation disorder | | | 4 | 7 | 898 | 36 | 29 | 20 | 5 | 11 | 2 | |
| Eczema | | | 2 | 2 | | 1,041 | | | 3 | | | |
| Superficial infection/infestation | | | 13 | | 29 | | 859 | | 2 | | | |
| Inflammation disorder | 3 | | | 9 | | 2 | | 690 | | | | |
| Not grouped | 9 | | 3 | 7 | 23 | 68 | | 34 | 94 | | 3 | 3 |
| Benign tumor | | 1 | | | 11 | | | | 1 | 1,488 | | 0 |
| Malignant tumor | | | | | 4 | | 15 | | 2 | 20 | 108 | 4 |
| Pre-malignant | | | | 3 | | | 2 | | 3 | 29 | 1 | 101 |

*Values of the color shade are the true positive results.*

**TABLE 4** | Confusion matrices for referrals and level of priority using GoogLeNet architecture.

| | | Results predicted by AI | | |
|---|---|---|---|---|
| | **Referral** | **Teledermatology** | **Dermatotolgy** | **Biopsy** |
| Dermatologists' Choice (ground truth) | Teledermatology | 6,013 | 36 | 10 |
| | Dermatology | 149 | 471 | 4 |
| | Biopsy | 75 | 3 | 214 |
| | Total | 6,237 | 510 | 228 |
| | Priority | Low | Moderate | High |
| | Low | 3,354 | 364 | 12 |
| | Moderate | 64 | 2,887 | 2 |
| | High | 61 | 17 | 214 |
| | Total | 3,479 | 3,268 | 228 |

obtained the best performance out of all using the RI approach, with 90.62% accuracy.

## Second Experiment

The GoogLeNet network, using IR weight initialization was, then, tested in 6,945 images, obtaining an accuracy of 89.72%. **Table 3** shows the confusion matrix in the diagnostic accuracy of the test in different categories of dermatoses.

Observing the distribution of errors in **Table 3**, a regularity can be noticed in the number of errors and hits for each class except for "ungrouped," which shows not only a smaller number of hits among the lesions but also in a greater number of classes classified as other lesions with this label.

An analysis was conducted of the referral and its priority proposed by the algorithm regardless of the lesion category. Regarding referrals, eight groups (6,237 images) indicated referral for teledermatology, two groups (510 images) for face-to-face dermatologist appointments and two groups (228 images) for biopsy. Among the 12 groups of lesions assessed in the test dataset, up to six had low priority (3,479 images), four had moderate service priority (3.268 images), and two had high priority calls (228 images). The distribution of the priority indication of the service and the routing suggested in the classification of the images are presented in **Table 4**.

The overall accuracy was 96.03% (6,013+471+214 = 6,698/6,975) for the referral of the patient and 92.54% (3,354+2,887+214 = 6,455/6,975) for the priority definition task. The referral confusion matrix showed equivalent specificity percentages in all possible outcomes, 96.41% (6,013/6,237) for referral to the teledermatologist, 92.35% (471/510) to attend dermatologist in person and 93.86% (214/228) for biopsy. As for the priority, it was noted that 93.86% (214/228) high priority lesions received a pertinent indication in the algorithm. However, 78 cases classified as high priority by the dermatologists were classified as low (61) and moderate (17), determining a specificity of 73.23% (214/292).

# DISCUSSION AND CONCLUSIONS

The present study tested 27 scenarios of deep-learning algorithms to determine the most efficient one for classifying common skin lesions in primary care attention into one of the predefined categories, reaching an accuracy of 90.6% in the validation phase and 89.7% in the test phase for 6,975 cases. These results were considered good compared to those in the literature. One of the studies in the literature aimed to use deep neural networks to classify 26 common dermatoses in primary care, with an overall accuracy of 0.66 in 963 cases (15). In another study, 3,501 cases were tested (using two different validation sets) for 134 classes of skin lesions, showing an accuracy of 56.7% in one test group and 44.8% in the other (16). In another research with 5,014 validated cases, AI obtained 76.9% accuracy in classifying 40 common dermatoses (17). Further, in a recently conducted study, 340 teledermatology images were tested for 174 different dermatological diseases, obtaining an accuracy of 41.2% (18).

Currently, a large number of articles show the development of algorithms for diagnostic support of diseases such as melanoma or a group of disorders such as skin cancer mainly using dermoscopic images (19–21). However, the use of dermoscopy may not be feasible on a large scale such as public health. For this reason, the present study used clinical images. Notably, the definitive diagnosis of malignant lesions to date is obtained by histopathology examination, i.e., through the microscopic analysis of the lesion in part or in totality after its surgical excision (biopsy). Therefore, although physicians or an algorithm may suggest skin cancer, the diagnosis is only confirmed by histopathology. Thus, if the biopsy referral is correct, this may be more significant than the diagnosis *per se*. An added advantage, especially in cases where the wait is sometimes as long as 6 months or more, can be if the priority of the disease is determined in addition to providing the correct referral. In cases of skin cancer, if the algorithm correctly points to high priority, it can benefit the patient as well as the health system as a whole. Thus, we consider our results with an accuracy of 96.0% for referrals and 92.5% for priority to be significant, as this data has not yet been reported in the literature.

Another fundamental aspect of the current study is the search for a simpler and low-cost means to obtain images: those clicked by health technicians using the standard photographic camera of a smartphone in regular offices. The use of common technology, with easy access and operability makes it viable to scale the present study. As the images and data were obtained by health technicians, the demand for the physician's specialized workforce is reduced, possibly also lowering costs in the public system.

In terms of the development of neural networks, several challenges were identified in the present study such as the labeling of skin lesions by dermatologists which was done through ICD-10. Initially, it was expected that the present work would be able to create a classifier that can identify the ICD of each lesion. However, after the reports were extracted, it was found that, in addition to the large number of classes ($n = 210$), some ICD codes had a limited number of copies—around two or three images—disabling the training of an algorithm for their identification. Another situation was the low number of cases ($n = 2,200$) in the premalignant category, for which the same images had to be used for both validation and testing. Although this situation is against the basic rules of deep learning algorithm development, we used the same images for validation and test datasets because we did not have enough number of cases in the pre-malignant class to divide it into the different datasets, as we had in the other classes in order to prevent imbalance among the classes.

Also, the category "not grouped" performed poorly in accuracy due to the greater heterogeneity of the images that make up this data set. This class encompassed images showing no lesions at times, or lesions which did not characterize a specific classification, and nail disorders that could not be specified in other groups (**Supplementary Table 1**). Thus, less similarity was observed between the images in the data set and, in some cases, with lesions of other classes.

There are limitations to our work. Our study population was confined to individuals with chronic skin conditions and, therefore, it has limited value as a triage tool because it has not been tested for acute conditions and might not not work in this setting. It is also important to note that the algorithm was in no way intended to take over the physician's role. Its objective lies only in the screening of chronic dermatological lesions, offering health professionals a supporting tool in the confirmation of clinical diagnosis and increasing their productivity in the evaluation of patients. This can optimize medical access for the more severe, surgical, or complex cases and direct them to the right referral and priority.

There are several future possibilities based on the present study. For clinical research, the most obvious pathway will be to apply the algorithm in real-life settings to compare its performance with that of physicians and assess its degree of accuracy. Second, in case of good performance, the use of the algorithm should be verified as this tool would modify medical management. In the field of computing, many possibilities are present for increasing the algorithm's accuracy: use of other network architectures such as ResNeXT, DenseNet and SE-Net; use of demographic data and clinical history of patients; and use of data augmentation for groups of dermatoses with less representation.

## ETHICS STATEMENT

The studies involving human participants were reviewed and approved by Ethics Committee of the Hospital Israelita Albert Einstein (project number: 3541-18). Written informed consent from the participants' legal guardian/next of kin was not required to participate in this study in accordance with the national legislation and the institutional requirements.

## AUTHOR CONTRIBUTIONS

MG-B was responsible for study's design, data collection, and writing and reviewing the article. AS was responsible for study's design, data collection, and performing the experiments and reviewing. EC was responsible for study's design, data collection, and reviewing the article. All authors contributed to the article and approved the submitted version.

## REFERENCES


1. Giavina-Bianchi M, Santos AP, Cordioli E. Teledermatology reduces dermatology referrals and improves access to specialists. *EClin Med.* (2020) 29–30:100641. doi: 10.1016/j.eclinm.2020.100641
2. Vieira R, Lima TMN, Gazzinelli A. The waiting time for specialized medical consultations in a small municipality of Minas Gerais, Brazil. *Rev Mineir Enfermagem.* (2015) 19:65–71. doi: 10.5935/1415-2762.20150006
3. Schmitt JV, Miot HA. Distribution of Brazilian dermatologists according to geographic location, population and HDI of municipalities: an ecological study. *An Bras Dermatol.* (2014) 89:1013–5. doi: 10.1590/abd1806-4841.20143276
4. Giavina-Bianchi M, Sousa R, Cordioli E. Part I: accuracy of teledermatology in inflammatory dermatoses. *Front Med.* (2020) 7:585792. doi: 10.3389/fmed.2020.585792
5. Giavina-Bianchi M, Azevedo MFD, Sousa RM, Cordioli E. Part II: accuracy of teledermatology in skin neoplasms. *Front Med.* (2020) 7:598903. doi: 10.3389/fmed.2020.598903
6. Levin YS, Warshaw EM. Teledermatology: a review of reliability and accuracy of diagnosis and management. *Dermatol Clin.* (2009) 27:163–76, vii. doi: 10.1016/j.det.2008.11.012
7. Shrivastava VK, Londhe ND, Sonawane RS, Suri JS. Computer-aided diagnosis of psoriasis skin images with HOS, texture and color features: a first comparative study of its kind. *Comp Meth Prog Biomed.* (2016) 126:98–109. doi: 10.1016/j.cmpb.2015.11.013
8. Han SS, Kim MS, Lim W, Park GH, Park I, Chang SE. Classification of the clinical images for benign and malignant cutaneous tumors using a deep learning algorithm. *J Invest Dermatol.* (2018) 138:1529–38. doi: 10.1016/j.jid.2018.01.028
9. Han SS, Park GH, Lim W, Kim MS, Na JI, Park I, et al. Deep neural networks show an equivalent and often superior performance to dermatologists in onychomycosis diagnosis: automatic construction of onychomycosis datasets by region-based convolutional deep neural network. *PLoS ONE.* (2018) 13:e0191493. doi: 10.1371/journal.pone.0191493
10. Tschandl P, Codella N, Akay BN, Argenziano G, Braun RP, Cabo H, et al. Comparison of the accuracy of human readers versus machine-

learning algorithms for pigmented skin lesion classification: an open, web-based, international, diagnostic study. *Lancet Oncol.* (2019) 20:938–47. doi: 10.1016/S1470-2045(19)30333-X
11. Tschandl P, Rinner C, Apalla Z, Argenziano G, Codella N, Halpern A, et al. Human-computer collaboration for skin cancer recognition. *Nat Med.* (2020) 26:1229–34. doi: 10.1038/s41591-020-0942-0
12. Marchetti MA, Codella NCF, Dusza SW, Gutman DA, Helba B, Kalloo A, et al. Results of the 2016 international skin imaging collaboration international symposium on biomedical imaging challenge: comparison of the accuracy of computer algorithms to dermatologists for the diagnosis of melanoma from dermoscopic images. *J Am Acad Dermatol.* (2018) 78:270–7.e1. doi: 10.1016/j.jaad.2017.08.016
13. Mahbod A, Schaefer G,Wang C, Ecker R, Ellinger I. Skin lesion classification using hybrid deep neural networks. In: *Presented at: 44th International Conference on Acoustics, Speech, and Signal Processing (ICASSP 2019).* Brighton (2017).
14. Simonyan K, Zisserman A. Very deep convolutional networks for large-scale image recognition. In: *Presented at: Computer Vision and Pattern Recognition (csCV).* San Diego, CA (2014).
15. Liu Y, Jain A, Eng C, Way DH, Lee K, Bui P, et al. A deep learning system for differential diagnosis of skin diseases. *Nat Med.* (2020) 26:900–8. doi: 10.1038/s41591-020-0842-3
16. Han SS, Park I, Lim W, Kim MS, Park GH, Chae JB, et al. Augment intelligence dermatology : deep neural networks empower medical professionals in diagnosing skin cancer and predicting treatment options for 134 skin disorders. *J Invest Dermatol.* (2020) 140:1753–61. doi: 10.1016/j.jid.2020.01.019
17. Pangti R, Mathur J, Chouhan V, Kumar S, Rajput L, Shah S, et al. A machine learning-based, decision support, mobile phone application for diagnosis of common dermatological diseases. *J Eur Acad Dermatol Venereol.* (2020) 35:536–45. doi: 10.1111/jdv.16967
18. Muñoz-López C, Ramírez-Cornejo C, Marchetti MA, Han SS, Del Barrio-Díaz P, Jaque A, et al. Performance of a deep neural network in teledermatology: a single-centre prospective diagnostic study. *J Eur Acad Dermatol Venereol.* (2020) 35:546–53. doi: 10.1111/jdv.16979
19. Chu YS, An HG, Oh BH, Yang S. Artificial intelligence in cutaneous oncology. *Front Med.* (2020) 7:318. doi: 10.3389/fmed.2020.00318
20. Esteva A, Kuprel B, Novoa RA, Ko J, Swetter SM, Blau HM, et al. Corrigendum: dermatologist-level classification of skin cancer with deep neural networks. *Nature.* (2017) 546:686. doi: 10.1038/nature22985
21. Han SS, Moon IJ, Lim W, Suh IS, Lee SY, Na JI, et al. Keratinocytic skin cancer detection on the face using region-based convolutional neural network. *JAMA Dermatol.* (2019) 1:29–37. doi: 10.1001/jamadermatol.2019.3807

3

# Teledermatology Adaptations in the COVID-19 Era

*Harrison A. Edwards* [1,2,3]*, *Xiaohua Shen* [1] *and H. Peter Soyer* [1,3]

[1] Princess Alexandra Hospital, Woolloongabba, QLD, Australia, [2] School of Public Health, University of Queensland, Herston, QLD, Australia, [3] Dermatology Research Centre, The University of Queensland Diamantina Institute, The University of Queensland, Brisbane, QLD, Australia

***Correspondence:**
Harrison A. Edwards
harrison.edwards@health.qld.gov.au

The COVID-19 pandemic has required health services worldwide to adapt to dramatically changing healthcare needs and risks across all medical specialties. In the dermatology department at Princess Alexandra Hospital, Brisbane, Australia, we developed and implemented a teledermatology system with 1 week's notice to help reduce infection risk bidirectionally, while saving patients many hours of travel and waiting time with acceptable technological substitutes for the clinical encounters. In this study, we report the efficacy and tolerability of our telephone consultation and store and forward imaging system, including patient experience from validated survey data. Our design, implementation and usage of a remote-default system provides experience and lessons to draw upon in developing future telemedicine systems to address dermatology service maldistribution – an issue affecting large areas of Australia – as well as preparedness for future infection mitigation requirements.

**Keywords: teledermatology, telemedicine, COVID-19 pandemic, infection control, clinical epidemiology, health services research [MeSH], clinical pathways, performance and evaluation**

## INTRODUCTION

The COVID-19 pandemic has required health services worldwide to adapt to dramatically changing healthcare needs and risks across all medical specialties.

In the dermatology department at Princess Alexandra Hospital, Brisbane, Australia we developed, and instituted a teledermatology system with 1 week's notice. This system comprised of appointments conducted by telephone, and the capacity to receive images by email. Here, we discuss the successes and lessons of implementing this simple system which helped reduce in-person patient numbers and infection risk bidirectionally, while saving patients many hours of travel and waiting time.

Our department has experience in managing a live interactive telehealth dermatology service to treat patients in remote locations (1), as well as a same-day store and forward emergency teledermatology service (2, 3). However, until the current pandemic, face-to-face assessment had been the modality for nearly all routine and urgent appointments and thus comprised the vast majority of patient care.

When the COVID-19 pandemic struck in March 2020 in Brisbane, Australia, and strict lockdown measures were enacted, our dermatology department faced the decision between closing entirely and leaving our catchment of over a million people without a dermatology service, or quickly developing a way that we could continue to serve our patients.

The pre-existing videoconferencing arrangement is limited in that it takes place in the hospital's telehealth center and can only be allocated limited space and time (one session per week), as it uses dedicated hardware and requires a clinic-to-clinic format. Video calls using smartphones would have required either the doctors to use their personal mobile phones and phone numbers, or for the department to acquire and setup additional hardware. These options unfortunately were not feasible, especially in the short time frame and in the context of institutional IT rules.

This study reports on the clinical efficacy and patient experience of a new remote consultation system we devised.

# METHOD

## Clinic Process

The system devised consisted of administrative staff checking in the patients by phone and confirming their phone number and email address in the hour prior to their booked appointment, which saves doctors time. Additionally, because most patients are waiting comfortably at home rather than in the clinic waiting room, they are less inconvenienced by waiting to be seen.

Patient files are queued by nursing staff, and the medical staff call the patients by phone. An email address with shared staff access was approved and created to receive clinical photos from patients to support the phone consultations when indicated. The images were then incorporated into the usual electronic medical record, Millennium (Cerner Corporation; North Kansas City, Missouri, United States).

Prescriptions and investigation forms are physically mailed to the patient's home address, and urgent prescriptions are faxed directly to the patient's pharmacy for rapid preparation and dispensing (**Figure 1**).

## System Implementation

This system was developed by nursing and administrative staff in the department with input and feedback from the doctors, and was instituted on 23rd March 2020 after a week of preparation.

At first, dermatology trainees were tasked with determining which upcoming appointments would be suitable for remote consultation. Factors evaluated included patient location, diagnosis, and current management if the appointment was for a review, and expected risk of deterioration and ability to evaluate without in-person examination.

Subsequently, we changed to a system whereby phone consultation was the default. If issues arose during the consultation that would require in-person review (such as an inability to adequately examine the patient using photos, a requirement for discussion of complex management decisions, or urgent physical treatments), a subsequent in-person appointment was made. Patients located nearby could sometimes attend the clinic in-person the same day; for other cases, an appointment would be arranged within a week.

This system of teledermatology by default and escalation when required increased the numbers of consultations conducted remotely and eliminated the time requirement of dermatology trainees assessing appropriateness for teledermatology prior to the appointment.

As the year progressed and government lockdown rules were reduced, more appointments were conducted in-person. In June to September, review appointments could be booked as in-person or teledermatology depending on doctors' clinical judgment and patient preference, whereas appointments for new patients were booked for teledermatology. During this period, appointments conducted in-person approached 50%.

By November, in-person appointments became the default, and subsequently ~20% of appointments were conducted by teledermatology.

## Evaluation

To assess the implementation of this system, clinic appointment counts were assessed and compared with the same period in the calendar year prior, appointments requiring a language interpreter were noted, and a count of cases in the email system was conducted.

For the patient perspective, a survey was conducted by phone of 100 patients of the ~2,000 patients who had a phone appointment between 23rd March 2020 and 15th January 2021. To minimize recall bias and to elicit the most accurate and detailed responses, this sample of patients was taken from those who had a phone appointment within the recent time frame of 18th November 2020 to 15th January 2021.

A validated survey tool, the Telehealth Usability Questionnaire (TUQ), was used to comprehensively cover the domains of usefulness, ease of use and learnability, interface quality, interaction quality, reliability, satisfaction and

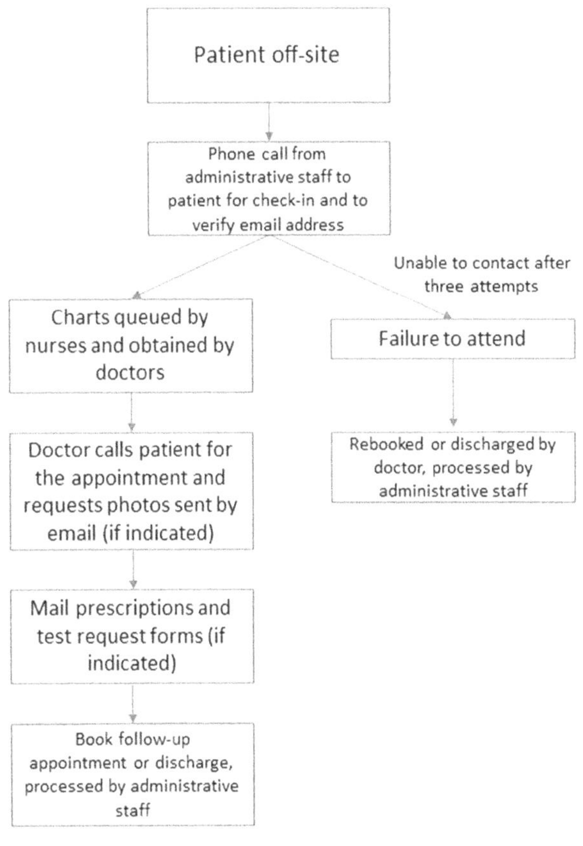


**FIGURE 1** | Clinic workflow in the teledermatology system.

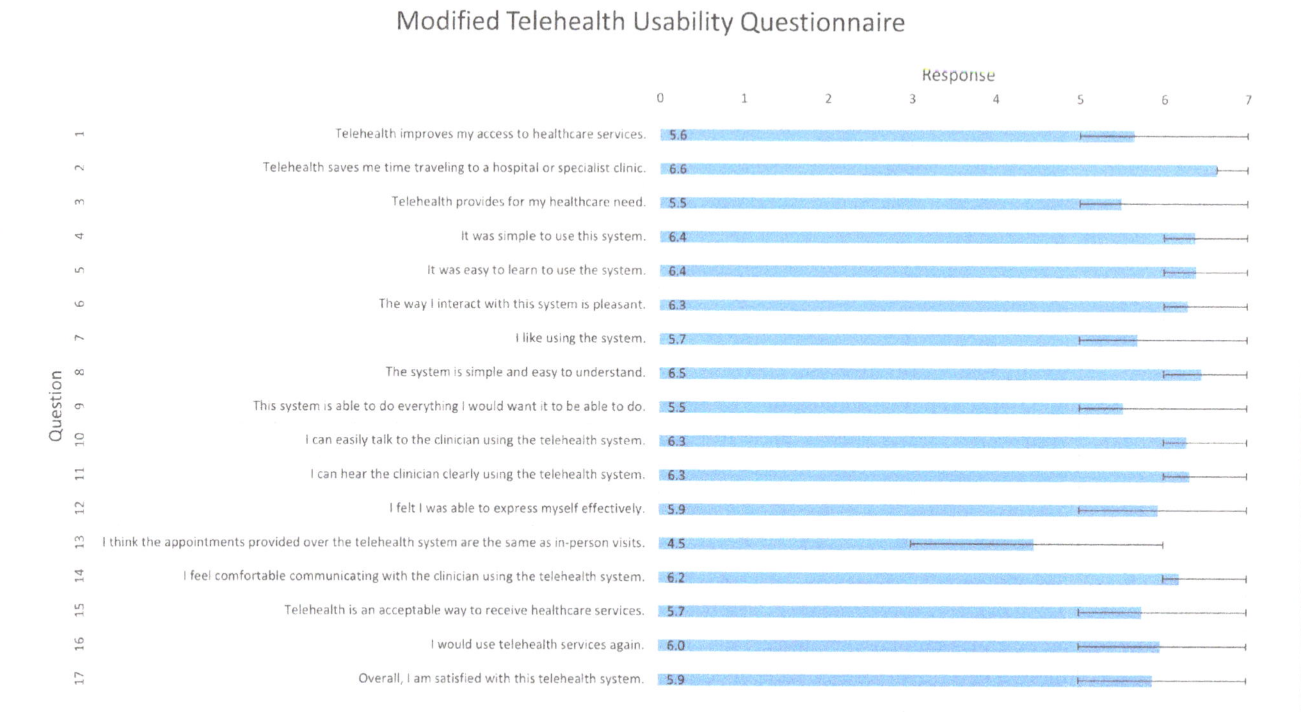


**FIGURE 2** | Modified Telehealth Usability Questionnaire, responses to quantitative questions. Likert scale; 1 (disagree) to 7 (agree); mean and interquartile range.

future use. The TUQ has demonstrated strong validity and reliability across various telecommunication systems, whereas most other questionnaires apply primarily to special purpose videoconferencing hardware or other single modalities (4).

The TUQ was modified to exclude questions that were not applicable to our context. Consequently, a set of 17 questions (based on a 7-point Likert scale) and an open-ended feedback question were used.

## RESULTS

Through this system, in-person clinic attendance was reduced by 95% at the initial peak of the pandemic while maintaining high clinical throughput: a sample of medical dermatology clinic sessions in the first 2 months of the teledermatology system showed higher patient numbers than the same period the year prior.

However, surgical clinic sessions were more negatively impacted by the pandemic: although appointment counts under the teledermatology system were only 11% lower than usual, these appointments served only as a safety check – urgent, complex lesions were subsequently booked for in-person management; patients were otherwise advised to see their general practitioner for other skin concerns.

A language interpreter was required in 5% of cases, and surprisingly, an evaluation of the email system in the first 3 weeks demonstrated that photos were required in only 36.5% (152/417) of appointments. When photos were required, patients could usually manage to send them by email to the shared inbox described above, and photos were generally of suitable quality. The proportion of consultations over the same period that required escalation to an in-person encounter was low, at 2.4% (10/417).

The major benefits identified from the survey (**Figure 2**) were saving travel time (Q2) and that it is simple and easy to understand and use (Q4, Q5, Q8).

Comparatively low scores were given for questions that asked about clinical equivalence to in-person appointments (Q3, Q9, Q13). However, most patients responded indicating that they were satisfied with the service and that they would use it again (Q16, Q17).

Based on 74 responses to the open-ended feedback question, certain benefits and drawbacks were identified. Some patients (5%), especially the elderly, identified difficulty with taking and emailing photos. Some patients (3%) whose phone appointment was not clinically adequate and required a subsequent in-person appointment were unhappy about the double handling and delay.

Many patients (20%) emphasized the benefit of eliminating travel time and reducing the interruption to their day, but many (27%) also felt that dermatology was particularly challenging for telemedicine due to the primacy of visual examination. Relatedly, a contingent of patients (7%), including some of those who reported overall satisfaction with the teledermatology system, stated a desire for periodic in-person appointments.

Despite the reduction in travel time, several patients (9%) expressed inconvenience regarding the unreliable appointment wait times on the day of their appointment. A surprisingly small number of patients (4%) commented on infection risk mitigation as a benefit of the teledermatology system.

# DISCUSSION

## Strengths

Our simple conventional phone-based teledermatology system has worked well, allowing patients to still receive clinical care while avoiding bidirectional infection risk. Although existing literature on teledermatology essentially always involves remote visual examination (either synchronously or asynchronously) (5, 6), our finding that images were required only in a minority of cases suggests that a large proportion of teledermatology, more feasibly follow-up appointments, could be conducted without visual examination. This may be due to the department's new:review ratio of 1:4; however, image requirement by appointment type could not be extracted to confirm this.

Administrative workload has been mostly unchanged in the new, remote system, and time-consuming steps such as patient and staff movement between waiting rooms and consultation rooms have been avoided.

This system is advantageous for reducing infection risk for the general patient population, but is especially protective for our many patients who are on immunosuppressive therapies. As well as reducing bidirectional infection risk, teledermatology reduces the need for personal protective equipment, helping to maintain supplies for clinical encounters where it is necessary.

As a department of a public hospital, we have the advantage that we do not rely on private health insurance or Medicare billing, and therefore issues related to those aspects can be avoided in our teledermatology process.

## Weaknesses

Many patients were able to send clinical photos through the email system, but as described above, 33% of survey respondents either found the email system technically challenging (5%) or felt it was inferior compared to in-person visual examination (27%). Email was used to receive photos from patients, even though it is not an institutionally approved way of communicating with patients outside of emergency conditions such as the COVID-19 pandemic. The other store and forward methods requested by patients, Facebook Messenger and Multimedia Messaging Service (MMS), would have carried additional issues of privacy and difficulty of shared staff access.

Evaluation of patients for skin cancer is problematic in this teledermatology system, because of the difficulty of replicating examination electronically and the significant consequences of incorrect skin cancer diagnosis. Each lesion on a patient poses new diagnostic uncertainty, and biopsies cannot be done remotely. Consequently, skin cancer patients requiring urgent biopsy comprised many of the patients needing to be seen in-person. Generally, patients were advised that their skin cancer examination would be delayed and that they should see their GP in the meantime.

Appointments requiring a language interpreter were sometimes complicated. These were arranged either as a consultation with an interpreter co-located with the doctor and the patient on the phone, or as a three-way phone conversation with the doctor in the clinic and the interpreter and patient on the phone. If the dermatology consultant needed to be involved, the three-way call between the doctor, patient and interpreter would need to be ended and later reconnected to relay the consultant's input, which was cumbersome and time consuming.

# CONCLUSION

This system was put in place after only 1 week of development, reduced the number of patients in the clinic by 95%, allowing us to greatly reduce the infection risk for both patients and staff, reduce PPE requirement, and also save patients travel time and waiting time.

The necessity of telemedicine systems to minimize infection risk during the current pandemic has been recognized in Australia and overseas. Health systems worldwide have responded by declaring that in-person medical care should be limited to only the most urgent patients. To facilitate this, they have reduced administrative and security requirements for telemedicine, allowing healthcare providers to serve patients through everyday communications technologies such as phone, email, instant messaging, and video chat software (7, 8).

Dermatology departments in the United States (9–11), China (12), and Europe (13–15) have accordingly restricted their in-person clinical encounters due to the recognized risk of SARS-CoV-2 transmission. Similarly, the Australian government has adapted administrative billing requirements for telemedicine by general practitioners and all medical specialists (16).

Our experience of urgently designing and implementing a teledermatology system was broadly positive, due to the benefits of infection risk reduction, reduced patient travel and waiting times, and acceptability to patients and doctors of in-person history and examination substitutes.

In the United States, The Society of Dermatology Hospitalists developed an algorithm to triage teledermatology consults. A high rate of teledermatology suitability was found, with only four out of the 35 patients sampled (11%) requiring escalation to in-person consultation (17), which accords with our result of 2.4%.

As before the COVID-19 pandemic, there is legitimate concern regarding technological security and patient privacy regarding teledermatology. Our imperfect but successful design, implementation and usage of a remote-default system using phone for consultations with supporting images sent by email provides experience and lessons to draw upon in developing future robust telemedicine systems to address dermatology service provision, taking into consideration specialist maldistribution in Australia as well as preparedness for future infection mitigation requirements.

# ETHICS STATEMENT

The studies involving human participants were reviewed and approved by Metro South Health Human Research Ethics Committee. Written informed consent for participation was not required for this study in accordance with the national legislation and the institutional requirements.

## AUTHOR CONTRIBUTIONS

HE and XS contributed to data acquisition. HE and HS contributed to data analysis. All authors contributed equally to the concept, design, and contributed to the drafting and critical revision of the manuscript.

## REFERENCES

1. Miller BJ, Finnane A, Vun Y, Halloran S, Stapelberg A, Soyer HP, et al. Real-time teledermatology clinics in a tertiary public hospital: a clinical audit. *Australas J Dermatol.* (2020) 61:e383–7. doi: 10.1111/ajd.13322
2. Finnane AR, Siller G, Soyer HP. Teledermatologists' management of emergency skin conditions. *Med J Aust.* (2015) 203:286. doi: 10.5694/mja15.00362
3. Finnane A, Siller G, Mujcic R, Soyer HP. The growth of a skin emergency teledermatology service from 2008 to 2014. *Australas J Dermatol.* (2016) 57:14–8. doi: 10.1111/ajd.12411
4. Parmanto B, Lewis AN, Graham KM, Bertolet MH. Development of the Telehealth Usability Questionnaire (TUQ). *Int J Telerehabil.* (2016) 8:3–10. doi: 10.5195/ijt.2016.6196
5. Finnane A, Dallest K, Janda M, Soyer HP. Teledermatology for the diagnosis and management of skin cancer a systematic review. *JAMA Dermatol.* (2017) 153:319–27. doi: 10.1001/jamadermatol.2016.4361
6. Lee JJ, English JC. Teledermatology: a review and update. *Am J Clin Dermatol.* (2018) 19:253–60. doi: 10.1007/s40257-017-0317-6
7. United States Centers for Medicare & Medicaid Services. *President Trump Expands Telehealth Benefits for Medicare Beneficiaries During COVID-19 Outbreak.* Available online at: https://www.cms.gov/newsroom/press-releases/president-trump-expands-telehealth-benefits-medicare-beneficiaries-during-covid-19-outbreak/ (accessed April 9, 2020).
8. Lee I, Kovarik C, Tejasvi T, Pizarro M, Lipoff JB. Telehealth: helping your patients and practice survive and thrive during the COVID-19 crisis with rapid quality implementation. *J Am Acad Dermatol.* (2020) 82:1213–4. doi: 10.1016/j.jaad.2020.03.052
9. Pathoulas JT, Stoff BK, Lee KC, Farah RS. Ethical outpatient dermatology care during the coronavirus (COVID-19) pandemic. *J Am Acad Dermatol.* (2020) 82:1272–3. doi: 10.1016/j.jaad.2020.03.047
10. Kwatra SG, Sweren RJ, Grossberg AL. Dermatology practices as vectors for COVID-19 transmission: a call for immediate cessation of nonemergent dermatology visits. *J Am Acad Dermatol.* (2020) 82:e179–80. doi: 10.1016/j.jaad.2020.03.037
11. Price KN, Thiede R, Shi VY, Curiel-Lewandrowski C. Strategic dermatology clinical operations during COVID-19 pandemic. *J Am Acad Dermatol.* (2020) 82:e207–9. doi: 10.1016/j.jaad.2020.03.089
12. Chen Y, Pradhan S, Xue S. What are we doing in the dermatology outpatient department amidst the raging of the 2019 novel coronavirus? *J Am Acad Dermatol.* (2020) 82:1034. doi: 10.1016/j.jaad.2020.02.030
13. Wollina U. Challenges of COVID-19 pandemic for dermatology. *Dermatol Ther.* (2020) 33:e13430. doi: 10.1111/dth.13430
14. Radi G, Diotallevi F, Campanati A, Offidani A. Global coronavirus pandemic (2019-nCOV): implication for an Italian medium size dermatological clinic of a II level hospital. *J Eur Acad Dermatol Venereol.* (2020) 34:e213–4. doi: 10.1111/jdv.16386
15. Wang R, Helf C, Tizek L, Neuhauser R, Eyerich K, Zink A, et al. The impact and consequences of SARS-CoV-2 pandemic on a Single University Dermatology Outpatient Clinic in Germany. *Int J Environ Res Public Health.* (2020) 17:6182. doi: 10.3390/ijerph17176182
16. Medical Benefits Schedule. *COVID-19 Temporary MBS Telehealth Services.* Australian Government Department of Health. Available online at: http://www.mbsonline.gov.au/internet/mbsonline/publishing.nsf/Content/Factsheet-TempBB (accessed February 25, 2021).
17. Salamon M. *A Decade of Telemedicine Policy Has Advanced in Just 2 Weeks* [Internet]. Medscape (2020). Available online at: http://www.medscape.com/viewarticle/928038

# 4

# Artificial Intelligence in Cutaneous Oncology

*Yu Seong Chu*[1], *Hong Gi An*[1], *Byung Ho Oh*[2*] *and Sejung Yang*[1*]

[1] *Department of Biomedical Engineering, Yonsei University, Wonju, South Korea,* [2] *Department of Dermatology and Cutaneous Biology Research Institute, Yonsei University College of Medicine, Seoul, South Korea*

***Correspondence:**
*Byung Ho Oh*
*obh505@gmail.com*
*Sejung Yang*
*syang@yonsei.ac.kr*

Skin cancer, previously known to be a common disease in Western countries, is becoming more common in Asian countries. Skin cancer differs from other carcinomas in that it is visible to our eyes. Although skin biopsy is essential for the diagnosis of skin cancer, decisions regarding whether or not to conduct a biopsy are made by an experienced dermatologist. From this perspective, it is easy to obtain and store photos using a smartphone, and artificial intelligence technologies developed to analyze these photos can represent a useful tool to complement the dermatologist's knowledge. In addition, the universal use of dermoscopy, which allows for non-invasive inspection of the upper dermal level of skin lesions with a usual 10-fold magnification, adds to the image storage and analysis techniques, foreshadowing breakthroughs in skin cancer diagnosis. Current problems include the inaccuracy of the available technology and resulting legal liabilities. This paper presents a comprehensive review of the clinical applications of artificial intelligence and a discussion on how it can be implemented in the field of cutaneous oncology.

**Keywords: artificial intellegence, cutaneous oncology, skin cancer, machine learning, deep learning**

## INTRODUCTION

The increasing incidence of skin cancer is a global trend. Skin cancer, which was previously known to be a common disease in Western countries, is occurring more frequently in South Korea. According to the Korean Statistical Information Service[1], the number of patients with non-melanoma skin cancer in 2015 was 4,804 (9.4 people per 100,000), an increase over the 1,960 in 2005 and 3,270 in 2010. The increase in incidence rate is thought to be due to the aging population, the increased popularity of outdoor activities, increased ultraviolet exposure, improved access to medical services, and increased awareness of skin cancer among patients (1).

Skin biopsy and histopathologic evaluation are essential in confirming skin cancer. However, it is impossible to confirm all pigmented lesions by biopsy due to pain and scar development. Therefore, it is first necessary to establish whether or not a biopsy is required through a visual inspection performed by an experienced dermatologist. Furthermore, dermatologist needs a device that can detect changes over time in skin lesions and record the lesions in detail so that wrong-site surgery does not occur (2, 3).

With the development of imaging technologies, methods and devices for recording and analyzing what doctors see have progressed rapidly. Universally, dermoscopic imaging irradiates light onto the upper dermal layer, to observe and record more detailed pigment changes. In recent years, development of high-resolution non-invasive diagnostic devices (e.g., confocal microscopy, multiphoton microscopy, etc.) that can detect cellular levels of the skin lesions without biopsy has also been enriched (4–6). In addition, diagnoses of such skin images using artificial intelligence

[1]http://kosis.kr/statHtml/statHtml.do?orgId=117&tblId=DT_117N_A00025&conn_path=I2

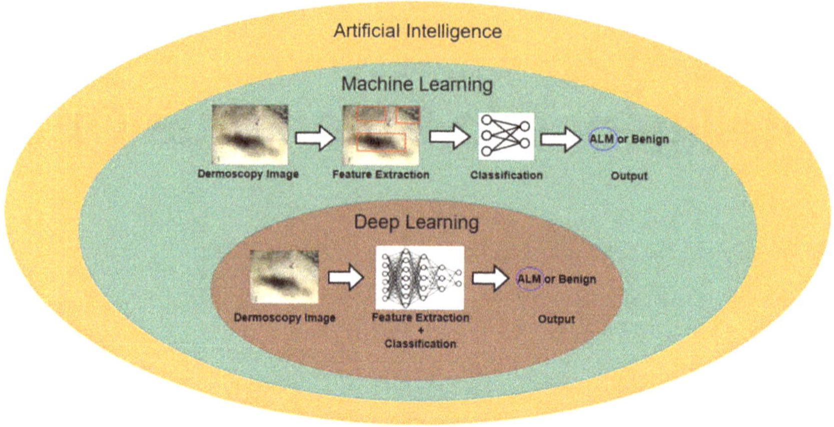


**FIGURE 1** | Relationship between artificial intelligence, machine learning, and deep learning.

(AI) have been shown to outperform the average diagnosis performances of doctors. These developments are expected to have a significant impact on the diagnosis of skin cancer, the accurate recording of changes in suspicious lesions, and the effectiveness of follow-up skin cancer surgery. For user convenience, applications suitable for general smartphones have become available; however, these are not sufficiently supported by scientific evidence.

In this review, we introduce the basic concepts and clinical applications of AI via a literature review and discuss how these can be implemented in the field of dermatological oncology.

## BASIC CONCEPTS OF ARTIFICIAL INTELLIGENCE

AI is a field of computer science that solves problems by imitating human intelligence, these problems typically require the recognition of patterns in various data. Conventional machine learning refers to machine learning methods that do not involve deep learning; these methods extract features such as those relating to colors, textures, and edges. In conventional machine learning, precise engineering knowledge and extensive experience are required to design feature extractors capable of extracting suitable features. Using these features, conventional machine learning can derive various results and identify correlations.

Deep learning uses deep neural networks to learn features, which are obtained by designing simple but non-linear modules for each layer. Using deep neural networks, very complex functions can be learned. For example, in the field of computer vision, a deep neural network's first layer typically learns the presence of edges at particular orientations and locations within the image. Larger combinations of such edges are identified in the next layer. As the layers become deeper, they learn larger and more specific features (7).

**Figure 1** shows the relationship between AI, machine learning, and deep learning. Deep learning falls within the category of machine learning, which falls within the category of AI. In this figure, the examples for conventional machine learning and deep learning are classifications of acral lentiginous melanoma (ALM) and benign nevus (BN) in dermoscopy images. Conventional machine learning extracts specific features from dermoscopy images; for example, the gray-level co-occurrence matrix (GLCM) is used to extract texture features (8). The conventional machine learning method then trains classifiers, using the extracted features to classify ALM and BN. However, deep learning methods learn by extracting various features through deep neural networks. The main difference between conventional machine learning and deep learning is that deep learning extracts various features per layer, without human intervention (9).

We divided the cutaneous oncology publications into those evaluating malignant skin cancers and non-melanoma skin cancers. In addition, each publication was divided into machine learning (excluding deep learning), deep learning, and hybrid methods (a combination of machine learning and deep learning) (**Figure 2**).

In terms of machine learning methods, most publications use a feature extractor to extract a feature from an image, they then train the classifier model using these features

---

**Abbreviations:** ACC, accuracy; AI, artificial intelligence; ALM, acral lentiginous melanoma; AUC, area under the curve; BCC, basal cell carcinoma; BN, benign nevus; BoF, bag of features; CLAHE, contrast-limited adaptive histogram equalization; CNN, convolutional neural network; DCNN, deep convolution neural network; DI, dice score; DLNN, deep learning-based neural network; FFOCT, full-field optical coherence tomography; GAC, geodesic active contour; GLCM, gray-level co-occurrence matrix; ICA, independent component analysis; ILSVRC, ImageNet large-scale visual recognition challenge; ISBI, International Symposium on Biomedical Imaging; ISIC, International Skin Imaging Collaboration; JA, Jaccard index; KNN, k-nearest neighbor; LFN, lesion feature network; LICU, lesion index calculation unit; LIN, lesion indexing network; MLP, multi-layer perceptron; MM, malignant melanoma; NPV, negative predictive values; OCT, optical coherence tomography; PCA, principal component analysis; PPV, positive predictive values; PS-OCT, polarization-sensitive optical coherence tomography; RF, random forest; SCC, squamous cell carcinoma; SGNN, self-generating neural network; SK, seborrheic keratosis; Sen, sensitivity; Spe, specificity; SVM, support vector machine.

(e.g., malignant melanoma (MM) vs. BN). Recently, deep convolution neural network (DCNN) have been implemented in many medical-imaging studies (10–12). DCNN use convolution operations to compensate for the problems that arise through neglecting the correlations and pixel localities of multi-layer perceptron (MLP). Thus, deep learning can be used to train a robust classifier model with a variety of data. **Figure 3** shows an example of a DCNN for classifying ALMs and BNs in dermoscopic images. The DCNN feature extractor repeatedly applies convolution and max-pooling (to obtain the largest activation for each region) operations to the layer input. This process generates a feature map. The feature map is inputted to a classifier via global average pooling for each channel. The classifier finally determines probabilities for ALM and BN. The result is then compared with the actual label, and the parameters are updated via backpropagation. However, DCNN operations require highly powerful graphics processing units to manage the complex computations and large datasets involved. Although DCNN learning capacities can be limited by insufficient medical-image data, it is possible to fine-tune state-of-art deep learning models that show high performance in ImageNet large-scale visual recognition challenge (ILSVRC), making them suitable for medical purposes (13). In the hybrid method, an ensemble classifier is designed by combining a conventional machine learning method and a deep learning method. For example, after extracting the features of an image using a conventional machine learning method, these extracted features are used as inputs for a DCNN. Another example is that of training a support vector machine (SVM) using a feature map obtained through a DCNN (14). One publication showed that hybrid models outperform both deep learning and conventional machine learning models (15), another publication highlighted the limitations of deep learning and stated a need for hybrid models to overcome these limitations (16). Thus, these two methods can be used effectively to create more accurate models.

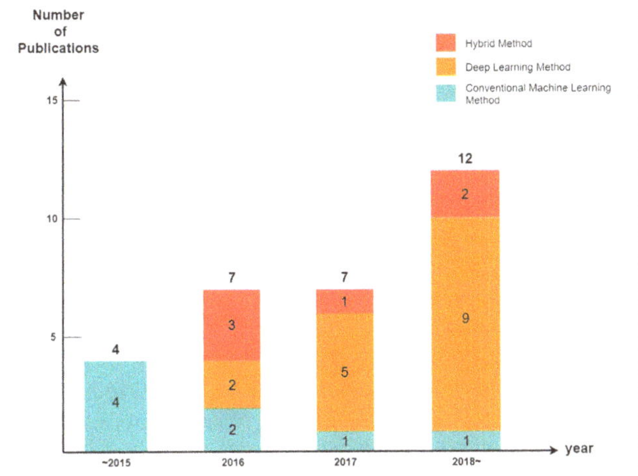


**FIGURE 2 |** Number of publications employing artificial intelligence in cutaneous oncology.

Every year, the number of articles describing AI implementations in the field of cutaneous oncology increases. By observing the trends of the discipline, it can be seen that studies using conventional machine learning have been decreasing in popularity since 2015 (five publications in 2015, three publications from 2016 to 2017, and one publication after 2018); however, the number of studies conducted using deep learning methods has increased significantly since 2015 (zero publications in 2015, seven publications from 2016 to 2017, and nine publications after 2018). These tendencies are a result of the increasing availability of big data and powerful GPUs. Since 2015, state-of-art deep learning models such as ResNet have also been studied [ResNet competed for the first time in the 2015 ILSVRC (17); it surpassed the human error rate of 5%, achieving an error rate of 3.6%].

## APPLICATION OF ARTIFICIAL INTELLIGENCE IN THE DIAGNOSIS OF MALIGNANT SKIN CANCERS

### Melanoma

A total of 18 publications were identified, six of these described the use of conventional machine learning, nine publications

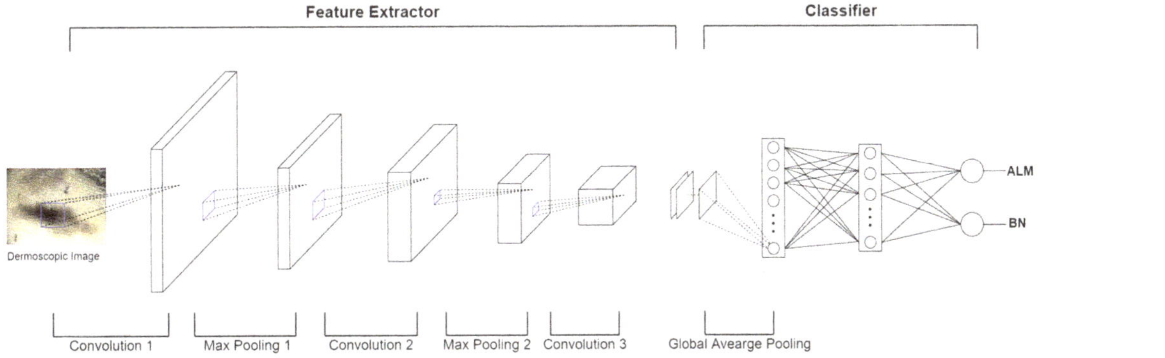


**FIGURE 3 |** Example of DCNN for classifying ALM and BN in dermoscopic images. In the feature extractor, each layer performs a convolution operation on the input data and then performs a max-pooling operation, thereby reducing the image size and increasing the number of channels. The feature extractor generates a feature map by repeating this process for each layer. After the global average pooling operation, the feature map is used as the input of the classifier layer (fully-connected layer). Finally, the output of the fully-connected layer appears as a probability of ALM or BN.

showed the use of deep learning, and two publications presented the use of hybrid models. Among the total 18 publications, 14 used dermoscopic images as the dataset, and the remainder used unspecified or clinical images; nine used more than 500 datasets, and the remainder used <500 datasets. Moreover, in five of the publications, other skin lesion data such as seborrheic keratosis (SK) and basal cell carcinoma (BCC) were used alongside malignant melanomas and nevus. Seven publications presented the area under the curve (AUC) as a performance indicator of the model and the remainder presented accuracy (Acc), sensitivity (Sen), and specificity (Spe) (**Tables 1–3**).

### Deep Learning

Among the deep learning algorithms discussed in the literature, five were fine-tuned using pre-trained models. The remainder were fully trained with new models. In four publications, preprocessing was performed prior to model training. In addition, two publications performed lesion segmentation and classification or segmentation of dermoscopic features. To measure the model performance, one publication (Tschandl, Kittler et al.) compared the results of final-year medical students with those of the model; two publications (Yang et al. and Lee et al.) used the results of dermatological experts as the comparison. From these, Lee et al. showed that experienced dermatologists and inexperienced dermatologists improved their decision making with the help of deep learning models. One publication (Premaladha and Ravichandran) compared the conventional machine learning method 'Hybrid Adaboost-SVM' and a deep learning-based neural network on the same dataset; they showed that the deep learning-based neural network delivered superior performance. Moreover, one publication (Cui et al.) demonstrated that when more data was used, the results of deep learning outperformed conventional machine learning methods.

### Conventional Machine Learning

From the conventional machine learning publications, four of the five publications performed feature extraction and then created a classifier. Two of these publications used SVM for the classifier, one used multivariable linear regression, and one used a layered model. In three publications, artifact removal or lesion segmentation were performed prior to feature extraction. On the other hand, one publication (Marchetti, Codella et al.) presented a new model using a fusion method, developed by 25 teams participating in International Symposium on Biomedical Imaging (ISBI) 2016.

### Hybrid (Deep Learning + Machine Learning)

In the publications using hybrid methods, one publication (Jafari, Nasr-Esfahani et al.) preprocessed the input images, extracted the patches, and performed segmentation using a convolutional neural network (CNN). In one publication (Xie, Fan et al.), segmentation was performed after preprocessing, using a neural network called self-generating neural network (SGNN); they then presented an ensemble network by designing a feature extractor and classifier. Furthermore, in one publication (Sabbaghi et al.), a deep auto-encoder combined with bag of features (BoF) outperformed the model using a BoF or deep auto-encoder alone.

## Non-melanoma Skin Cancer: BCC, Squamous Cell Carcinoma (SCC)

We identified seven deep learning publications, three machine learning publications and three hybrid publications on non-melanoma skin cancer. Several publications discussed MM; however, all of them discussed BCC and three publications discussed SCC, thus we classified the publications into these categories. The results are organized in **Tables 4–6**.

The results of all publications were presented using an accuracy indicator, and some of these publications using a variety of indicators, such as specificity, sensitivity, precision, and F1 score. The datasets used in each publication were different, making it impossible to compare them directly.

### Deep Learning

Rezvantalab et al. compared the abilities of deep learning against the performances of highly trained dermatologists. This publication presented outcomes from various deep learning models. In the BCC classification, the highest AUC of the publication was reported as 99.3%, using DenseNet 201. When compared against dermatologists (AUC 88.82%), the results of deep learning were found superior.

Five publications used datasets of dermoscopic images. One used full-field optical coherence tomography (FFOCT) images, and Jordan Yap et al. used different forms of data including metadata, macroscopic images, and dermoscopic images. Next, they trained a deep learning model using fusion techniques, in which image feature vectors were concatenated with the metadata feature vectors. Two publications by Zhang et al. written in 2017 and 2018, showed interesting results; the 2018 publication improved the previous year's algorithm for utilizing medical information. Their results showed an average improvement of 0.7% over those of the previous year.

### Conventional Machine Learning

We identified four publications that used only machine learning techniques. Three publications used dermoscopic images and one used polarization-sensitive optical coherence tomography (PS-OCT) images. Each author used different methods and features.

Marvdashti et al. performed feature extraction and classification using multiple machine learning methods [SVM, k-nearest neighbor (KNN)]. Kharazmi et al. segmented vascular structures using independent component analysis (ICA) and k-means clustering, then classified them using a random forest classifier. Kefel et al. introduced automatically generated borders using geodesic active contour (GAC) and Otsu's threshold for the detection of pink blush features, known as a common feature of BCCs. Subsequently, they classified using logistic regression, based on features such as smoothness and brightness.

### Hybrid (Deep Learning + Machine Learning)

Three publications implementing hybrids were identified. Each publication used a different dataset. One publication used optical coherence tomography (OCT) images and another used

**TABLE 1** | Melanoma skin cancer publications using deep learning method.

| Publication | End-point | Results | Method | Dataset |
|---|---|---|---|---|
| Li et al. (18) | – Lesion segmentation (task1)<br>– Lesion dermoscopic feature extraction (task2)<br>– Lesion classification (task3) | Task 1: JA : 0.710 (LIN)<br>Task 2 :AUC : 0.848 (LFN)<br>Task 3 :AUC : 0.912 (LIN with LICU) | – Task 1 and Task 3<br>Preprocessing:<br>Center crop + Resize(320*320)<br>Data augmentation<br>Task 1 used LIN<br>Task 3 used LIN with LICU<br>– Task 2<br>Pre-processing:<br>Superpixel extraction<br>Data augmentation<br>Random sample<br>Patch rotation<br>Using LFN | ISIC 2017 dataset ($n = 2000$)<br>The dataset contains melanoma, SK and nevus |
| Pour et al. (19) | – Lesion segmentation<br>– Lesion dermoscopic feature segmentation (streak and globule features) | Lesion segmentation:<br>Sen : 0.91<br>Spe : 0.95<br>Acc : 0.94<br>JA : 0.83<br>DI : 0.89<br>Lesion dermoscopic feature segmentation:<br>Sen: 0.119<br>Spe: 0.997<br>Acc: 0.991<br>JA: 0.60<br>DI: 0.108 | Data Augmentation<br>– Lesion segmentation : Deeper model with 16 conv. layers, augmentation by flipping and cropping (7200 training images)<br>– Lesion dermoscopic feature segmentation:<br>Similar convolutional layers initialized with a pre-trained model from lesion segmentation phase. This architecture is followed by two parts, each contains two convolutional layers and four deconvolutional layers to predict masks for both streak and globule features. | ISBI 2016 challenge dataset<br>The dataset contains a representative mix of images of both MM and BN<br>– Lesion segmentation:<br>Train_Images ($n = 900$)<br>Test_Images ($n = 379$)<br>– Lesion dermoscopic feature segmentation:<br>Train_Images ($n = 807$)<br>Test_Images ($n = 335$) |
| Yu et al. (20) | Classification (ALM and BN) | Group A<br>– CNN<br>Sen: 92.57%<br>Spe: 75.39%<br>Acc: 83.51%<br>PPV: 77.14%<br>NPV: 91.88%<br>– Expert<br>Sen: 94.88%<br>Spe: 68.72%<br>Acc.: 81.08%<br>PPV: 73.13%<br>NPV: 93.71% | – Training<br>Data augmentation : 12 patches cropping, rotation, and flipping<br>CNN: 5-layer convolution network + FC<br>– Testing<br>Cropping 12 patches per test image and when one or more images were predicted as containing melanoma, the corresponding test image was interpreted as containing melanoma | Dermoscopic images<br>ALM ($n = 350$) and BN ($n = 374$)<br>– Group A<br>ALM ($n = 175$) and BN ($n = 187$) |
| Nasr-Esfahani et al. (21) | Classification (melanoma and nevus) | Sen: 81%<br>Spe: 80%<br>Acc: 81%<br>PPV: 75%<br>NPV: 86% | Pre-processing : Removal of noise and illumination artifacts<br>CNN: 2-layer convolution network (20 feature maps and 50 feature maps) + FC | Clinical images<br>Melanoma ($n = 70$) and nevus ($n = 100$)<br>Train_Images (80%)<br>Test_Images (20%) |
| Premaladha et al. (22) | Classification (MM and BN)<br>Best model : DLNN | Sen. 94.83%<br>Spe. 90.46%<br>Acc. 92.89% | Pre-processing : CLAHE and median filter<br>Segmentation : Normalized Otsu's segmentation (NOS)<br>Classifier : Compared DLNN and hybrid Adaboost-SVM. Best model was DLNN | Dermoscopy images<br>Train_Images (85%)<br>Test_Images (15%) |
| Matsunaga et al. (23) | Classification (melanoma, nevus and SK) | – ISBI 2017 challenge dataset<br>AUC : 0.958<br>– ISBI 2016 challenge dataset<br>AUC : 0.874 | Pre-processing : luminance and color balance of input images are normalized exploiting color constancy<br>CNN :<br>Fine-tuned 50-layer ResNet MM classifier and SK classifier<br>Ensemble classifier made by merging two classifiers | ISBI 2017 challenge dataset<br>Train_Images : provided data (374 MM, 254 SK, 1372 nevi) + external data (409 MM, 66 SK, 969 nevi)<br>Test_Images ($n = 150$) |

(Continued)

**TABLE 1** | Continued

| Publication | End-point | Results | Method | Dataset |
|---|---|---|---|---|
| Tschandl et al. (24) | Classification (melanoma, BCC, dermatofibroma, melanocytic naevi, seborrheic keratoses and vascular lesion) | - CNN<br>Sen: 90%<br>Spe: 71%<br>AUC: 91%<br>- Students<br>Sen: 86%<br>Spe: 79%<br>AUC: 85% | All images from the students' training session were also used to retrain the last layer of the "GoogLeNet Inception v3" neural network, without any kind of test-set augmentation (4,000 epochs, learning rate 0.001, batch size 50). | Dermoscopic images (*n* = 348)<br>Train_Images (*n* = 298):<br>melanoma (*n* = 62), BCC (*n* = 40), dermatofibroma (*n* = 7), melanocytic naevi (*n* = 129), SK (*n* = 38), and vascular lesion (*n* = 22)<br>Test_Images (30%):<br>melanoma (*n* = 10), BCC (*n* = 10), dermatofibroma (*n* = 2), melanocytic naevi (*n* = 14), SK (*n* = 9) and vascular lesion (*n* = 5) |
| Esteva et al. (25) | Classification (757 diseases) | - 3-way classification<br>Dermatologist 1 Acc: 65.6%<br>Dermatologist 2 Acc: 66.0%<br>CNN Acc: 69.4 ± 0.8%<br>CNN – partitioning algorithm Acc: 72.1 ± 0.9%<br>- 9-way classification<br>Dermatologist 1 Acc: 53.3%<br>Dermatologist 2 Acc: 55.0%<br>CNN Acc: 48.9 ± 1.9%<br>CNN – partitioning algorithm Acc: 55.4 ± 1.7% | - Training Using Google Inception v3 CNN architecture pretrained on the ImageNet dataset (1.28 million images of over 1,000 generic object classes) and fine-tuned on their own dataset of 129,450 skin lesions comprising 2,032 different diseases. The 757 training classes were defined using a novel taxonomy of skin diseases and a partitioning algorithm that maps diseases into training classes.<br>- Testing Author developed an algorithm to partition diseases into fine-grained training classes (for example, amelanotic melanoma and acral lentiginous melanoma). During inference, the CNN outputs a probability distribution over these fine classes. To recover the probabilities for coarser-level classes of interest (for example, melanoma) they summed the probabilities of their descendants | Dermoscopic and conventional images (*n* = 129,450)<br>Train_Images (*n* = 127,463)<br>Test_Images (*n* = 1,942) |
| Lee et al. (26) | Classification (ALM and BN) | - CNN<br>Sen: 90.2%<br>Spe: 93.8%<br>AUC: 97.6%<br>- Board-certified dermatologists<br>Sen: 87.0%<br>Spe: 71.4%<br>Acc: 79.2% | Data augmentation : four center-overlapping patches<br>CNN :<br>Fine-tuned 50-layer ResNet<br>Made an ensemble model [merging Model 2 (intermediate tumor in BN set) and Model 3 (intermediate tumor in ALM set)] | Dermoscopy images<br>ALM (*n* = 500), BN (*n* = 500) and intermediate tumor (*n* = 72)<br>Train_Images (*n* = 872):<br>ALM (*n* = 400), BN (*n* = 400) and intermediate tumor (*n* = 72)<br>Test_Images (*n* = 200):<br>ALM (*n* = 100), BN (*n* = 100) |
| Cui et al. (27) | Classification (melanoma and non-melanoma) | - CNN<br>(best model: Inception V3)<br>Acc: 93.70%<br>Sen: 95.30%<br>Spe: 92.10% | CNN:<br>Fine-tuned CNNs (AlexNet, VGG16, VGG19, Inception V3) and compared CNNs (best model was Inception V3) | Dermoscopy images<br>deep learning dataset (*n* = 2,200):<br>melanoma (*n* = 564) and non-melanoma (*n* = 1,636) |

dermoscopic images. Unusually, the third publication used data downloaded from the Internet, not directly taken.

Annan Li et al. used deep learning for feature extraction, then classified images using the principal component analysis (PCA) and SVM machine learning techniques. They compared deep learning models and assessed the differences in dimensions of the PCA features. Sarkar et al. applied Gaussian blurring to denoise the images and then used the contrast-limited adaptive histogram equalization (CLAHE) algorithm to enhance them. Unlike previous publications, deep learning was used for classification.

## IMPLEMENTATION IN SMARTPHONES

With the spread of smartphones, the mobile application market has expanded rapidly. Applications can be used in various fields, particularly in the field of dermatology through the use of smartphone cameras. In particular, due to the ubiquity of smartphones, easily accessible mobile apps can make it more efficient to detect and monitor skin cancers during the early stages of development. In addition, with the recent development of smartphone processors and cameras, machine learning techniques can be applied, and skin cancer diagnoses

**TABLE 2** | Melanoma skin cancer publications using conventional machine learning method.

| Publication | End-point | Results | Method | Dataset |
|---|---|---|---|---|
| Sabouri et al. (28) | Classification (MM and BN) | Sen: 89.28%<br>Spe: 100%<br>(best model: cascade classifier) | Pre-processing:<br>Artifact removal (hair artifact removal)<br>Cropping (512*512) and lesion segmentation (border segmentation)<br>Feature extraction:<br>Color features: RGB and HSV<br>Texture features: using GLCM<br>Classifier: compared many models (KNN, MLP, Naïve Bayes, RF, SVM). Best model was cascade SVM Classifier (SVM #1 using normalized HSV, SVM #2 using a combination of color and texture features) | Unspecified images<br>Train_Images ($n = 370$):<br>MM ($n = 175$) and BN ($n = 195$)<br>Test_Images ($n = 42$):<br>MM ($n = 16$) and BN ($n = 26$) |
| Kaur et al. (29) | Pink lesion classification within MM or BN | AUC: 0.879 (all features) | Relative color thresholds<br>Segment of 3 shades of pink (light, dark and orange pink)<br>Quintile overlays<br>Feature extraction:<br>Blob features (5 per shade)<br>Color features for each pink shade over entire lesion (15 per shade)<br>Texture features derived from lesion histogram (24 per shade)<br>Location features (6 per shade)<br>Classifier : multivariate analysis using linear regression was performed using the Proc Logistic function in SAS | Dermoscopic images.<br>Train_Images ($n = 60$):<br>Only MM containing visible pink areas within the lesion<br>Test_Images ($n = 132$):<br>MM ($n = 54$), benign dysplastic, and congenital nevi ($n = 78$) |
| Shimizu et al. (30) | 4-class classification (melanoma, nevus, BCC, SK) Best model: Layered model | Acc: 0.904<br>AUC: 0.864<br>(AUC denotes the area of the receiver-operating characteristic (ROC) curve between %M and min (%N, %B, %S).) | Border detection : The core of the algorithm was color thresholding, removal of artifacts such as microscope border and hair, and inclusion of bright area seen specifically in NoMSLs (BCC and SK)<br>Feature extraction:<br>Color-related Features : calculating ten statistics for the intensity of six color channels (RGB, HSV)<br>Subregion-related features : describing geometrical distribution of the color.<br>Texture-related features : by adopting GLCM<br>Classifier: compared layered model and flat model. | Dermoscopic images<br>Train_Images (not described)<br>Test_Images ($n = 964$):<br>melanoma ($n = 105$), nevi ($n = 692$), and SK ($n = 98$), BCC ($n = 69$) |
| Abedini et al. (31) | Classification (MM and BN) | Acc: 0.90<br>(accuracy continues to improve with some fluctuation before converging at approximately 90% after 150 responses.) | One feature of the system enables the domain expert to improve previously built models.<br>Classifier with a stochastic gradient descent SVM and a feedback mechanism.<br>Eventually, as more feedback is provided (more training examples), the SVM accuracy improves. | Dermoscopic images<br>Train_Image ($n = 100$)<br>Test_Image ($n = 5$):<br>melanoma ($n = 3$) and normal skin ($n = 2$) |
| Marchetti et al. (32) | Classification (MM and BN)<br>Best model: greedy fusion | – Greedy fusion<br>Sen: 58%<br>Spe: 92%<br>AUC: 86%<br>– Average dermatologist<br>Sen: 82%<br>Spe: 59%<br>AUC: 71% | Compared five methods of fusing all automated predictions from the 25 participating teams in the ISBI challenge into a single prediction (three machine learning methods and two non-learned approaches) | ISBI 2016 challenge dataset<br>The dataset contains a representative mix of images of both MM ($n = 248$) and BN ($n = 1,031$)<br>Train_Images ($n = 900$)<br>Test_Images ($n = 379$)<br>Reader study images ($n = 100$):<br>MM ($n = 50$) and BN ($n = 50$) |

**TABLE 3 |** Melanoma skin cancer publications using hybrid method.

| Publication | End-point | Results | Method | Dataset |
|---|---|---|---|---|
| Jafari et al. (33) | Lesion segmentation | Sen: 95.2%<br>Spe: 99%<br>Acc: 98.7% | - Training<br>Pre-processing:<br>edge-preserving smoothing<br>Patch selection:<br>Lesion patch selection<br>Border patch selection<br>Normal skin patch selection<br>CNN: local texture analysis + general structure analysis<br>- Testing<br>Pre-processing:<br>edge-preserving smoothing<br>Patch selection:<br>Global and local patch definition<br>CNN: local texture analysis + general structure analysis<br>Post-processing : selecting largest connected component, dilation and hole filling | Clinical images ($n = 126$)<br>MM ($n = 66$) and non-MN ($n = 60$)<br>Train_Images (75%)<br>Test_Images (25%) |
| Xie et al. (34) | Classification (melanoma and nevus) | - Xanthous race dataset<br>Sen: 95%<br>Spe: 93.75%<br>Acc: 94.17%<br>- Caucasian race dataset<br>Sen: 83.33%<br>Spe: 95%<br>Acc: 91.11% | Pre-processing : hair removal (using partial differential equation)<br>Segmentation: using SGNN<br>Feature extraction:<br>Region division on dermoscopy images<br>Description of color, texture and border features<br>Feature normalization and dimensionality reduction<br>Classifier: meta-ensemble model of multiple neural network ensembles<br>Ensemble 1: single-hidden-layer BP nets with same structures<br>Ensemble 2: single-hidden-layer BP nets and fuzzy nets<br>Ensemble 3: double-hidden-layer BP nets with different structures | Dermoscopy images<br>- Xanthous race dataset ($n = 240$): MM ($n = 80$) and BN ($n = 160$)<br>- Caucasian race dataset (n = 360): MM ($n = 120$) and BN ($n = 240$) |
| Sabbaghi et al. (35) | Classification (MM and BN) | Sen: 95.5%<br>Spe: 94.9%<br>Acc: 95%<br>(Deep auto-encoder with BoF) | Each RGB dermoscopy image from a training set is converted to BoF mode Then, the generated BoF (scale-invariant feature transform (SIFT) + color) are fed into the stack auto-encoder for training | Dermoscopic images.<br>MM ($n = 174$) and BN ($n = 640$)<br>Train_Images ($n = 570$)<br>Test_Images ($n = 244$) |

can be conducted through smartphones. **Table 7** shows that a lot of research and development on smartphone implementation is carried out. AI technology relevant to skin cancer diagnosis is anticipated to eventually be implemented in smartphones, enabling the reduction of unnecessary hospital visits. Many types of mobile health application are already available.

## Types and Accuracies of Diagnostic Applications Using a Smartphone

According to a recent review (53, 54), numerous applications have already been released, seven of which use image analysis algorithms. Four of the seven applications are not supported by scientific evidence, and these four have been deleted from the app store since the review was conducted; the other three apps are still available. **Table 7** provides a summary of the apps. SkinScan, SkinVision, and SpotMole are currently available. SkinVision uses machine learning algorithms and SkinScan and SpotMole use the ABCDE rule (that is asymmetry, border irregularity, color that is not uniform, diameter >6 mm, and evolving size, shape or color). Only one application employs a machine learning technique. The sensitivity and specificity of these applications are shown in the table.

Most diagnosis applications are not accurate (55). Furthermore, only a few inform users using image analysis and machine learning. Most apps are not supported by scientific evidence and require further research.

## Problems and Possible Solutions

Inaccuracies in medical applications can result in problems of legal liability. In addition, the transmission of patient information may correspond to telemedicine practices, for which there are certain legal restrictions; these include

**TABLE 4** | Non-melanoma skin cancer publications using deep learning method.

| Publication | End-point | Results | Method | Dataset |
|---|---|---|---|---|
| Rezvantalab et al. (36) | Compare ability of deep learning with the performance of highly trained dermatologists | - Melanoma AUC<br>82.26% (Dermatologist)<br>93.80% (DenseNet 201)<br>94.40% (ResNet 152)<br>93.40% (Inception v3)<br>93.20% (Inception ResNet v2)<br>- Basal cell carcinoma AUC<br>88.82% (Dermatologist)<br>99.30% (DenseNet 201)<br>99.10% (ResNet 152)<br>98.60% (Inception v3)<br>98.60% (Inception ResNet v2) | Pre-trained Inception v3, Inception ResNet v2, ResNet 152, DenseNet 201 | $n$ = 10,015 dermoscopic images.<br>Melanoma (1,113 samples)<br>Melanocytic nevi (6,705 samples)<br>BCC (514 samples)<br>Actinic keratosis and intraepithelial carcinoma (327 samples)<br>Benign keratoses (1,099 samples)<br>Dermatofibroma (115 samples)<br>Vascular lesions (142 samples)<br>n_train = 70%<br>n_val, n_test = 15% |
| Zhang et al. (37) | Automatically classify dermoscopic images for clinical decision support | - Dataset A<br>Acc: 86.54%<br>- Dataset B<br>Acc: 85.86% | GoogLeNet Inception v3<br>Pre-trained on over 1.28 million images and adjusted the final layer to input own datasets using transfer learning | $n$ = 1,067 dermoscopic images<br>Dataset A<br>418 (Nevus)<br>291 (SK)<br>132 (BCC)<br>226 (Psoriasis)<br>Dataset B<br>132 (Nevus, SK, BCC, Psoriasis)<br>n_train = 80%<br>n_val, n_test = 10% |
| Vander Putten et al. (38) | Demonstrate a sensitivity and specificity that could make neural networks a realistic tool for dermatologists | Classification layer<br>53 layers<br>AUC 0.92, Sen 0.98, Spe 0.95<br>98 layers<br>AUC 0.89, Sen 0.98, Spe 0.94<br>152 layers<br>AUC 0.93, Sen 0.97, Spe 0.96 | 1. Segmentation (deep residual network)<br>2. Classification (very deep residual network) | Two independent sources (BCC) Dermoscopic images<br>1. "Skin Lesion Analysis Toward Melanoma Detection" competition released with ISBI 2016<br>2. International Skin Imaging Collaboration (ISIC) Archive |
| Mandache et al. (39) | Propose exploiting FFOCT images | AUC: 95.93%<br>Sen: 95.2%<br>Spe: 96.54% | **Feature extractor**<br>- Convolutional blocks<br>- Dropout layer<br>- ReLU<br>**Classifier**<br>- Fully connected layer<br>- Dropout layer | $n$ = 40 FFOCT images<br>10 (BCC) |
| Zhang et al. (40) | Machine learning algorithms need to be combined with sufficient clinical expertise in order to achieve an optimal result | - Dataset A<br>Acc: 87.25%<br>- Dataset B<br>Acc: 86.63% | Developed algorithm based on pre-trained GoogLeNet Inception v3<br>In order to facilitate decision-making and improve the accuracy algorithm, this summarized classification/diagnosis scenarios based on domain expert knowledge and semantically represented them in a hierarchical structure | $n$ = 1,067 dermoscopic images<br>Dataset A<br>418 (Nevus)<br>291 (SK)<br>132 (BCC)<br>226 (Psoriasis)<br>Dataset B<br>132 (Nevus, SK, BCC, Psoriasis)<br>n_train = 80%<br>n_val, n_test = 10% |
| Yap et al. (41) | A method which combines multiple imaging modalities together with patient metadata | - Melanoma<br>AUC: 86.1%<br>- Cancer<br>AUC: 88.8% | Used pre-trained modified ResNet-50 architecture (to extract image features)<br>Using a late fusion technique<br>Image feature vectors were concatenated together with the metadata feature vectors and sent through the embedding network | $n$ = 2,917 (metadata + macroscopic images + dermoscopic images)<br>1,127 (Nevus)<br>727 (All cutaneous melanomas except mucosal and ocular)<br>647 (BCC)<br>273 (SCC)<br>143 (BKL) |

information protection regulations to prevent third parties accessing data during the transmission process. Even if the accuracy is improved, the advertisements embedded in the application suggest that the technology could be used for commercial advertisements; for example, to attract patients.

**TABLE 5** | Non-melanoma skin cancer publications using conventional machine learning method.

| Publication | End-point | Results | Method | Dataset |
|---|---|---|---|---|
| Marvdashti et al. (42) | Fully automated procedure to detect BCC in *ex-vivo* human skin from PS-OCT images | AUC: 97.2%<br>Sen: 95.4%<br>Spe: 95.4% | Extracting image features from the two complementary image contrasts offered by PS-OCT, intensity and phase retardation (PR) using machine learning<br>Then, classify image features using SVM with linear and Gaussian kernels, KNN, and RF | $n$ = 520 PS-OCT<br>260 (Healthy, 26 patients)<br>260 (BCC, 26 patients) |
| Kharazmi et al. (43) | Detection and segmentation of cutaneous vasculature from dermoscopy images and extracted vascular features are explored for skin cancer classification | - BCC AUC: 96.5%<br>- Non-BCC AUC: 96.5% | Segment vascular structures by decomposing the image using ICA, k-means clustering<br>Then, a vessel mask is generated as a result of global thresholding<br>Vascular features fed into an RF classifier (decision tree) | $n$ = 659 dermoscopy images<br>299 (BCC)<br>360 (Non-BCC) |
| Kefel et al. (44) | Automatic method for detection of pink blush<br>(common feature in BCC)<br>Manually created borders vs. automatic created borders | Manual<br>AUC: 87.8%<br>Automatic<br>AUC: 87.7% | Border detection by GAC and modified Otsu's threshold<br>Classification:<br>logistic regression by Proc Logit of SAS (smoothness, brightness) | $n$ = 2,266 dermoscopic images<br>manually created borders<br>n_train = 354<br>n_test = 1,024<br>GAC<br>n_train = 888<br>n_test = 1,024 |

To solve this problem, a supervisory institution in which doctors participate is required, along with a connection to remote medical care services. The United States has been steadily attempting to promote telemedicine in its early stages, to address the issue of access to healthcare. Since the establishment of the American Telemedicine Association (ATA)—a telemedicine research institute—in 1993, legislation, including the Federal Telemedicine Act, has been established. It has been applied to more than 50 detailed medical subjects, including heart diseases, and has been successfully implemented in rural areas, prisons, homes, and schools (56).

To obtain good results, it is necessary to focus on securing high-quality data, to form a consensus between the patient and the doctor, and to actively participate in development.

In summary, the evidence for the diagnostic accuracy of smartphone applications is still lacking because few mHealth apps offer services. In addition, because the rate of service or algorithm change is faster than the peer-review publishing process, it is difficult to compare different apps accurately.

## Risks of Smartphone Applications

Smartphone applications pose some risk to users, especially if the algorithm returns negative results and delays the detection and treatment of undiagnosed skin cancer. It is very difficult to study false-negative rates because there is no histological evidence. Users may not be able to assess all skin lesions, especially if they are located in areas difficult to reach or to see. Given the generally low specificity of current applications, there would be a few false positives. This would put unnecessary stress on the user and result in unnecessary visits to the dermatologist. Furthermore, through limited trust and awareness, the user may not follow the advice provided by the smartphone application.

Chao et al. described the ethical and privacy issues of smartphone applications (57). Whilst applications have the potential to improve the provisions of medical services, there are important ethical concerns regarding patient confidentiality, informed consent, transparency in data ownership, and protection of data privacy. Many apps require users to agree to their data policies; however, the methods in which patient data are externally mined, used, and shared are often not transparent. Therefore, if a patient's data are stored on a cloud server or released to a third party for data analysis, assessing liability in the event of a breach of personal information is a challenge. In addition, it is unclear how the responsibilities for medical malpractice will be determined if the patient is injured as a result of inaccurate information.

# CONCLUSION

In this review, we analyzed a total of 35 publications. Studies on skin lesions were divided into those assessing malignant melanomas and non-melanoma skin cancers. In addition, studies involving clinical data and OCT images were used alongside those involving the dermoscopic images widely used in dermatology. Because the considered datasets differed between the publications, it was impossible to determine how best to perform the analysis. However, as seen in the publication by Cui et al. deep learning methods obtain better results than conventional machine learning methods if the dataset is large. Also, certain publications have reported comparable or superior results to dermatologist. In

**TABLE 6** | Non-melanoma skin cancer publications using Hybrid method.

<table>
<tr><th>Publication</th><th>End-point</th><th>Results</th><th>Method</th><th>Dataset</th></tr>
<tr><td>Annan et al. (45)</td><td>Propose BCC detection method</td><td>Proposed method AUC (Best model : VGG-16)
<table>
<tr><th>ConvNet</th><th>Ori</th><th colspan="4">Dimension of PCA feature</th></tr>
<tr><th></th><th></th><th>100</th><th>200</th><th>500</th><th>1,000</th></tr>
<tr><td>AlexNet</td><td>0.916</td><td>0.897</td><td>0.915</td><td>0.897</td><td>0.917</td></tr>
<tr><td>GoogLeNet</td><td>0.744</td><td>0.744</td><td>0.744</td><td>0.744</td><td>0.744</td></tr>
<tr><td>VGG-16</td><td>0.935</td><td>0.858</td><td>0.913</td><td>0.928</td><td>0.931</td></tr>
<tr><td>VGG-19</td><td>0.891</td><td>0.798</td><td>0.824</td><td>0.863</td><td>0.894</td></tr>
</table></td><td>1. Graph based skin surface segmentation<br>2. Surface flattening<br>3. Deep feature extraction (pre-trained AlexNet, GoogLeNet, VGG-16, VGG-19)<br>BCC classification (PCA, SVM)</td><td>$n = 5{,}040$ OCT images 1,875 (lesion or irregular structure)</td></tr>
<tr><td>Sarkar et al. (46)</td><td>Novel state of the art deep neural network for skin carcinoma detection</td><td>- BCC<br>AUC: 97.9%<br>Spe: 97.5%<br>Sen: 98.3%<br>Precision: 96.7%<br>F1 score: 97.5%<br>- Benign<br>AUC: 97.9%<br>Spe: 98.6%<br>Sen: 96.6%<br>Precision: 98.3%<br>F1 score: 97.5%</td><td>Pre-processing:<br>Denoising of images by Gaussian blurring<br>Enhancement of images by CLAHE algorithm and use parallel deep residual network (RMSprop optimizer) for classification</td><td>n = 700 dermoscopic images<br>300 (BCC positive)<br>100 (augmented set of SCC positive)<br>300 (benign skin lesion)<br>n_train = 560<br>n_val = 140</td></tr>
<tr><td>Dorj et al. (47)</td><td>Focus on the task of the classifying skin cancer</td><td><table>
<tr><th>Cancer</th><th>AUC, %</th><th>Sen, %</th><th>Spe, %</th></tr>
<tr><td>Actinic Keratoses</td><td>92.3</td><td>98.9</td><td>91.67</td></tr>
<tr><td>Basal cell carcinoma</td><td>91.8</td><td>97.7</td><td>86.73</td></tr>
<tr><td>Squamous cell carcinoma</td><td>95.1</td><td>96.9</td><td>94.17</td></tr>
<tr><td>Melanoma</td><td>94.2</td><td>97.83</td><td>90.74</td></tr>
</table></td><td>Pre-trained AlexNet is used to extract training features and the obtained convolutional neural network features are classified into four groups using error-correcting output codes (ECOC), SVM</td><td>$n = 3{,}753$ collected from the internet<br>Actinic Keratoses<br>- 712 (Train), 185 (Test)<br>BCC<br>- 728 (Train), 193 (Test)<br>SCC<br>- 777 (Train), 200 (Test)<br>Melanoma<br>768 (Train), 190 (Test)</td></tr>
</table>

**TABLE 7** | Smartphone applications.

| Application name | Algorithm | Evidence | Performance | | References |
|---|---|---|---|---|---|
| DermaCompare (removed) | Machine learning | Not found | Not found | | [1] |
| Lubax (removed) | Content-based image retrieval (compare), KNN (classification) | One peer-reviewed supporting publication | Sensitivity (95% CI) 90% (86–94) | Specificity (95% CI) 92% (85–95) | (48) [2] |
| MskinDoctor (removed) | Grab cut algorithm (segmentation), SVM (classification) | Not found | Not found | | [3] |
| MySkinMap (removed) | Machine learning | Not found | Not found | | [4] |
| SkinScan | Image processing technique, ABCDE rule | Not found | Not found | | [5] |
| SkinVision | Conditional generative adversarial neural network (segmentation) and SVM (classification) | Two peer-reviewed supporting publications, evaluated in independent publications | Sensitivity (95% CI) iOS: 50% (22–78) Android: 72%(58–87) | Specificity (95% CI) iOS: 50% (22–78) Android: 27% (1–56) | (49–52) [6] |
| SpotMole | Image processing techniques, ABCDE rule | Evaluated in independent publications | Sensitivity (95% CI) 43% (28–58) | Specificity (95% CI) 80% (60–100) | (52) [7] |

*[1]AppAdvice. Derma Compare by Emerald Medical Applications. Available online at: https://appadvice.com/app/derma-compare/982517772.*
*[2]AppAdvice. Lubax - Skin Lesion ID Using Image Recognition by Lubax, Inc. Available online at: https://appadvice.com/app/lubax-skin-lesion-id-using-image-recognition/956423382.*
*[3]AppBrain. mSkin Doctor Mobile Application for Skin Cancer Detection by Aleem Technologies. Available online at: https://www.appbrain.com/app/mskin-doctor/com.maleemtaufiq.mSkinDoctor.*
*[4]AppAdvice. MySkinMap by Xyrupt Technologies, LLC. Available online at: https://appadvice.com/app/myskinmap/1151655127.*
*[5]AppAdvice. SkinScan by TeleSkin ApS. Available online at: https://appadvice.com/app/skinscan/1025190936.*
*[6]SkinVision. Available online at: https://www.skinvision.com/.*
*[7]Google Play. SpotMole. Available online at: https://play.google.com/store/apps/details?id=com.spotmole&hl=nl.*

particular, recent publications have reported that dermatologists have improved diagnostic accuracy with the help of deep learning (26, 58). Therefore, in the future, computer-aided diagnostics in dermatology will show greater reliance on deep learning methods.

For the convenience of users, the use of a smartphone is necessary. However, an accuracy limitation occurs when applied to smartphones. This problem is due to the limitations of hardware, which used conventional machine learning techniques such as SVM rather than deep learning. However, MobileNet has recently made it possible to use deep learning methods in IoT devices, including smartphones (59). This enables deep learning to be applied to IoT devices for faster performances than large networks, which will lead to more active research into skin lesion detection using applications.

Application inaccuracies can lead to legal problems. To solve this problem, doctors and patients must participate together in the development stage, and an institution for managing and supervising this process is also required.

## AUTHOR CONTRIBUTIONS

BO and SY: contributed conception and design of the study, wrote sections of the manuscript, and contributed to manuscript revision. YC and HA: collected data and wrote the first draft of the manuscript. All authors read and approved the submitted version.

## REFERENCES

1. Ha SM, Ko DY, Jeon SY, Kim KH, Song HK. A clinical and statistical study of cutaneous malignant tumors in Busan City and the eastern Gyeongnam Province over 15 years (1996-2010). *Korean J Dermatol.* (2013) 51:167–72.
2. Alam M, Lee A, Ibrahimi OA, Kim N, Bordeaux J, Chen K, et al. A multistep approach to improving biopsy site identification in dermatology: physician, staff, and patient roles based on a Delphi consensus. *JAMA Dermatol.* (2014) 150:550–8. doi: 10.1001/jamadermatol.2013.9804
3. St. John J, Walker J, Goldberg D, Maloney EM. Avoiding medical errors in cutaneous site identification: a best practices review. *Dermatol Surg.* (2016) 42:477– 84. doi: 10.1097/DSS.0000000000000683
4. Cinotti E, Couzan C, Perrot J, Habougit C, Labeille B, Cambazard F, et al. *In vivo* confocal microscopic substrate of grey colour in melanosis. *J Eur Acad Dermatol Venereol.* (2015) 29:2458–62. doi: 10.1111/jdv.13394

5. Dubois A, Levecq O, Azimani H, Siret D, Barut A, Suppa M, et al. Line-field confocal optical coherence tomography for high-resolution noninvasive imaging of skin tumors. *J Biomed Opt.* (2018) 23:106007. doi: 10.1117/1.JBO.23.10.106007
6. Oh B-H, Kim KH, Chung K-Y. Skin Imaging Using Ultrasound Imaging, Optical Coherence Tomography, Confocal Microscopy, and Two-Photon Microscopy in Cutaneous Oncology. *Front Med.* (2019) 6:274. doi: 10.3389/fmed.2019.00274
7. LeCun Y, Bengio Y, Hinton G. Deep learning. *Nature.* (2015) 521:436–44. doi: 10.1038/nature14539
8. Mohanaiah P, Sathyanarayana P, GuruKumar L. Image texture feature extraction using GLCM approach. *Int J Sci Res Publications.* (2013) 3:1–5.
9. Krizhevsky A, Sutskever I, Hinton EG. Imagenet classification with deep convolutional neural networks. In: Pereira F, Burges CJC, Bottou L, Weinberger K, editors. *Advances in Neural Information Processing Systems (NIPS)*, Vol. 25. Lake Tahoe, NV (2012). p. 1097–105. doi: 10.1145/3065386
10. Chilamkurthy S, Ghosh R, Tanamala S, Biviji M, Campeau NG, Venugopal VK, et al. Deep learning algorithms for detection of critical findings in head CT scans: a retrospective study. *Lancet.* (2018) 392:2388–96. doi: 10.1016/S0140-6736(18)31645-3
11. Li X, Zhang S, Zhang Q, Wei X, Pan Y, Zhao J, et al. Diagnosis of thyroid cancer using deep convolutional neural network models applied to sonographic images: a retrospective, multicohort, diagnostic study. *Lancet Oncol.* (2019) 20:193–201. doi: 10.1016/S1470-2045(18)30762-9
12. Bejnordi BE, Veta M, Van Diest PJ, Van Ginneken B, Karssemeijer N, Litjens G, et al. Diagnostic assessment of deep learning algorithms for detection of lymph node metastases in women with breast cancer. *JAMA.* (2017) 318:2199–210. doi: 10.1001/jama.2017.14585
13. Tajbakhsh N, Shin JY, Gurudu SR, Hurst RT, Kendall CB, Gotway MB, et al. Convolutional neural networks for medical image analysis: full training or fine tuning? *IEEE Trans Med Imaging.* (2016) 35:1299–312. doi: 10.1109/TMI.2016.2535302
14. Tang Y. Deep learning using linear support vector machines. *arXiv [Preprint].* arXiv:1306.0239. (2013).
15. Szarvas M, Yoshizawa A, Yamamoto M, Ogata J. Pedestrian detection with convolutional neural networks. In: *IEEE Proceedings. Intelligent Vehicles Symposium 2005.* Las Vegas, NV: IEEE (2005). doi: 10.1109/IVS.2005.1505106
16. O'Mahony N, Campbell S, Carvalho A, Harapanahalli S, Hernandez GV, Krpalkova L, et al. Deep Learning vs. Traditional Computer Vision. In: O'Mahony N, editor. Cham: Springer International Publishing (2020). p. 128–144.
17. He K, Zhang X, Ren S, Sun J. Deep residual learning for image recognition. In: *Proceedings of the IEEE Conference on Computer Vision and Pattern Recognition.* Las Vegas, NV: IEEE (2016).
18. Li Y, Shen L. Skin lesion analysis towards melanoma detection using deep learning network. *Sensors.* (2018) 18:556. doi: 10.3390/s18020556
19. Pour MP, Seker H, Shao L. Automated lesion segmentation and dermoscopic feature segmentation for skin cancer analysis. In: *2017 39th Annual International Conference of the IEEE Engineering in Medicine and Biology Society (EMBC).* Seogwipo: IEEE (2017). doi: 10.1109/EMBC.2017.8036906
20. Yu C, Yang S, Kim W, Jung J, Chung K-Y, Lee SW, et al. Acral melanoma detection using a convolutional neural network for dermoscopy images. *PLoS ONE.* (2018) 13:e0193321. doi: 10.1371/journal.pone.0196621
21. Nasr-Esfahani E, Samavi S, Karimi N, Soroushmehr SMR, Jafari MH, Ward K, et al. Melanoma detection by analysis of clinical images using convolutional neural network. In: *2016 38th Annual International Conference of the IEEE Engineering in Medicine and Biology Society (EMBC).* Orlando, FL: IEEE (2016). doi: 10.1109/EMBC.2016.7590963
22. Premaladha J, Ravichandran K. Novel approaches for diagnosing melanoma skin lesions through supervised and deep learning algorithms. *J Med Syst.* (2016) 40:96. doi: 10.1007/s10916-016-0460-2
23. Matsunaga K, Hamada A, Minagawa A, Koga H. Image classification of melanoma, nevus and seborrheic keratosis by deep neural network ensemble. *arXiv [Preprint].* arXiv:1703.03108. (2017).
24. Tschandl P, Kittler H, Argenziano G. A pretrained neural network shows similar diagnostic accuracy to medical students in categorizing dermatoscopic images after comparable training conditions. *Br J Dermatol.* (2017) 177:867–9. doi: 10.1111/bjd.15695
25. Esteva A, Kuprel B, Novoa RA, Ko J, Swetter SM, Blau HM, et al. dermatologist-level classification of skin cancer with deep neural networks. *Nature.* (2017) 542:115–18. doi: 10.1038/nature 21056
26. Lee S, Chu Y, Yoo S, Choi S, Choe S, Koh S, et al. Augmented decision making for acral lentiginous melanoma detection using deep convolutional neural networks. *J Eur Acad Dermatol Venereol.* (2020) doi: 10.1111/jdv.16185. [Epub ahead of print].
27. Cui X, Wei R, Gong L, Qi R, Zhao Z, Chen H, et al. Assessing the effectiveness of artificial intelligence methods for melanoma: a retrospective review. *J Am Acad Dermatol.* (2019) 81:1176–80. doi: 10.1016/j.jaad.2019.06.042
28. Sabouri P, GholamHosseini H, Larsson T, Collins J. A cascade classifier for diagnosis of melanoma in clinical images. In: *2014 36th Annual International Conference of the IEEE Engineering in Medicine and Biology Society.* Chicago, IL: IEEE. (2014). doi: 10.1109/EMBC.2014.6945177
29. Kaur R, Albano PP, Cole JG, Hagerty J, LeAnder RW, Moss RH, et al. Real-time supervised detection of pink areas in dermoscopic images of melanoma: importance of color shades, texture and location. *Skin Res Technol.* (2015) 21:466–73. doi: 10.1111/srt.12216
30. Shimizu K, Iyatomi H, Celebi ME, Norton K-A, Tanaka M. Four-class classification of skin lesions with task decomposition strategy. *IEEE Trans Biomed Eng.* (2014) 62:274–83. doi: 10.1109/TBME.2014.2348323
31. Abedini M, von Cavallar S, Chakravorty R, Davis M, Garnavi R. A cloud-based infrastructure for feedback-driven training and image recognition. *Stud Health Technol Inform.* (2015) 216:691–5. doi: 10.3233/978-1-61499-564-7-691
32. Marchetti MA, Codella NC, Dusza SW, Gutman DA, Helba B, Kalloo A, et al. Results of the 2016 international skin imaging collaboration international symposium on biomedical imaging challenge: comparison of the accuracy of computer algorithms to dermatologists for the diagnosis of melanoma from dermoscopic images. *J Am Acad Dermatol.* (2018) 78:270–77.e1. doi: 10.1016/j.jaad.2017.08.016
33. Jafari MH, Nasr-Esfahani E, Karimi N, Soroushmehr SR, Samavi S, Najarian K. Extraction of skin lesions from non-dermoscopic images for surgical excision of melanoma. *Int J Comput Assist Radiol Surg.* (2017) 12:1021–30. doi: 10.1007/s11548-017-1567-8
34. Xie F, Fan H, Li Y, Jiang Z, Meng R, Bovik A. Melanoma classification on dermoscopy images using a neural network ensemble model. *IEEE Trans Med Imaging.* (2016) 36:849–58. doi: 10.1109/TMI.2016.2633551
35. Sabbaghi S, Aldeen M, Garnavi R. A deep bag-of-features model for the classification of melanomas in dermoscopy images. In: *2016 38th Annual International Conference of the IEEE Engineering in Medicine and Biology Society (EMBC).* Orlando, FL: IEEE (2016). doi: 10.1109/EMBC.2016.7590962
36. Rezvantalab A, Safigholi H, Karimijeshni S. Dermatologist level dermoscopy skin cancer classification using different deep learning convolutional neural networks algorithms. *arXiv [Preprint].* arXiv:1810.10348. (2018).
37. Zhang X, Wang S, Liu J, Tao C. Computer-aided diagnosis of four common cutaneous diseases using deep learning algorithm. In: *2017 IEEE International Conference on Bioinformatics and Biomedicine (BIBM).* Kansas, MO: IEEE. (2017). doi: 10.1109/BIBM.2017.8217850
38. Vander Putten E, Kambod A, Kambod M. Deep residual neural networks for automated basal cell carcinoma detection. In: *2018 IEEE EMBS International Conference on Biomedical & Health Informatics (BHI).* Las Vegas, NV: IEEE. (2018). doi: 10.1109/BHI.2018.8333437
39. Mandache D, Dalimier E, Durkin J, Boceara C, Olivo-Marin J-C, Meas-Yedid V. Basal cell carcinoma detection in full field OCT images using convolutional neural networks. In: *2018 IEEE 15th International Symposium on Biomedical Imaging (ISBI 2018).* Washington, DC: IEEE (2018) doi: 10.1109/ISBI.2018.8363689
40. Zhang X, Wang S, Liu J, Tao C. Towards improving diagnosis of skin diseases by combining deep neural network and human knowledge. *BMC Med Inform Decis Making.* (2018) 18:59. doi: 10.1186/s12911-018-0631-9
41. Yap J, Yolland W, Tschandl P. Multimodal skin lesion classification using deep learning. *Exp Dermatol.* (2018) 27:1261–67. doi: 10.1111/exd.13777
42. Marvdashti T, Duan L, Aasi SZ, Tang JY, Ellerbee Bowden AK. Classification of basal cell carcinoma in human skin using machine learning and quantitative features captured by polarization sensitive optical coherence

tomography. *Biomed Opt Express.* (2016) 7:3721–35. doi: 10.1364/BOE.7.003721

43. Kharazmi P, AlJasser MI, Lui H, Wang ZJ, Lee KT. Automated detection and segmentation of vascular structures of skin lesions seen in Dermoscopy, with an application to basal cell carcinoma classification. *IEEE J Biomed Health Inform.* (2016) 21:1675–84. doi: 10.1109/JBHI.2016.2637342
44. Kefel S, Pelin Kefel S, LeAnder R, Kaur R, Kasmi R, Mishra N, et al. Adaptable texture-based segmentation by variance and intensity for automatic detection of semitranslucent and pink blush areas in basal cell carcinoma. *Skin Res Technol.* (2016) 22:412–22. doi: 10.1111/srt.12281
45. Annan L, Jun C, Ai Ping Y, Srivastava R, Wong DW, Hong Liang T, et al. Automated basal cell carcinoma detection in high-definition optical coherence tomography. *Conf Proc IEEE Eng Med Biol Soc.* (2016) 2016:2885–88. doi: 10.1109/EMBC.2016.7591332
46. Sarkar R, Chatterjee CC, Hazra A. A novel approach for automatic diagnosis of skin carcinoma from dermoscopic images using parallel deep residual networks. In: *International Conference on Advances in Computing and Data Sciences.* (Springer) (2019). doi: 10.1007/978-981-13-9939-8_8
47. Dorj U-O, Lee K-K, Choi J-Y, Lee M. The skin cancer classification using deep convolutional neural network. *Multimedia Tools Appl.* (2018) 77:9909–24. doi: 10.1007/s11042-018-5714-1
48. Chen RH, Snorrason M, Enger SM, Mostafa E, Ko JM, Aoki V, et al. Validation of a skin-lesion image-matching algorithm based on computer vision technology. *Telemed e-Health.* (2016) 22:45– 50. doi: 10.1089/tmj.2014.0249
49. Udrea A, Lupu C. Real-time acquisition of quality verified nonstandardized color images for skin lesions risk assessment—A preliminary study. In: *2014 18th International Conference on System Theory, Control and Computing (ICSTCC).* Sinaia: IEEE (2014) doi: 10.1109/ICSTCC.2014.6982415
50. Maier T, Kulichova D, Schotten K, Astrid R, Ruzicka T, Berking C, et al. Accuracy of a smartphone application using fractal image analysis of pigmented moles compared to clinical diagnosis and histological result. *J Eur Acad Dermatol Venereol.* (2015) 29:663– 7. doi: 10.1111/jdv.12648
51. Thissen M, Udrea A, Hacking M, von Braunmuehl T, Ruzicka T. mHealth app for risk assessment of pigmented and nonpigmented skin lesions—a study on sensitivity and specificity in detecting malignancy. *Telemed e-Health.* (2017) 23:948–54. doi: 10.1089/tmj.2016.0259
52. Ngoo A, Finnane A, McMeniman E, Tan JM, Janda M, Soyer PH. Efficacy of smartphone applications in high-risk pigmented lesions. *Austr J Dermatol.* (2018) 59:e175–e182. doi: 10.1111/ajd.12599
53. Kassianos A, Emery J, Murchie P, Walter MF. Smartphone applications for melanoma detection by community, patient and generalist clinician users: a review. *Br J Dermatol.* (2015) 172:1507– 18. doi: 10.1111/bjd.13665
54. de Carvalho TM, Noels E, Wakkee M, Udrea A, Nijsten T. Development of smartphone apps for skin cancer risk assessment: progress and promise. *JMIR Dermatol.* (2019) 2:e13376. doi: 10.2196/13376
55. Wolf JA, Moreau JF, Akilov O, Patton T, English JC, Ho J, et al. Diagnostic inaccuracy of smartphone applications for melanoma detection. *JAMA Dermatol.* (2013) 149:422–6. doi: 10.1001/jamadermatol.2013.2382
56. Jo JW, Jeong DS, Kim YC. Analysis of trends in dermatology mobile applications in korea. *Korean J Dermatol.* (2020) 58:7– 13.
57. Chao E, Meenan CK, Ferris KL. Smartphone-based applications for skin monitoring and melanoma detection. *Dermatol Clin.* (2017) 35:551–7. doi: 10.1016/j.det.2017.06.014
58. Han SS, Park I, Chang SE, Lim W, Kim MS, Park GH, et al. Augmented Intelligence Dermatology. Deep neural networks empower medical professionals in diagnosing skin cancer and predicting treatment options for 134 skin disorders. *J Invest Dermatol.* (2020). doi: 10.1016/j.jid.2020.01.019. [Epub ahead of print].
59. Howard AG, Zhu M, Chen B, Kalenichenko D, Wang W, Weyand T, et al. Mobilenets: efficient convolutional neural networks for mobile vision applications. *arXiv [Preprint].* arXiv:1704.04861. (2017).

5

# Dermoscopic Features Summarization and Comparison of Four Types of Cutaneous Vascular Anomalies

*Jing Gao[1†], Wenmin Fei[2,3,4†], Changbing Shen[5,6†], Xue Shen[7], Minghui Sun[1], Ning Xu[5,6], Qing Li[1], Cong Huang[5,6], Tingfang Zhang[1], Randy Ko[8], Yong Cui[2,3,4*] and Chunjun Yang[1*]*

*[1] Department of Dermatology, The Second Affiliated Hospital, Anhui Medical University, Hefei, China, [2] Department of Dermatology, China-Japan Friendship Hospital, Beijing, China, [3] Institute of Skin Health, China-Japan Friendship Hospital, Beijing, China, [4] Graduate School, Peking Union Medical College and Chinese Academy of Medical Sciences, Beijing, China, [5] Department of Dermatology, Peking University Shenzhen Hospital, Shenzhen, China, [6] Shenzhen Key Laboratory for Translational Medicine of Dermatology, Shenzhen Peking University–The Hong Kong University of Science and Technology Medical Center, Shenzhen, China, [7] Department of Dermatology, Chengdu Second People's Hospital, Chengdu, China, [8] Division of Molecular Medicine, Department of Internal Medicine, University of New Mexico Health Sciences Center, Albuquerque, NM, United States*

***Correspondence:**
*Yong Cui*
*wuhucuiyong@vip.163.com*
*Chunjun Yang*
*yangchunjun9@163.com*

*† These authors have contributed equally to this work*

**Objective:** Dermoscopic features of cutaneous vascular anomalies have been reported, but the described features currently known are limited and not well-understood. The aim of this study is to comprehensively summarize and compare the dermoscopic features of the four different types of cutaneous vascular anomalies [infantile hemangiomas (IH), cherry angioma (CA), angiokeratomas (AK), and pyogenic granuloma (PG)] in the Chinese Han population.

**Materials and Methods:** Dermoscopic features of 31 IH, 172 CA, 31 AK, and 45 PG were collected based on the contact non-polarized mode of dermoscopy at 20-fold magnification. Dermoscopic features including background, lacunae, vessel morphology and distribution were collected and summarized. Additionally, we compared these features by age stage, gender, and anatomical locations in CA.

**Results:** The dermoscopic features of IH included the red lacunae, red/red-blue/red-white backgrounds, and vessel morphology such as linear curved vessels, serpiginous vessels, coiled vessels. For CA, the lacunae appeared reddish brown to reddish blue or only red. In terms of vascular morphology, serpentine vessels, coiled vessels, looped vessels, and curved vessels could be seen in the lesions. A few lesions were black or presented with a superficial white veil. There were statistical differences in red background ($P = 0.021$), unspecific vessel distribution ($P = 0.030$), black area ($P = 0.029$), and white surface ($P = 0.042$) among different age groups. Red-brown lacunae ($P = 0.039$), red-blue ($P = 0.013$), red-white background ($P = 0.015$), black area ($P = 0.016$), and white surface ($P = 0.046$) were of statistical difference in terms of the locations of lesions. Lacunae were also observed in AK, which presented with red, dark purple, dark blue, black. Global dermoscopic patterns that were characterized by a homogeneous area were obvious in all PG lesions, among which 30 (66.7%) were red-white and 15 (33.3%) were red. As for local features, "white rail" lines were detected in 19 (42.2%) lesions and white collarette was seen in 34 (75.6%) lesions.

**Conclusions:** Dermoscopy is an applicable diagnostic tool for the diagnosis of cutaneous vascular anomalies. It is necessary to take into account the age stage and lesion location when we diagnose CA using dermoscopy.

**Keywords: dermoscopy, features, cutaneous vascular anomalies, summarization, comparison**

## INTRODUCTION

Vascular anomalies account for a considerable number of patients in the dermatology and surgical outpatient departments, which can be grouped into vascular tumors and vascular malformations. Some vascular tumors are proliferative and have the potential to fade away spontaneously, while vascular malformations normally stay stagnant over a long period of time (1). Timely and accurate diagnosis of vascular anomalies are essential for treatment and management, but remains a challenge for clinicians (2). Infantile hemangioma (IH), pyogenic granuloma (PG), angiokeratoma (AK), and cherry angiomas (CA) are common cutaneous vascular anomalies. According to the latest classification for vascular anomalies by the International Society for Vascular Anomalies (ISSVA), IH and PG are classified into the benign vascular tumors, angiokeratoma (AK) is classified into provisionally unclassified vascular anomalies (3). However, CA are not included in the current classification by the latest ISSVA (4).

IH is one of the most common cutaneous vascular anomalies present in infants, with the affected population being approximately 2–4.5% (5). The majority of IHs can be identified by clinical features, but some cases may still be misdiagnosed. CA, also known as cherry hemangiomas, adult hemangiomas, or senile angiomas as their number tends to increase with age, are cherry-red papules on the skin containing abnormal growth of blood vessels. CA are the most common vascular anomalies in adults, and elderly patients are especially concerned about the possible progression to malignancy. AK is a rare vascular malformation of the upper dermis that tends to have a distinct clinical presentation without self-limiting behavior. Clinically, the presentation of AK is often a dark nodule or macule which may be easily confused with malignant tumors, such as malignant melanomas, or pigmented basal cell carcinomas. A previous study reported that 20% of AK lesions were clinically diagnosed as melanomas (6). PG is a common and benign vascular tumor that can be diagnosed correctly by medical history and appearance. However, a survey indicated that 38% of the clinical diagnosis of PG proved to be inaccurate (7).

Dermoscopy has been widely accepted as a useful non-invasive diagnostic tool for various pigmented and non-pigmented skin disorders for increasing the diagnostic accuracy and avoiding unnecessary biopsies (8–12). The dermoscopic features of the above four types of cutaneous vascular anomalies have been previously reported in a few cases (6, 7, 12–17). However, dermoscopic features described in these studies are limited and not well-understood. Hence, this study aimed to comprehensively summarize the dermoscopic features of the four types of cutaneous vascular anomalies in the Chinese Han population.

## MATERIALS AND METHODS

### Study Design

This study was a morphological study carried out at the Second Affiliated Hospital of Anhui Medical University and China-Japan Friendship Hospital from June 1st, 2017 to October 31st, 2020. Approval was granted by the two institutions' ethics committees and conformed to the Declaration of Helsinki. All patients or their guardians provided informed consents. All lesions were clinically diagnosed by two associate chief physicians or chief physicians. If there was a disagreement between the two experts, the lesion would be discussed by an additional chief physician. The exclusion criteria included the use of: topical beta blocker, or intra-lesion injection, or laser treatment in the past 2 weeks, or a history of hematological malignancy. One lesion of each patient was selected to undergo dermoscopic examination.

### Imaging Procedure

Dermoscopic examinations were performed with a digital dermoscopy system (Medicam 800HD, FotoFinder Systems GmbH, Birbach, Germany) at a 20-fold magnification. The contact non-polarized mode of dermoscopy was utilized. In order to acquire better visualization, minimal pressure was applied and ultrasound gel was used to preserve vessels' morphology. Dermoscopic images were evaluated by two independent dermatologists (JG and WF). Any poor-quality images were excluded. We developed a list of features based from literature review and preliminary observation which included lacunae, background, vessel morphology and distribution. Two dermatologists (WF and XS) completed the list independently and also supplemented new items features beyond the list if necessary. If there was a disagreement between the two experts or any supplementary information, a consensus meeting with other experts was held to settle any discrepancies. The dermoscopic features described in this study refer to the standardized dermoscopic terminology from an expert consensus on behalf of the International Dermoscopy Society (18, 19).

### Divisions of Body Locations and Age Stages

Previous studies showed that there were differences of dermoscopic features and patterns in different age stages, gender, body location of lesions (20, 21). General information such as age, gender, anatomical locations were collected in

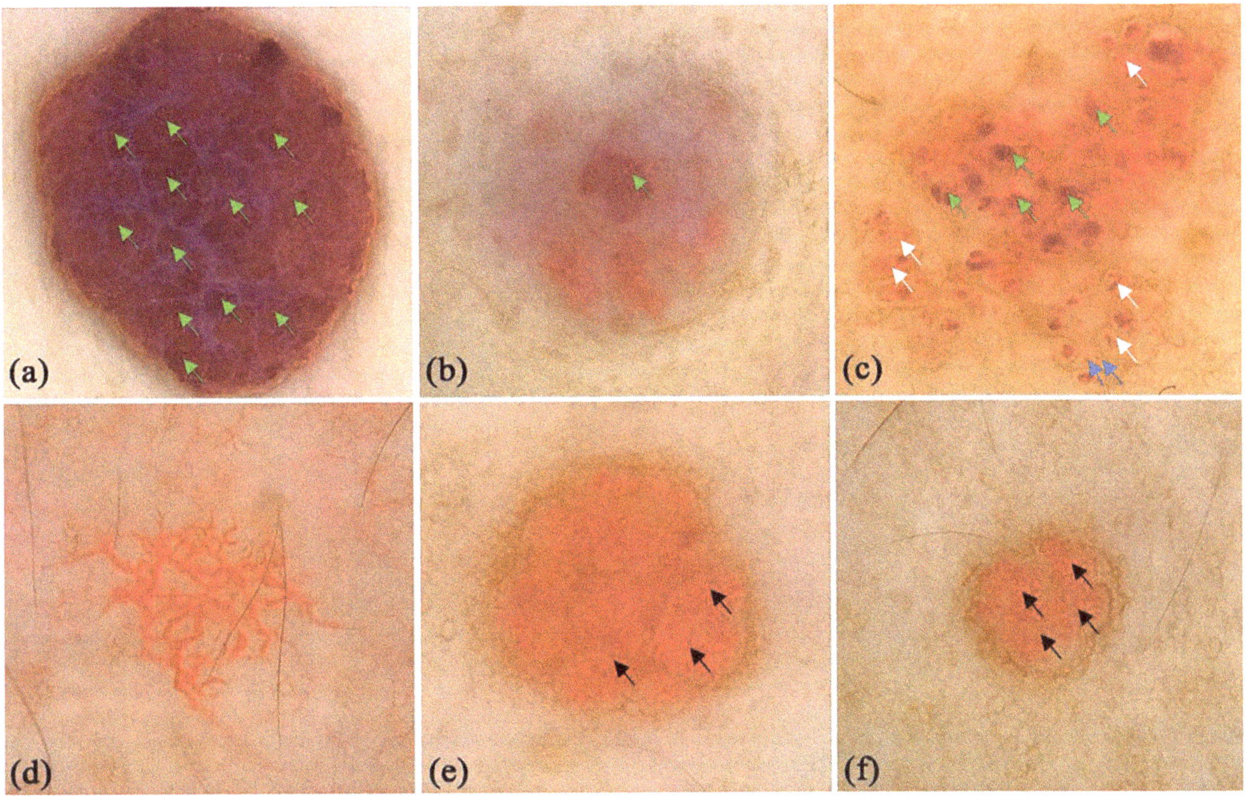


**FIGURE 1** | Dermoscopic features of infant hemangiomas. **(a)** red-blue background, clustered red lacunae (green arrows); **(b)** red-white background, red lacunae (green arrows); **(c)** red background, red lacunae (green arrows), red globules (blue arrows) and helical vessels (white arrows); **(d)** reticular vessel distribution; **(e)** clustered serpentine vessels (black arrows); **(f)** serpentine vessels (black arrows).

this study. The body locations were divided into four groups, including upper limbs, lower limbs, head and neck, and trunk. The hips were classified into the lower limbs category, and the perineum was categorized into the lower trunk. Gender, age, and location difference were analyzed in CA. For the CA patients, we divided the patients' age into three stages: <18 years old group (children), 18–60 years old group (adults), and >60 years old group (elders).

## Statistical Analysis

The continuous data are represented as mean (M) ± standard deviation (SD), and the categorical data are shown as number (N) and percentage (%). The categorical variables were compared by utilizing the Chi-square test. Regarding the Chi-square test in R x C contingency tables, if the expected count (T) of any grid in the R x C contingency tables were <1, or the number of grids with $1 \leq T < 5$ exceed 20% of the total number of grids, then Fisher's exact test was used to calculate the $P$-value. Statistical package for social science (SPSS), version 22.0 (IBM Corp., Armonk, NY, USA) was used for all analysis. A two-sided $P$-value $< 0.05$ was considered statistically significant in all analysis.

# RESULTS

There were 31 patients with IH, including 8 male and 23 female infants. The lesions were located on the upper limbs ($n = 2$, 6.5%), lower limbs ($n = 4$, 12.9%), head and neck ($n = 12$, 38.7%), and trunk ($n = 13$, 41.9%). Red lacunae was seen in 10 (32.3%) lesions. Red, red-blue, and red-white backgrounds were seen in 19 (61.3%), 1 (3.2%), and 4 (12.9%) lesions, respectively. There were definitive vascular structures besides lacunae in some lesions. Linear curved vessels could be discovered in 2 (6.5%) lesions, serpiginous vessels in 9 (29.0%) lesions, and coiled vessels in 6 (19.4%) lesions. In the lesions that contained multiple structures, reticular vessel distribution was seen in 9 (29.0%) lesions, 12 (38.7%) lesions with unspecific vessel distribution, while 9 (29.0%) lesions with clustered vessel distribution. Some of the classical and specifical dermoscopic features were showed in **Figure 1**.

A total of 172 CA patients (92 males and 80 females, mean age was 39.38 ± 18.41 years old) were included in the study. There were 41 (23.8%) lesions located on the upper limbs, 28 (16.3%) lesions on the lower limbs, 52 (30.2%) lesions on the head and neck, and 51 (29.7%) lesions on the trunk. Typical lacunae existed in 127 (73.84%) lesions, among which red lacunae were seen in 78 (45.3%) lesions, red-brown lacunae in 24 (14.0%) lesions, and red-blue lacunae in 42 (24.4%) lesions. Different colored backgrounds were identified in 158 (91.86%) lesions. Among the lesions, 77 (44.8%) were red, 52 (30.2%) were red-blue, and 34 (19.8%) were red-white. Regarding the vessel morphology, linear curved vessels were found in 29 (16.9%) lesions, serpiginous vessels in 27 (15.7%)

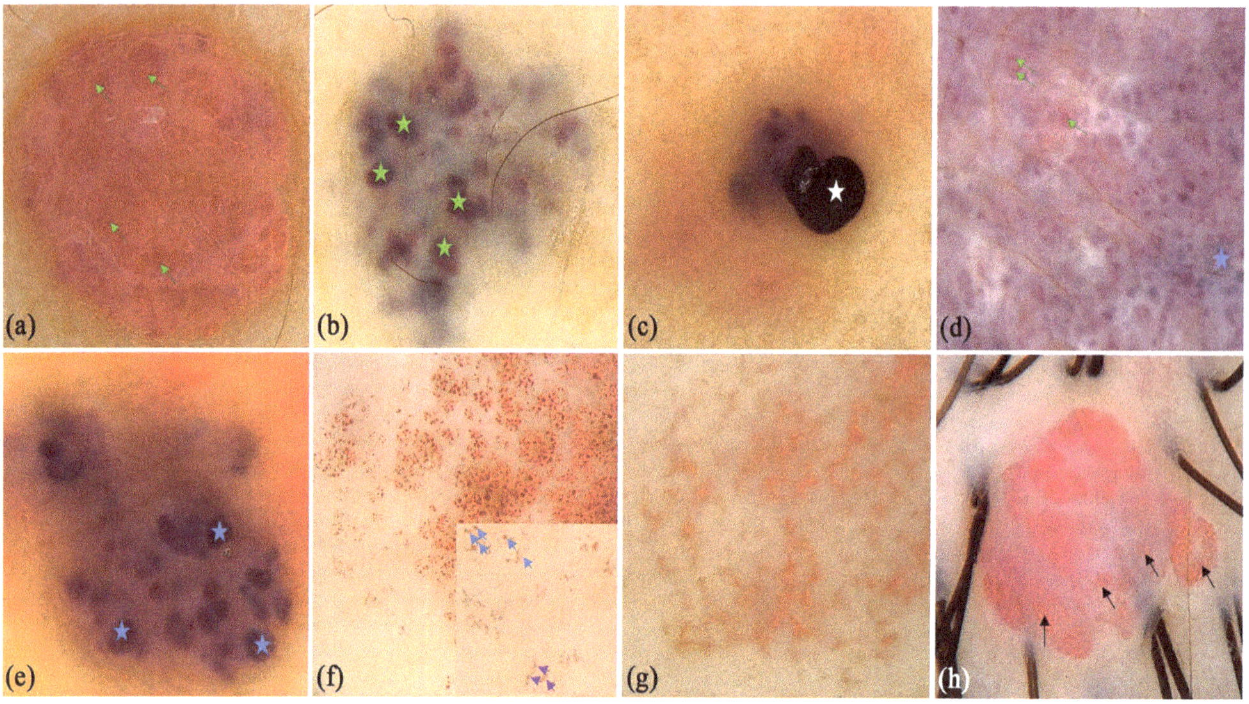


**FIGURE 2** | Dermoscopic features of cherry angioma. **(a)** Typical dermoscopic appearance: red background, clustered red lacunae (green arrows), white surface; **(b)** red-white background, red-brown lacunae (green stars); **(c)** red background and black area (white star); **(d)** red-blue background, clustered red (green arrows) and red-blue lacunae (blue stars), white surface; **(e)** red-blue background, red-blue lacunae (blue stars), white surface; **(f)** red background, red globules (blue arrows) and curved vessels (purple arrows), clearer in the small box; **(g)** reticular vessel distribution; **(h)** clustered serpentine vessels (black arrows).

lesions, coiled vessels in 33 (19.2%) lesions, looped vessels in 7 (4.1%) lesions, and dotted vessels in 14 (8.1%) lesions. For the vessel distribution, reticular distribution in 12 (7.0%) lesions, 58 (33.7%) lesions with clustered vessel distribution, and 70 (40.7%) lesions with unspecific vessel distribution. A black area was seen in 24 (14.0%) lesions, and superficial white veil was seen in 63 (36.6%) lesions. Other infrequent vessel morphology in CA, included linear ($n = 12$, 6.98%), looped ($n = 6$, 3.49%), helical ($n = 6$, 3.49%), coiled ($n = 7$, 4.07%), serpiginous ($n = 1$, 0.58%), and branched ($n = 1$, 0.58%) vessels. Some classical and specifical dermoscopic features are shown in **Figure 2**.

We conducted comparisons of the dermoscopic features of CA (**Table 1**). There was no difference of dermoscopic features were observed between males and females. There were statistical differences in the red background ($P = 0.021$), clustered vessel distribution ($P = 0.03$), black area ($P = 0.029$), and white surface features ($P = 0.042$) among different age groups. Red-brown lacunae ($P = 0.039$), red-blue ($P = 0.013$), red-white background ($P = 0.015$), black area ($P = 0.016$), and white surface ($P = 0.046$) were of statistical difference in terms of the body locations of the lesions. Red lacunae were most common in head and neck, red background was most common in lower limbs, while a black area was most common in trunk.

We also collected 31 patients (16 males and 15 females) with AK, whereas the mean age was 33.29 (SD = 18.03) years old. Some of the classical and specifical dermoscopic features are shown in **Figure 3**. There were 5 (16.1%), 14 (45.2%), and 12 (38.7%) lesions that were located on the upper limbs, lower limbs, head and neck, respectively. Red lacunae could be seen in 13 (41.9%) lesions, dark purple lacunae in 25 (80.6%) lesions, dark blue in 3 (9.7%) lesions, and black lacunae in 4 (12.9%) lesions. A superficial white veil feature was found in 24 (77.4%) lesions, bleeding in 6 (19.4%) lesions, hemorrhagic crusts in 4 (12.9%) lesions, and scales in 7 (22.6%) lesions. Peripheral redness was seen in 7 (22.6%) lesions and peripheral pigment network in 2 (6.5%) lesions.

There were 45 patients (29 males and 16 females) with PG in this study, whereas the mean age was 44.11 (SD = 16.47) years old. Some of the classical and specifical dermoscopic features are shown in **Figure 4**. There were 26 (64.4%) lesions located on the upper limbs, 3 (6.7%) lesions on lower limbs, 15 (33.3%) lesions on head and neck, and only 1 (2.2%) lesion located on trunk. Global dermoscopic patterns that were characterized by a homogeneous area were obvious in all lesions, among which 30 (66.7%) were red-white and 15 (33.3%) were red. As for local features, "white rail" lines were detected in 19 (42.2%) lesions and white collarette in 34 (75.6%) lesions. Furthermore, vascular structures were observed in 19 (42.2%) lesions. Other atypical dermoscopic features included superficial ulcer ($n = 2$, 4.4%), thick crust ($n = 10$, 22.2%), bleeding ($n = 4$, 8.9%), scale ($n = 13$, 28.9%), and a central white veil ($n = 2$, 4.4%).

**TABLE 1** | Summarization and comparison of dermoscopic features of cherry angioma.

| Groups / Features | Sex | | | Age stage | | | | Anatomical location | | | | |
|---|---|---|---|---|---|---|---|---|---|---|---|---|
| | Male ($n = 92$) | Female ($n = 80$) | *P* | <18 years old ($n = 26$) | 18–60 years old ($n = 120$) | >60 years old ($n = 26$) | *P* | Upper limbs ($n = 41$) | Lower limbs ($n = 28$) | Head and neck ($n = 52$) | Trunk ($n = 51$) | *P* |
| **Lacunae** | | | | | | | | | | | | |
| Red | 48 (52.2) | 30 (37.5) | 0.054 | 11 (42.3) | 55 (45.8) | 12 (46.2) | 0.944 | 17 (41.5) | 8 (28.6) | 28 (53.8) | 25 (49.0) | 0.156 |
| Red-brown | 13 (14.1) | 11 (13.8) | 0.943 | 6 (23.1) | 14 (11.7) | 4 (15.4) | 0.303 | 6 (14.6) | 9 (32.1) | 3 (5.8) | 6 (11.8) | 0.013 |
| Red-blue | 24 (26.1) | 18 (22.5) | 0.585 | 4 (15.4) | 30 (25.0) | 8 (30.8) | 0.419 | 4 (9.8) | 8 (28.6) | 12 (23.1) | 18 (35.3) | 0.039 |
| **Background** | | | | | | | | | | | | |
| Red | 41 (44.6) | 36 (45.0) | 0.954 | 7 (26.9) | 62 (51.7) | 8 (30.8) | 0.021 | 21 (51.2) | 13 (46.4) | 20 (38.5) | 23 (45.1) | 0.668 |
| Red-blue | 26 (28.3) | 26 (32.5) | 0.546 | 10 (38.5) | 31 (25.8) | 11 (42.3) | 0.155 | 11 (26.8) | 14 (50.0) | 12 (23.1) | 15 (29.4) | 0.082 |
| Red-white | 22 (23.9) | 12 (15.0) | 0.143 | 3 (11.5) | 22 (18.3) | 9 (34.6) | 0.087 | 5 (12.2) | 1 (3.6) | 16 (30.8) | 12 (23.5) | 0.015 |
| **Vessel morphology** | | | | | | | | | | | | |
| Linear curved | 18 (19.6) | 11 (13.8) | 0.310 | 5 (19.2) | 21 (17.5) | 3 (11.5) | 0.739 | 9 (22.0) | 1 (3.6) | 10 (19.2) | 9 (17.6) | 0.211 |
| Serpiginous | 14 (15.2) | 13 (16.3) | 0.853 | 2 (7.7) | 22 (18.3) | 3 (11.5) | 0.395 | 8 (19.5) | 2 (7.1) | 6 (11.5) | 11 (21.6) | 0.261 |
| Globules | 19 (20.7) | 14 (17.5) | 0.601 | 3 (11.5) | 28 (23.3) | 2 (7.7) | 0.140 | 9 (22.0) | 5 (17.9) | 8 (15.4) | 11 (21.6) | 0.824 |
| Looped | 4 (4.3) | 3 (3.8) | > 0.99* | 0 (0.0) | 6 (5.0) | 1 (3.8) | 0.835 | 3 (7.3) | 0 (0.0) | 2 (3.8) | 2 (3.9) | 0.583* |
| Dots | 9 (9.8) | 5 (6.3) | 0.398 | 1 (3.8) | 9 (7.5) | 4 (15.4) | 0.347 | 7 (17.1) | 2 (7.1) | 2 (3.8) | 3 (5.9) | 0.135* |
| **Vessel distribution** | | | | | | | | | | | | |
| Reticular | 4 (4.3) | 8 (10.0) | 0.147 | 4 (15.4) | 5 (4.2) | 3 (11.5) | 0.058 | 4 (9.8) | 3 (10.7) | 2 (3.8) | 3 (5.9) | 0.567* |
| Clustered | 33 (35.9) | 25 (31.3) | 0.523 | 4 (15.4) | 41 (34.2) | 13 (50.0) | 0.030 | 10 (24.4) | 8 (28.6) | 16 (30.8) | 24 (47.1) | 0.103 |
| Unspecific | 36 (39.1) | 34 (42.5) | 0.654 | 11 (42.3) | 49 (40.8) | 10 (38.5) | 0.959 | 23 (56.1) | 7 (25.0) | 21 (40.4) | 19 (37.3) | 0.068 |
| **Black area** | 16 (17.4) | 8 (10.0) | 0.163 | 6 (23.1) | 18 (15.0) | 0 (0.0) | 0.029 | 4 (9.8) | 7 (25.0) | 2 (3.8) | 11 (21.6) | 0.016 |
| **White surface** | 34 (37.0) | 29 (36.3) | 0.924 | 7 (26.9) | 41 (34.2) | 15 (57.7) | 0.042 | 9 (22.0) | 8 (28.6) | 25 (48.1) | 21 (41.2) | 0.046 |

*Fisher's exact test was used to calculate the P-values.*

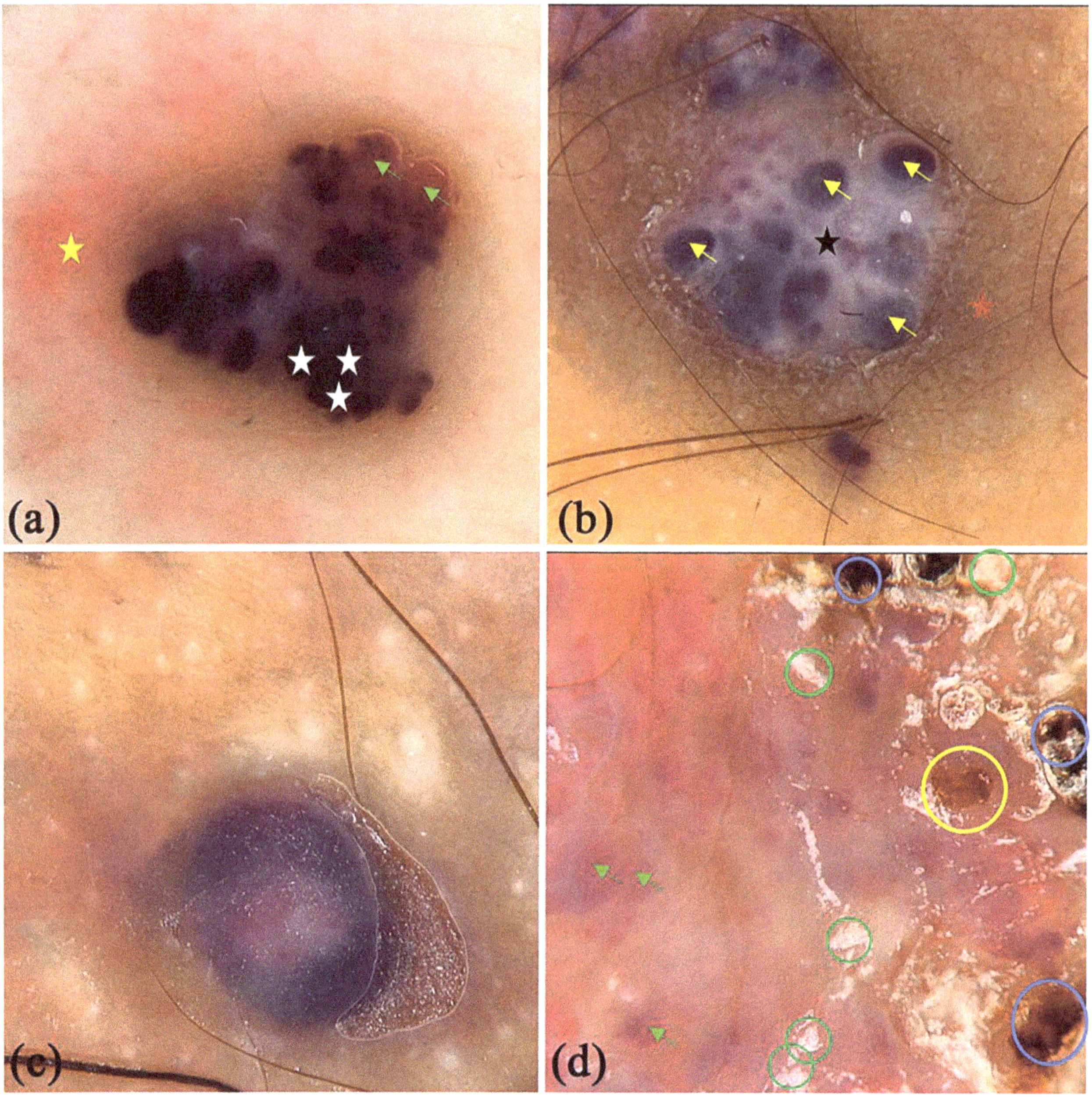


**FIGURE 3 |** Dermoscopic features of angiokeratoma. **(a)** clustered black area (white star) and red lacunae (green arrows), light white curtain, peripheral redness (yellow star); **(b)** dark purple lacunae (yellow arrows), light white curtain (black star), peripheral pigment network (red star); **(c)** dark blue lacuna; **(d)** red lacunae (green arrows), white scales (green circles), dark red scabs (blue circles) and bleeding (yellow circle).

## DISCUSSION

Early and accurate diagnosis represents the safest strategy in the treatment of cutaneous vascular anomalies. This may reduce disease-related mortality, avoid unnecessary surgery, relieve the suffering of patients and ease potential financial burden. However, it can be difficult to manage as a result of the atypical clinical presentation and the progression being similar to malignancy. Dermoscopy is a non-invasive tool that has been applied clinically to support the diagnosis and differential diagnosis of skin tumors (22–25), here we present the dermoscopic differential diagnosis of four types of cutaneous vascular anomalies from other skin disorders (25–31) (**Table 2**). With dermoscopy, predominant vascular structures and other recognizable concomitant features can be observed. This may lead to improved accurate diagnosis of cutaneous vascular anomalies that originate from cutaneous vessels, if promptly recognized. This study describes the dermoscopic

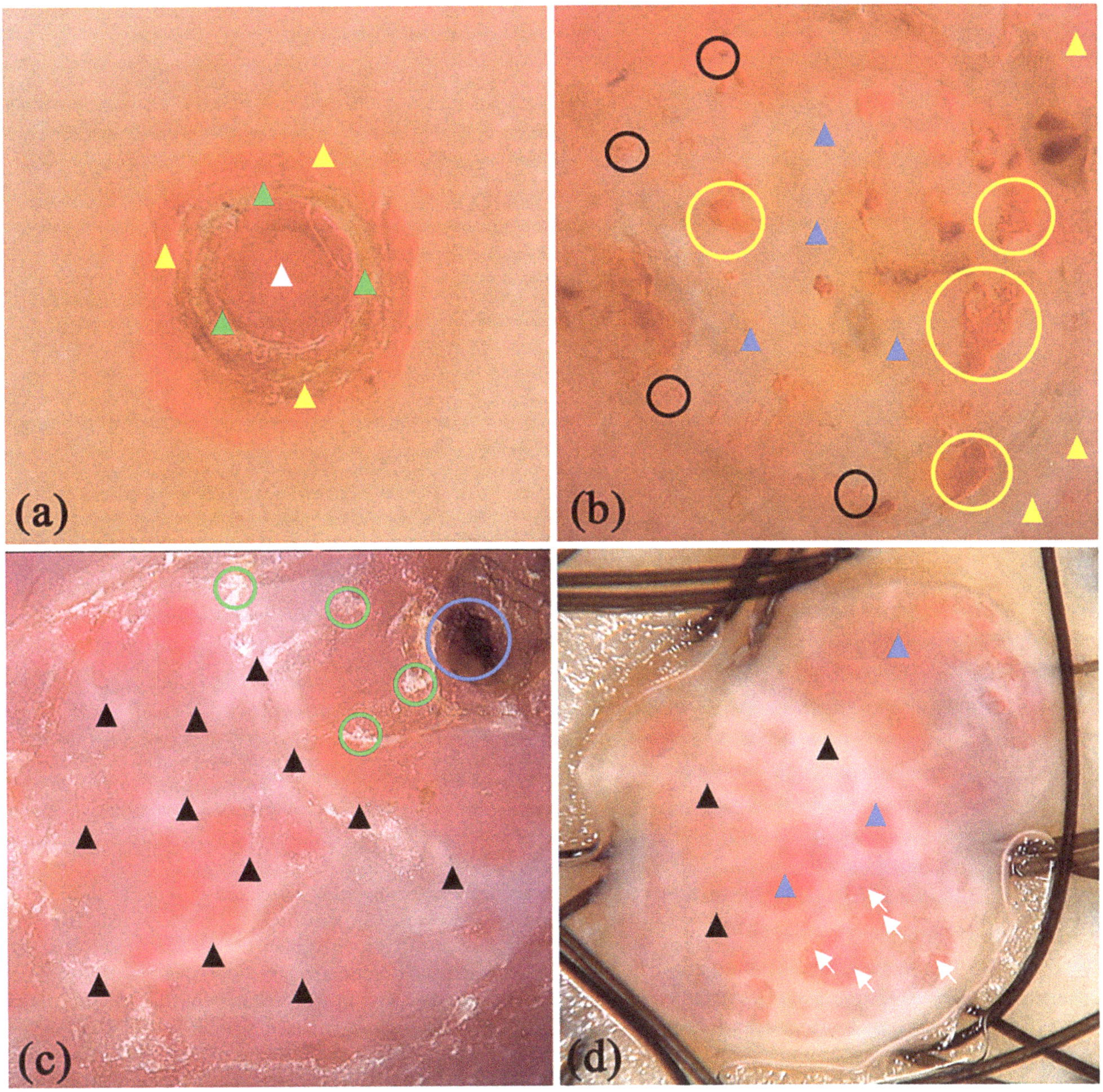


**FIGURE 4** | Dermoscopic features of pyogenic granuloma. **(a)** red homogeneous area (white triangle), yellow scabs (green triangles), collar pattern (yellow triangles); **(b)** red-white homogeneous area (blue triangles), white collar pattern (yellow triangles), vascular structures (black circles) and bleeding (yellow circles); **(c)** "white rail" lines (black triangles), dark red scabs (blue circles) and white scales (green circles); **(d)** red-white homogeneous area (blue triangles) and "white rail" lines (black triangles), serpentine vessels (white arrows).

features of four types of cutaneous vascular anomalies in 279 patients.

Our study indicated that nearly three quarters of the lesions showed lacunae, which is regarded as a diagnostic clue for IH and CA (32). Lacunae corresponded to dilated vessels that are filled with red blood cells in the dermal papillae. Although lacunae appear in a variety of colors, their overall hue is red. The overall hue of backgrounds in IH and CA were red as well and the observed three colors in our study were consistent with a previous study (17). Besides lacunae, there are other vessels structures in IH and CA. The arrangement of vessels includes reticular, clustered, and unspecific vessel distributions, and the last one is the most common. It is worth noting that some lesions contain only one structure, and the possibilities of IH or CA should be taken into consideration when this is observed. In the vascular structures that have been reported before, we found that coiled vessel features were the most common. The appearance of a well-defined black area corresponds to thrombogenesis under histopathology (33). The superficial white veil feature, which were detected frequently, histopathologically resulted

**TABLE 2 |** Dermoscopic differential diagnosis of four types of cutaneous vascular anomalies from other skin disorders.

| Category | Diseases | Common dermoscopic features |
|---|---|---|
| Four types of cutaneous vascular anomalies | IH | Red/red-blue/red-white background, clustered red lacunae; polymorphous vascular structures: red globular and helical vessels; clustered serpentine vessels (25). |
| | CA | Red/red-white/red-blue background, red/red-blue/dark lacunae, white surface; red globular and curved vessels, clustered serpentine, blue-whitish veil, ulceration, rainbow pattern. |
| | AK | Clustered black to dark red or purple-blue lacunae and whitish veil, peripheral redness; peripheral pigment network; white scales, dark red scabs and bleeding, blue whitish veil, ulceration, rainbow pattern (16). |
| | PG | Reddish homogeneous area, white collarette, "white rail" lines that intersect the lesion and ulceration (15). Red or white homogeneous area, surrounded by a white collar-like structure, thick tortuous blood vessels can be seen in the skin lesions. reddish homogeneous areas associated with "white rail" lines (17). |
| Other differential skin disorders | Foreign body granuloma | Orange background, white or blue-gray homogeneous areas; branched vessels (12). |
| | Verruca vulgaris | Multiple tightly packed papillae with red, brown dots, linear or looped vessels; white halos around looped vessels in some cases; irregular red, black, brown bleeding or scabs (12, 29, 30). |
| | Malignant melanoma | Negative or atypical pigment network; atypical streaks (radial streaming or pseudopods); blue-whitish veil; irregular dots or globules; irregular blotch; polychromatic; shiny white streaks; vascular pattern: pink areas, irregular dots or looped vessels (12). |
| | Spitz nevus | Starburst pattern, pink or pigment homogeneous pattern, globular pattern, atypical pattern, reticular pattern (12, 31). |
| | Bowenoid papulosis | Scattered dot, curved, looped, or coiled vessels; blue-gray or gray-brown homogeneous area (12, 27). |
| | Kaposi sarcoma | Bluish-reddish coloration including purple; multicolored areas showing various colors of the rainbow spectrum; scaly surface; small brown globule or blotch; reticular coarse vessels; shiny white streaks (12, 28). |
| | Dermatofi-brosarcoma protuberan | Topographic pattern background (pink, buff or tan); branched vessels (clustered or disseminated); shiny white streaks; delicate pigment network; structureless area or hypopigmented area (12). |
| | Proliferating trichilemmal tumor | Pink background, shiny white streaks, irregular and crown vessels, (sometimes) with hairs and ulceration (12, 26). |

from the presence of an acanthotic epidermis with compact hyperkeratosis (34).

Typical dermoscopic features of AK include a well-demarcated, round lacunae and a whitish veil, whose histopathological basis are consistent with their equivalents in IH and CA (35). The overall hue of lacunae in AK is dark, with dark purple being the most common one in our study. Dark blue, purple, or a black color corresponds to vascular spaces that are partially or completely thrombosed. Peripheral redness, which likely represents inflammation of the lesion and erythrocyte extravasation in the papillary dermis, were seen in seven lesions. Two lesions presented a peripheral pigment network due to hyperpigmented rete ridges, which is akin to the network observed in dermatofibromas (36). Hemorrhagic crusts were detected in 12.9% lesions, which is far lower than the 53% reported in previous study (16). Scale features, which have been reported in previous study (6), were discovered in 22.6% lesions (7 of 31). Also, scale is a clinical manifestation of AK.

From our observation, a homogeneous area including reddish and red-whitish features, were the most frequent dermoscopic structure associated with PG, which is consistent with a previous study (7). The histopathological correlation of a homogeneous area may be attributed to the presence of numerous small capillaries or proliferating vessels which served as a foundation for various vascular structures. The white collarette, which was seen in 75.6% of lesions in our study, corresponds to the hyperplastic adnexal epithelium that partially or totally surrounds the lesion at the periphery of PG. This frequency of the white collarette is similar to previous study (7). The "white rail" lines may correspond to the fibrous septa that surround the capillary tufts or lobules (15), but it was not so common as white collarette features. The "white rail" lines can be observed in dermatofibromas and fully regressive melanomas when a polarized mode is used (37, 38). Erosion, bleeding, and scabbing are common clinical features of PG. These often lead to a misdiagnosis as malignant tumors which present as a dark-red or black homogeneous structure, hemorrhagic crusts, or ulceration revealed with dermoscopy. Serous exudation present explains the observation of orange-yellow crusts.

Other than the reported features in previous literatures, we observed some other dermoscopic findings in these cutaneous vascular anomalies. In IH and CA, some other morphology features include irregular linear, looped, helical, coiled, serpiginous, and branched vessels which were detected in our study. These features seem to be associated with dilated and proliferated vessels in the upper dermis and some of them had diagnostic specificity for some malignant tumors. For example, coiled vessels in Bowen's disease (39). In our experience, scales and partial whitish veil features can also be seen in PG, which had never been described previously. These two features could appear in multiple diseases, for instance, scales may be present in inflammatory skin diseases and whitish veil in skin tumors.

We analyzed differences in gender, age stage, and location of the lesions. Red lacunae was more commonly observed in females. They may be linked to the higher levels of estrogen in female patients (40). Red-blue background and lacunae were more common in adults, which may be a signs of thrombi within the vascular spaces (17). This may also explain why black areas were more common in older patients. Additionally, dilated vessels in CA were veins, with the addition of some vessels in deeper dermis which may contribute to the color of red-blue in the adult. Another age-related dermoscopic feature was the presence of a superficial whitish veil, which may be explained as IH is self-limited while CA is not. In relation to anatomical areas, the feature of a black area, red-brown lacunae, and red-white background were the most prevalent in the trunk region.

It should be noted especially that there are some limitations of our study. One is that the diagnosis of four types of cutaneous vascular anomalies were based on clinical and dermoscopic features by two dermatologists and no histopathological examination was performed. The variations in anatomical sites and some newly discovered features have not been well-studied by histological analysis. Another one is the limited study sample size of IH, AK, and PG; many more numbers of these three cutaneous vascular anomalies patients should be recruited for a future study.

## CONCLUSION

Dermoscopic evaluation is an easy, applicable, and ancillary diagnostic tool for the diagnosis of cutaneous vascular anomalies. In clinical practice, when dermatologists diagnose CA with dermoscopy, it is necessary to consider that dermoscopic features vary in age stages and different anatomical sites.

## ETHICS STATEMENT

The studies involving human participants were reviewed and approved by The Second Affiliated Hospital of Anhui Medical University and China-Japan Friendship Hospital. Written informed consent in this study was provided by participants or the participants' legal guardian/next of kin.

## AUTHOR CONTRIBUTIONS

CY and YC designed this study. WF, XS, JG, CS, MS, NX, QL, and TZ collected the clinical and dermoscopic data. CS, JG, RK, and WF analyzed of data and interpreted the analysis results. JG, WF, CS, and XS prepared the manuscript. RK, CH, CS, CY, and YC revised this manuscript. All authors contributed to the article and approved the submitted version.

## REFERENCES


1. Johnson EF, Davis DM, Tollefson MM, Fritchie K, Gibson LE. Vascular tumors in infants: case report and review of clinical, histopathologic, and immunohistochemical characteristics of infantile hemangioma, pyogenic granuloma, noninvoluting congenital hemangioma, tufted angioma, and kaposiform hemangioendothelioma. *Am J Dermatopathol.* (2018) 40:231–9. doi: 10.1097/DAD.0000000000000983
2. Grazzini M, Stanganelli I, Rossari S, Gori A, Oranges T, Longo AS, et al. Dermoscopy, confocal laser microscopy, and hi-tech evaluation of vascular skin lesions: diagnostic and therapeutic perspectives. *Dermatol Ther.* (2012) 25:297–303. doi: 10.1111/j.1529-8019.2012.01547.x
3. International Society for the Study of Vascular Anomalies. *ISSVA classification for Vascular Anomalies [EB/OL].* Available online at: http://www.issva.org/UserFiles/file/ISSVA-Classification-2018.pdf (accessed May 17, 2021).
4. Qadeer HA, Singal A, Patel BC. *Cherry Hemangioma, StatPearls, StatPearls Publishing Copyright © 2021.* (2021). Treasure Island (FL): StatPearls Publishing LLC.
5. Anderson KR, Schoch JJ, Lohse CM, Hand JL, Davis DM, Tollefson MM. Increasing incidence of infantile hemangiomas (IH) over the past 35 years: correlation with decreasing gestational age at birth and birth weight. *J Am Acad Dermatol.* (2016) 74:120–6. doi: 10.1016/j.jaad.2015.08.024
6. Kim JH, Kim MR, Lee SH, Lee SE, Lee SH. Dermoscopy: a useful tool for the diagnosis of angiokeratoma. *Ann Dermatol.* (2012) 24:468–71. doi: 10.5021/ad.2012.24.4.468
7. Zaballos P, Carulla M, Ozdemir F, Zalaudek I, Bañuls J, Llambrich A, et al. Dermoscopy of pyogenic granuloma: a morphological study. *Br J Dermatol.* (2010) 163:1229–37. doi: 10.1111/j.1365-2133.2010.10040.x
8. Braun RP, Rabinovitz HS, Oliviero M, Kopf AW, Saurat JH. Dermoscopy of pigmented skin lesions. *J Am Acad Dermatol.* (2005) 52:109–21. doi: 10.1016/j.jaad.2001.11.001
9. Fargnoli MC, Kostaki D, Piccioni A, Micantonio T, Peris K. Dermoscopy in the diagnosis and management of non-melanoma skin cancers. *Eur J Dermatol.* (2012) 22:456–63. doi: 10.1684/ejd.2012.1727
10. Shen X, Yu RX, Shen CB, Li CX, Jing Y, Zheng YJ, et al. Dermoscopy in China: current status and future prospective. *Chin Med J (Engl).* (2019) 132:2096–104. doi: 10.1097/CM9.0000000000000396
11. Wang ZY, Shen CB, Fei WM, Shen X, Li CX, Jing Y, et al. Accuracy of dermoscopic and reflectance confocal microscopic criteria for diagnosis of psoriasis. *Chin Med J (Engl).* (2020) 133:3010–2. doi: 10.1097/CM9.0000000000001198
12. Meng RS, Cui Y. *Multimodal Medical Imaging Atlas of Dermatology.* Beijing: People's Medical Publishing House (2021).
13. Lee JS, Mun JH. Dermoscopy of venous lake on the lips: a comparative study with labial melanotic macule. *PLoS ONE.* (2018) 13:e0206768. doi: 10.1371/journal.pone.0206768
14. Jassi R, Sanke S, Chander R. Dermoscopic evaluation of infantile hemangioma treated with topical timolol. *Dermatol Pract Concept.* (2020) 10:e2020073. doi: 10.5826/dpc.1004a73
15. Zaballos P, Llambrich A, Cuéllar F, Puig S, Malvehy J. Dermoscopic findings in pyogenic granuloma. *Br J Dermatol.* (2006) 154:1108–11. doi: 10.1111/j.1365-2133.2006.07193.x
16. Zaballos P, Daufí C, Puig S, Argenziano G, Moreno-Ramírez D, Cabo H, et al. Dermoscopy of solitary angiokeratomas: a morphological study. *Arch Dermatol.* (2007) 143:318–25. doi: 10.1001/archderm.143.3.318
17. Wolf IH. Dermoscopic diagnosis of vascular lesions. *Clin Dermatol.* (2002) 20:273–5. doi: 10.1016/S0738-081X(02)00222-5

18. Errichetti E, Zalaudek I, Kittler H, Apalla Z, Argenziano G, Bakos R, et al. Standardization of dermoscopic terminology and basic dermoscopic parameters to evaluate in general dermatology (non-neoplastic dermatoses): an expert consensus on behalf of the International Dermoscopy Society. *Br J Dermatol.* (2020) 182:454–67. doi: 10.1111/bjd.18125
19. Kittler H, Marghoob AA, Argenziano G, Carrera C, Curiel-Lewandrowski C, Hofmann-Wellenhof R, et al. Standardization of terminology in dermoscopy/dermatoscopy: results of the third consensus conference of the International Society of Dermoscopy. *J Am Acad Dermatol.* (2016) 74:1093–106. doi: 10.1016/j.jaad.2015.12.038
20. Piazza CD, Yamada S, Marcassi AP, Maciel MG, Seize MP, Cestari SCP. Dermoscopic patterns of melanocytic nevi in children and adolescents: a cross-sectional study. *An Bras Dermatol.* (2017) 92:340–4. doi: 10.1590/abd1806-4841.20175209
21. Cheng CY, Su HJ, Kuo TT. Dermoscopic features and differential diagnosis of sebaceous carcinoma. *J Dermatol.* (2020) 47:755–62. doi: 10.1111/1346-8138.15384
22. Darmawan CC, Jo G, Montenegro SE, Kwak Y, Cheol L, Cho KH, et al. Early detection of acral melanoma: a review of clinical, dermoscopic, histopathologic, and molecular characteristics. *J Am Acad Dermatol.* (2019) 81:805–12. doi: 10.1016/j.jaad.2019.01.081
23. Yélamos O, Braun RP, Liopyris K, Wolner ZJ, Kerl K, Gerami P, et al. Usefulness of dermoscopy to improve the clinical and histopathologic diagnosis of skin cancers. *J Am Acad Dermatol.* (2019) 80:365–77. doi: 10.1016/j.jaad.2018.07.072
24. Shen CB, Shen X, Li CX, Meng RS, Cui Y. Assessment of imaging diagnosis ability of skin tumors in Chinese dermatologists. *Chin Med J (Engl).* (2019) 132:2119–20. doi: 10.1097/CM9.0000000000000389
25. Natsis NE, Gordon SC, Kaushik A, Seiverling EV. A practical review of dermoscopy for pediatric dermatology part II: vascular tumors, infections, and inflammatory dermatoses. *Pediatr Dermatol.* (2020) 37:798–803. doi: 10.1111/pde.14284
26. Miyachi H, Togawa Y, Yamamoto Y, Oguma R, Suehiro K, Matsue H. Proliferating trichilemmal tumour: a comparison of dermoscopic, ultrasonographic and histopathological features. *Eur J Dermatol.* (2016) 26:400–2. doi: 10.1684/ejd.2016.2795
27. Chan SL, Watchorn RE, Panagou E, Panou E, Ong EL, Heelan K, et al. Dermatoscopic findings of penile intraepithelial neoplasia: bowenoid papulosis, Bowen disease and erythroplasia of Queyrat. *Australas J Dermatol.* (2019) 60:e201–7. doi: 10.1111/ajd.12981
28. Hu SC, Ke CL, Lee CH, Wu CS, Chen GS, Cheng ST. Dermoscopy of Kaposi's sarcoma: areas exhibiting the multicoloured 'rainbow pattern'. *J Eur Acad Dermatol Venereol.* (2009) 23:1128–32. doi: 10.1111/j.1468-3083.2009.03239.x
29. Tognetti L, Cartocci A, Cinotti E, Moscarella E, Farnetani F, Carrera C, et al. Dermoscopy of early melanomas: variation according to the anatomic site. *Arch Dermatol Res.* (2021). doi: 10.1007/s00403-021-02226-x. [Epub ahead of print].
30. Kato J, Horimoto K, Sato S, Minowa T, Uhara H. Dermoscopy of melanoma and non-melanoma skin cancers. *Front Med (Lausanne).* (2019) 6:180. doi: 10.3389/fmed.2019.00180
31. Lallas A, Apalla Z, Ioannides D, Lazaridou E, Kyrgidis A, Broganelli P, et al. Update on dermoscopy of Spitz/Reed naevi and management guidelines by the International Dermoscopy Society. *Br J Dermatol.* (2017) 177:645–55. doi: 10.1111/bjd.15339
32. Oiso N, Kawada A. The dermoscopic features in infantile hemangioma. *Pediatr Dermatol.* (2011) 28:591–3. doi: 10.1111/j.1525-1470.2011.01385.x
33. Moscarella E, Zalaudek I, Buccini P, Cota C, Catricalà C, Argenziano G. Dermoscopy and confocal microscopy of thrombosed hemangiomas. *Arch Dermatol.* (2012) 148:410. doi: 10.1001/archdermatol.2011.1027
34. Massi D, De Giorgi V, Carli P, Santucci M. Diagnostic significance of the blue hue in dermoscopy of melanocytic lesions: a dermoscopic-pathologic study. *Am J Dermatopathol.* (2001) 23:463–9. doi: 10.1097/00000372-200110000-00013
35. Jha AK, Sonthalia S, Jakhar D. Dermoscopy of angiokeratoma. *Indian Dermatol Online J.* (2018) 9:141–2. doi: 10.4103/idoj.IDOJ_278_17
36. Cuestas D, Perafan A, Forero Y, Bonilla J, Velandia A, Gutierrez A, et al. Angiokeratomas, not everything is Fabry disease. *Int J Dermatol.* (2019) 58:713–21. doi: 10.1111/ijd.14330
37. Bories N, Dalle S, Debarbieux S, Balme B, Ronger-Savlé S, Thomas L. Dermoscopy of fully regressive cutaneous melanoma. *Br J Dermatol.* (2008) 158:1224–9. doi: 10.1111/j.1365-2133.2008.08501.x
38. Zaballos P, Llambrich A, Ara M, Olazarán Z, Malvehy J, Puig S. Dermoscopic findings of haemosiderotic and aneurysmal dermatofibroma: report of six patients. *Br J Dermatol.* (2006) 154:244–50. doi: 10.1111/j.1365-2133.2005.06844.x
39. Yang Y, Lin J, Fang S, Han S, Song Z. What's new in dermoscopy of Bowen's disease: two new dermoscopic signs and its differential diagnosis. *Int J Dermatol.* (2017) 56:1022–5. doi: 10.1111/ijd.13734
40. Sun ZY, Yang L, Yi CG, Zhao H, Han DL, Yang T, et al. Possibilities and potential roles of estrogen in the pathogenesis of proliferation hemangiomas formation. *Med Hypotheses.* (2008) 71:286–92. doi: 10.1016/j.mehy.2008.02.015

6

# Attitudes Toward Artificial Intelligence within Dermatopathology

*Sam Polesie[1,2]*, Phillip H. McKee[3], Jerad M. Gardner[4], Martin Gillstedt[1,2], Jan Siarov[2,5], Noora Neittaanmäki[2,5] and John Paoli[1,2]*

*[1] Department of Dermatology and Venereology, Institute of Clinical Sciences, Sahlgrenska Academy, University of Gothenburg, Gothenburg, Sweden, [2] Region Västra Götaland, Sahlgrenska University Hospital, Department of Dermatology and Venereology, Gothenburg, Sweden, [3] Retired, Boston, MA, United States, [4] Department of Laboratory Medicine, Geisinger Medical Center, Danville, PA, United States, [5] Department of Pathology, Institute of Biomedicine, Sahlgrenska Academy, University of Gothenburg, Gothenburg, Sweden*

***Correspondence:***
*Sam Polesie*
*sam.polesie@vgregion.se*

**Background:** Artificial intelligence (AI) has recently surfaced as a research topic in dermatology and dermatopathology. In a recent survey, dermatologists were overall positive toward a development with an increased use of AI, but little is known about the corresponding attitudes among pathologists working with dermatopathology. The objective of this investigation was to make an inventory of these attitudes.

**Participants and Methods:** An anonymous and voluntary online survey was prepared and distributed to pathologists who regularly analyzed dermatopathology slides/images. The survey consisted of 39 question divided in five sections; (1) AI as a topic in pathology; (2) previous exposure to AI as a topic in general; (3) applications for AI in dermatopathology; (4) feelings and attitudes toward AI and (5) self-reported tech-savviness and demographics. The survey opened on March 13, 2020 and closed on May 5, 2020.

**Results:** Overall, 718 responders (64.1% females) representing 91 countries were analyzed. While 81.5% of responders were aware of AI as an emerging topic in pathology, only 18.8% had either good or excellent knowledge about AI. In terms of diagnosis classification, 42.6% saw strong or very strong potential for automated suggestion of skin tumor diagnoses. The corresponding figure for inflammatory skin diseases was 23.0% ($P_{adj}$ <0.0001). For specific applications, the highest potential was considered for automated detection of mitosis (79.2%), automated suggestion of tumor margins (62.1%) and immunostaining evaluation (62.7%). The potential for automated suggestion of immunostaining (37.6%) and genetic panels (48.3%) were lower. Age did not impact the overall attitudes toward AI. Only 6.0% of the responders agreed or strongly agreed that the human pathologist will be replaced by AI in the foreseeable future. For the entire group, 72.3% agreed or strongly agreed that AI will improve dermatopathology and 84.1% thought that AI should be a part of medical training.

**Conclusions:** Pathologists are generally optimistic about the impact and potential benefit of AI in dermatopathology. The highest potential is expected for narrow specified tasks rather than a global automated suggestion of diagnoses. There is a strong need for education about AI and its use within dermatopathology.

**Keywords: artificial intelligence, attitude, dermatopathology, machine learning, online survey**

## INTRODUCTION

Even though artificial intelligence (AI) has been discussed for decades, the unprecedented computer processor development, storage availability, and universal internet access including cloud services have contributed to the recent accelerated research interest in AI in several domains of medicine including pathology (1). AI and machine learning (ML) have recently pervaded every aspect of medical image analysis at an extraordinary pace (2).

While historically restricted to traditional microscopes and glass slides, pathology has recently transitioned to become a more digitally oriented specialty. Within the past decade, the use of whole slide imaging (WSI) has been validated for surgical pathology and dermatopathology (3, 4). Although WSI has not uniformly been well-received among dermatopathologists (5), the diagnostic modality has proven non-inferior to traditional microscopes for most diagnostic classes, except for a subset of melanocytic lesions, in a recent intra-observer validation investigation (6). With the rise of whole slide scanner technology (7), and free-hand smartphone photography (8), large numbers of tissue slides are being captured and archived digitally. For dermatopathology specifically, closed online forums now represent an important piece of continuing medical education and attract thousands of users from multiple countries across the world in all age groups (9). In many centers, all glass slides are routinely scanned and are made available digitally. While the primary diagnosis might still be made by pathologists using traditional microscopes, ancillary diagnoses by ML-based software might only be a few computer maneuvers away, fundamentally changing pathology as we know it.

The immense accumulation of online dermatopathology images represents a substantial resource not only for education, but also for ML research purposes. Recently, Schaumberg et al. presented the first pan-tissue and pan-disease ML-method for predicting disease as well as immunostaining (10). The training set consisted of thousands of images obtained through social media and PubMed articles and was prospectively tested in public on social media. Although in its early stages, the potential seen for ML in dermatopathology have been demonstrated both pertaining to specific tasks as well as diagnosis (11–13). The use of ML within dermatopathology has recently been listed as one of the important dermatological applications of AI (14). Nonetheless, little is known about dermatopathologists' attitudes toward an increased use of AI within their field. In a recent study, including 1,271 dermatologists, investigating the attitudes toward AI within dermatology, the majority of responders were positive toward a development with an increased use of AI. Moreover, only a minority expressed fear toward an increased use. Interestingly, a majority of responders (58.1%) saw either strong or very strong potential for automated detection of skin diseases based on dermatopathology images (15).

Dermatopathology and dermatology depend on one another and collaboration between our disciplines is essential for clinical-pathological correlation. In order to prepare for a future with an increased use of AI, it is our belief that a first inventory of dermatopathologists' views on the topic is important. Ultimately, it is our hope that dermatopathologists together with dermatologists should be the ones who guide and lead the development in our fields. Thus, the following study was performed as an exploratory survey with the aim to specifically address feelings and attitudes toward AI among dermatopathologists.

## MATERIALS AND METHODS

An anonymized and voluntary English online survey was prepared and distributed through SurveyMonkey® (www.surveymonkey.com, San Mateo, CA, USA). The survey started with a brief introduction followed by 39 questions (Q1–Q39). The first baseline question (Q1) tested for eligibility (i.e., if the responders worked as a pathologist who regularly analyzed dermatopathology slides/images). If a responder answered "no" to this first question, the survey ended. The rest of the survey questions were divided into five sections: (1) AI as a topic in pathology (Q2-Q3); (2) previous exposure to AI as a topic in general (Q4-Q7); (3) applications for AI in dermatopathology (Q8-Q14); (4) feelings and attitudes toward AI (Q15-Q25) and (5) self-reported tech-savviness and demographics (Q26-Q39). Most of the response options were prepared as Likert-type scales (16). The complete survey as displayed to the responder is available in the **Supplementary Material**. Answers to all questions were required for the survey to be considered complete.

The survey opened on March 13, 2020 and closed on May 5, 2020 (53 survey days). The survey link was advertised on a closed Facebook® (Menlo Park, CA, USA) group called McKee Derm, which is frequently visited by international pathologists, dermatopathologists and dermatologists and has ~15,000 members (17). The group opened in May 2017 and its main purpose is to share and discuss dermatopathology cases. The survey link was also shared publicly by one of the authors (JMG) on their public Facebook page and Twitter account. Since all responses were obtained voluntarily and anonymously from professional colleagues, the study was exempt from approval by an ethics review board.

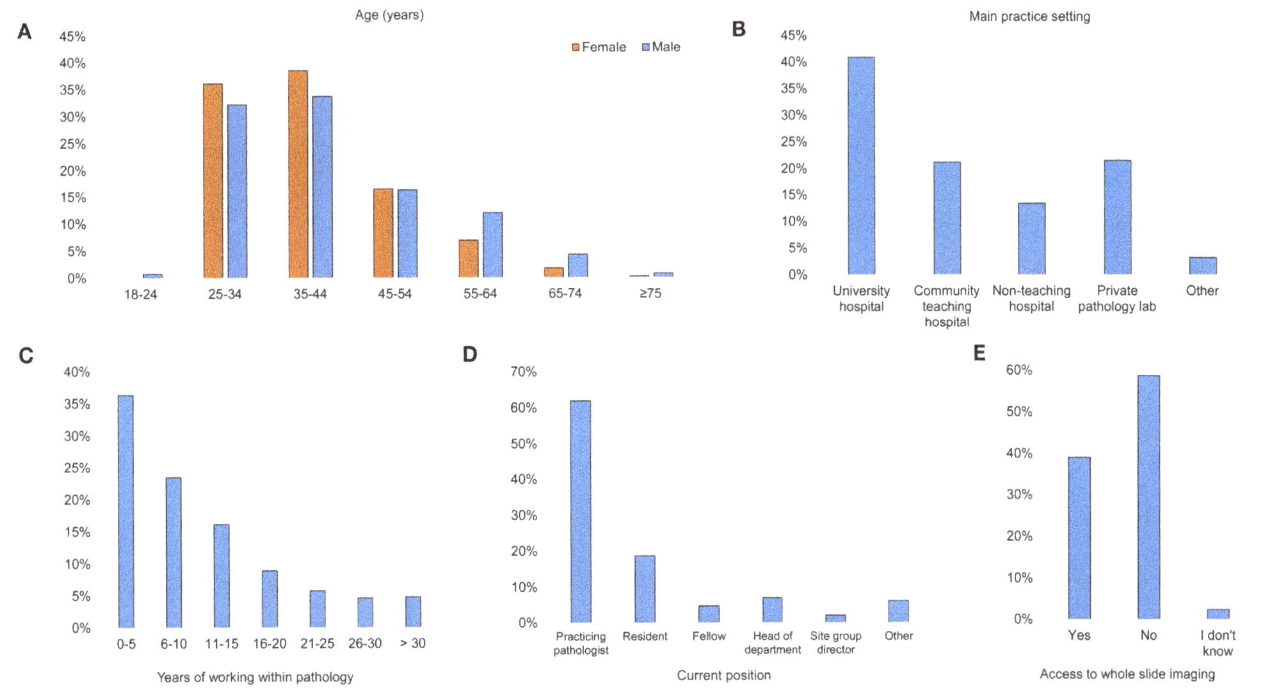


**FIGURE 1** | Responder characteristics. **(A)** Age distribution for each sex. **(B)** Proportion in each type of practice setting. **(C)** Distribution of the number of years working within pathology. **(D)** Current position. **(E)** Access to whole slide imaging at work.

## Statistical Analysis

All data were analyzed using R version 3.5.3 (https://www.r-project.org/). Fisher's exact test and Wilcoxon's rank sum test were used for two-sample tests. Wilcoxon's signed rank test was used for paired tests. For questions with dichotomous answers, logistic regression was used with *"no"*/*"yes"* as the dependent variable and sex and age group as independent variables. For questions with non-dichotomous answers, linear regression models were used to correlate answers to sex and age group using a score for the answers, for example: *"Strongly disagree"* = 1, *"Disagree"* = 2, *"Neither agree nor disagree"* = 3, *"Agree"* = 4 and *"Strongly agree"* = 5. The age groups (20-24, 25-34, 35-44, 45-54, 55-64, 65-74, and ≥75 years) were used as numeric values in the regression models, i.e., numbers ranging from 1 to 7. P-values were adjusted ($P_{adj}$) for multiple comparisons using the Holm method (18). All tests were two-sided and $P_{adj} < 0.05$ was considered as statistically significant.

## RESULTS

Of 1,263 surveys received, 848 responders worked as pathologists who regularly analyzed dermatopathology slides/images in a clinical setting. Among these, 718 completed the survey resulting in an 84.7% response rate among the eligible audience and these responses were further analyzed. The median time to complete the survey was 6.1 min (interquartile range, 4.7–8.5 min). All aggregated result summaries for Q1-Q38 are available in **Supplementary Material**. An overview of the age and sex distribution of the responders as well as other demographic data are presented in **Figure 1**. Practicing specialists and residents in pathology constituted 80.5% of the responders. The median age (range) was 38 years (22–79 years), 64.1% ($n$ = 460) were females and 39.0% ($n$ = 280) had access to WSI at work. The great majority of the surveyed dermatopathologists mainly used traditional microscopes for routine diagnostic dermatopathology while only 4% (29 of 718) of the responders mainly used digitally scanned slides. Overall, 91 different countries were represented. The three countries where most responders worked were India ($n$ = 96, 13.4%), USA ($n$ = 80, 11.1%) and United Kingdom ($n$ = 35, 4.9%).

While 81.5% of responders were aware of AI as an emerging topic in pathology, only 18.8% had either good or excellent knowledge about AI within pathology. Younger responders (<40 years) were equally aware of the recent development compared to older responders (≥40 years) with 322 of 400 (80.5%) vs. 263 of 318 (82.7%) claiming awareness ($P = 0.50$, $P_{adj} = 1$). A higher percentage of responders mainly working in a university hospital (255 of 293, 87.0%) were aware of the AI development within pathology compared to those working in other settings (330 of 425, 77.6%) ($P = 0.0017$, $P_{adj} = 0.073$). Males generally had a higher self-reported level of knowledge about AI than females (26.0 vs. 14.8%, $P = 0.003$, $P_{adj} = 0.12$).

Among all responders, 22.3% had used AI as a diagnostic aid in real life within pathology and 11.0% had used AI within dermatopathology in particular. Use of AI was not associated with age nor sex (**Table 1**). Physicians with access to WSI and those with previous use of AI within pathology

**TABLE 1** | Distribution of answers to questions regarding background knowledge about AI.

| Question | Yes | No | | | | log(OR) for age -group (95% CI) | *P-value* | Holm corrected *P*-value | log(OR) for sex (95% CI) [Ref. Female] | *P*-value | Holm corrected *P*-value |
|---|---|---|---|---|---|---|---|---|---|---|---|
| AI is a topic that has become of interest for the pathology community. Were you already aware of this topic in pathology? | 585 (81.5%) | 133 (18.5%) | | | | 0.10 (−0.08, 0.28) | 0.28 | 1 | −0.03 (-0.42, 0.37) | 0.89 | 1 |
| Have you read any medical publications regarding AI within dermatopathology? | 181 (25.2%) | 537 (74.8%) | | | | 0.12 (−0.03, 0.27) | 0.12 | 1 | 0.29 (−0.06, 0.63) | 0.11 | 1 |
| Have you used AI as a diagnostic aid in real life within pathology? | 160 (22.3%) | 558 (77.7%) | | | | 0.09 (−0.07, 0.25) | 0.29 | 1 | −0.18 (−0.55, 0.19) | 0.35 | 1 |
| Have you used AI as a diagnostic aid in real life within dermatopathology? | 79 (11.0%) | 639 (89.0%) | | | | 0.18 (−0.03, 0.38) | 0.087 | 1 | −0.07 (−0.56, 0.42) | 0.78 | 1 |
| | **I have never heard about it** | **I have heard about it, but not more** | **Basic knowledge** | **Good knowledge** | **Excellent knowledge** | **Score increase per age interval (95% CI)** | ***P-value*** | **Holm corrected *P*-value** | **Sex; Score difference (95% CI) [Ref. Female]** | ***P*** | **Holm corrected *P*-value** |
| Which degree of knowledge would you say you have when it comes to AI within pathology? | 25 (3.5%) | 275 (38.3%) | 283 (39.4%) | 111 (15.5%) | 24 (3.3%) | 0.06 (0.01, 0.12) | **0.034** | 1 | 0.20 (0.07, 0.33) | **0.003** | 0.12 |

*For the questions with dichotomous answers, log-odds ratios, 95% CI and P-values for the logistic regression model (no=0 and yes=1) containing both sex and age group (20-24, 25-34, 35-44, 45-54, 55-64, 65-74, and ≥75 years) are included. The age groups are used as numeric values in the regression model, i.e., numbers ranging from 1 to 7. For the final question with five possible answers, the answer was transformed to a numeric score (1–5) and a linear regression model with both sex and age group was used with the coefficients, 95% CI and P-values included in the table. AI, artificial intelligence; CI, confidence interval; OR, odds ratio. Bold values indicates the singificant values $P < 0.05$.*

and dermatopathology were more knowledgeable about the technique (**Supplementary Table 1**).

Responders with ≤10 years of experience within pathology (339 of 423, 80.1%) were equally aware of the AI development as responders with >10 years of experience (237 of 285, 83.2%) ($P = 0.33$, $P_{adj} = 1$). In the tech-savvy group, 99 of 376 responders (26.3%) reported either good or excellent knowledge about AI within pathology compared to 36 of 342 non-tech-savvy responders (10.5%) ($P < 0.0001$, $P_{adj} < 0.0001$).

When responders were asked about previous exposure to AI as a topic in general (Q4-Q7), 71.0, 74.9, 53.5, and 65.5% had heard about AI from the media, social media, lectures and friends, respectively. Social media and friends were more common sources for younger age groups. Other media was a more common source among men compared to females (**Table 2**).

The aggregated results from Q8-Q14 about seven applications for AI within dermatopathology are summarized in **Figure 2**. In terms of classification of diagnoses, 42.6% ($n = 306$) saw strong or very strong potential for automated suggestion of skin tumor diagnoses. The corresponding figure for inflammatory skin diseases was 23.0% ($n = 165$) ($P < 0.0001$, $P_{adj} < 0.0001$). For specific applications, the highest potential was considered for automated detection of mitosis (79.2%), automated suggestion of tumor margins (62.1%) and immunostaining evaluation (62.7%). The potential for automated suggestion of immunostaining (37.6%) and genetic panels (48.3%) were lower.

Results for feelings and attitudes toward AI (Q15-Q25) are presented in **Table 3**. Age did not impact the overall attitudes toward AI. Males displayed more excitement and less fear about the use of AI within dermatopathology as well as within medicine in general. The level of fear toward a development with an increased use of AI within dermatopathology did not differ between dermatopathologists working mainly at a university hospital compared to those who mainly worked in another setting (16.7 vs. 15.8%, $P = 0.76$, $P_{adj} = 1$). Among 280 responders with known access to WSI, 14.6% ($n = 41$) expressed fear toward a development with an increase use of AI within dermatopathology, which did not differ significantly to expressed fears among 74 of 421 responders without such access (17.6%) ($P = 0.35$, $P_{adj} = 1$). Furthermore, tech-savviness did not influence expressed levels of fear (data not shown). The attitudes toward AI among those with and without access to WSI did not differ, whereas those with previous use of the technique in dermatopathology had generally more positive attitudes (**Supplementary Table 2**).

Only 6.0% (43 of 718) of the responders agreed or strongly agreed that the human pathologist will be replaced by AI in the foreseeable future. Among tech-savvy responders, the corresponding figure was 7.7% (29 of 376, $P = 0.086$, $P_{adj} = 1$). For the entire group, 72.3% agreed or strongly agreed that AI will improve dermatopathology and 84.1% thought that AI should be a part of medical training.

## DISCUSSION

Our results indicate a generally positive attitude toward AI within dermatopathology among surveyed pathologists. The majority of responders have not yet used AI tools as a diagnostic aid within dermatopathology, underlining that such tools are still under development and a broad implementation to a large extent still is pending.

Age did not influence the results and, while males generally expressed more excitement and less fear compared to female responders, the differences were small in absolute terms. Nonetheless, some of the differences between the genders, might be due to systematic gaps in confidence levels between men and women (19, 20). The majority of the responders were not afraid of being replaced by AI and felt that AI will improve dermatopathology making it more exciting. Only 4% of the responders mainly worked with digital pathology which could explain the low usage of AI tools. Interestingly, only 25% of the responders

**TABLE 2** | Distribution of answers to questions regarding sources about AI applications.

| Other applications we use in daily life already use AI (e.g., speech recognition, spam filters, recommendation algorithms). Have you been made aware of the use of AI in such applications? | Yes | No | log(OR) for age -group (95% CI) | *P*-value | Holm corrected *P*-value | log(OR) for sex (95% CI) [Ref. Female] | *P*-value | Holm corrected *P*-value |
|---|---|---|---|---|---|---|---|---|
| From the media | 510 (71.0%) | 208 (29.0%) | 0.07 (−0.08, 0.23) | 0.37 | 1 | 0.53 (0.18, 0.88) | **0.003** | 0.14 |
| From social media | 538 (74.9%) | 180 (25.1%) | −0.30 (−0.46, −0.15) | **0.0001** | **0.004** | 0.27 (−0.10, 0.63) | 0.15 | 1 |
| From lectures | 384 (53.5%) | 334 (46.5%) | 0.11 (−0.03, 0.25) | 0.12 | 1 | 0.17 (−0.14, 0.48) | 0.27 | 1 |
| From friends | 470 (65.5%) | 248 (34.5%) | −0.16 (−0.30, −0.02) | **0.029** | 1 | 0.37 (0.04, 0.70) | **0.029** | 1 |

*A logistic regression model (no = 0 and yes = 1) containing both sex and age group (20-24, 25-34, 35-44, 45-54, 55-64, 65-74, and ≥75 years) was used. The age groups are used as numeric values in the regression model, i.e., numbers ranging from 1 to 7. Log-odds ratios, 95% CI and P-values for the coefficients are included. AI, artificial intelligence; CI, confidence interval; OR, odds ratio. Bold values indicates the singificant values P < 0.05.*

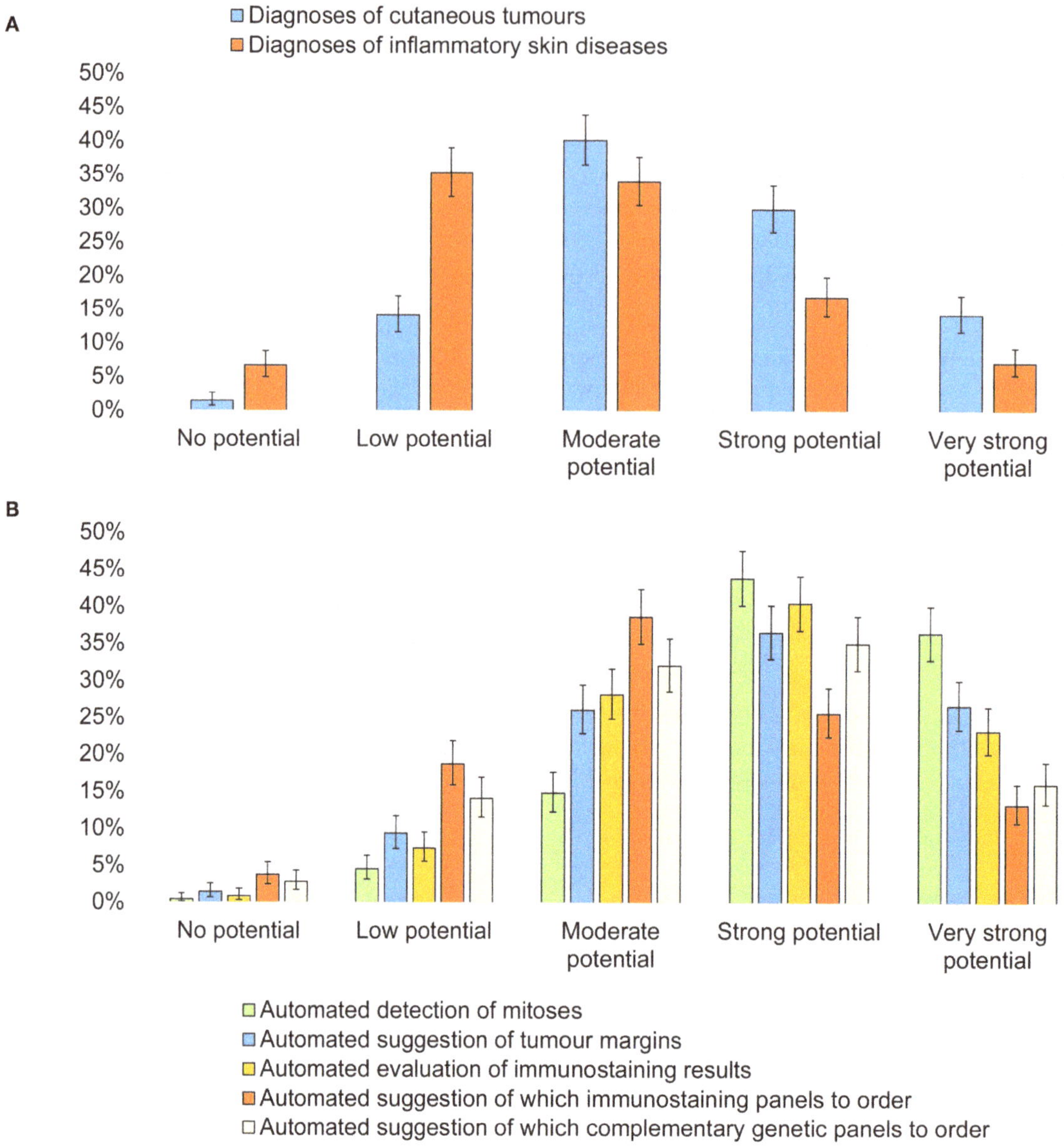


**FIGURE 2 |** Potential seen for AI within dermatopathology. Regardless of whether you have thought about this before, which potential do you personally see for AI for dermatopathology images regarding each of the following. **(A)** Potential seen for automated suggestion of diagnoses of cutaneous tumors and inflammatory skin diseases. **(B)** Potential seen for specific tasks including; automated detection of mitoses; automated suggestion of tumor margins; automated evaluation of immunostaining results; automated suggestion of which immunostaining panels to order; automated suggestion of which complementary genetic panels to order.

had read a medical publication regarding AI within dermatopathology which may reflect that studies in this field are still rare.

Narrow tasks such as automated detection of mitoses and tumor margins were seen to have higher potential compared to automated diagnosis of both cutaneous tumors and inflammatory skin disorders. This is not surprising since several studies have shown AI's potential in detecting mitoses while evidence in diagnostic use is still rare (21, 22). In regards to AI-driven automated diagnostics, its usefulness for tumors was considered more likely than for dermatoses. In fact, a few studies have shown the potential of AI in differentiating skin tumors in WSI (12, 23). AI has even outperformed pathologists in the classification of melanoma (24). Melanocytic lesions in specific have proven particularly difficult for dermatopathologists, where significant levels of inter- and intra-observer variability have been reported (25). ML-based solutions likely hold strong promise in this domain.

The responders reported a high potential for automated suggestion of tumor margins. Such benefits were observed in a recent study in which fluorescence lifetime imaging and ML

**TABLE 3** | Distribution of answers to questions regarding attitudes and feelings about AI.

| Question | Strongly disagree | Disagree | Neither agree nor disagree | Agree | Strongly agree | I don't know | Score increase per age interval (95% CI) | *P*-value | Holm corrected *P*-value | Sex; Score difference (95% CI) [Ref. Female] | *P*-value | Holm corrected *P*-value |
|---|---|---|---|---|---|---|---|---|---|---|---|---|
| AI will revolutionize Medicine in general. | 3 (0.4%) | 59 (8.2%) | 122 (17.0%) | 405 (56.4%) | 129 (18.0%) | 0 (0.0%) | 0.02 (−0.04, 0.071) | 0.56 | 1 | 0.21 (0.08, 0.33) | **0.001** | **0.046** |
| AI will revolutionize dermatopathology. | 7 (1.0%) | 64 (8.9%) | 190 (26.5%) | 322 (44.8%) | 113 (15.7%) | 22 (3.1%) | 0.02 (−0.04, 0.08) | 0.52 | 1 | 0.16 (0.02, 0.30) | **0.023** | 0.80 |
| AI will revolutionize dermatopathology more than other subfields within pathology. | 22 (3.1%) | 217 (30.2%) | 304 (42.3%) | 96 (13.4%) | 37 (5.2%) | 42 (5.8%) | −0.01 (−0.07, 0.05) | 0.79 | 1 | −0.02 (−0.16, 0.12) | 0.74 | 1 |
| In the foreseeable future all physicians will be replaced by AI. | 250 (34.8%) | 342 (47.6%) | 70 (9.7%) | 26 (3.6%) | 17 (2.4%) | 13 (1.8%) | 0.01 (−0.06, 0.07) | 0.84 | 1 | −0.01 (−0.15, 0.13) | 0.91 | 1 |
| The human pathologist will be replaced by AI in the foreseeable future. | 248 (34.5%) | 337 (46.9%) | 66 (9.2%) | 30 (4.2%) | 14 (1.9%) | 23 (3.2%) | 0.03 (−0.03, 0.09) | 0.28 | 1 | 0.09 (−0.05, 0.22) | 0.23 | 1 |
| A development with an increased use of AI in dermatopathology frightens me. | 78 (10.9%) | 320 (44.6%) | 204 (28.4%) | 93 (13.0%) | 23 (3.2%) | 0 (0.0%) | −0.01 (−0.08, 0.05) | 0.65 | 1 | −0.17 (−0.32, −0.03) | **0.022** | 0.79 |
| A development with an increased use of AI in dermatopathology makes dermatopathology more exciting to me. | 12 (1.7%) | 69 (9.6%) | 210 (29.2%) | 340 (47.4%) | 87 (12.1%) | 0 (0.0%) | −0.03 (−0.09, 0.03) | 0.35 | 1 | 0.18 (0.05, 0.31) | **0.009** | 0.34 |
| A development with an increased use of AI makes medicine in general more exciting to me. | 8 (1.1%) | 60 (8.4%) | 186 (25.9%) | 371 (51.7%) | 93 (13.0%) | 0 (0.0%) | 0.01 (−0.05, 0.07) | 0.73 | 1 | 0.17 (0.05, 0.30) | **0.008** | 0.33 |
| AI will improve dermatopathology | 6 (0.8%) | 36 (5.0%) | 126 (17.5%) | 425 (59.2%) | 94 (13.1%) | 31 (4.3%) | 0.01 (−0.04, 0.06) | 0.64 | 1 | 0.20 (0.09, 0.32) | **0.001** | **0.034** |
| AI will improve medicine in general. | 3 (0.4%) | 20 (2.8%) | 93 (13.0%) | 464 (64.6%) | 116 (16.2%) | 22 (3.1%) | 0.00 (−0.04, 0.05) | 0.84 | 1 | 0.26 (0.15, 0.36) | **<0.0001** | **<0.0001** |
| AI should be part of medical training. | 6 (0.8%) | 19 (2.6%) | 72 (10.0%) | 441 (61.4%) | 163 (22.7%) | 17 (2.4%) | 0.06 (0.01, 0.11) | **0.017** | 0.62 | 0.10 (−0.01, 0.21) | 0.081 | 1 |
| I consider myself well-informed about the use of modern technology, especially computers. | 3 (0.4%) | 59 (8.2%) | 122 (17.0%) | 405 (56.4%) | 129 (18.0%) | 0 (0.0%) | −0.03 (−0.09, 0.03) | 0.31 | 1 | 0.18 (0.05, 0.30) | **0.0064** | 0.26 |

*The five possible answers were transformed to a numeric score (1–5) used as the dependent variable and a linear regression model with both sex and age group as predictors was used with the coefficients, 95% CI and P-values included in the table. The age groups are used as numeric values in the regression model, i.e., numbers ranging from 1 to 7. All "I don't know" answers were excluded from the regression model. AI, artificial intelligence; CI, confidence interval. Bold values indicates the singificant values $P < 0.05$.*

were used to visualize tumor margins in excised breast specimens showing high specificity and sensitivity (26). In a previous survey about general pathologists' attitudes toward AI, 75% of the pathologists showed interest or excitement about AI as a diagnostic tool and the vast majority felt it could increase diagnostic efficiency (27). This is in line with the findings in our survey.

As the fields of dermatology and dermatopathology are getting ready for a tremendous transition, we believe inventories of attitudes toward AI are important since it will clarify the potential in specific domains and hopefully unify the community to try to work together. Future ML tools will probably make use of several sources of information simultaneously and parallel systems might provide an even more accurate output. Recently, online dermatopathology forums have collected large amounts of digital cases. This online educational resource could potentially be used to train convolutional neural networks. Ideally, these tools should be available through a web-browser and should be freely available to all users. We believe that pathologists must engage in this development in order to take a leading position in AI. The positive attitudes presented here could certainly help promote this development. Nonetheless, this survey also illustrates that the majority (61.0%) of responders don't yet have access to WSI. A broad implementation of WSI is most likely a prerequisite for an increased use of AI in dermatopathology.

When interpreting our results, it is imperative to remember that the majority of responders received the survey invitation via their social media interest in dermatopathology. The possibility of a selection bias exists and physicians with positive attitudes may have been more likely to have completed the survey. Moreover, AI is a new technique and different responders might have varying ideas of what it includes and represents, particularly since the processes between input and output by the algorithms are not usually clearly defined, and the methods and variable combinations may differ from our own decision-making.

Setting up an online link rather than solely inviting pathologists from a predetermined mailing list also makes it difficult to obtain an exact survey response rate. We acknowledge that attitudes toward new technologies including AI can be fluid and have a tendency to change over time. Therefore, it will also be interesting to reassess attitudes toward AI in follow-up investigations. Moreover, we recognize the inherent difficulties in analyzing and merging the results of attitudes. Undoubtedly, the same question and answer options can represent different meanings to different responders who also have different baseline knowledge about the technology. Finally, ethical and legal aspects, which may vary between countries, were not addressed in our survey.

## CONCLUSION

In summary, our results demonstrate an overall optimistic attitude toward AI in dermatopathology among surveyed physicians. Nonetheless, our data also highlight the need for education about AI for pathologists. Surveyed pathologists predict greater potential for automated suggestion of skin tumor diagnoses than for inflammatory skin diseases. The greatest potential of AI in dermatopathology was predicted for automated detection of mitoses and tumor margins as well as for immunostaining evaluation.

## ETHICS STATEMENT

Ethical review and approval was not required for the study on human participants in accordance with the local legislation and institutional requirements. Written informed consent for participation was not required for this study in accordance with the national legislation and the institutional requirements.

## AUTHOR CONTRIBUTIONS

SP and JP contributed to study concept and design, supervised the project, and wrote the manuscript. SP carried out the implementation, data collection, analysis, and statistics with contributions from MG. MG provided biostatistical advice. PM, JG, JS, and NN contributed to design and distribution of the questionnaire. All authors critically reviewed and edited the questionnaire and the manuscript.

## SUPPLEMENTARY MATERIAL

**Supplementary Material 1 |** Complete survey text.

**Supplementary Material 2 |** Aggregated survey responses.

**Supplementary Table 1 |** Distribution of answers to questions regarding background knowledge about AI. Proportions of answers to questions on the specific rows stratified according to access to WSI, previous use of AI in pathology and previous use of AI in dermatopathology. P-values are computed with Fisher's exact test.

**Supplementary Table 2 |** Distribution of answers to questions regarding attitudes and feelings about AI. Proportions of answers to questions on the specific rows stratified according to access to WSI, previous use of AI in pathology and previous use of AI in dermatopathology. P-values are computed with Fisher's exact test.

## REFERENCES

1. Tizhoosh HR, Pantanowitz L. Artificial intelligence and digital pathology: challenges and opportunities. *J Pathol Inform.* (2018) 9:38. doi: 10.4103/jpi.jpi_53_18
2. Litjens G, Kooi T, Bejnordi BE, Setio AAA, Ciompi F, Ghafoorian M, et al. A survey on deep learning in medical image analysis. *Med Image Anal.* (2017) 42:60–88. doi: 10.1016/j.media.2017.07.005
3. Bauer TW, Schoenfield L, Slaw RJ, Yerian L, Sun Z, Henricks WH. Validation of whole slide imaging for primary diagnosis in surgical

pathology. *Arch Pathol Lab Med.* (2013) 137:518–24. doi: 10.5858/arpa.2011-0678-OA
4. Fertig RM, Sangueza O, Gaudi S, Gamret AC, Cervantes J, Jukic DM. Whole Slide Imaging. *Am J Dermatopathol.* (2018) 40:938–9. doi: 10.1097/DAD.0000000000001008
5. Onega T, Reisch LM, Frederick PD, Geller BM, Nelson HD, Lott JP, et al. Use of digital whole slide imaging in dermatopathology. *J Digit Imaging.* (2016) 29:243–53. doi: 10.1007/s10278-015-9836-y
6. Kent MN, Olsen TG, Feeser TA, Tesno KC, Moad JC, Conroy MP, et al. Diagnostic accuracy of virtual pathology vs traditional microscopy in a large dermatopathology study. *JAMA Dermatol.* (2017) 153:1285–91. doi: 10.1001/jamadermatol.2017.3284
7. Madabhushi A, Lee G. Image analysis and machine learning in digital pathology: challenges and opportunities. *Med Image Anal.* (2016) 33:170–5. doi: 10.1016/j.media.2016.06.037
8. Morrison AS, Gardner JM. Smart phone microscopic photography: a novel tool for physicians and trainees. *Arch Pathol Lab Med.* (2014) 138:1002. doi: 10.5858/arpa.2013-0425-ED
9. Gardner JM, McKee PH. Social media use for pathologists of all ages. *Arch Pathol Lab Med.* (2019) 143:282–6. doi: 10.5858/arpa.2018-0431-ED
10. Schaumberg AJ, Juarez-Nicanor WC, Choudhury SJ, Pastrián LG, Pritt BS, Prieto Pozuelo M, et al. Interpretable multimodal deep learning for real-time pan-tissue pan-disease pathology search on social media. *Modern Pathol.* (2020). doi: 10.1038/s41379-020-0540-1. [Epub ahead of print].
11. Lang UE, Torres R, Cheung C, Vladar EK, McCalmont TH, Kim J, et al. Ciliation index is a useful diagnostic tool in challenging spitzoid melanocytic neoplasms. *J Invest Dermatol.* (2020) 140:1401–9.e2. doi: 10.1016/j.jid.2019.11.028
12. Olsen TG, Jackson BH, Feeser TA, Kent MN, Moad JC, Krishnamurthy S, et al. Diagnostic performance of deep learning algorithms applied to three common diagnoses in dermatopathology. *J Pathol Inform.* (2018) 9:32. doi: 10.4103/jpi.jpi_31_18
13. Fouad S, Randell D, Galton A, Mehanna H, Landini G. Unsupervised morphological segmentation of tissue compartments in histopathological images. *PLoS ONE.* (2017) 12:e0188717. doi: 10.1371/journal.pone.0188717
14. Gomolin A, Netchiporouk E, Gniadecki R, Litvinov IV. Artificial intelligence applications in dermatology: where do we stand? *Front Med.* (2020) 7:100. doi: 10.3389/fmed.2020.00100
15. Polesie S, Gillstedt M, Kittler H, Lallas A, Tschandl P, Zalaudek I, et al. Attitudes towards artificial intelligence within dermatology: an international online survey. *Br J Dermatol.* (2020) 183:159–61. doi: 10.1111/bjd.18875
16. Likert R. A technique for the measurement of attitudes. *Arch Psychol.* (1932)
17. *McKee Derm* [Last accessed 10 September 2020]. Available online at: https://www.facebook.com/groups/mckeederm/
18. Holm S. A simple sequentially rejective multiple test procedure. *Scand J Stat.* (1979) 65–70.
19. Vajapey SP, Weber KL, Samora JB. Confidence gap between men and women in medicine: a systematic review. *Curr Orthopaed Pract.* (2020) 31:494–502. doi: 10.1097/BCO.0000000000000906
20. Nomura K, Yano E, Fukui T. Gender differences in clinical confidence: a nationwide survey of resident physicians in Japan. *Acad Med.* (2010) 85:647–53. doi: 10.1097/ACM.0b013e3181d2a796
21. Andres C, Andres-Belloni B, Hein R, Biedermann T, Schäpe A, Brieu N, et al. iDermatoPath - a novel software tool for mitosis detection in H&E-stained tissue sections of malignant melanoma. *J Eur Acad Dermatol Venereol.* (2017) 31:1137–47. doi: 10.1111/jdv.14126
22. Nielsen PS, Spaun E, Riber-Hansen R, Steiniche T. Automated quantification of MART1-verified Ki-67 indices: useful diagnostic aid in melanocytic lesions. *Hum Pathol.* (2014) 45:1153–61. doi: 10.1016/j.humpath.2014.01.009
23. Campanella G, Hanna MG, Geneslaw L, Miraflor A, Werneck Krauss Silva V, Busam KJ, et al. Clinical-grade computational pathology using weakly supervised deep learning on whole slide images. *Nat Med.* (2019) 25:1301–9. doi: 10.1038/s41591-019-0508-1
24. Hekler A, Utikal JS, Enk AH, Solass W, Schmitt M, Klode J, et al. Deep learning outperformed 11 pathologists in the classification of histopathological melanoma images. *Eur J Cancer.* (2019) 118:91–6. doi: 10.1016/j.ejca.2019.06.012
25. Elmore JG, Barnhill RL, Elder DE, Longton GM, Pepe MS, Reisch LM, et al. Pathologists' diagnosis of invasive melanoma and melanocytic proliferations: observer accuracy and reproducibility study. *BMJ.* (2017) 357:j2813. doi: 10.1136/bmj.j2813
26. Unger J, Hebisch C, Phipps JE, Lagarto JL, Kim H, Darrow MA, et al. Real-time diagnosis and visualization of tumor margins in excised breast specimens using fluorescence lifetime imaging and machine learning. *Biomed Opt Express.* (2020) 11:1216–30. doi: 10.1364/BOE.381358
27. Sarwar S, Dent A, Faust K, Richer M, Djuric U, Van Ommeren R, et al. Physician perspectives on integration of artificial intelligence into diagnostic pathology. *NPJ Digital Med.* (2019) 2:28. doi: 10.1038/s41746-019-0106-0

# 7

# Artificial Intelligence in Skin Cancer Diagnostics: The Patients' Perspective

*Tanja B. Jutzi[1†], Eva I. Krieghoff-Henning[1†], Tim Holland-Letz[2], Jochen Sven Utikal[3,4], Axel Hauschild[5], Dirk Schadendorf[6], Wiebke Sondermann[6], Stefan Fröhling[1], Achim Hekler[1], Max Schmitt[1], Roman C. Maron[1] and Titus J. Brinker[1*]*

*[1] Division of Translational Oncology, National Center for Tumor Diseases (NCT), German Cancer Research Center (DKFZ), Heidelberg, Germany, [2] Division of Biostatistics, German Cancer Research Center, Heidelberg, Germany, [3] Department of Dermatology, Heidelberg University, Mannheim, Germany, [4] Skin Cancer Unit, German Cancer Research Center, Heidelberg, Germany, [5] Department of Dermatology, University Hospital Schleswig-Holstein, Kiel, Germany, [6] Department of Dermatology, University Hospital Essen, Essen, Germany*

***Correspondence:**
*Titus J. Brinker*
*titus.brinker@nct-heidelberg.de*

*[†] These authors have contributed equally to this work*

**Background:** Artificial intelligence (AI) has shown promise in numerous experimental studies, particularly in skin cancer diagnostics. Translation of these findings into the clinic is the logical next step. This translation can only be successful if patients' concerns and questions are addressed suitably. We therefore conducted a survey to evaluate the patients' view of artificial intelligence in melanoma diagnostics in Germany, with a particular focus on patients with a history of melanoma.

**Participants and Methods:** A web-based questionnaire was designed using LimeSurvey, sent by e-mail to university hospitals and melanoma support groups and advertised on social media. The anonymous questionnaire evaluated patients' expectations and concerns toward artificial intelligence in general as well as their attitudes toward different application scenarios. Descriptive analysis was performed with expression of categorical variables as percentages and 95% confidence intervals. Statistical tests were performed to investigate associations between sociodemographic data and selected items of the questionnaire.

**Results:** 298 individuals (154 with a melanoma diagnosis, 143 without) responded to the questionnaire. About 94% [95% CI = 0.91–0.97] of respondents supported the use of artificial intelligence in medical approaches. 88% [95% CI = 0.85–0.92] would even make their own health data anonymously available for the further development of AI-based applications in medicine. Only 41% [95% CI = 0.35–0.46] of respondents were amenable to the use of artificial intelligence as stand-alone system, 94% [95% CI = 0.92–0.97] to its use as assistance system for physicians. In sub-group analyses, only minor differences were detectable. Respondents with a previous history of melanoma were more amenable to the use of AI applications for early detection even at home. They would prefer an application scenario where physician and AI classify the lesions independently. With respect to AI-based applications in medicine, patients were concerned about insufficient data protection, impersonality and susceptibility to errors, but expected faster, more precise and unbiased diagnostics, less diagnostic errors and support for physicians.

**Conclusions:** The vast majority of participants exhibited a positive attitude toward the use of artificial intelligence in melanoma diagnostics, especially as an assistance system.

**Keywords: artificial intelligence, patients view, melanoma, diagnostics, acceptance, skin cancer, online survey**

## INTRODUCTION

Systems based on artificial intelligence, particularly on deep learning, are entering the medical field at an impressive pace. Layered mathematical models process large datasets to perform a specific task, for example automatic pattern recognition (1). Image analysis is one of the areas in which the fastest progress is currently achieved (2), for instance in the detection and quantification of lung nodules on radiological images (3), image-based detection of potential strokes (4) or breast cancer screening (5).

In the field of dermatology, Artificial intelligence-based tools are being developed to evaluate the severity of psoriasis (6) or to distinguish between onychomycosis and healthy nails (7, 8). In experimental settings, the sensitivity and specificity of AI-based algorithms in discriminating melanomas from nevi were similar to or better than those of dermatologists (9–11). Since the detection of melanomas at an early stage greatly improves prognosis and the distinction between melanomas and harmless lesions is often not trivial, AI-based classification systems might yield enormous benefits for patients with suspicious skin lesions.

However, there is still some controversy surrounding the use of AI for diagnostics in "real life" clinical settings. Concerns include the possibility of biases, the lack of transparency and explainability, scalability, data integration and interoperability, reliability, safety, privacy and ethics of aggregated digital data (12, 13).

The success of AI applications in clinical diagnostics depends on acceptance by both physicians and patients, which is driven by their understanding of the potential benefits and harms of AI. Patients' needs regarding medicinal aspects, but also data security, may differ from experts' expectations (14, 15). Therefore, physicians and patients have to be involved in the AI research agenda at an early stage to ensure that their needs are addressed adequately during the development of such applications.

A recent study in Korea has shown that in general, Korean medical doctors have a positive attitude toward AI in medicine (16). Similar results were obtained in a large international survey among dermatologists, indicating that AI is well-accepted in the dermatology field: The majority of participants agreed or strongly agreed that AI will improve dermatology and felt that AI should be a part of medical training (17). A survey on computer-assisted diagnosis of melanomas with dermatofluoroscopy also showed a high acceptance of that technology among patients (18). A Swedish survey among participants in a breast cancer screening program about AI-based automated mammogram analysis showed a high level of confidence in computer-aided decision making (19). A study on skin cancer-related apps revealed that around 43% of the participants thought that these apps might be able to supplement the professional skin examination. However, almost all patients had never used skin cancer-related apps or could not remember (20).

Here, we report the results of a survey-based cross-sectional study designed to investigate the hopes and fears of patients with and without a history of melanoma toward the use of AI in skin lesion diagnostics, especially with respect to the classification of melanoma.

## METHODS

### Survey

We conducted an anonymous online survey, using the open source software LimeSurvey (Version 3.17.3.). The questionnaire was designed de novo as we were not aware of any validated survey tools for the objective of our study. After conducting a literature review we designed a questionnaire addressing the main topics and follow-up questions. These questionnaires were sent to dermato-oncological experts for annotation. After revisions, we tested the survey on five volunteers who had no professional background in artificial intelligence to review the comprehensibility and consistency, and revised it further. In addition to sociodemographic questions (age, sex, previous history of melanoma diagnosis, educational level), the questionnaire contained various items dealing with expectations and concerns regarding the use of artificial intelligence in melanoma diagnostics in general and in different application scenarios. For most questions, there were multiple choice response options, few questions were designed to fill in free text. This strategy ensures high interpretability, comprehensibility, and consistency in representation.

The survey was conducted from November 2019 to January 2020. We used an online survey to avoid the influence of study directors and to ensure anonymity (21).

As we wanted to compare the attitudes and opinions of patients with and without a history of melanoma the questionnaire was distributed via email to our dermatological university hospital cooperation partners and melanoma support groups with the request for further dissemination. In addition, it was advertised on social media. We did not do any formal hypothesis testing in the paper, and therefore also did not do a power calculation in the original sense. However, the sample size of at least 250 was planned in order to obtain standard errors of +/−2.5% or, equivalently, confidence intervals of about +/−5% for our rate estimates (see section "Data Analysis"). We closed the online LimeSurvey when we had surpassed that number of full-answer sets.

Participation was voluntary and anonymity was ensured by design. This might lead to an increased motivation to answer the questions thoroughly and truthfully and thereby enhance the intrinsic data quality. Every participant agreed with LimeSurvey's privacy policy. All data were stored at DKFZ. Participants were informed that the results of the survey would be used for scientific publication. All questions were optional and were available in German only. The survey received approval by the board of data protection at the German Cancer Research Center (DKFZ). For most questions, there were 5 response options: "agree entirely," "rather agree," "unsure," "rather disagree," and "disagree entirely." Questions regarding concerns and expectations were designed to fill in free text (see questionnaire in the **Appendix** in German).

## Data Analysis

Three hundred and sixty one data sets were generated. Sixty three data sets were excluded in the analysis as they were only filled in to an extremely limited extent (less than half of the questions answered). Two hundred and ninety eight data sets were included in the data analysis: 292 of them were completed up to the end, 6 were completed except for the last page (last two questions). All questions were optional, 140 participants answered every question.

Descriptive analysis was performed with interpretation of categorical variables as percentages. For simplified descriptive statistics, the categories "rather agree" and "agree entirely" were summarized as agreement while "rather disagree" and "disagree entirely" were summarized as disagreement. The category "unsure" was reported separately. For statistical analyses on associations between sociodemographic data and selected items of the questionnaire, the original categories were preserved, in order to obtain a better differentiation to best reflect the comparison between the subgroups. We pre-specified sub-group analyses on age, education, gender, and participants with and without a history on melanoma and collected these personal data in the anonymous survey. Subgroup analyses were conducted for each question. In the results section, we report only those in detail where there was a significant difference.

Ninety five percentage confidence intervals were computed for the main results using the normal distribution approximation.

The margin of error (standard error) for percentage rates estimated from $n = 298$ participants is $+/-2.5$ percentage points at rates of about 80%.

Statistical analysis was done using Microsoft Excel and SigmaPlot. Comparison of the distribution of responses across sub-groups was performed using the Wilcoxon signed rank or the chi$^2$ test. In data analyses with chi$^2$ tests, participants with no answer to the relevant question were not included. A $p < 0.05$ was regarded as statistically significant.

# RESULTS

## Baseline Characteristics of the Study Population

Over a 10 week period, a total of 298 individuals responded to the questionnaire. About half of the respondents reported a previous melanoma diagnosis, almost three quarters were female and almost two thirds graduated from high school with German "Abitur" or had a university degree (**Table 1**). This is not representative for the situation in the general population.

**TABLE 1** | Baseline characteristics of the study population.

| | | % ($n = 298$) |
|---|---|---|
| **Gender** | | |
| Female | 218 | 73.2 |
| Male | 73 | 24.5 |
| Diverse/Not reported | 7 | 2.3 |
| **Previous diagnosis of melanoma** | | |
| Yes | 154 | 51.7 |
| No | 143 | 48 |
| Not reported | 1 | 0.3 |
| **Age** | | |
| ≤30 | 41 | 13.8 |
| 31–45 | 102 | 34.2 |
| 46–60 | 123 | 41.3 |
| 61–75 | 27 | 9.1 |
| >75 | 4 | 1.3 |
| Not reported | 1 | 0.3 |
| **Education** | | |
| Graduated from general secondary school ("Hauptschulabschluss") | 19 | 6.4 |
| Graduated from intermediate secondary school ("Realschulabschluss") | 77 | 25.8 |
| Higher school certificate qualifying for university admission ("Abitur") | 77 | 25.8 |
| University degree | 121 | 40.6 |
| Not reported | 4 | 1.3 |

## General Awareness of and Attitude Toward the Use of AI

Of all respondents, 88% had already heard of artificial intelligence and had a general idea on what AI signifies (3% did not, 6% were uncertain, 3% did not answer the question). Less respondents (80%) had explicitly heard of examples of AI in use in medical applications (12% did not, 6% were uncertain, 2% did not answer this question). The vast majority of the respondents (94, 95% CI = 0.91−0.97) stated that they would support the use of AI in medicine. Only 1.3% explicitly did not agree with the statement that AI should be used to support physicians to make skin cancer diagnostics even more reliable (91% agreement, 4% uncertain, 3.7% no answer). Eighty eight percent [95% CI = 0.85–0.92] claimed that they would even make their own health data anonymously available for the further development of AI-based medical applications (5% disagreement, 6% uncertain, 1% no answer). If an AI-based system was able to distinguish well between images of nevi and melanoma, a vast majority of respondents would be willing to use AI for early detection of skin cancer in some way. In particular, 94% [95% CI = 0.92–0.97] would endorse the use of AI as assistance system at the physician's (2% disagreement, 3% uncertain, 1% no answer). At least 41% [95% CI = 0.35–0.46] would also consider its use at

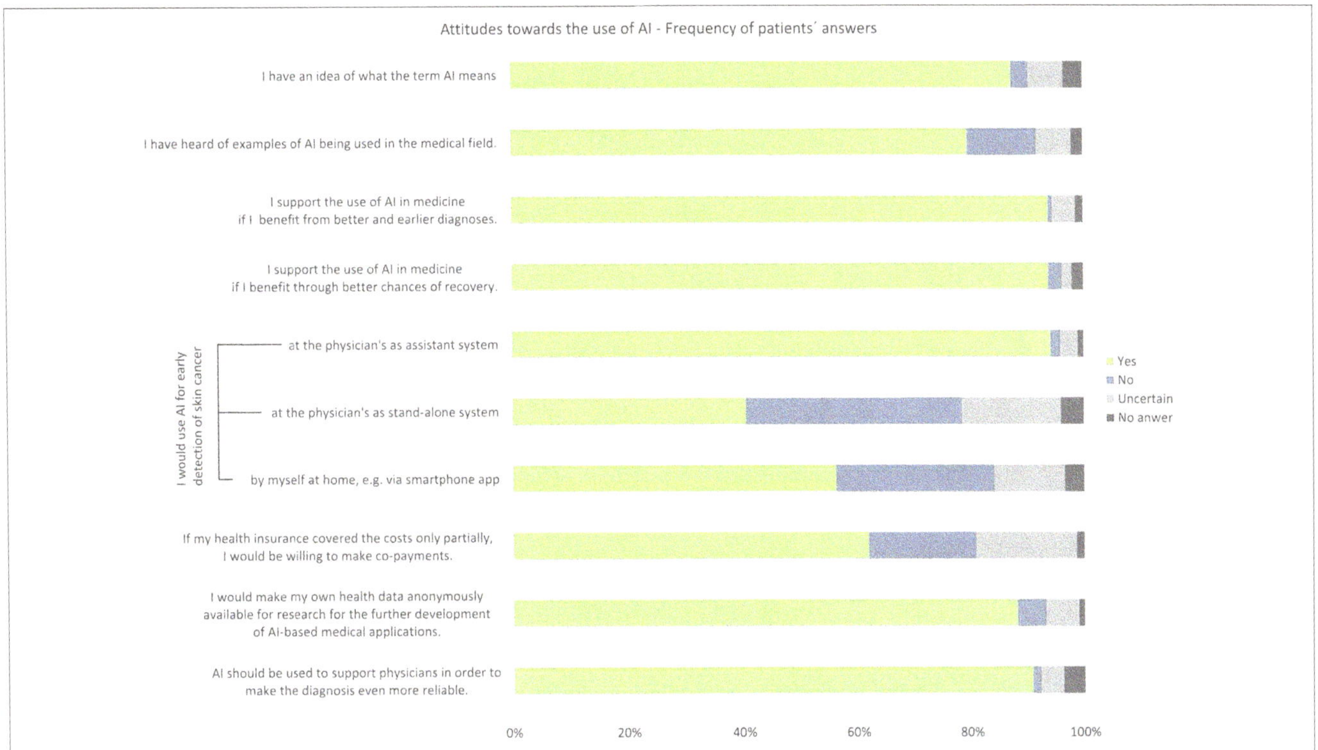


**FIGURE 1** | General attitude toward the use of Artificial Intelligence (AI) in the medical field. Bar chart shows distribution of participants' answers regarding their awareness of and attitude toward AI in medical use, provided that the AI-based system can distinguish well between images of harmless moles and melanoma.

the physician's as a stand-alone system (38% disagreement, 17% uncertain, 4% no answer) and 56% stated that they might use AI-based applications even at home, e.g., as a diagnostic smartphone app (28% disagreement, 13% unsure, 3% no answer, **Figure 1**).

## Confidence in Artificial Intelligence vs. Medical Doctors

If the AI-based classification of pigmented skin lesions was proven to be equally accurate as that of physicians, respondents had slightly more confidence in the physician's decisions than in those of the AI algorithm. If the physician considered a tissue biopsy or an excision necessary, but the algorithm did not, 89% of respondents would agree to the operation (the disagreement was <1%, around 7% were unsure, 4% did not answer the question), whereas 85% would do so in the reverse case (3% disagreement, 8% unsure, 4% no answer). However, if it was proven that AI-based classification systems were more accurate than physicians, most respondents would rely on the algorithm rather than on the physician: 91% of respondents would agree to a biopsy/excision if the algorithm rated this as necessary and the physician did not (2% disagreement, 3% uncertain, 4% no answer), whereas only 80% would do so in the reverse case (4% disagreement, 11% uncertain, 5% no answer). Overall, most participants responded that they would have the lesion biopsied or excised in any case (> 80%, **Figure 2**).

## Concerns Regarding AI

Questions regarding concerns and expectations were designed to fill in free text.

The concerns most frequently voiced in this survey were related to data protection, impersonality and susceptibility to errors.

Participants feared that their data might not be anonymized, and hence might be misused to their disadvantage by health and other insurance companies or employers. Also, there was a concern that personal data might be published by hackers.

Another common concern regarding the use of AI was a diminished physician-patient relationship—consultations could become more sterile, with no personal conversation with the physician and less time for questions. Respondents were also worried that physicians might be tempted to rely on the AI-based algorithm so much that they would lose their own expertise and diagnostic skills. This would reduce their ability to classify lesions without the assistance system as well as their ability to notice obvious mistakes or malfunctioning of the algorithm itself, which could occur due to various technical problems or even deliberate manipulation by hackers.

Further perceived problems that were mentioned were the non-traceability of the decision algorithms and the missing transparency of the applied systems. In addition, the risk of unequal opportunities due to potential high costs not covered by standard health insurance was pointed out.

## Hopes and Expectations Regarding Artificial Intelligence

Participants expected that by integrating AI algorithms into skin cancer diagnostics, waiting time due to the requirement for tissue

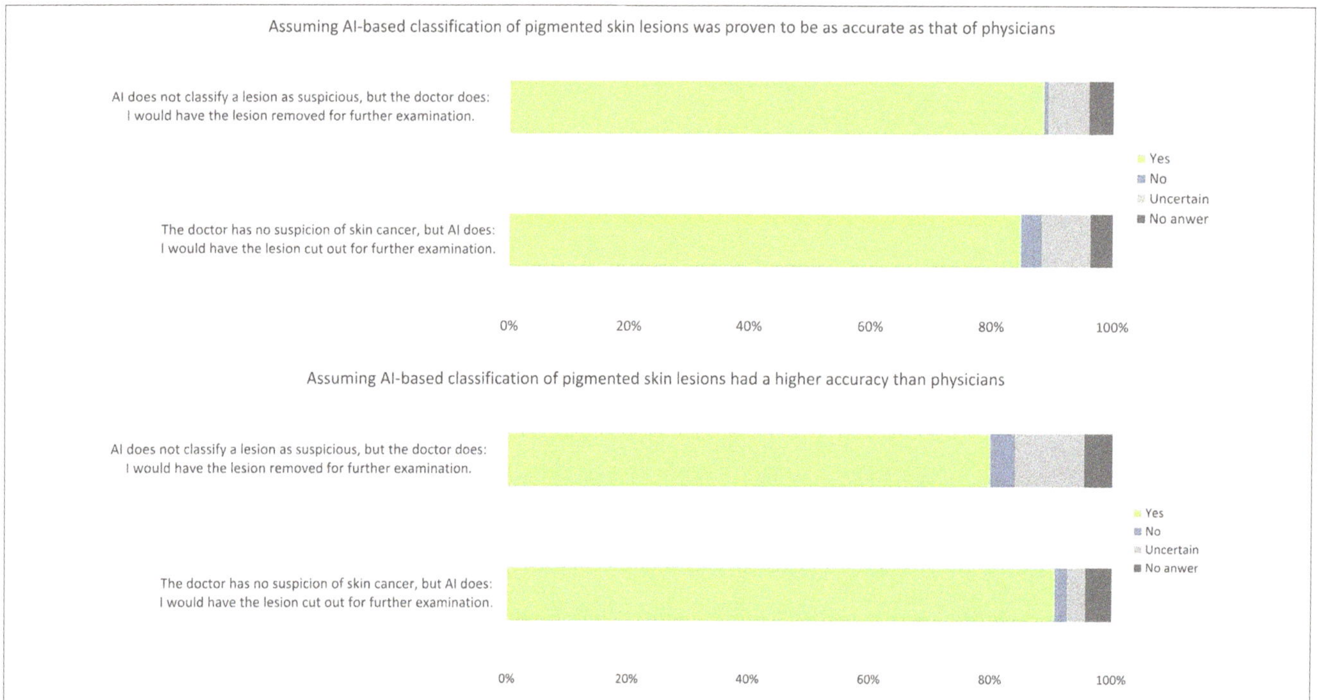


**FIGURE 2** | Confidence in AI. Bar chart shows the frequency of participants' answers.

analysis by the pathologist might be reduced. Many participants also hoped that AI would lead to earlier detection of skin cancers, maybe even at the precursor stage, thereby decreasing the required therapeutic intensity for those lesions. Moreover, they stated that the use of AI might lead to more reliable and less subjective diagnoses, which might lead to fewer unnecessary biopsies and less overlooked malignant lesions. As AI offers the possibility of evaluating large amounts of data in the context of diagnosis, its use might increase quality and ensure objectivity of skin cancer diagnostics. AI algorithms can be trained with larger amounts of image data than even an experienced dermatologist can assess, which may increase the accuracy of the algorithm relative to physicians.

If used as an assistance tool, participants expected AI to be able to reduce error rates in diagnoses especially for less experienced physicians. They hoped that physicians would even be able to learn from the AI-based systems. In their opinion, the direct comparison might also motivate specialists to strive continuously to improve their own performance.

The use of AI-based tools might save time that physicians could use for more personal contact to the patient. Conversely, AI could allow first self-tests at home without visiting a physician—which could become even more important due to the increasing paucity of physicians. AI was also expected to improve processes, and to reduce the burden on healthcare by helping to avoid unnecessary diagnostics and treatments.

Participants also assumed that using AI in skin cancer diagnosis might ultimately result in more transparency, if AI-based tools were able to objectively quantify the likelihood of a lesion being malignant objectively in a way that patients could comprehend.

## Attitudes Toward Different Application Scenarios and Participation

Nearly half of all participants could envisage a diagnostic routine in which physicians and an AI-based assistance system classify the same lesion independently of each other and a tissue sample is taken when either of them rates the lesion as requiring further investigation. One third stated that they would like the physician to include the result of AI always in his or her diagnosis. Altogether, more than 90% of the participants endorsed the use of AI as supporting tool for the physician. Only a very small proportion, 3% of all participants, claimed that they would prefer not to incorporate AI in skin cancer diagnostics at all (**Figure 3A**).

When asked about their attitude toward shared decision-making, the vast majority of the patients (82%) stated that they would like to take their decision together with the physician on the basis of the results of the examination. About 10% would prefer to get all information and to take the decision on their own and only 4% of the participants would prefer to not be involved in the decision making at all (**Figure 4**).

## Associations Between Sociodemographic Data on Attitude and Awareness Toward AI: Subgroup Analyses

We prespecified sub-group analyses on age, education, gender, and participants with and without a history on melanoma. Subgroup analyses were conducted for each question for

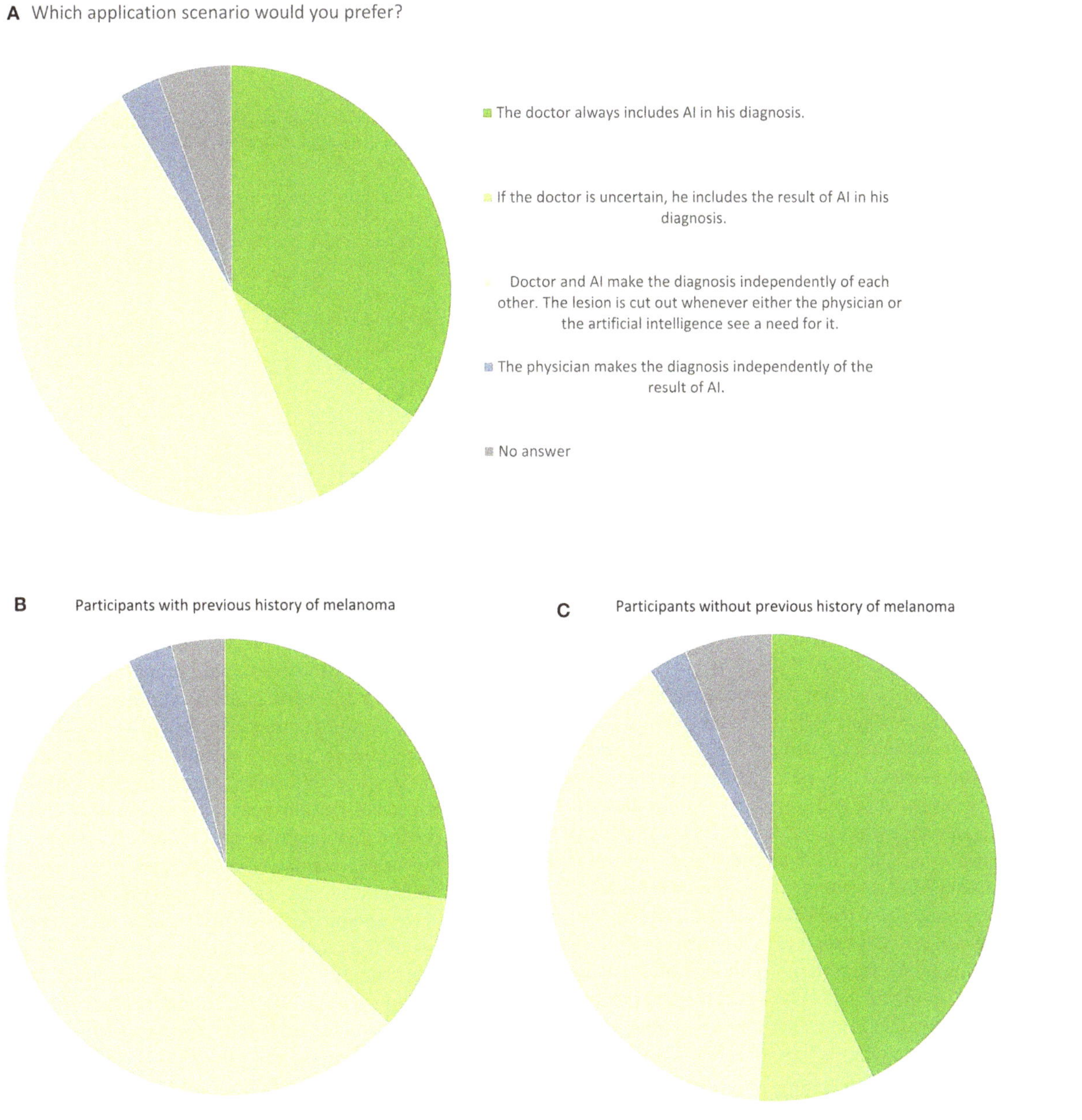


**FIGURE 3 |** Attitudes toward different application scenarios. **(A)** Pie chart shows the percentages of all participants' preferences. **(B)** Pie chart shows the percentages of melanoma patients' preferences. **(C)** Pie chart shows the percentages of preferences of participants without previous history of melanoma.

every subgroup. Overall, only minor differences were identified in the attitudes toward AI in medical use between the evaluated subgroups. Most of these differences appeared between participants with and without a history of melanoma.

There was no significant difference between age groups. Numerical differences between participants with higher and lower education levels were not statistically significant.

Sub-group analyses showed that more female than male participants would have the lesion removed if either the physician or the AI algorithm rated this as necessary (83–93% vs. 70–83%, $p < 0.02$).

Significantly more (about 97%) respondents with a previous history of melanoma would support the use of AI in medicine compared to non-melanoma patients (~91%) ($p = 0.03$). Moreover, they would be considerably more open to using AI applications for early detection even at home (around 66% compared to 46%, $p = 0.004$). Moreover, the majority of melanoma patients preferred an application scenario in which AI and the physician take the decision on a lesion independently from each other, whereas the majority of the non-melanoma patient respondents preferred the inclusion of AI results into the diagnosis by the physician ($p = 0.027$, see **Figures 3B,C**).

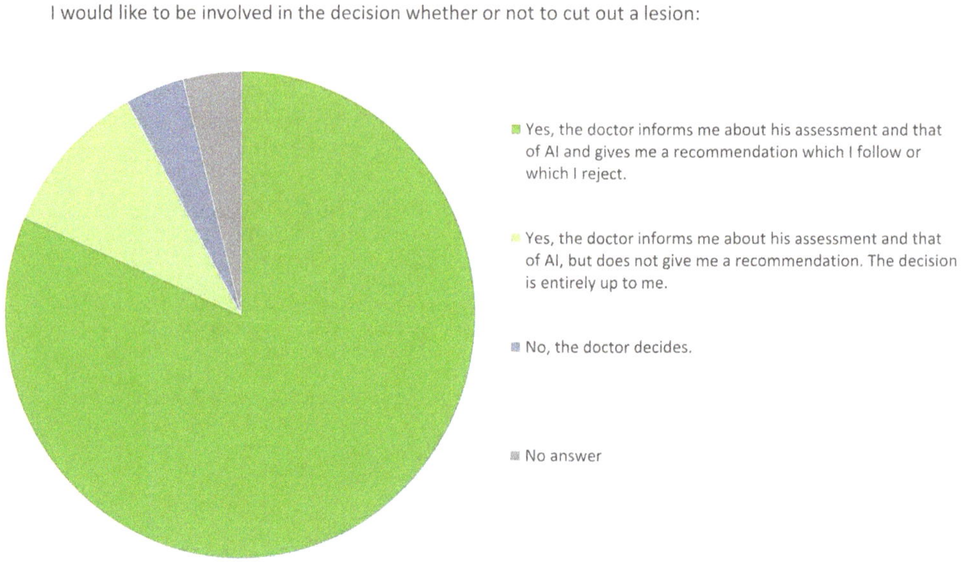


**FIGURE 4 |** Attitudes toward patients' participation. Pie chart shows the percentages of participants' preferences.

## DISCUSSION

As the use of AI might lead to more precise, impartial and faster diagnostics, experts consider it likely that AI-driven technology will increasingly be implemented in the medical field in the near future, in particular in skin cancer diagnostics. A lack of acceptance by patients and physicians would have severely curtailed this development. In our survey amongst patients and putative patients regarding their attitudes and their awareness toward the use of AI in melanoma diagnostics, we found that the overwhelming majority of participants support the use of AI for medical applications. They expressed a high level of confidence in decision-making by AI. Importantly, although most participants in our survey thought that AI can contribute to improve diagnostic accuracy, they also believed that it cannot and should not replace the dermatologist. This ambivalence might reflect a general fear that AI might supplant the expertise and diagnostic skills of physicians and is concordant with the desire for personal contact with the treating physician, impersonal consultations were among the most common concerns mentioned in the survey. This may imply that AI-based applications as stand-alone systems in diagnosis would probably not be accepted. Along the same lines, the majority of German undergraduate medical students don't think that human radiologists will be replaced by AI (22).

While some participants also hope that the use of AI in diagnosis will lead to fewer unnecessary biopsies, many participants apparently see the biggest advantage of additional AI-based diagnostics in the detection of malignant lesions that might otherwise be overlooked by the physician performing the examination. This result is mainly triggered by the preference of the participants with previous history of melanoma to obtain separate assessment results from both the AI-based system and the physician about a pending biopsy. This might mean that additional diagnostic tools would primarily lead to more biopsies, a burden that the participants would accept for safety reasons. Although avoiding unnecessary biopsies is obviously also an important goal in melanoma early detection, it is important to take this into account when determining the optimal relationship between sensitivity and specificity and suitable cut-off values for an algorithm that might be applied in clinics. However, this result may not be representative of the situation in the general public, since our results also show that a previous cancer diagnosis may have altered patients' preferences in some respects. The answers of the participants could help to decide how such an algorithm should be implemented in the clinic, but they ought to be supplemented with the results of another survey targeting individuals with little previous contact with the skin cancer topic.

Either positioning the physician or the AI-based tool first, have advantages and disadvantages (23). But independent decisions could provide the benefits of both, increased sensitivity while maintaining current clinical workflows, provide an automated second opinion, reduce excessive dependence on AI, and take note of a possible discrepancy between AI and physician.

Somewhat surprisingly, more than half of the participants would be amenable to the use of AI at home, e.g., via a smartphone app. However, incorrect use, flawed or scientifically unsound applications or incomprehensible outputs and a lack of personal contact with the physician might increase rather than reduce stress and anxiety levels for users and the misclassifications of both benign and malignant lesions (24). Thus, AI-based diagnostic apps will have to be evaluated very carefully to determine their potential for benefits and harms. With people's desire for empowerment and autonomy through self-management in mind, it might be indispensable to develop digital end devices that enable independent, quality-assured and always available support without spatial and temporal barriers. If an AI-based skin diagnostics app did pass the required tests, patients might profit considerably from its use.

To encompass the requirement for transparent and comprehensible treatment decisions, it will be necessary to work on strategies that allow the results of AI to be interpreted and verified (at least in part). Due to the high complexity of the algorithms, a complete transparency of AI will probably not be possible, but it might be possible to explain the decisive influencing factors on individual decision steps within the algorithms (25, 26).

Altogether, most participants see the use of AI in the medical field in general and particularly in skin cancer diagnostics as a gain, especially for those areas that exceed human capabilities. However, they envisage it mainly as an assisting system that supports and complements a decision made by a human provider. Although the survey in this form may mainly reflect the view of people who have concerned themselves with the topic of skin cancer, the results may be valuable knowledge for the transfer of the diagnosis algorithms from research into clinical practice and further studies using AI in medical applications.

## LIMITATIONS

The sample size of this study ($n = 298$) is still relatively small. Also, more of the respondents were predominantly female, and more respondents had a high or very high educational level. Since half of the questionnaires were filled in by (former) melanoma patients and via self-help organizations, we cannot exclude the risk of sampling bias and the results that we obtained are probably not fully generalizable to the general population. Our approach was chosen to be able to gain a first impression of the difference between the attitudes given by melanoma patients or –survivors and those of participants without a history of melanoma. Since none of the survey questions was mandatory, not every participant answered every question. Some responders also did not reveal their sociodemographic data, so those data couldn't be included into the statistics in subgroup analyses.

## CONCLUSION

Most of the participants in our survey, both with and without a previous melanoma diagnosis, had a positive attitude toward the use of AI in the medical field in general and melanoma diagnostics in particular, especially when AI was applied as assistant system for the treating physician.

## ETHICS STATEMENT

Ethics approval for the online survey was waived by the Ethics Committee of the University of Heidelberg due to the fact that all of the participants remained anonymous. Ethical approval for this study was not required in accordance with local legislation and national guidelines. The survey received approval by the Board of Data Protection at the German Cancer Research Center (DKFZ).

## AUTHOR CONTRIBUTIONS

TJ, EK-H, AHe, and TB contributed to study concept and design. TJ carried out the implementation, data collection, analysis and statistics with contributions from EK-H and AHe. TH-L provided biostatistical advice. TJ and EK-H wrote the manuscript. AHe, MS, and RM contributed to design and distribution of the questionnaire. SF and TB supervised the project and obtained the funding. JU, AHa, DS, and WS and all other co-authors critically reviewed and edited the questionnaire and the manuscript.

## ACKNOWLEDGMENTS

We thank Prof. E. Breitbart of Hautkrebs-Netzwerk Deutschland e. V. and Astrid Doppler and Katharina Kaminski of Melanom-Info Germany for distribution of the questionnaire.

## REFERENCES


1. Miller DD, Brown EW. Artificial intelligence in medical practice: the question to the answer? *Am J Med.* (2018) 131:129–33. doi: 10.1016/j.amjmed.2017.10.035
2. Kulkarni S, Seneviratne N, Baig MS, Khan AHA. Artificial intelligence in medicine: where are we now?" *Acad Radiol.* (2019) 27:62–70. doi: 10.1016/j.acra.2019.10.001
3. Prayer F, Röhrich S, Pan J, Hofmanninger J, Langs G, Prosch HJD, et al. Artificial intelligence in lung imaging. *Radiologe.* (2019) 60:42–7. doi: 10.1007/s00117-019-0 0611-2
4. Petrone JJNB. FDA approves stroke-detecting AI software. *Nat Biotechnol.* (2018) 36:290. doi: 10.1038/nbt0418-290
5. McKinney SM, Sieniek M, Godbole V, Godwin J, Antropova N, Ashrafian H, et al. International evaluation of an AI system for breast cancer screening. *Nature.* (2020) 577:89–94. doi: 10.1038/s41586-019-1799-6
6. Shrivastava VK, Londhe ND, Sonawane RS, Suri JS. A novel and robust Bayesian approach for segmentation of psoriasis lesions and its risk stratification. *Comput Methods Prog Biomed.* (2017) 150:9–22. doi: 10.1016/j.cmpb.2017.07.011
7. Han SS, Park GH, Lim W, Kim MS, Im Na J, Park I, et al. Deep neural networks show an equivalent and often superior performance to dermatologists in onychomycosis diagnosis: automatic construction of onychomycosis datasets by region-based convolutional deep neural network. *PLoS ONE.* (2018) 13:e0191493. doi: 10.1371/journal.pone.0191493
8. Hogarty DT, Su JC, Phan K, Attia M, Hossny M, Nahavandi S, et al. Artificial intelligence in dermatology—where we are and the way to the future: a review. *Am J Clin Dermatol.* (2019) 21:41–4. doi: 10.1007/s40257-019-00462-6
9. Esteva A, Kuprel B, Novoa RA, Ko J, Swetter SM, Blau HM, et al. Dermatologist-level classification of skin cancer with deep neural networks. *Nature.* (2017) 542:115. doi: 10.1038/nature21056
10. Brinker TJ, Hekler A, Enk AH, Berking C, Haferkamp S, Hauschild A, et al. Deep neural networks are superior to dermatologists in melanoma image classification. *Eur J Cancer.* (2019) 119:11–7. doi: 10.1016/j.ejca.2019.05.023

11. Brinker TJ, Hekler A, Enk AH, Klode J, Hauschild A, Berking C, et al. Deep learning outperformed 136 of 157 dermatologists in a head-to-head dermoscopic melanoma image classification task. *Eur J Cancer.* (2019) 113:47–54. doi: 10.1016/j.ejca.2019.04.001
12. Lau AY, Staccini P. Artificial intelligence in health: new opportunities, challenges, and practical implications. *Yearb Med Inform.* (2019) 28:174–8. doi: 10.1055/s-0039-1677935
13. Cath C. Governing artificial intelligence: ethical, legal and technical opportunities and challenges. *Phil Trans R Soc A.* (2018) 376:20180080. doi: 10.1098/rsta.2018.0080
14. Grande D, Asch DA, Wan F, Bradbury AR, Jagsi R, Mitra N. Are patients with cancer less willing to share their health information? *Privacy Sensitiv Soc Purpose.* (2015) 11:378–83. doi: 10.1200/JOP.2015.004820
15. Bartlett G, Macgibbon B, Rubinowicz A, Nease C, Dawes M, Tamblyn R. The importance of relevance: willingness to share eHealth data for family medicine research. *Front Public Health.* (2018) 6:255. doi: 10.3389/fpubh.2018.00255
16. Oh S, Kim JH, Choi S-W, Lee HJ, Hong J, Kwon SH. Physician confidence in artificial intelligence: an online mobile survey. *J Med Internet Res.* (2019) 21:e12422. doi: 10.2196/12422
17. Polesie S, Gillstedt M, Kittler H, Lallas A, Tschandl P, Zalaudek I, et al. Attitudes towards artificial intelligence within dermatology: an international online survey. *BJD.* (2020) doi: 10.1111/bjd.18875. [Epub ahead of print].
18. Fink C, Uhlmann L, Hofmann M, Forschner A, Eigentler T, Garbe C, et al. Patient acceptance and trust in automated computer-assisted diagnosis of melanoma with dermatofluoroscopy. *J Dtsch Dermatol Ges.* (2018) 16:854–9. doi: 10.1111/ddg.13562
19. Jonmarker O, Strand F, Brandberg Y, Lindholm P. The future of breast cancer screening: what do participants in a breast cancer screening program think about automation using artificial intelligence? *Acta Radiol Open.* (2019) 8:2058460119880315. doi: 10.1177/2058460119880315
20. Steeb T, Wessely A, Mastnik S, Brinker TJ, French LE, Niesert AC, et al. Patient attitudes and their awareness towards skin cancer-related apps: cross-sectional survey. *JMIR mHealth uHealth.* (2019) 7:e13844. doi: 10.2196/13844
21. Bryant SM, Hunton JE, Stone DN. Internet-based experiments: prospects and possibilities for behavioral accounting research. *Behav Res Account.* (2004) 16:107–29. doi: 10.2308/bria.2004.16.1.107
22. Pinto dos Santos D, Giese D, Brodehl S, Chon SH, Staab W, Kleinert R, et al. Medical students' attitude towards artificial intelligence: a multicentre survey. *Eur Radiol.* (2019) 29:1640–6. doi: 10.1007/s00330-018-5601-1
23. Janda M, Soyer HP. Can clinical decision making be enhanced by artificial intelligence? *Br J Dermatol.* (2019) 180:247–8. doi: 10.1111/bjd.17110
24. Lucivero F, Jongsma KR. A mobile revolution for healthcare? Setting the agenda for bioethics. *J Med Ethics.* (2018) 44:685–9. doi: 10.1136/medethics-2017-104741
25. Bach S, Binder A, Montavon G, Klauschen F, Müller K-R, Samek WJPO. On pixel-wise explanations for non-linear classifier decisions by layer-wise relevance propagation. *PLoS ONE.* (2015) 10:e0130140. doi: 10.1371/journal.pone.0130140
26. van der Maaten L, Hinton G. Visualizing data using t-SNE. *J Mach Learn Res.* (2008) 9:2579–605. Available online at: http://www.jmlr.org/papers/volume9/vandermaaten08a/vandermaaten08a.pdf

8

# High-Frequency Ultrasonography and Evaporimetry in Non-invasive Evaluation of the Nail Unit

*Marta Szymoniak-Lipska [1†], Adriana Polańska [2*†], Dorota Jenerowicz [1], Adam Lipski [3], Ryszard Żaba [2], Zygmunt Adamski [1] and Aleksandra Dańczak-Pazdrowska [1]*

*[1] Department of Dermatology, Poznan University of Medical Sciences, Poznan, Poland, [2] Department of Dermatology and Venereology, Poznan University of Medical Sciences, Poznan, Poland, [3] Department of Urology, Poznań University of Medical Sciences, Poznan, Poland*

***Correspondence:***
*Adriana Polańska*
*adriana-polanska@wp.pl*

*† These authors have contributed equally to this work and share first authorship*

**Background:** The nail unit (NU) is a complex structure that performs a number of functions, including protection, defense, manipulation, and palpation. Non-invasive research methods can facilitate the recognition of NU structure and function. Evaporimetry and HF-USG due to their availability of equipment and low research costs seem to be particularly noteworthy, but so far have been assessed to a limited extent. The aim of the presented study was to check the usefulness of TOWL and HF-USG in examination of NU.

**Materials and Methods:** A total of 58 volunteers aged 25–65 years (mean age: $41 \pm 10.16$ years) were qualified for the study. The subjects did not present symptoms of clinically evident onychopathy and did not suffer from any dermatoses associated with lesions occurring within the NU. Additionally, the patients did not suffer from systemic diseases that could affect NU (including heart, lung, and endocrine diseases). In all volunteers, the measurement of TOWL and 20 MHz ultrasonography [high-frequency ultrasonography (HF-USG)] with the special emphasis on determination of nail plate thickness were performed.

**Results:** Analysis of 464 HF-USG images revealed that the nail plate presented as two hyperechoic, parallel streaks (railway sign) with a linear hypoechoic middle layer between them. Matrix was visualized as a hypoechoic structure with blurred boundaries, mostly within the fourth and fifth fingers and more often in women. We found statistically significant correlations between the type of a finger and the thickness of the nail plate both in the entire study group and taking into account gender. In the dominant hand, the results were $r = -0.341$; $p < 0.001$; $r = -0.417$, $p < 0.001$; and $r = 0.337$; $p = 0.001$ (for the whole group, for women, and for men, respectively). In the non-dominant hand, the results were $r = -0.465$; $p < 0.001$; $r = -0.493$, $p < 0.01$; and $r = -0.503$; $p < 0.01$ (for the whole group, for women, and for men, respectively). There were statistically significant differences in the thickness of the nail plates of the corresponding types of fingers between female and male NUs. Statistically significant correlations were found between the type of a finger and the TOWL value in the whole group and taking into account gender ($p < 0.05$), except for the non-dominant hand in men. There were no statistically significant differences in the

TOWL values of the corresponding types of fingers between male and female NUs ($p > 0.05$). There was no statistically significant correlation between the TOWL value and the nail plate thickness in any of the tested NUs, apart from the one statistically significant correlation in nd5 ($r = 0.390$, $p = 0.021$).

**Conclusions:** To sum up, non-invasive methods, such as HF-USG and TOWL, enable assessment of the NU and are useful in examination of its structure and function. HF-USG shows characteristic elements of NUs that can be distinguished because of differences in their echogenicity. The thickness of the nail plate and TOWL depend on the type of finger, and show a relationship with gender.

**Keywords: HF-USG, High frequency ultrasonography, TOWL, transonychial water loss, nail plate thickness, nail, nail unit**

## INTRODUCTION

The nail unit (NU) is a complex structure that performs a number of functions, including protection, defense, manipulation, and palpation (1). Nowadays special attention is also paid to the aesthetic function of NU (2), and deterioration in its appearance may negatively affect the quality of life (3). For those reasons, diseases of NU seem to be hot topics for researchers around the world (4, 5). There is a significant tendency to look for non-invasive research methods that facilitate the recognition of NU structure and function. Among these methods, evaporimetry and HF-USG seem to be particularly noteworthy, due to the availability of equipment, and low research costs that so far have been assessed to a limited extent (6).

Transepidermal water loss (TEWL) measurement is used to indirectly assess the function of the epidermal barrier function and is applied mostly in studies conducted among patients with atopic dermatitis (AD) (7–9). The modification of this procedure adapted to NU is a transonychial water loss (TOWL). TOWL values have been reported in single studies and are many times higher than the TEWL values, which can be related to NU composition (10). The possibility of imaging NU in real time can be achieved using ultrasound examination (USG). With the application of frequencies dedicated for dermatological applications [high-frequency ultrasound (HF-USG)] (11), there is the possibility to visualize the NU structure. To date, in single reports, NU pathological processes like abscesses, hematomas (12), glomeruli, and mucous cysts were described with the use of HF-USG, and the utility of this method in differentiation of psoriasis (13) and onychomycosis (14) was presented. However, studies evaluating usefulness of HF-USG in examination of complete finger NU structure in regards to sex, age, and dominant hand are still lacking. The relationship between TOWL value and thickness of the nail plate was assessed only to a small extent in few reports (6, 15, 16), using a variety of research methodology. Thus, there is a need for detailed, global ultrasonographic assessment of NU, the knowledge of which could translate into a better understanding of the pathological processes occurring within this appendage.

The aim of the presented study was to explore the utility of TOWL and HF-USG in examination of NU as well as to obtain the ultrasonographic features of NU with special emphasis on non-invasive measurement of the nail plate thickness.

## MATERIALS AND METHODS

### Examined Group

A total of 58 volunteers aged 25–65 years (mean age: 41 ± 10.16 years) were qualified for the study. Thirty-five women (mean age: 41.49 ± 9.80 years) and 23 men were examined (mean age: 40.26 ± 10.86 years). All of the participants have given their written consent. The subjects did not present symptoms of clinically evident onychopathy and did not suffer from any dermatoses associated with lesions occurring within the NU. All subjects were right-handed and non-smokers. In two cases, two NU of the thumbs were excluded from the study due to the condition after mechanical trauma.

The tests were performed in standardized conditions at the temperature of 20–24°C. At least 30 days prior to examination, volunteers had to stop using any nail polish or varnish and performing manicure, except nail clipping. Subjects were asked not to use detergents and disinfectants for a minimum of 20 min before tests. First, TOWL measurement was performed, followed by HF-HSG. The above order was determined by necessity to use a medium in the form of an ultrasound gel for HF-USG examination. We were aware that its application to the nail plate could cause a change in NU hydration and make TOWL results unreliable.

The letter designation was adopted for the description of NU: "d" for the finger of the dominant hand and "nd" for the non-dominant one. The number describes the type of finger, and so the number (1), corresponded to the thumb; (2), the index finger; (3), the middle finger; (4), the ring finger; and (5), little finger.

### HF-USG

The HF-USG examination was performed with the use of The Dermascan C device (version 3) by Cortex Technology (Hadsund, Denmark) equipped with a linear head 20 MHz (11). The probe was covered with a layer of ultrasound gel and then placed on the NU to obtain sagittal sections. The transducer was positioned in the midline to include the proximal nail fold and 1/2 proximal to the nail plate in the imaging. The axial

**TABLE 1** | Percentage results of imaged matrixes.

| **Whole group** | | | | | | | | |
|---|---|---|---|---|---|---|---|---|
| Type of finger | d2 | d3 | d4 | d5 | nd2 | nd3 | nd4 | nd5 |
| % of visible matrixes (%) | 12 | 9 | 19 | 22 | 21 | 22 | 28 | 24 |
| **Women** | | | | | | | | |
| Type of finger | d2 | d3 | d4 | d5 | nd2 | nd3 | nd4 | nd5 |
| % of visible matrixes (%) | 14 | 11 | 29 | 29 | 29 | 31 | 37 | 20 |
| **Men** | | | | | | | | |
| Type of finger | d2 | d3 | d4 | d5 | nd2 | nd3 | nd4 | nd5 |
| % of visible matrixes (%) | 9 | 4 | 4 | 13 | 9 | 9 | 13 | 30 |

*nd, the finger of the non-dominant hand; d, the finger of the dominant hand; number, type of finger; i.e., 2, index finger.*

resolution was 80 μm, and the lateral resolution was 200 μm. The ultrasonic wave propagated through the tissues at a speed of 2,480 m/s. The B-mode presentation was used to qualitatively evaluate the images. The A-mode presentation was used to carry out the measurements of the thickness of the nail plate, which was measured in each examined finger three times in the area between the proximal 1/3 and middle 1/3. Then, the arithmetic mean was calculated.

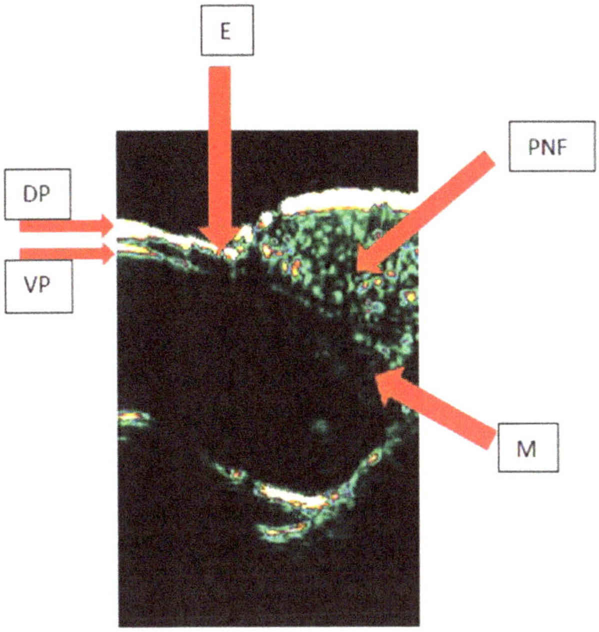


**FIGURE 1** | The HF-USG image of the nail unit.

## TOWL

TOWL measurements were conducted using a Tewameter® TM 300 Courage-Khazaka (Köln, Germany), with a reduction diaphragm recommended by the manufacturer (diameter 2 mm) for testing small areas (Z00812) according to the guidelines originally established for TEWL (17). The Tewameter® TM 300 was connected to the Cutometer® MPA 580. The device was placed in the middle on the nail plate within its proximal 1/3 and central part. An attempt was made to achieve the comparable pressure. In case of each examined NU, 20 measurements were performed at 1 s intervals. An arithmetic mean was then calculated. The results were presented in conventional units (c.u.).

## Statistical Analysis

For the values of parameters such as plate thickness and TOWL, appropriate descriptive statistics were determined: arithmetic mean with the corresponding standard deviation, minimum, and maximum values. The differences between the groups were assessed using the non-parametric Mann–Whitney *U* test. The relationships between the parameters were investigated using Spearman's correlation. Values at $p < 0.05$ were considered statistically significant. The calculations were made with the use of the STATISTICA v 13.3 statistical package.

## RESULTS

### Analysis of HF-USG Results

Finally, HF-USG 464 images of NU were taken into consideration, which was related to the repeated unsuccessful attempts to visualize NU in the thumbs. The difficulties were associated with the inability to fit an ultrasound head for anatomical curvatures of NU within d1 and nd1 and the gained images had insufficient quality. Therefore, analysis of them was abandoned.

In all analyzed fingers, the nail plate presented as two hyperechoic, parallel streaks (railway sign). Between them, a linear hypoechoic middle layer was visible. The abovementioned hyperechoic bands were, respectively, the dorsal and ventral lamina of the nail plate. The cuticle was located proximally to the described structures and its echogenicity was similar to the echogenicity of the dorsal and ventral plates. Moving further, proximal nail fold, with an echogenicity lower than the mentioned dorsal and ventral plates, occurred. Matrix was visualized as a hypoechoic structure with blurred boundaries, adjacent to the nail fold and the proximal part of the abdominal plate. It was visible in a minority of respondents, and the number of visualized matrixes varied in different types of finger. The matrix was seen more often in the fourth and fifth fingers and more often in women. The detailed percentage results of imaged matrixes are presented in **Table 1**. **Figure 1** shows the sagittal section of HF-USG of the NU with its characteristic elements.

The average thickness of the nail plate in the whole group ranged from 0.36 mm in nd5 to 0.43 mm in nd2. The thinnest nail plate was observed in the group of women in nd5 (0.25 mm), and the thickest was observed in the group of men in nd2 (0.54 mm). The mean thickness of the nail plate in the group of women ranged from 0.35 mm in nd5 to 0.40 mm d2. The greatest thickness in this group was observed in nd2 (0.51 mm). The average thickness of the nail plate in the group of men ranged from 0.39 mm in nd5 to 0.45 mm in nd2. The lowest thickness in this group was noted in nd4 (0.30 mm). The thickness of nail plates is presented in **Table 2**.

**TABLE 2** | The thickness of nail plates in the whole group and in the group of women and men.

| Type of finger | | Mean ± SD [mm] | Min [mm] | Max [mm] |
|---|---|---|---|---|
| **Whole group** | | | | |
| 2 | D | 0.42 ± 0.05 | 0.33 | 0.52 |
| | Nd | 0.43 ± 0.04 | 0.35 | 0.54 |
| 3 | D | 0.41 ± 0.05 | 0.30 | 0.51 |
| | Nd | 0.40 ± 0.05 | 0.29 | 0.50 |
| 4 | D | 0.39 ± 0.04 | 0.29 | 0.49 |
| | Nd | 0.38 ± 0.05 | 0.28 | 0.52 |
| 5 | D | 0.38 ± 0.05 | 0.27 | 0.48 |
| | Nd | 0.36 ± 0.04 | 0.25 | 0.45 |
| **WOMEN** | | | | |
| Type of finger | | Mean ± SD [mm] | Min [mm] | Max [mm] |
| 2 | D | 0.40 ± 0.04 | 0.33 | 0.49 |
| | Nd | 0.41 ± 0.04 | 0.35 | 0.51 |
| 3 | D | 0.39 ± 0.04 | 0.30 | 0.46 |
| | Nd | 0.39 ± 0.04 | 0.29 | 0.48 |
| 4 | D | 0.37 ± 0.04 | 0.29 | 0.44 |
| | Nd | 0.37 ± 0.04 | 0.28 | 0.43 |
| 5 | D | 0.36 ± 0.04 | 0.27 | 0.44 |
| | Nd | 0.35 ± 0.04 | 0.25 | 0.42 |
| **MEN** | | | | |
| Type of finger | | Mean ± SD [mm] | Min [mm] | Max [mm] |
| 2 | D | 0.45 ± 0.05 | 0.35 | 0.52 |
| | Nd | 0.45 ± 0.04 | 0.36 | 0.54 |
| 3 | D | 0.43 ± 0.05 | 0.34 | 0.51 |
| | Nd | 0.43 ± 0.04 | 0.36 | 0.50 |
| 4 | D | 0.41 ± 0.04 | 0.34 | 0.49 |
| | Nd | 0.41 ± 0.06 | 0.30 | 0.52 |
| 5 | D | 0.41 ± 0.04 | 0.33 | 0.48 |
| | Nd | 0.39 ± 0.03 | 0.33 | 0.45 |

*nd, the finger of the non-dominant hand; d, the finger of the dominant hand; number, type of finger; i.e., 2, index finger.*

We found statistically significant correlations between the type of a finger and the thickness of the nail plate both in the entire study group and taking into account gender. In the dominant hand, the results were as follows: $r = -0.3$; $p < 0.001$; $r = -0.4$, $p < 0.001$; and $r = 0.3$; $p = 0.001$ (for the whole group, for women, and for men, respectively). In the non-dominant hand, the results were $r = -0.5$; $p < 0.001$; $r = -0.5$, $p < 0.01$; and $r = -0.5$; $p < 0.01$ (for the whole group, for women, and for men, respectively). There were statistically significant differences in the thickness of the nail plates of the corresponding types of fingers between female and male NUs (**Table 3**).

There were no statistically significant differences in the thickness of the nail plates of the corresponding fingers of the dominant and non-dominant hand, both in the whole group and taking into account gender ($p > 0.05$).

The statistically significant correlation between the age and the thickness of the nail plate was observed only in the d5 fingers in the entire study group and in the group of men ($r = -0.3$, $p = 0.027$; $r = -0.4$, $p = 0.043$, respectively).

**TABLE 3** | *p*-values for differences in the thickness of the nail plates of the corresponding types of fingers between female and male NUs.

| Type of finger | d2 | d3 | d4 | d5 | nd2 | nd3 | nd4 | nd5 |
|---|---|---|---|---|---|---|---|---|
| *P* | <0.001 | 0.002 | 0.002 | <0.001 | <0.001 | 0.001 | 0.026 | <0.001 |

*nd, the finger of the non-dominant hand; d, the finger of the dominant hand; number, type of finger; i.e., 2, index finger.*

## Analysis of TOWL Values

The mean TOWL value in the entire group ranged from 5.02 c.u. in d1 to 7.41 c.u. in d5. The lowest measured TOWL value was recorded in the group of men in d1 (1.10 c.u.), and the highest value, also observed in the group of men, in nd3 (17.60 c.u.). The mean value of TOWL in the group of women ranged from 5.1 c.u. in d1 to 7.30 c.u. in d5. In this group, the minimal value of TOWL was observed in d1 (2.70 c.u.), and the highest value (12.80 c.u.) was obtained in d5. The mean value of TOWL in the group of men ranged from 4.90 c.u. in d1 to 7.58 c.u. in d5.

The TOWL value for each type of NU are presented in the **Table 4**

Statistically significant correlations were found between the type of a finger and the TOWL value in the whole group and taking into account gender ($p < 0.05$), except for the non-dominant hand in men ($r = 0.8$, $p = 0.068$) (**Table 5**).

There were no statistically significant differences in the TOWL values of the corresponding fingers of the dominant and non-dominant hand, both in the whole group and taking into account gender ($p > 0.05$). There were no statistically significant differences in the TOWL values of the corresponding types of fingers between male and female NUs ($p > 0.05$). The statistically significant correlation between the age and the TOWL value was observed only in the group of men in d3 finger ($r = -0.5$, $p = 0.031$).

## Analysis of Correlations Between HF-USG Results and TOWL Values

There was no statistically significant correlation between the TOWL value and the nail plate thickness in any of the tested NUs, neither in the whole group and in the group of men. The significant correlations were not detected in the majority of fingers in women's group, the only statistically significant correlation was pointed in nd5 ($r = 0.4$, $p = 0.021$).

# DISCUSSION

To our knowledge, our study presents for the first time a detailed characteristic of a NU achieved with the use of non-invasive tools in subjects with no evident onychopathy, taking into account all fingers of both hands in relation to volunteers' gender and age.

## HF-USG

Similarly to previous studies (12), we found that the normal nail plate is a trilaminar structure with the first and third layer being hyperechoic, while the second layer is anechoic. The nail matrix is a hypoechoic area that is placed proximally within NU.

**TABLE 4 |** The values of TOWL measurements in the whole group, in the group of women, and in the group of men.

| Whole group | | | | |
|---|---|---|---|---|
| **Type of finger** | | **Mean ± SD [c.u.]** | **Min [c.u.]** | **Max [c.u.]** |
| 1 | D | 5.02 ± 1.50 | 1.10 | 8.00 |
| | Nd | 5.33 ± 1.72 | 2.90 | 11.60 |
| 2 | D | 6.13 ± 1.80 | 3.30 | 10.90 |
| | Nd | 6.41 ± 2.27 | 2.10 | 12.80 |
| 3 | D | 6.64 ± 2.70 | 2.30 | 16.80 |
| | Nd | 6.43 ± 2.39 | 3.10 | 17.60 |
| 4 | D | 6.74 ± 2.00 | 2.90 | 12.50 |
| | Nd | 6.52 ± 2.24 | 3.30 | 16.30 |
| 5 | D | 7.41 ± 2.50 | 3.10 | 13.30 |
| | Nd | 6.53 ± 2.13 | 1.80 | 11.80 |
| **WOMEN** | | | | |
| **Type of finger** | | **Mean ± SD [c.u.]** | **Min [c.u.]** | **Max [c.u.]** |
| 1 | D | 5.10 ± 1.20 | 2.70 | 8.00 |
| | Nd | 5.39 ± 1.55 | 2.90 | 9.90 |
| 2 | D | 5.92 ± 1.73 | 3.70 | 10.60 |
| | Nd | 6.40 ± 1.93 | 3.30 | 11.50 |
| 3 | D | 6.36 ± 1.64 | 3.90 | 12.00 |
| | Nd | 6.07 ± 1.40 | 3.50 | 8.50 |
| 4 | D | 7.03 ± 1.95 | 3.60 | 12.50 |
| | Nd | 6.50 ± 2.02 | 3.30 | 10.70 |
| 5 | D | 7.30 ± 2.41 | 3.50 | 12.80 |
| | Nd | 6.61 ± 1.87 | 3.90 | 11.10 |
| **MEN** | | | | |
| **Type of finger** | | **Mean ± SD [c.u.]** | **Min [c.u.]** | **Max [c.u.]** |
| 1 | D | 4.90 ± 1.91 | 1.10 | 8.00 |
| | Nd | 5.24 ± 1.99 | 3.00 | 11.60 |
| 2 | D | 6.46 ± 1.90 | 3.30 | 10.90 |
| | Nd | 6.43 ± 2.75 | 2.10 | 12.80 |
| 3 | D | 7.08 ± 3.80 | 2.30 | 16.80 |
| | Nd | 6.97 ± 3.36 | 3.10 | 17.60 |
| 4 | D | 6.31 ± 2.03 | 2.90 | 10.40 |
| | Nd | 3.55 ± 2.58 | 3.40 | 16.30 |
| 5 | D | 7.58 ± 2.67 | 3.10 | 13.30 |
| | Nd | 6.41 ± 2.51 | 1.80 | 11.80 |

*Nd, the finger of the non-dominant hand; d, the finger of the dominant hand; number, type of finger; i.e., 2, index finger; c.u., conventional units.*

**TABLE 5 |** Values of *r* and *p* for correlations between the type of a finger and the TOWL value.

| **Dominant hand** | ***R*** | ***P*** |
|---|---|---|
| Whole group | 0.3 | <0.001 |
| Women | 0.4 | <0.001 |
| Men | 0.3 | 0.003 |
| Non-dominant hand | *R* | *P* |
| Whole group | 0.2 | 0.002 |
| Women | 0.2 | 0.012 |
| Men | 0.8 | 0.068 |

In our study, matrix was visible in a minority of respondents, and the number of visualized matrixes varied in different types of fingers. The matrix was seen more often in the fourth and fifth fingers and more often in women. It may be due to the fact that in these fingers, the nail plate is the thinnest and the visualization of deeper NU structures is easier. The other reason could be that the curvature of mentioned NUs is the slightest and USG probe adheres better, therefore giving higher chances to obtain good quality images. Unfortunately, in our study images gained from d1 and nd1 had insufficient quality, although repeated attempts to visualize these NU were performed. The difficulties were related to the limitations of our probe (inability to fit the ultrasound head for anatomical curvatures of thumbs). Finally, HF-USG 464 images of NU of fingers two to five were taken into consideration.

Literature data regarding NU USG in healthy volunteers are scarce and most researchers focus on NU pathologies (particularly psoriasis) (18–20). The pioneers of a nail plate thickness analysis using ultrasound transmission time were Finlay et al. (21). They compared acquired data with micrometer measurements and concluded that ultrasounds can be useful to determine nail thickness. In our study, we used A-mode to estimate the nail plate thickness. The average thickness of the nail plate in the whole group ranged from 0.36 mm in nd5 to 0.43 mm in nd2. Estimated borderline values suggest that the thinnest nail plate was observed in female volunteers in nd5 (0.25 mm), and the thickest was observed in males in nd2 (0.54 mm). Similar results were obtained by Wollina et al. (22)—according to their analysis, the thickness of the nail plate ranged between 0.481 mm (right hand thumb) and 0.397 mm (fifth finger of the left hand).

We observed statistically significant correlations between finger type and the thickness of the nail plate (in both the dominant and non-dominant hand) in the whole group and taking gender into account ($p < 0.05$). The average thickness of the nail plate was lower the further the finger was from the thumb. We assume that those observations arise from the more frequent use of the radially located fingers in everyday activities. The greater exposure to mechanical stimuli requires more effective protection of the fingertips and hence the appearance of thicker nail plates in index fingers than in the little fingers.

In our study, gender-related differences between nail thickness were observed—men presented with thicker nail plates. Wollina et al. (22) also showed differences in nail and matrix volume, also with higher levels in the male.

The results of our study showed that there is no significant difference between NU in the dominant and non-dominant hand. However, we would rather suspect that the dominant hand, as being more exposed to external factors, would have showed a higher thickness of NUs as an adaptation to more frequent exposure to destructive environmental factors and help in manipulation. Ruan et al. (23), however, also did not obtain data, suggesting differences between mentioned NU.

In our study, we found inverse statistically significant correlation between the age and the thickness of the nail plate only in the d5 in the whole study group and in the group of men ($r = -0.3$, $p = 0.027$; $r = -0.4$, $p = 0.043$, respectively), whereas there were no such observations in case of other fingers. Those correlations are most likely random statistical results. In general, in examined subjects with no evident onychopathy, there were no significant changes in nail thickness, which is commonly described in the elderly (24, 25).

## TOWL

Although the TEWL measurement is a well-recognized parameter reflecting the function of the stratum corneum (SC), this measurement in relation to the entirely keratinized structure of the nail plate, known as TOWL, is still not fully understood. There are just single reports regarding TOWL measurement within healthy NU, which present different methodology (6, 16, 26).

We have made an attempt to analyze the value of TOWL, taking into account various variables. We did not observe the relations of TOWL to age and sex, and the value of TOWL did not differ between the right and the left hand. We found that the lowest measured TOWL value was recorded in the group of men in d1 (1.10 c.u.), and the highest value was also observed in the group of men in nd3 (17.60 c.u.). Statistically significant correlations were found between finger type and TOWL value in the whole group and taking into account gender ($p < 0.05$) except of the non-dominant hand in men. In general, the further from the thumb the NU is, the higher TOWL values are obtained. We suspect that these findings may be linked to a better adaptation to preserve water in thumb and index, because of their utility in everyday activities. The results obtained in male non-dominant hand should be considered as random statistical discovery.

We observed moderate statistically significant correlation between the age and TOWL value only in the male group in the d3 finger ($r = -0.5$, $p = 0.031$) and we did not gain any statistically significant differences in the TOWL values of the corresponding types of fingers between male and female NUs. Jemec et al. (6) also showed no differences in case of TOWL—gender relation, but suggested that with aging TOWL, value decreases. However, they published data based on examination of thumbs' TOWL of 21 healthy volunteers (12 female, nine male; 22–71 years, median 32). We presume that differences between sexes may be related to the thicker nail plates in men; however, this observation was not confirmed by our research. Also, age may act as a factor deteriorating the function of water resistance within the NUs, although obtained data (TOWL value of only one type of NUs in men inversely correlated with age) suggest that it could be a random statistical finding.

We did not observe any significant statistical differences between NUs of the dominant and non-dominant hand. However, our suspicion was that the dominant hand (being highly exposed to external factors) would show a difference, with higher TOWL values. Murdan et al. measured TOWL values in only three volunteers using an evaporimeter with a closed condensation chamber with a dedicated adapter and showed that there are differences in the TOWL values in the same person in the corresponding fingers of the left and right hand and the left and right foot. However, the authors did not define if the extremities were dominant or non-dominant (16).

Also, the study of Sattler et al. (27) faces limitations considering the number of analyzed NUs—only a middle finger of the dominant and non-dominant hand was examined. The number of participants was higher than in previously mentioned studies; however, the group of 30 volunteers would benefit from broadening. In their study the authors used an open-chamber evaporimeter with holding ring. The researchers did not observe statistically significant differences in the TOWL values of the middle finger of the dominant and non-dominant hand, as it was presented in our study.

An equipment is definitely an important factor influencing acquired results. According to The European Group on Efficacy Measurement and Evaluation of Cosmetics and other Products (EEMCO) guidance for TEWL (17), three different measurement methods may be applied: open-chamber methods, semiopen methods (open-chamber method with wind shield incorporated in probe), and closed-chamber methods. Open-chamber evaporimeters are still the preferred techniques to measure TEWL. However, because of their susceptibility to environmental factors, they have been supplemented with semiopen- and closed-chamber probes, which are more convenient to use and more applicable to field studies. Closed-chamber methods interfere with evaporation and cannot be used for continuous monitoring. The authors suggest that validation of methods with respect to intra- and inter-instrument variation is still a challenge (17). Still, no guidelines related to TOWL measurement exist.

## Correlation Between HF-USG Results and TOWL Values

The results of previous studies based on assessment of correlation between nail plate thickness and water loss (measured using various methods) are inconclusive and based on small groups (6, 15, 16).

We found that thickness of the nail plate is not correlated with TOWL value in most cases. There was no statistically significant correlation between the TOWL value and the thickness of the nail plate measured with HF-USG in any of the tested NUs. A similar observation was also made by Jemec et al. (6); however, they assessed only thumbs. Moreover, Spruit (15) investigated the specific permeability of the nail plate to water. The thickness of all NUs was measured with a caliper in only one volunteer. The author concluded that in a healthy volunteer, the loss of water is independent of the thickness of the nail plate. On the other hand, different results, partially obtained *in vitro*, were presented by Murdan et al. They showed a relationship between TOWL value and plate thickness assessed by measuring cut nails with a micrometer (16).

According to previous research, TEWL is not affected by skin thickness (28). It is worth considering if, similarly, the water permeability of nail plates, either does not depend on the thickness of the SC. However, the differences in chemical composition may be the factor influencing permeability of SC in the skin (29). Is it true for the NU? More research is required. Certainly, it would be necessary to continue research in this area with a larger number of NU.

## CONCLUSIONS

To sum up, non-invasive methods, such as high-frequency ultrasonography and TEWL, enable assessment of the NU and are useful in examination of its structure and function. High-frequency ultrasonography shows characteristic elements of NU that can be distinguished because of differences in their echogenicity. The thickness of the nail plate and TEWL depend on the type of finger, and show a relationship with gender.

## ETHICS STATEMENT

The studies involving human participants were reviewed and approved by Bioethical Commission. The patients/participants provided their written informed consent to participate in this study.

## AUTHOR CONTRIBUTIONS

RŻ and ZA assistance in writing article and performing research. AL statistical analysis. DJ supervision over writing thesis and English style analysis. AD-P assistance in conducting and interpreting research and supervision over writing thesis. AP originator of the research, assistance in conducting and interpreting research, author of the text on a par with the MS-L and AP. MS-L performer of research and analysis and author of the text on a par with the AP. All authors contributed to the article and approved the submitted version.

## REFERENCES


1. de Berker DA, André J, Baran R. Nail biology and nail science. *Int J Cosmet Sci.* (2007) 29:241–75. doi: 10.1111/j.1467-2494.2007.00372.x
2. Rich P. Nail cosmetics and esthetics. *Skin Pharmacol Appl Skin Physiol.* (1999) 12:144–5. doi: 10.1159/000029869
3. Belyayeva E, Gregoriou S, Chalikias J, Kontochristopoulos G, Koumantaki E, Makris M, et al. The impact of nail disorders on quality of life. *Eur J Dermatol.* (2013) 23:366–71. doi: 10.1684/ejd.2013.2048
4. Ruben BS. Pathology of the nail unit. *Dermatol Clin.* (2021) 39:319–36. doi: 10.1016/j.det.2020.12.009
5. Rigopoulos D, Rompoti N, Gregoriou S. Management of nail psoriasis. *Dermatol Clin.* (2021) 39:211–20. doi: 10.1016/j.det.2020.12.014
6. Jemec GB, Agner T, Serup J. Transonychial water loss: relation to sex, age and nail-plate thickness. *Br J Dermatol.* (1989) 121:443–6. doi: 10.1111/j.1365-2133.1989.tb15511.x
7. Agner T. Noninvasive measuring methods for the investigation of irritant patch test reactions. A study of patients with hand eczema, atopic dermatitis and controls. *Acta Derm Venereol Suppl (Stockh).* (1992) 173:1–26.
8. Polańska A, Dańczak-Pazdrowska A, Silny W, Jenerowicz D, Osmola-Mańkowska A, Olek-Hrab K. Evaluation of selected skin barrier functions in atopic dermatitis in relation to the disease severity and pruritus. *Postep Derm Alergol.* (2012) 29:373–77. doi: 10.5114/pdia.2012.31492
9. Alexander H, Brown S, Danby S, Flohr C. Research techniques made simple: transepidermal water loss measurement as a research tool. *J Invest Dermatol.* (2018) 138:2295–300.e1. doi: 10.1016/j.jid.2018.09.001
10. Jacobi O. Die Nägel des lebenden Menschen und die Perspiration insensibilis. *Arch. klin. exp. Derm.* (1962) 214:559–72. doi.org/10.1007/BF00483524
11. Wortsman X, Alfageme F, Roustan G, Arias-Santiago S, Martorell A, Catalano O, et al. Guidelines for performing dermatologic ultrasound examinations by the DERMUS group. *J Ultrasound Med.* (2016) 35:577–80. doi: 10.7863/ultra.15.06046
12. Wortsman X, Jemec GB. Ultrasound imaging of nails. *Dermatol Clin.* (2006) 24:323–8. doi: 10.1016/j.det.2006.03.014
13. Gutierrez M, Wortsman X, Filippucci E, De Angelis R, Filosa G, Grassi W. High-frequency sonography in the evaluation of psoriasis: nail and skin involvement. *J Ultrasound Med.* (2009) 2:1569–74. doi: 10.7863/jum.2009.28.11.1569
14. Essayed SMA, Al-Shatouri MA, Allah YSN, Atwa MA. Ultrasonographic characterization of the nails in patients with psoriasis and onychomycosis. *Egypt J Radiol Nuc Med.* (2015) 46:733–39. doi: 10.1016/j.ejrnm.2015.04.009
15. Spruit D. Measurement of water vapor loss through human nail *in vivo*. *J Invest Dermatol.* (1971) 56:359–61. doi: 10.1111/1523-1747
16. Murdan S, Hinsu D, Guimier M. A few aspects of transonychial water loss (TOWL): inter-individual, and intra-individual inter-finger, inter-hand and inter-day variabilities, and the influence of nail plate hydration, filing and varnish. *Eur J Pharm Biopharm.* (2008) 70:684–9. doi: 10.1016/j.ejpb.2008.05.018
17. Berardesca E, Loden M, Serup J, Masson P, Rodrigues LM. The revised EEMCO guidance for the *in vivo* measurement of water in the skin. *Skin Res Technol.* (2018) 24:351–8. doi: 10.1111/srt.12599
18. Marina ME, Solomon C, Bolboaca SD, Bocsa C, Mihu CM, Tătaru AD. High-frequency sonography in the evaluation of nail psoriasis. *Med Ultrason.* (2016) 18:312–7. doi: 10.11152/mu.2013.2066.183.hgh
19. Idolazzi L, Gisondi P, Fassio A, Viapiana O, Giollo A, Rossini M, et al. Ultrasonography of the nail unit reveals quantitative and qualitative alterations in patients with psoriasis and psoriatic arthritis. *Med Ultrason.* (2018) 20:177–84. doi: 10.11152/mu-1327
20. Naredo E, Janta I, Baniandrés-Rodríguez O, Valor L, Hinojosa M, Bello N, et al. To what extend is nail ultrasound discriminative between psoriasis, psoriatic arthritis and healthy subjects? *Rheumatol Int.* (2019) 39:697–705. doi: 10.1007/s00296-018-4222-y
21. Finlay A, Moseley H, Duggan TC. Ultrasound transmission time: an *in vivo* guide to nail thickness. *Br J Dermatol.* (1987) 117:765–70. doi: 10.1111/j.1365-2133.1987.tb07358.x
22. Wollina U, Berger M, Karte K. Calculation of nail plate and nail matrix parameters by 20 MHz ultrasound in healthy volunteers and patients with skin disease. *Skin Res Technol.* (2001) 7:60–4. doi: 10.1034/j.1600-0846.2001.007001060.x
23. Ruan J, Wang XM, Xia MN. The evaluation of nail heath conditions with skin ultrasound. *Cutan Ocul Toxicol.* (2012) 31:318–22. doi: 10.3109/15569527.2011.645099
24. Abdullah L, Abbas O. Common nail changes and disorders in older people: diagnosis and management. *Can Fam Physician.* (2011) 57:173–81.
25. Baran R. The nail in the elderly. *Clin Dermatol.* (2011) 29:54–60. doi: 10.1016/j.clindermatol.2010.07.008
26. Krönauer C, Gfesser M, Ring J, Abeck D. Transonychial water loss in healthy and diseased nails. *Acta Derm Venereol.* (2001) 81:175–7. doi: 10.1080/000155501750376249
27. Sattler EC, Poloczek K, Kästle R, Welzel J. Confocal laser scanning microscopy and optical coherence tomography for the evaluation of the kinetics and quantification of wound healing after fractional laser therapy. *J Am Acad Dermatol.* (2013) 69:e165–73. doi: 10.1016/j.jaad.2013.04.052
28. Elias PM, Cooper ER, Korc A, Brown BE. Percutaneous transport in relation to stratum corneum structure and lipid composition. *J Invest Dermatol.* (1981) 76:297–301. doi: 10.1111/1523-1747.ep12526137
29. Hattingh J. The correlation between transepidermal water loss and the thickness of epidermal components. *Comp Biochem Physiol A Comp Physiol.* (1972) 43:719–22. doi: 10.1016/0300-9629(72)90140-5

9

# The Differential Diagnosis of Hypopigmented Mycosis Fungoides and Vitiligo with Reflectance Confocal Microscopy

*Huaxu Liu [1], Leilei Wang [2], Yan Lin [1], Xiaofeng Shan [1] and Min Gao [2]**

*[1] Shandong Provincial Institute of Dermatology and Venereology, Shandong First Medical University & Shandong Academy of Medical Sciences, Jinan, China, [2] Shandong Cancer Hospital and Institute, Shandong First Medical University & Shandong Academy of Medical Sciences, Jinan, China*

***Correspondence:***
*Min Gao*
*gmlhx@163.com*

**Objective:** To investigate the role of reflectance confocal microscopy (RCM) in the differential diagnosis of hypopigmented mycosis fungoides (HMF) and vitiligo.

**Methods:** Cases with persistent hypopigmented patches, suspicious of early stage vitiligo, or HMF were imaged with RCM. The melanin contents and inflammatory conditions of the epidermis and superficial dermis of the lesions were compared with the same layers of the adjacent skin, and then, the imaged lesions were biopsied and analyzed by histology.

**Results:** 15 cases were enrolled in this study, and based on the RCM findings, there was just slight or moderate reduction of melanin but no melanin absence in the basal cell layer of HMF lesions. The finding of monomorphous weakly refractile, oval to round cells on the basis of vesicle-like dark space was clearly elucidated in the epidermis of the lesions by RCM, which indicates the Pautrier's microabscesses on histopathology. Among those 15 cases, 13 cases were identified as HMF, and the other two cases were vitiligo, based on RCM findings, which were confirmed by histology analysis.

**Conclusions:** The RCM findings correlated well with histology results in the screening of HMF, which indicates the RCM is an important tool in the early detection and differential diagnosis of HMF.

**Keywords: imaging, reflectance confocal microscopy (RCM), detection, vitiligo, hypo-pigmented mycosis fungoides, differential daignosis**

## INTRODUCTION

Mycosis fungoides (MF), the most common primary cutaneous T-cell lymphoma, is a neoplastic disease characterized by classical non-infiltrated lesions (patches), plaques, tumors, and erythrodermic stages (1). Several distinct clinical forms of MF have been described, among which, the granulomatous, pustular, purpuric, hyperkeratotic and verrucous, bullous, invisible, and hypopigmented variants of the disease were included (1). The hypopigmented mycosis fungoides (HMF) was first described by (2, 3). It is an atypical and often misdiagnosed variant of MF characterized by persistent hypopigmented-to-achromic patches, with a vitiligo-like aspect, which is mainly distributed on the trunk and proximal portions of the extremities (1, 3). Unlike conventional MF, which is regarded as a disease most commonly found in the fifth to sixth decades of life, HMF most commonly affects the pediatric population, especially in Asians (1, 3). Clinically, thc diagnosis of HMF is commonly delayed, which may have a potential negative effect on the treatment and prognosis because it is rare, and it may resemble early vitiligo and other hypopigmentary skin disorders (4–6).

Reflectance confocal microscopy (RCM) is a non-invasive imaging technique that provides high-resolution cellular imaging of the epidermis and superficial dermis (7), which has been used in the diagnosis and differential diagnosis of skin tumors and inflammatory diseases for more than two decades with high sensitivity and specificity (8). Agero et al. (9) first investigated the characteristics of MF in the imaging of RCM. The Pautrier's microabscesses in epidermis on histopathology correlated with the vesicle-like dark space filled with collections of monomorphous weakly refractile oval to round cells in epidermis on the RCM images. Other studies (10) verified the correlation of RCM image and histology analysis in the diagnosis of MF.

In this study, we aimed to investigate the role of RCM in the early detection and differential diagnosis of HMF.

## MATERIALS AND METHODS

The study was approved by the Ethics Committee of Shandong Provincial Institute of Dermatology and Venereology. The cases with persistent round-to-oval hypopigmentation with mild scales or not, which distributed on the trunk, arms, and legs, wood lamp examination (±) and clinically suspicious of HMF and early vitiligo, were enrolled in the study. Cases with comparatively typical vitiligo lesions were not included in the study.

After written informed consent obtained and the related history recorded, the clinical pictures were taken and the hypopigmentary lesions and adjacent normal skin were imaged with RCM. *In-vivo* RCM imaging was performed with a commercially available, near-infrared, reflectance mode confocal microscope (Vivascope 1500; Lucid Inc., Rochester, NY, USA). A detailed description of the technique and the device used has been published previously (7, 8). At least three areas of hypopigmented lesions were imaged for each case to compare the changes with the perilesional normal skin. The single (0.5*0.5 mm) or mosaic RCM images (2*2 mm, or 3*3 mm) were captured or saved. Then one of the lesions imaged were suggested to be biopsied and analyzed histologically. The excisions were fixed in formalin and embedded in paraffin. After routine processing, slides were stained with hematoxylin and eosin (H–E) and further stained with immune-chemistry methods to detect the changes of CD4 and CD8 molecules.

Based on the previous studies, the RCM features of the lesions were analyzed layer by layer and correlated to the findings of histology analysis.

## RESULTS

In total, 15 cases with RCM and histology results were enrolled in the study. Among those enrolled 15 cases, 13 cases were

**TABLE 1** | The details of the included cases.

| Case | Age | Sex | Main distribution | Duration of evolution (month) | Previous tretments | RCM findings | Pathology findings |
|---|---|---|---|---|---|---|---|
| 1 | 15 | M | Trunk and legs | 36 | Topical steroids | + | + |
| 2 | 20 | F | Trunk and legs | 40 | none | + | + |
| 3 | 14 | F | Trunk, arms, and legs | 32 | Topical steroids | + | + |
| 4 | 31 | F | Trunk and legs | 72 | none | + | + |
| 5 | 21 | F | Trunk and arms | 24 | Topical steroids | + | + |
| 6 | 15 | M | Trunk, arms, and legs | 12 | Topical steroids | + | + |
| 7 | 22 | F | Trunk, arms, and legs | 26 | Topical steroids | + | + |
| 8 | 21 | M | Trunk, arms, and legs | 31 | Topical steroids | + | + |
| 9 | 19 | F | Trunk, arms, and legs | 37 | Topical steroids | + | + |
| 10 | 17 | F | Trunk and legs | 16 | Topical steroids | + | + |
| 11 | 18 | F | Trunk, arms, and legs | 22 | Topical steroids | + | + |
| 12 | 20 | M | Trunk and arms | 28 | Topical steroids | + | + |
| 13 | 19 | F | Trunk, arms, and legs | 20 | none | + | + |
| 14 | 16 | M | Trunk | 5 | Topical steroids | Absence of melanin | vitiligo |
| 15 | 20 | F | Trunk | 3 | Topical steroids | Absence of melanin | vitiligo |
| Mean | 19.2 | | | 26.9 | | | |

*(1) The lesions were mainly located on the trunk and limbs. (2) The duration of evolution was calculated from the early onset of hypopigmented patches, according to the patients' medical histories. (3) The RCM findings was the slight melanin reduction, but not melanin absence in the basal cell layer, and the monomorphous weakly refractile, oval-to-round cells in epidermis and weakly refractive cells with a round-to-oval cellular contour scattered within the papillary dermis or inside dermal papillae rings were the positive findings (+). (4) The histology and immunochemistry findings to confirm those RCM features and diagnosed as HMF was the "+" in the table.*

diagnosed as HMF, while two cases as vitiligo, based on our RCM examination, and was demonstrated by histology results, which showed the excellent correlation between RCM and histology findings.

Five of the 15 cases were male, 10 were female, and the average age of the 15 cases was 19.2. The average duration of evolution of the lesions was 26.9 months. The details of the enrolled cases are listed in **Table 1**. Clinically, the persistent, round-to-oval hypopigmentation with mild scales or not were distributed on the trunk, arms, and legs (**Figures 1a–c**).

When the normal skin was imaged with RCM, there were no significant inflammatory condition changes in honeycomb pattern stratum spinosum (**Figure 2a**) and no melanin changes in basal cell layer (**Figure 2b**). While for the lesions of vitiligo, the significant reduction of melanin contents or melanin absence was observed (**Figure 2c**) compared with the adjacent normal skin, and sometimes the slight infiltration of phagocytes and inflammatory cells in the superficial dermis was also recorded. The histology picture (**Figure 2d**) demonstrated the RCM findings.

The HMF lesions showed different changes based on the RCM imaging, as there was only slight reduction of melanin contents but no melanin absence in the basal cell layer. And the other significant changes were founded in stratum spinosum. The finding of monomorphous weakly refractile, oval-to-round cells on the basis of vesicle-like dark space was clearly elucidated in epidermis of the lesions by RCM (**Figures 3a,b**), which indicates the Pautrier's microabscesses on histopathology (**Figure 3c**). And weakly reflective cells with a round-to-oval cellular contour scattered within the papillary dermis or inside dermal papillae rings in the lesions were also observed. Immunohistochemistry analysis (**Figure 3d**) demonstrated the HMF was characterized by CD8+ T cells residing predominantly in the dermal papillae. Thirteen cases with these findings by RCM were confirmed by pathology results.

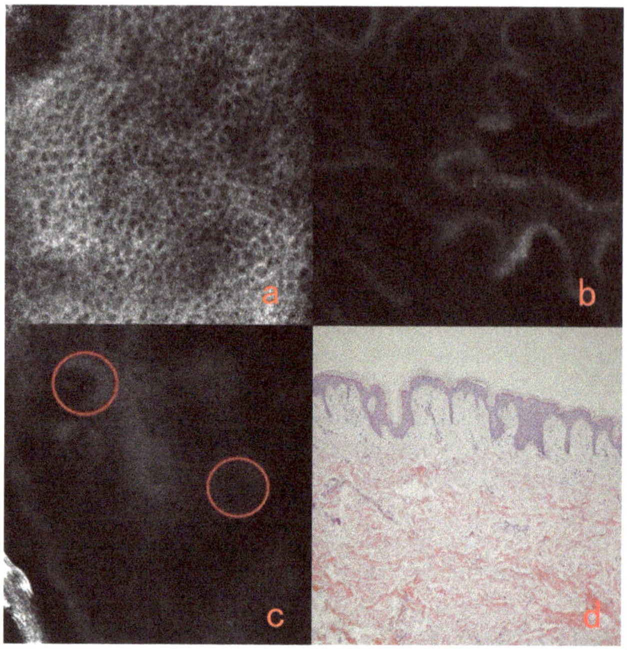


**FIGURE 2 |** The honeycomb pattern of stratum spinosum **(a)**, the normal basal cell layer, the dermal-epidermal junction of vitiligo **(c)** and the histology of vitiligo. There was no inflammation in the regular arranged honeycomb pattern of stratum spinosum **(a)**. There was no melanin reduction in the basal cell layer of normal DEJ **(b)**. The significant reduction or melanin absence (circles) in the basal cell layer of DEJ of vitiligo **(c)**. There is no melanin in basal cell layer of vitiligo **(d)**.

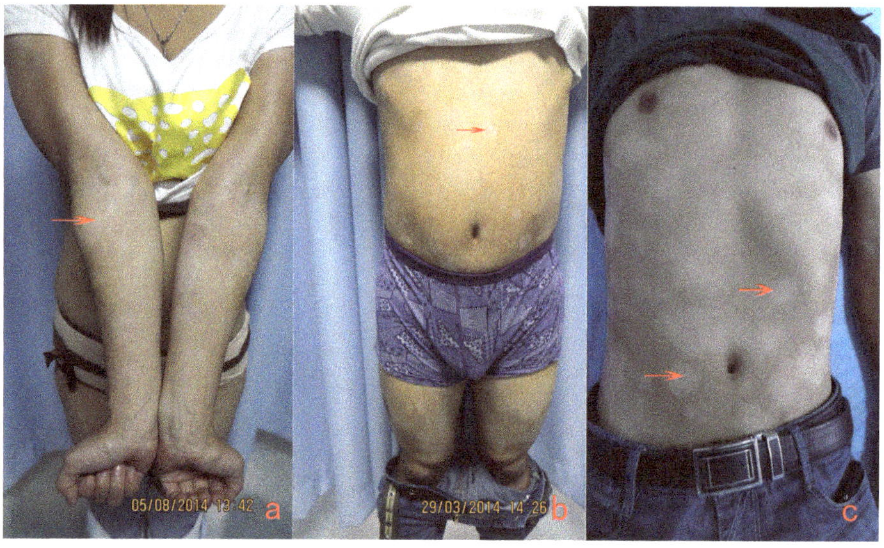


**FIGURE 1 |** The clinical image of three cases of HMF. An 18-year old woman with the hypopigmented patches for 2 years on arms **(a)** and legs, and a 25-year-old **(b)** and 19-year-old man **(c)**, with generalized lesions on bodies and limbs. The hypopigmentary patches were 2–5 cm in diameter, slightly scaly, with no infiltration (arrows).

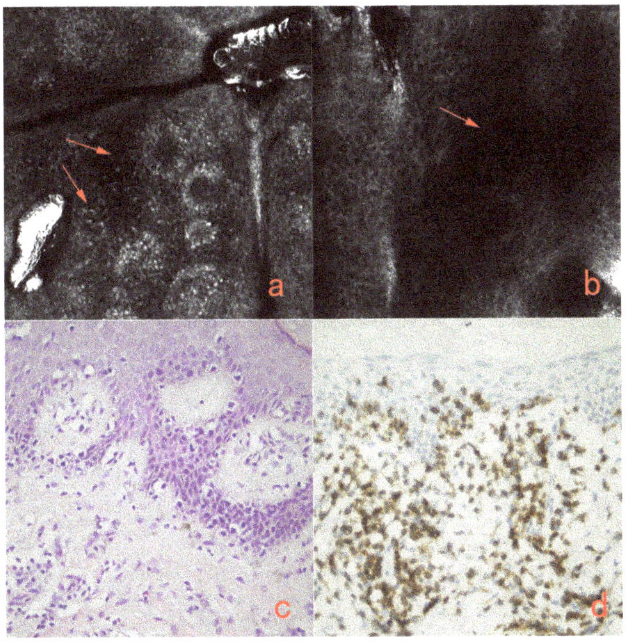


**FIGURE 3 |** The RCM image of HMF **(a,b)**, the histology of HMF **(c)** and immunochemistry-stained image of HMF **(d)**. The monomorphous weakly refractile, oval-to-round cells (**a,b**, arrows) on the basis of vesicle-like dark spaces were clearly elucidated in epidermis of the lesions by RCM, which indicates the Pautrier's microabscesses on histopathology **(c)**. Immunohistochemical analysis **(d)** demonstrated the HMF was characterized by CD8+ T cells residing predominantly in the dermal papillae.

## DISCUSSION

RCM imaging non-invasively shows nuclear and cellular-level morphology in human skin *in vivo* (11, 12). Imaging is based on the detection of single back-scattered photons from the optical section, and contrast is due to the relative variations in refractive indices and sizes of organelles and microstructures (11). Melanin is the natural and strongest contrast in the skin (11, 12), which indicates the significant role of RCM in the imaging of pigmented skin disorders. The cellular changes of the lesion in epidermis and superficial dermis could be imaged and compared with that of the adjacent normal skin. Ardigo et al. (13) first reported the characteristics of vitiligo in confocal images, and other related reports (14) revealed RCM is useful in the diagnosis and differential diagnosis of vitiligo and other hypopigmentary skin disorders. As previously mentioned, RCM has also been reported to be used in the screening of MF and showed relatively specific characteristics in confocal images (9, 10, 15, 16). The migration of abnormal inflammatory cells in the epidermis, the disorder of the basal cell layer, and infiltration of mononuclear inflammatory cells in superficial dermis of MF lesions could be imaged with RCM (15).

The pathology features of HMF are similar to MF. And the histology changes of HMF and vitiligo were located in epidermis and superficial dermis,which was within the penetration depth of RCM.

Our study revealed the melanin contents in the basal cell layer is different based on the RCM findings. Significant melanin reduction or melanin absence was found in vitiligo, while there was a slight reduction of melanin but not melanin loss in HMF. As reported previously, hypopigmentation of HMF may arise from a defect in the transfer of melanosomes from melanocytes to keratinocytes, with reversal of this defect after treatment (4). On the contrary, the significant reduction or total absence of melonosome and melanocytes is the characteristic in the vitiligo lesion (6). The other difference was focused on the stratum spinosum and superficial dermis. The finding of monomorphous weakly refractile, oval-to-round cells on the basis of vesicle-like dark space was regarded as the features of HMF by RCM, while commonly there were no changes in this layer in vitiligo. And weakly refractive cells with a round-to-oval cellular contour scattered within the papillary dermis or inside dermal papillae rings in HMF were also different with that of vitiligo because these changes were the characteristics of HMF in histology level. RCM and histology results had excellent correlation.

Our study highly indicated the role of RCM in the early detection and differential diagnosis of HMF and vitiligo. However, more cases with long time follow-up study were required to confirm our findings.

## ETHICS STATEMENT

The studies involving human participants were reviewed and approved by Ethics Committee of Shandong Provincial Institute of Dermatology and Venereology. Written informed consent to participate in this study was provided by the participants' legal guardian/next of kin. Written informed consent was obtained from the minor(s)' legal guardian/next of kin for the publication of any potentially identifiable images or data included in this article.

## AUTHOR CONTRIBUTIONS

HL and MG designed the study and prepared the manuscript. YL and LW collected the clinical and RCM data. XS collected the histology data. All authors contributed to the article and approved the submitted version.

## REFERENCES


1. Jawed SI, Myskowski PL, Horwitz S, Moskowitz A, Querfeld C. Primary cutaneous T-cell lymphoma (mycosis fungoides and Sézary syndrome): part I. Diagnosis: clinical and histopathologic features and new molecular and biologic markers. *J Am Acad Dermatol.* (2014) 70:205. doi: 10.1016/j.jaad.201307049
2. Ryan EA, Sanderson KV, Bartak P, Samman PD. Can mycosis fungoides begin in the epidermis? A hypothesis. *Br J Dermatol.* (1973) 88:419–29. doi: 10.1111/j.1365-2133.1973.tb15444.x
3. Muñoz-González H, Molina-Ruiz AM, Requena L. Clinicopathologic variants of mycosis fungoides. *Actas Dermosifiliogr.* (2017) 108:192–208. doi: 10.1016/j.adengl.201702010
4. Furlan FC, Sanches JA. Hypopigmented mycosis fungoides: a review of its clinical features and pathophysiology. *An Bras Dermatol.* (2013) 88:954–60. doi: 10.1590/abd1806-484120132336
5. Ardigó M, Borroni G, Muscardin L, Kerl H, Cerroni L. Hypopigmented mycosis fungoides in Caucasian patients: a clinicopathologic study of 7 cases. *J Am Acad Dermatol.* (2003) 49:264–70. doi: 10.1067/S0190-9622(03)00907-1
6. El-Darouti MA, Marzouk SA, Azzam O, Fawzi MM, Abdel-Halim MR, Zayed AA, et al. Vitiligo vs. hypopigmented mycosis fungoides (histopathological and immunohistochemical study, univariate analysis). *Eur J Dermatol.* (2006) 16:17–22.
7. Liu H, Lin Y, Nie X, Chen S, Chen X, Shi B, et al. Histological classification of melasma with reflectance confocal microscopy: a pilot study in Chinese patients. *Skin Res Technol.* (2011) 17:398–403. doi: 10.1111/j.1600-0846.201100517x
8. Rajadhyaksha M, Marghoob A, Rossi A, Halpern AC, Nehal KS. Reflectance confocal microscopy of skin *in vivo*: from bench to bedside. *Lasers Surg Med.* (2017) 49:7–19. doi: 10.1002/lsm22600
9. Agero AL, Gill M, Ardigo M, Myskowski P, Halpern AC., González S. *In vivo* reflectance confocal microscopy of mycosis fungoides: a preliminary study. *J Am Acad Dermatol.* (2007) 57:435–41. doi: 10.1016/j.jaad.200702026
10. Mancebo SE, Cordova M, Myskowski PL, Flores ES, Busam K, Jawed SI., et al. Reflectance confocal microscopy features of mycosis fungoides and Sézary syndrome: correlation with histopathologic and T-cell receptor rearrangement studies. *J Cutan Pathol.* (2016) 43:505–15. doi: 10.1111/cup12708
11. Rajadhyaksha M, Grossman M, Esterowitz D, Webb RH, Anderson RR. *In vivo* confocal scanning laser microscopy of human skin: melanin provides strong contrast. *J Invest Dermatol.* (1995) 104:946–52. doi: 10.1111/1523-1747ep12606215
12. Rajadhyaksha M, González S, Zavislan JM, Anderson RR, Webb RH. *In vivo* confocal scanning laser microscopy of human skin II: advances in instrumentation and comparison with histology. *J Invest Dermatol.* (1999) 113:293–303. doi: 10.1046/j.1523-1747.199900690x
13. Ardigo M, Malizewsky I., Dell'anna ML, Berardesca E, Picardo M. Preliminary evaluation of vitiligo using *in vivo* reflectance confocal microscopy. *J Eur Acad Dermatol Venereol.* (2007) 21:1344–50. doi: 10.1111/j.1468-3083.200702275x
14. Lai LG, Xu AE. *In vivo* reflectance confocal microscopy imaging of vitiligo, nevus depigmentosus and nevus anemicus. *Skin Res Technol.* (2011) 17:404–10. doi: 10.1111/j.1600-0846.201100521x
15. Zhu M, Yu W, Wang P, Liu J, Li Z, Dai H, et al. Reflectance confocal microscopy may be included as part of the diagnostic algorithm of early-stage mycosis fungoides. *Skin Res Technol.* (2020) 26:591–598. doi: 10.1111/srt12840
16. Melhoranse Gouveia B, Wells J, Kim J, Consuegra G, Longo C, Fernandez-Penas P. Systematic review and proposal of an *in vivo* reflectance confocal microscopy assessment tool for cutaneous lymphoma. *J Cutan Pathol.* (2020) 47:295–304. doi: 10.1111/cup13598

10

# Review of Machine Learning in Predicting Dermatological Outcomes

*Amy X. Du*[1*], *Sepideh Emam*[2†] *and Robert Gniadecki*[1†]

[1] *Division of Dermatology, Faculty of Medicine and Dentistry, University of Alberta, Edmonton, AB, Canada,* [2] *Information Services and Technology, University of Alberta, Edmonton, AB, Canada*

***Correspondence:***
*Amy X. Du*
*xdu@ualberta.ca*

† *These authors share senior authorship*

Artificial intelligence is a broad branch of computer science that has garnered significant interest in the field of medicine because of its problem solving, decision making and pattern recognition abilities. Machine learning, a subset of artificial intelligence, hones in on the ability of computers to receive data and learn for themselves, manipulating algorithms as they organize the information they are processing. Dermatology is at a particular advantage in the implementation of machine learning due to the availability of large clinical image databases that can be used for machine training and interpretation. While numerous studies have implemented machine learning in the diagnostic aspect of dermatology, less research has been conducted on the use of machine learning in predicting long-term outcomes in skin disease, with only a few studies published to date. Such an approach would assist physicians in selecting the best treatment methods, save patients' time, reduce treatment costs and improve the quality of treatment overall by reducing the amount of trial-and-error in the treatment process. In this review, we aim to provide a brief and relevant introduction to basic artificial intelligence processes, and to consolidate and examine the published literature on the use of machine learning in predicting clinical outcomes in dermatology.

**Keywords: artificial intelligence, machine learning, dermatology, prediction, clinical outcomes**

## INTRODUCTION

Artificial intelligence (AI) is a broad branch of computer science that has garnered significant interest in the field of medicine because of its problem solving, decision making, and pattern recognition abilities. Machine learning (ML), a subset of AI, hones in on the ability of computers to receive data and learn for themselves, manipulating algorithms as they organize the information they are processing. Dermatology is at a particular advantage in the implementation of ML due to the availability of large clinical image databases that can be used for machine training and interpretation. In fact, studies have already demonstrated the successful use of ML in classification and diagnosis of skin diseases, such as skin cancer (1, 2), eczema (3), psoriasis (4), onychomycosis (5) at a performance level equal or superior to board-certified dermatologists.

While numerous studies have implemented ML in the diagnostic aspect of dermatology (6), less research has been conducted on the use of ML in predicting long-term outcomes in skin disease, with only a few studies published to date. In an era of personalized medicine, there is a push toward a data-driven approach allowing for accurate prediction of long-term clinical outcomes for individual patients (7–9). Such an approach would assist physicians in selecting the best treatment methods, save patients' time, reduce treatment costs and improve the quality of treatment overall by reducing the amount of trial-and-error in the treatment process (8).

Machine learning techniques are very good at managing large amounts of high-level data from patient databases, such as electronic medical records, and are often able to detect sophisticated data patterns that traditional statistical methods are unable to delineate (7–9). These approaches have been used with increasing success to predict patient prognoses in many other areas of medicine, such as the risk of readmission after hospital discharge (10), cancer progression (11), diabetic complications (12, 13), cardiovascular mortality (14), and many others (15–17).

In this review, we aim to provide a brief and relevant introduction to basic AI processes, and to consolidate and examine the published literature on the use of ML in predicting clinical outcomes in dermatology.

## BRIEF OVERVIEW OF PRINCIPLES IN ARTIFICIAL INTELLIGENCE

Artificial intelligence can be subdivided in a number of ways, but in its simplest form, it can be broken into two main categories: strong AI and weak AI (**Figure 1**).

Strong AI refers to a programmed machine that takes on human-level cognition, with the capacity for consciousness, self-awareness and ethical decision-making (18). The machine has the competence to learn, on its own, to simultaneously conduct a number of complex tasks, and the capability of learning more based on what it already knows (19). Currently, strong AI does not exist outside the realm of science fiction.

Weak AI, on the other hand, does currently exist and is the process by which we train a machine to complete a specific, designated task. The machine simply acts upon and is bound by the rules and algorithms that are set for it. It does not have the capacity, unlike strong AI, to think and act beyond those parameters (19).

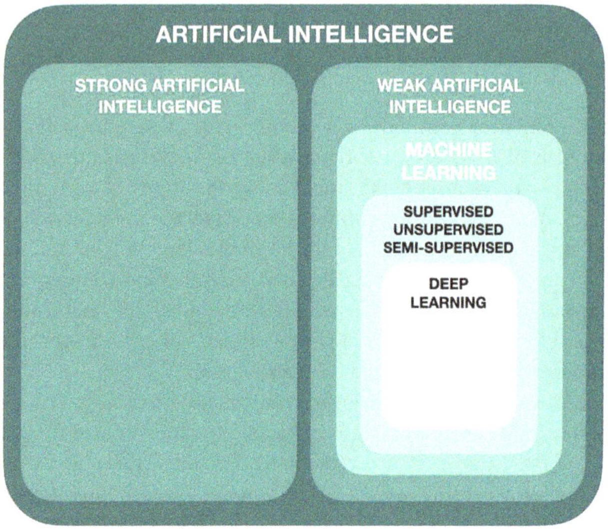


**FIGURE 1** | Subdivisions of artificial intelligence.

### Machine Learning

Machine learning is a subdivision of AI in which algorithmic models are trained to perform specific tasks by recognizing and learning patterns from the data it sees, rather than through explicit computer programming by a human expert. This process can be categorized as supervised, semi-supervised or unsupervised, with the most common method being supervised (20).

Supervised learning occurs when the algorithm system gains experience through training with a labeled dataset, and is then expected to categorize a new, unfamiliar data point. For example, in the case of recognizing benign vs. malignant skin lesions, the computer system would be provided with many images of skin lesions that have already been labeled as either being benign or malignant. Once training with these images is completed, the algorithm would then be tested by being presented with novel, unlabeled images to classify as either being benign or malignant (21).

When no training dataset is available for the corresponding output data, it is known as unsupervised learning. Very much like supervised learning, the goal of this type of learning is to place input data into categories. The main difference is that, in unsupervised learning, the input data are not labeled, and therefore, the model aims to categorize data based on their inherent features. This method of machine learning allows us to take a more open-ended approach to learn about the underlying distribution of data that may have been missed otherwise (22).

Finally, a hybrid method of machine learning, known as semi-supervised machine learning, combines aspects of supervised and unsupervised learning. In this approach, a large amount of unlabeled inputs are combined with a small amount of labeled inputs in an effort to lessen the challenge of data labeling (22).

### Deep Learning

Deep learning is a further subdivision of ML and refers to a specific type of learning that involves the use of artificial neural networks (ANN) (23). It is often used for unsupervised learning, as it is capable of learning from data that is unstructured and unlabeled. It is able to detect patterns in datasets that it has not been previously trained on. Deep learning functions by imitating the neural connections made in the human brain and are connected in a network of nodes, forming multiple layers.

### Performance Analysis of Machine Learning Algorithms

In order to statistically evaluate the performance of learning approaches, and to best determine which approach predicts with the highest accuracy, machine learning algorithms are often assessed using the area under the curve receiver operating characteristic (AUC-ROC). This test quantifies how accurately a model is able to distinguish between categories, typically in medicine, "disease" vs. "no disease." The ROC curve is plotted with the true positive rate on the y-axis against the false positive rate on the x-axis. The closer the AUC is to 1.0 for any given model, the better and more accurate the performance of that model (22).

## METHODS

A literature search on Ovid MEDLINE® was conducted in January 2020 for papers published from 2000-2019, to focus on recently published literature. The database was searched with relevant keywords in combination with the Boolean operators "AND" and "OR." The search included keywords from each of the following lists: dermatology, skin disease, skin cancer, psoriasis, or atopic dermatitis, AND artificial intelligence, machine learning, deep learning, or neural network, AND prediction, predicting, or outcome.

Inclusion criteria included: English language, original studies, and focusing on the prognostic utility of artificial intelligence/machine learning in dermatology (i.e., predicting outcomes, risk stratification, selection of best treatment). Exclusion criteria included: reviews, animal studies, case reports, systematic reviews, studies not published in English. Any studies focusing on the diagnostic utility of artificial intelligence/machine learning in dermatology, focusing on a different medical field, or not using machine learning methods were also excluded.

Our literature search yielded a total of 73 articles, among which 6 were deemed relevant to this review based on our inclusion and exclusion criteria.

## APPLICATIONS OF MACHINE LEARNING IN PREDICTING DERMATOLOGICAL OUTCOMES

A total of six studies on the use of machine learning in predicting dermatological outcomes have been published to date (**Table 1**). One study focused on the risk of biologic discontinuation in psoriasis patients (24), two studies investigated the risk of developing non-melanoma skin cancer (25, 26), one study looked at response to wart treatment modalities (27), one study explored the complexity of reconstructive surgery after periocular basal cell carcinoma excision (28), and one final study examined the risk of developing chronic venous ulcers in patients with cardiovascular disease (29).

Five of the six studies used a supervised approach of machine learning in their training and validation. Wang et al. (25) used a semi-supervised approach. Generally, the results of each study were presented with varying outcomes, but AUC was reported as the primary outcome in five of the six studies. Other outcomes reported included sensitivity and specificity (25, 26), accuracy (27), and positive and negative predictive values (28). Franciscis et al. reported outcomes in the form of "level-of-risk" (29). We are unable to directly compare the outcomes of all studies as the methodology of the studies vary.

**TABLE 1** | Summary of literature on the use of machine learning in predicting dermatological outcomes.

| Study | Type of supervision | End point | Results | Software(s) utilized | Data used |
|---|---|---|---|---|---|
| Emam et al. (24) | Supervised | Risk of discontinuation of biologic | AUC for predicted risk of discontinuation due to:<br>Any reason 0.95<br>Lack of efficacy 0.91<br>Adverse event 0.88<br>Other reasons 0.80 | Generalized linear model, support vector machine, decision tree, random forest, gradient boosted trees, deep learning | $n = 681$ psoriasis patients<br>13 clinically relevant features per patient |
| Wang et al. (25) | Semi-supervised | Risk of developing non-melanoma skin cancer | AUC 0.89<br>Sensitivity 83.1%<br>Specificity 82.3% | Convolutional neural network (deep learning) | $n = 9,494$, 1,829 non-melanoma skin cancer patients, 7,665 random non-cancer controls<br>20 clinically relevant features per patient |
| Roffman et al. (26) | Supervised | Risk of developing non-melanoma skin cancer | AUC 0.81<br>Sensitivity 86.2%<br>Specificity 62.7% | Artificial neural network (deep learning) | $n = 462,630$, 2,056 non-melanoma skin cancer patients, 460,574 non-cancer patients<br>13 clinically relevant features per patient |
| Khozeimeh et al. (27) | Supervised | Response to wart treatment method | Cryotherapy:<br>AUC 0.902, accuracy 80%<br>Immunotherapy:<br>AUC 0.813, accuracy 98% | Fuzzy logic and adaptive network-based fuzzy inference system (ANFIS) | $n = 180$, 90 patients in cryotherapy group, 90 patients in immunotherapy group<br>7 clinically relevant features per patient in the cryotherapy group, 8 in the immunotherapy group |
| Tan et al. (28) | Supervised | Complexity of reconstructive surgery after periocular basal cell carcinoma excision | Naïve Bayesian Classifier:<br>AUC 0.854<br>PPV 38.1%<br>NPV 94.1%<br>ADTree:<br>AUC 0.835<br>PPV 31%<br>NPV 97% | Decision table, Bayesian, tree-based methods, multivariate logistic regression, nearest neighbor classifier, support vector machine | $n = 156$ periocular BCC patients<br>7 clinically relevant features per patient |
| de Franciscis et al. (29) | Supervised | Risk of developing chronic venous ulcers in patients with chronic venous disease | CVU group level of risk $32.38 \pm 7.19\%$<br>Non-CVU group level of risk $8.34 \pm 3.38\%$ | Fuzzy logic to stratify CVD patients into CVU and non-CVU groups | $n = 77$, 40 patients with CVU, 37 patients without CVU<br>27 clinically relevant features |

Emam et al. considered seven different modeling techniques in evaluating a dataset of 681 psoriasis patients to determine which learner performed best in terms of accuracy, interpretability and runtime to predict risk of biologic discontinuation. Thirteen clinically relevant features per patient were analyzed. The Generalized Linear Model (GLM) outperformed the six other models that were tested. The AUC for predicted risk of discontinuation due to any reason was found to be 0.95, lack of efficacy was 0.91, adverse event was 0.88, and other reasons was 0.80 using the GLM (24).

Wang et al. and Roffman et al. used convolutional neural networks (CNN) (25) and artificial neural networks (ANN) (26), respectively, to delineate the risk of developing non-melanoma skin cancer. Both approaches are branches of deep learning and make use of the algorithm's ability to extract important classifying information at each node of a network of data. Both studies included data from non-melanoma skin cancer patients as well as an abundance of data from non-cancer patients. The system by Wang et al. analyzed data from a total of 9,494 patients, using 20 clinically relevant features per patient, and reported higher outcomes (AUC 0.89, sensitivity 83.1%, specificity 82.3%) than Roffman et al., which analyzed data from a total of 462,630 patients, using 13 clinically relevant features per patient (AUC 0.81, sensitivity 86.2%, specificity 62.7%).

Two studies used fuzzy rule-based systems to stratify patients into groups. Fuzzy logic is a flexible mathematical system that can model non-linear functions with arbitrary meaning. It is a system that very closely models human thinking and is able to handle a great degree of uncertainty (30). Khozeimeh et al. (27) aimed to predict patient responses to two wart treatment modalities: cryotherapy and immunotherapy. Important clinically relevant features were extracted from the dataset using the Apriori algorithm and converted into fuzzy rules for each group. Data from a total of 180 patients, 90 in each group, were analyzed. Seven fuzzy rules were generated for the cryotherapy group and eight fuzzy rules were generated for the immunotherapy group. The resulting AUC of the cryotherapy and immunotherapy datasets was 0.902 and 0.813, respectively. The accuracy of both datasets was 80 and 98%, respectively.

Franciscis et al. (29) also used fuzzy logic to stratify the risk factors for developing chronic leg ulcers in patients in patients living with chronic venous disease (CVD). Data from seventy-seven CVD patients, 40 patients with active ulceration, 37 without, was analyzed. Twenty-seven clinically relevant features were generated for each patient. Results of the study were reported as risk scores, with the group of CVD patients with active venous ulceration being 32.38 ± 7.19%, and the group of CVD patients without active venous ulceration being 8.34 ± 3.38%.

Finally, Tan et al. (28) considered ten machine learning algorithms to determine the most predictive model for surgical complexity post-periocular basal cell carcinoma (BCC) excision. Data from 156 periocular BCC patients was analyzed, with seven clinically relevant features per patient. The most predictive model was Naive Bayesian classifier, with an average AUC of 0.854, and positive (PPV) and negative predictive values (NPV) of 38.1 and 94.1%, respectively. The second-best model was Alternating Decision Tree, achieving an AUC of 0.835, PPV of 31% and NPV of 97%.

## DISCUSSION

Our review summarizes the current literature exploring the use of machine learning in predicting various dermatological outcomes. All studies conducted on this topic thus far have demonstrated promising outcomes. During a time where precision medicine is a focus of many clinicians, ML techniques provide a method for dermatologists to more accurately predict the clinical outcomes and prognoses of their patients in a variety of skin conditions.

When compared to traditional statistical methods, which focuses on inference, ML methodology focuses more on prediction (31). This is to say that ML methods aim to anticipate future behavior, rather than just drawing associations between data. ML is also particularly useful when looking at complex and detailed datasets with a large number of input variables. In fact, a larger sample size allows ML algorithms to better make associations within the data and thus, form more accurate outputs (32). Traditional statistical methods were designed to be most accurate and successful with a small to moderate number of input variables. As the number of inputs increases, the statistical models tend to become less precise.

While there are many benefits to the implementation of ML in a clinical dermatology setting, it is critical to discuss potential limitations to its implementation as well. One area of concern is the quantity of data required to operate ML algorithms. Some large dermatology patient registries do exist (33), however, there will need to be significantly more national and international collaboration to ensure that there is comprehensive coverage of dermatologic data.

Another limitation is the lack of ability for human operators to explain how ML algorithms make their conclusions. While there are methods to assess an algorithm's performance, there is no way to rationalize its decision. As such, they are often called "black box" technology (34). In this case, interpretation of the ML results by an experienced clinician is of utmost importance.

## FUTURE DIRECTIONS

Although early studies assessing the prognostic value of machine learning in dermatology have demonstrated promising outcomes, further research is needed. To address whether the use of ML in predicting outcomes is truly a worthwhile avenue for clinicians to explore, prospective randomized clinical trials are needed.

## CONCLUSION

Machine learning is a quickly advancing field in medicine and can be of great utility to clinicians in the near future, particularly in predicting the prognoses of complex dermatological conditions. As this technology advances, dermatologists will need to develop a foundational understanding of how it works and when it should be appropriately used in their clinical practice.

## AUTHOR CONTRIBUTIONS

AD, SE, and RG have all provided substantial contributions to the conception and design of the work. AD drafted the work, SE and RG revised it critically for important intellectual content. All authors provide approval for publication of the content and agree to be accountable for all aspects of the work in ensuring that questions related to the accuracy or integrity of any part of the work are appropriately investigated and resolved.

## REFERENCES


1. Esteva A, Kuprel B, Novoa RA, Ko J, Swetter SM, Blau HM, et al. Corrigendum: dermatologist-level classification of skin cancer with deep neural networks. *Nature.* (2017) 546:686. doi: 10.1038/nature 22985
2. Brinker TJ, Hekler A, Enk AH, Klode J, Hauschild A, Berking C, et al. A convolutional neural network trained with dermoscopic images performed on par with 145 dermatologists in a clinical melanoma image classification task. *Eur J Cancer.* (2019) 111:148–54. doi: 10.1016/j.ejca.2019. 02.005
3. Guzman LCD, De Guzman LC, Maglaque RPC, Torres VMB, Zapido SPA, Cordel MO. Design and evaluation of a multi-model, multi-level artificial neural network for eczema skin lesion detection. In: *2015 3rd International Conference on Artificial Intelligence, Modelling and Simulation (AIMS)* (Kota Kinabalu) (2015). doi: 10.1109/AIMS.2015.17
4. Shrivastava VK, Londhe ND, Sonawane RS, Suri JS. Computer-aided diagnosis of psoriasis skin images with HOS, texture and color features: A first comparative study of its kind. *Comput Methods Programs Biomed.* (2016) 126:98–109. doi: 10.1016/j.cmpb.2015.11.013
5. Han SS, Park GH, Lim W, Kim MS, Im Na J, Park I, et al. Deep neural networks show an equivalent and often superior performance to dermatologists in onychomycosis diagnosis: Automatic construction of onychomycosis datasets by region-based convolutional deep neural network. *PLoS ONE.* (2018) 13:e0191493. doi: 10.1371/journal.pone. 0191493
6. Ferris LK, Harkes JA, Gilbert B, Winger DG, Golubets K, Akilov O, et al. Computer-aided classification of melanocytic lesions using dermoscopic images. *J Am Acad Dermatol.* (2015) 73:28. doi: 10.1016/j.jaad.2015. 07.028
7. Shickel B, Tighe PJ, Bihorac A, Rashidi P. Deep EHR: a survey of recent advances in deep learning techniques for electronic health record (EHR) analysis. *IEEE J Biomed Health Inform.* (2018) 22:1589–604. doi: 10.1109/JBHI.2017.2 767063
8. Goldstein BA, Navar AM, Pencina MJ, Ioannidis JPA. Opportunities and challenges in developing risk prediction models with electronic health records data: a systematic review. *J Am Med Inform Assoc.* (2017) 24:198–208. doi: 10.1093/jamia/ocw042
9. Cheng Y, Wang F, Zhang P, Hu J. Risk prediction with electronic health records: a deep learning approach. In: *Proceedings of the 2016 SIAM International Conference on Data Mining Proceedings. (Society for Industrial and Applied Mathematics)* (Miami, FL) (2016). p. 432–40. doi: 10.1137/1.978161197 4348.49
10. Morgan DJ, Bame B, Zimand P, Dooley P, Thom KA, Harris AD, et al. Assessment of machine learning vs standard prediction rules for predicting hospital readmissions. *JAMA Netw Open.* (2019) 2:e190348. doi: 10.1001/jamanetworkopen.2019.0348
11. Kehl KL, Elmarakeby H, Nishino M, Van Allen EM, Lepisto EM, Hassett MJ, et al. Assessment of deep natural language processing in ascertaining oncologic outcomes from radiology reports. *JAMA Oncol.* (2019) 5:1421–9. doi: 10.1001/jamaoncol.2019.1800
12. Dagliati A, Marini S, Sacchi L, Cogni G, Teliti M, Tibollo V, et al. Machine Learning Methods to Predict Diabetes Complications. *J Diabetes Sci Technol.* (2018) 12:295–302. doi: 10.1177/19322968177 06375
13. Gulshan V, Peng L, Coram M, Stumpe MC, Wu D, Narayanaswamy A, et al. Development and validation of a deep learning algorithm for detection of diabetic retinopathy in retinal fundus photographs. *JAMA.* (2016) 316:2402–10. doi: 10.1001/jama.2016.17216
14. Motwani M, Dey D, Berman DS, Germano G, Achenbach S, Al-Mallah MH, et al. Machine learning for prediction of all-cause mortality in patients with suspected coronary artery disease: a 5-year multicentre prospective registry analysis. *Eur Heart J.* (2017) 38:500–7. doi: 10.1093/eurheartj/ ehw188
15. Hogarty DT, Mackey DA, Hewitt AW. Current state and future prospects of artificial intelligence in ophthalmology: a review. *Clin Exp Ophthalmol.* (2019) 47:128–39. doi: 10.1111/ceo.13381
16. Rajkomar A, Dean J, Kohane I. Machine Learning in Medicine. *N Eng J Med.* (2019) 380:1347–58. doi: 10.1056/NEJMra18 14259
17. Chen JH, Asch SM. Machine learning and prediction in medicine - beyond the peak of inflated expectations. *N Engl J Med.* (2017) 376:2507–9. doi: 10.1056/NEJMp1702071
18. Hildt E. Artificial intelligence: does consciousness matter? *Front Psychol.* (2019) 10:1535. doi: 10.3389/fpsyg.2019.01535
19. Flowers JC. Strong and weak ai: deweyan considerations. In: *AAAI Spring Symposium: Towards Conscious AI Systems.* Available online at: http://ceur-ws.org/Vol-2287/paper34.pdf.
20. Erickson BJ, Korfiatis P, Akkus Z, Kline TL. Machine learning for medical imaging. *Radiographics.* (2017) 37:505–15. doi: 10.1148/rg.20171 60130
21. Moore MM, Slonimsky E, Long AD, Sze RW, Iyer RS. Machine learning concepts, concerns and opportunities for a pediatric radiologist. *Pediatr Radiol.* (2019) 49:509–16. doi: 10.1007/s00247-018-4277-7
22. Chartrand G, Cheng PM, Vorontsov E, Drozdzal M, Turcotte S, Pal CJ, et al. Deep learning: a primer for radiologists. *Radiographics.* (2017) 37:2113–31. doi: 10.1148/rg.2017170077
23. Hogarty DT, Su JC, Phan K, Attia M, Hossny M, Nahavandi S, et al. Artificial intelligence in dermatology-where we are and the way to the future: a review. *Am J Clin Dermatol.* (2020) 21:41–7. doi: 10.1007/s40257-019-00462-6
24. Emam S, Du AX, Surmanowicz P, Thomsen SF, Greiner R, Gniadecki R. Predicting the Long-term Outcomes of Biologics in Psoriasis Patients using Machine Learning. *Br J Dermatol.* (2020) 182:1305–7. doi: 10.1111/bjd. 18741
25. Wang H-H, Wang Y-H, Liang C-W, Li Y-C. Assessment of deep learning using nonimaging information and sequential medical records to develop a prediction model for nonmelanoma skin cancer. *JAMA Dermatol.* (2019) 155:1277–83. doi: 10.1001/jamadermatol.2019.2335
26. Roffman D, Hart G, Girardi M, Ko CJ, Deng J. Predicting non-melanoma skin cancer via a multi-parameterized artificial neural network. *Sci Rep.* (2018) 8:1701. doi: 10.1038/s41598-018-19907-9
27. Khozeimeh F, Alizadehsani R, Roshanzamir M, Khosravi A, Layegh P, Nahavandi S. An expert system for selecting wart treatment method. *Comput Biol Med.* (2017) 81:167–5. doi: 10.1016/j.compbiomed.2017.01.001
28. Tan E, Lin F, Sheck L, Salmon P, Ng S. A practical decision-tree model to predict complexity of reconstructive surgery after periocular basal cell carcinoma excision. *J Eur Acad Dermatol Venereol.* (2017) 31:14012. doi: 10.1111/jdv.14012
29. de Franciscis S, Fregola S, Gallo A, Argirò G, Barbetta A, Buffone G, et al. PredyCLU: a prediction system for chronic leg ulcers based on fuzzy logic; part I - exploring the venous side. *Int Wound J.* (2016) 13:12529. doi: 10.1111/iwj.12529
30. Phuong NH, Kreinovich V. Fuzzy logic and its applications in medicine. *Int J Med Inform.* (2001) 62:5 doi: 10.1016/S1386-5056(01)00160-5

31. Bzdok D, Altman N, Krzywinski M. Statistics versus machine learning. *Nat Methods.* (2018) 15:233–4. doi: 10.1038/nmeth.4642
32. Miotto R, Li L, Kidd BA, Dudley JT. Deep patient: an unsupervised representation to predict the future of patients from the electronic health records. *Sci Rep.* (2016) 6:26094. doi: 10.1038/srep26094
33. DiMarco G, Hill D, Feldman SR. Review of patient registries in dermatology. *J Am Acad Dermatol.* (2016) 75:824–9. doi: 10.1016/j.jaad.2016.03.020
34. Wang F, Kaushal R, Khullar D. Should health care demand interpretable artificial intelligence or accept "black box" medicine? *Ann Intern Med.* (2020) 172:59. doi: 10.7326/M19-2548

# 11

# Ultra-High-Frequency Ultrasound in the Evaluation of Paediatric Pilomatricoma Based on the Histopathologic Classification

*Li Li*[1†], *Jiaosheng Xu*[2*†], *Siwei Wang*[3] *and Jun Yang*[4]

*[1] Department of Dermatology, Plastic Surgery Hospital, Chinese Academy of Medical Sciences and Peking Union Medical College, Beijing, China, [2] Department of Dermatology, Beijing Children's Hospital, National Center for Children's Health, Capital Medical University, Beijing, China, [3] Department of Radiology, Beijing Children's Hospital, National Center for Children's Health, Capital Medical University, Beijing, China, [4] Institute of Biomedical Engineering, Chinese Academy of Medical Sciences, Tianjin, China*

***Correspondence:**
*Jiaosheng Xu*
*xujiaosheng@sina.com*

*[†] These authors have contributed equally to this work*

**Background:** Pilomatricoma (PM) is one of the most common benign tumours in children. However, the inaccuracy of preoperative diagnosis and evaluation is high. Non-invasive examinations, including dermoscopy and ultrasound are helpful for diagnosing and evaluating PM. To date, ultra-high-frequency ultrasonographic features of PM have been rarely studied.

**Objective:** We aimed to investigate the ultra-high frequency ultrasonographic features of PM in a large paediatric cohort and to determine the associations of these features with the clinical features of different histological subtypes of PM.

**Methods:** This was a retrospective study. Patients who had both preoperative ultra-high-frequency ultrasonographic evaluation and pathological diagnosis of PM were enrolled. A series of infantile haemangiomas and cutaneous cysts during the same period were included as controls. Histological findings, including the stage, calcifying type, and ultrasonographic features of each lesion, were described.

**Results:** A total of 133 patients with PM were included, and 147 PM lesions were analysed. The male-to-female ratio was 1:1.58, and the median age of onset was 91 (range: 10–188) months. On ultra-high-frequency ultrasonography, PM presented as heterogeneous (144/147, 98.0%), well-demarcated (143/147, 97.3%), and hypoechoic (126/147, 85.7%) tumours located between the deep dermis and subcutaneous tissue (139/147, 94.6%). The most common features were internal echogenic foci (135/147, 91.8%), hypoechoic rim (133/147, 90.5%), and posterior acoustic shadowing (94/147, 63.9%). Fourteen (9.5%) lesions were histologically categorized in the early stage, 58 (39.5%) in the fully developed stage, 65 (44.2%) in the early regressive stage and 10 (6.8%) in the late regressive stage. Three calcifying types, including scattered dots, clumps and arcs, were observed on histologic examination, which corresponded well with grey-scale imaging on ultra-high-frequency ultrasonography. Each calcifying type was significantly different in various histological stages ($P$ = 0.001), among which scattered dots were mainly present in the early and fully developed stage and arc-shaped calcifying were present in the regressive stages. Calcification was observed in skin cysts, while there was more frequent posterior enhancement, less frequent posterior shadowing, and hypoechoic rim than PM. Haemangioma also presented as a hypoechoic tumour on grey-scale imaging. However, haemangioma was homogeneous and rarely calcifying.

**Conclusions:** PM is a heterogeneous, well-demarcated, hypoechoic tumour located between the deep dermis and the subcutis on ultra-high-frequency ultrasonography. The most common features are internal echogenic foci (calcifying) and hypoechoic rim. Calcifying types can help in the staging of PM. Ultra-high-frequency ultrasound is a useful tool for the diagnosis and evaluation of PM.

**Keywords: pilomatricoma, ultrasound, ultra-high-frequency, diagnosis, paediatric, histopathologic**

## INTRODUCTION

Pilomatricoma (PM) is a benign, deep dermal or subcutaneous tumour that is derived from the hair cortex cell (1). It is also known as calcifying epithelioma of Malherbe (2). PM has a bimodal peak, first presenting in the first two decades and second in the sixth decade. It has a female predominance. Lesions mainly occur on the head, neck, and extremities, which range from 0.5 to 3 cm in size. On palpation, PM is characteristically hard and nodular or multinodular. The overlying skin can be bluish or reddish, which can mimic infantile haemangioma (3).

The typical histopathology of PM shows sheets of basaloid cells and masses of eosinophilic cornified material containing ghost cells. Calcification is mostly observed in the ghost cell regions. Based on morphological features, PM is classified into four stages (4). The first is the early stage and is typified by small cystic structures lined by squamoid and basaloid epithelium, and shadow cell formation. The second is the fully developed stage characterized by large neoplasms lined by basaloid epithelium at their periphery; within, it comprises clusters of shadow cells. The third is the early regressive stage with no apparent epithelial lining but has basaloid cell foci at the periphery; within, it comprises shadow cells surrounded by granulation tissue. The fourth is the late regressive stage, demonstrating no obvious parenchymal cells but irregularly shaped, partially confluent masses of faulty hair material, and calcification or ossification, with little or no inflammatory infiltrate.

The clinical diagnosis rate of PM is usually very low. Prior reviews have shown that preoperative diagnostic accuracy for PMs ranges from 21 to 32% (1, 5). The most common differential diagnoses are haemangiomas and several types of skin cysts (3, 6). Non-invasive techniques such as dermoscopy and ultrasonography have been increasingly used to aid in the diagnosis of skin tumours (7, 8). They are popular in paediatric patients because they are simple, quick, and non-invasive. Hughes et al. reported on the sonographic diagnosis of PM in childhood with a diagnostic accuracy of 80% (9). On ultrasound, PM is a heterogeneous tumour with inner echogenic foci and a hypoechoic rim or a completely echogenic mass with strong posterior acoustic shadowing in the subcutis (10). The reliable diagnostic features for PM are hypoechogenicity, heterogenicity, internal echogenic foci, hypoechoic rim, and posterior shadowing (11).

However, another study has demonstrated PM as a well-defined hyperechoic or calcific nodule in subcutaneous fat (12), probably because of the different frequencies of the transducer. Therefore, we used ultra-high-frequency ultrasound to explore the ultrasonographic features and determine the histopathological correlations of PM.

## MATERIALS AND METHODS

This was a retrospective study. From April 2016 to December 2020, paediatric patients with histopathologically proven PM after surgery at the Plastic Surgery Hospital, Chinese Academy of Medical Sciences and Peking Union Medical College and Beijing Children's Hospital, Capital Medical University, were included in this study with Institutional Review Board approval. Written informed consent for the procedure was obtained from all the patients' parents. A series of 91 infantile haemangiomas and 28 cutaneous cysts (including dermal and epidermal cysts) during the same period were included as controls.

### Ultra-High-Frequency Ultrasonography

Ultrasonographic examination was performed using an ultrasound skin scanner (MD-300S, MEDA, Co., Ltd., Tianjin, China) equipped with 50 MHz linear array transducers. The grey-scale images were captured by the bioscope (MD-300SII, MEDA, Co., Ltd., Tianjin, China) attached to the ultrasonograph. Each image was reviewed by an experienced radiologist and dermatologist. The analysis of ultrasonographic features included tumour location, margin, shape, size, echo texture, and echogenicity. The tumour echo texture was recorded as homogeneous or heterogeneous, and echogenicity as hyperechoic if the tumour echogenicity was higher than that of dermal connective tissues. The following ultrasonographic features were observed in the study: inner echogenic foci, posterior shadowing, hypoechoic rim, and peritumoral hyperechogenicity. Inner echogenic foci were defined as calcification regardless of posterior shadowing. The calcification mode was described as an arc, scattered dots, or clumps.

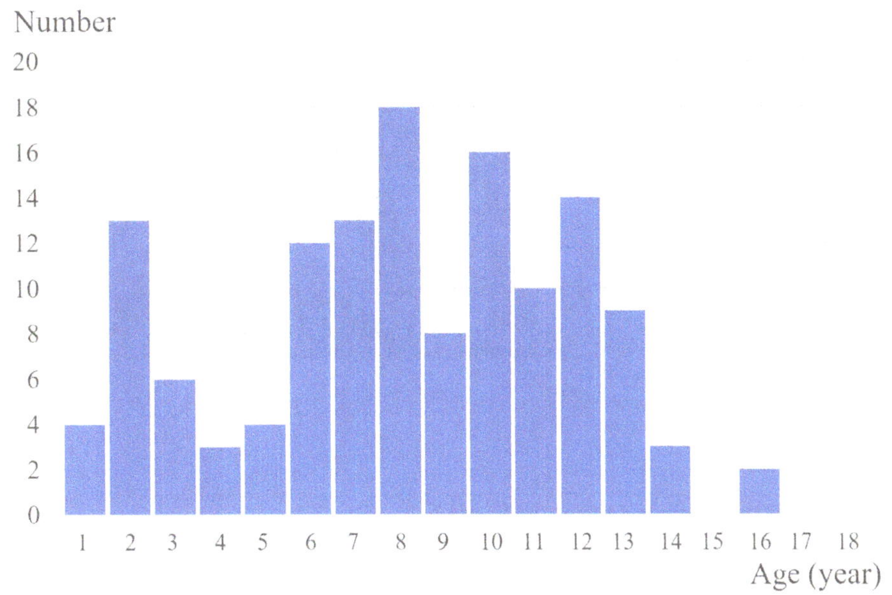


**FIGURE 1** | Population distribution with age in pediatric PM.

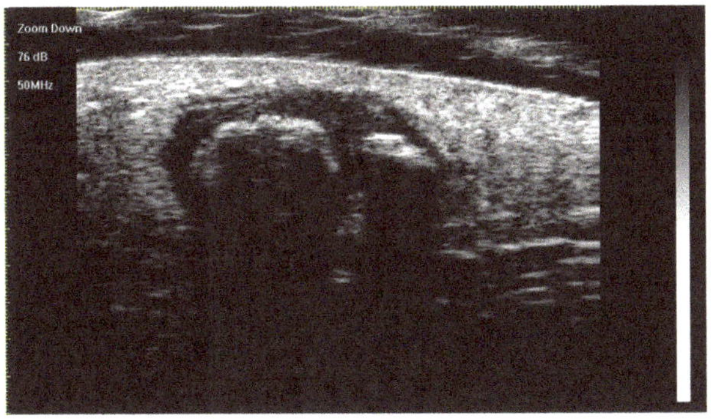


**FIGURE 2** | The lesion is a heterogeneous, well-demarcated, hypoechoic tumour located between the deep dermis and the subcutis with typical ultra-high-frequency ultrasonographic features, including internal echogenic foci, hypoechoic rim, and posterior acoustic shadowing.

## Histopathology

After ultrasonographic examination, the tumours were arranged for complete resection and routine histological examination. Each lesion was examined by the experienced pathologist and dermatologist. Based on the morphology of tumour and infiltrating cells, the histopathological stages were categorized into four stages as in a previous report (4): early, fully developed, early regressive, or late regressive stage. The calcification shape at low magnification was described as scattered dots, an arc, or clumps.

## Statistical Analyses

Descriptive statistics for categorical variables are presented as numbers. The differences between two independent categorical variables were evaluated using the chi-square test (Fisher exact test when necessary) and Kruskal-Wallis rank sum tests were performed for grouped data. SPSS Windows version 26.0 (SPSS Inc., Chicago, IL, USA) was used for the statistical analyses and $P < 0.05$ was considered statistically significant.

# RESULTS

All patients underwent preoperative ultra-high-frequency ultrasound examination and were histologically diagnosed with PM post-operatively.

## Clinical and Histopathological Findings of PM

A total of 133 patients with PM were included, and 147 PM lesions were analysed. The male-to-female ratio was 1:1.58. The median age of onset was 91 (range: 10–188) months, and two peaks were observed (ages 2 and 8) (**Figure 1**). The meantime from onset to diagnosis was 14.8 months (range: 0.5–132 months). One hundred and twenty-two patients had a solitary lesion, eight patients had two lesions, and three patients had three lesions (113 in the head and neck, 11 in the trunk and 23 in the extremities). The mean length of the largest tumour diameter was 0.8 (range: 0.3–7) cm. Fourteen (9.5%) lesions were histologically categorized in the early stage (**Figure 3A**), 58 (39.5%) in the fully developed stage (**Figure 4A**), 65 (44.2%) in the early regressive stage (**Figure 5A**), and 10 (6.8%) in the late regressive stage (**Figure 6A** and **Table 1**). Three calcifying types, including scattered dots, clumps and arcs, were observed on low power histologically. On high power, bone formation was noted in the arc-shaped calcification but not in the other two types.

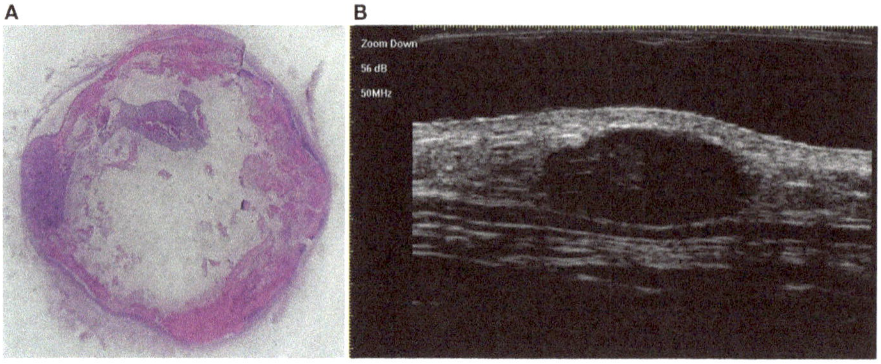


**FIGURE 3 |** The histological presentation [**(A)** HE, original magnification × 10] and ultra-high frequency ultrasound **(B)** of PM in the early stage, indicating no obvious calcification and cystic formation.

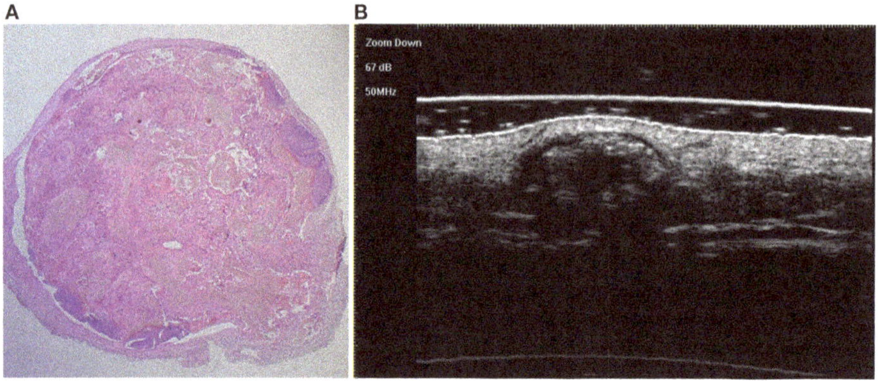


**FIGURE 4 |** The histological presentation [**(A)** HE, original magnification × 25] and ultra-high frequency ultrasound **(B)** of PM in the fully developed stage, indicating scattered dot calcification.

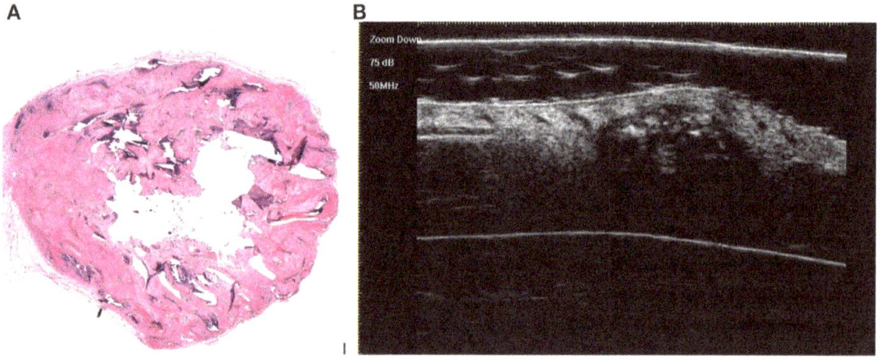


**FIGURE 5 |** The histological presentation [**(A)** HE, original magnification × 10] and ultra-high frequency ultrasound **(B)** of PM in the early regressive stage, indicating clump calcification.

## Ultrasonographic Features of PM and Its Clinical and Histological Correlations

On ultra-high frequency ultrasonography, PM manifested as heterogeneous (144/147, 98.0%), well-demarcated (143/147, 97.3%), and hypoechoic (126/147, 85.7%) tumours located between the deep dermis and subcutaneous tissue (139/147, 94.6%) (**Table 2**). The lesions were mostly arranged in a regular shape (oval or round), while a few were irregular in shape. The most common features were internal echogenic foci (135/147, 91.8%), hypoechoic rim (133/147, 90.5%), posterior shadowing (94/147, 63.9%), and peritumoral hyperechogenicity (45/147, 30.6%) (**Figure 2**). Three calcifying types, including

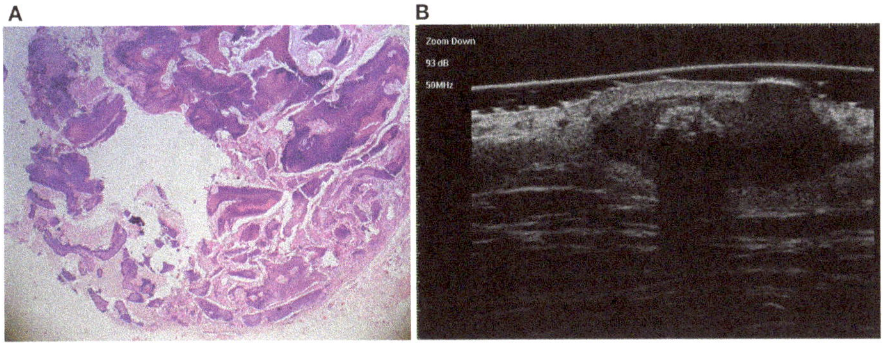


**FIGURE 6 |** The histological presentation [**(A)** HE, original magnification × 25] and ultra-high frequency ultrasound **(B)** of PM in the early regressive stage, indicating arc calcification.

**TABLE 1 |** Ultra-high-frequency ultrasonographic features in various histological stages.

| **Ultrasound features** | **Histological staging** | | | | **P*** |
|---|---|---|---|---|---|
| | **Early (*n* = 14)** | **Fully developed (*n* = 58)** | **Early regressive (*n* = 65)** | **Late regressive (*n* = 10)** | |
| **Echogenicity** | | | | | |
| Hyperechoic | 2 | 8 | 11 | 0 | |
| Hypoechoic | 12 | 50 | 54 | 10 | |
| **Echotexture** | | | | | |
| Homogeneous | 2 | 1 | 0 | 0 | |
| Heterogeneous | 12 | 57 | 65 | 10 | |
| **Margin** | | | | | 0.001 |
| Well | 13 | 57 | 63 | 10 | |
| Ill | 1 | 1 | 2 | 0 | |
| **Calcification** | 8 | 53 | 60 | 10 | |
| Scattered dots | 5 | 34 | 20 | 0 | |
| Clumps | 3 | 17 | 28 | 4 | |
| An arc | 0 | 2 | 12 | 6 | |
| **Hypoechoic rim** | 13 | 57 | 63 | 10 | |
| **Posterior shadowing** | 1 | 30 | 55 | 8 | |
| **Posterior enhancement** | 3 | 6 | 0 | 0 | |
| **Peritumoral hyperechogenicity** | 2 | 23 | 18 | 2 | |

*Kruskal-Wallis rank-sum test.

scattered dots, clumps, and arcs, were observed on ultra-high frequency ultrasonography corresponding well with the histological manifestations (**Figures 3B**, **4B**, **5B**, **6B**). Each calcifying type was significantly different in the various histological stages ($P < 0.05$), among which scattered dots were mainly presented in the early and developed stages, while arc-shaped calcifications were present in the regressive stages. The different stages were observed in one lesion (**Figure 7**). Posterior enhancement was observed only in the early (3/14) and fully developed (6/58) stages, when cystic architecture formation was detected histologically (**Table 2**).

## Comparison With PM From Infantile Haemangioma and Skin Cysts

A total of 91 patients with infantile haemangioma and 28 patients with skin cysts were enrolled as controls. The male-to-female ratio was 1:2.6 and 1:0.87, respectively. The mean age of onset was 3 (range: 1–20) months and 41 (range: 3–204) months, respectively. Infantile haemangioma also presented as a well-defined (81/91, 89.0%), and hypoechoic tumour (90/91, 98.9%) on grey-scale imaging. However, infantile haemangiomas were irregular (81/91, 89.0%) in shape and homogenous (88/91, 96.7%), rarely with calcification (2/91, 2.2%), and mostly located in the dermis (79/91, 86.8%). In addition, hypoechoic rim, posterior shadowing, posterior enhancement, and peritumoral hyperechogenicity were rarely observed in infantile haemangiomas. Calcification was observed in skin cysts (5/28, 17.9%), while there was more frequent posterior enhancement (24/28, 85.7%), less frequent posterior shadowing (3/28, 10.7%), and less hypoechoic rim (2/28, 7.1%) than in PM (**Table 2**).

# DISCUSSION

In our study of the paediatric population, PM had a predilection for girls and the lesions mostly presented as solitary nodules,

**TABLE 2 |** Comparison of PM with hemangioma and skin cysts on ultrasound.

| Ultrasonographic features | PM | Hemangioma | *P** | PM | Cysts | *P** |
|---|---|---|---|---|---|---|
| **Shape** | | | 0.001 | | | NS |
| Round/oval | 143 | 10 | | 143 | 26 | |
| Irregular | 4 | 81 | | 4 | 2 | |
| **Location** | | | 0.001 | | | 0.001 |
| Dermis | 8 | 79 | | 8 | 19 | |
| Dermis to subcutaneous layer | 139 | 12 | | 139 | 9 | |
| **Largest diameter (mean, mm)** | 0.8 (0.3–7) | 0.7 (0.6–8) | NS | 0.8 (0.3–7) | 0.6 (0.5–1.2) | NS |
| **Echogenicity** | | | 0.001 | | | NS |
| Hyperechoic | 21 | 1 | | 21 | 11 | |
| Hypoechoic | 122 | 90 | | 122 | 17 | |
| **Echotexture** | | | 0.001 | | | 0.001 |
| Homogeneous | 3 | 88 | | 3 | 19 | |
| Heterogeneous | 140 | 3 | | 140 | 9 | |
| **Margin** | | | 0.01 | | | 0.001 |
| Well | 143 | 81 | | 143 | 20 | |
| Ill | 4 | 10 | | 4 | 6 | |
| **Internal echogenic foci** | | 0.001 | | | 0.001 | |
| Scattered dots | 59 | 1 | | 59 | 4 | |
| Clumps | 52 | 1 | | 52 | 1 | |
| An arc | 20 | 0 | | 20 | 0 | |
| **Hypoechoic rim** | 140 | 1 | 0.001 | 143 | 2 | 0.001 |
| **Posterior shadowing** | 94 | 0 | 0.001 | 94 | 3 | 0.001 |
| **Posterior enhancement** | 9 | 1 | NS | 9 | 24 | 0.001 |
| **Peritumoral hyperechogenicity** | 45 | 1 | 0.001 | 45 | 2 | 0.001 |

*NS, not significant; PM, pilomatricoma.*
**Chi-square test.*

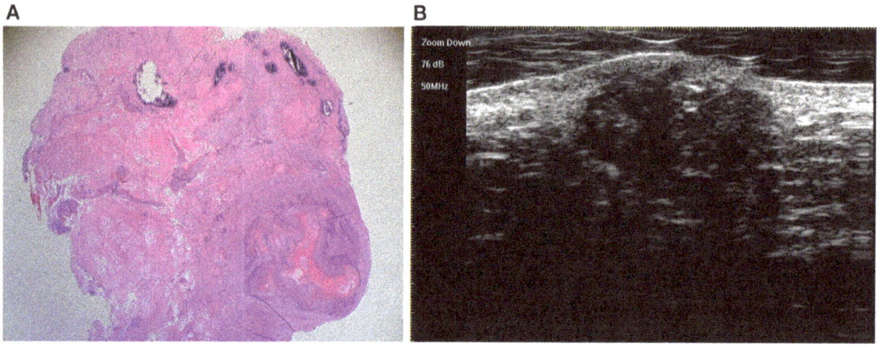


**FIGURE 7 |** The last three stages overlap in one lesion, which is detected by histology [**(A)** original magnification × 25] and ultra-high frequency ultrasound **(B)**.

mainly occurring in the head and neck area, as previously reported (12). However, two peaks of onset in paediatric population were observed in our study. PMs in children present a great challenge in clinical diagnosis and treatment, especially regarding the first peak onset age. Although PM is one of the most common skin tumours in children, its clinical diagnosis is very low (1, 6). The accurate diagnosis rate in accordance with post-operative histopathology is <35% (1). Ultrasonographic assessment can improve the diagnosis of PM (11, 13, 14).

The ultrasonographic features of PM have been described in several studies (9–13), and include calcification in the heterogeneous background of the hypoechoic area, posterior acoustic shadowing, hypoechoic rim, and peritumoral hyperechogenicity. The background of the hyperechoic areas was also described (12). These ultrasonographic features of PM were observed in the present study. According to our data, most of the cases were hypoechoic on ultra-high frequency ultrasonography. On histopathology, this hypoechoic area demonstrated infiltrates of basaloid, ghost cells, and reactive inflammation accordingly. The high ratio of hypoechogenicity was detected mainly due to the use of ultra-high-frequency transducers in our study, which improved the lesion tissue resolution (7).

The most common ultrasonographic features of PM are calcification and a hypoechoic rim compared with infantile haemangiomas and skin cysts. The ultra-high-frequency ultrasound is sensitive to display minimal calcification. Calcification on ultrasound mainly presented as scattered dots, clumps, and arcs, which is consistent with the previous reports (15). The morphology of the calcification is well-demonstrated on histopathology. Moreover, various histological stages notably displayed distinct calcifying types in our study. In the early and fully developed stages, scattered dots were the main type of calcification, whereas in the regressive stages, arc-shaped calcifications were the main type. Clumps can manifest in all the histological stages. Histopathologic examination reveals that the hypoechoic rim represents a connective tissue capsule surrounding the tumour. Unlike various types of skin cysts, there is no cystic wall in PM, which is lined with compact epithelial tissues. This annular connective loose connective tissue in PM was well-demonstrated characteristically on high frequency ultrasonography as a hypoechoic rim. The overall analysis of calcification and the hypoechoic rim can help in the diagnosis of PM. Moreover, the evolution of calcification reflects the PM process (4). The analysis of calcifying type on preoperative ultrasound may aid in the staging of PM.

Clinically, the overlying skin of some PMs may manifest as bruises or reddish hues. On ultrasound, infantile haemangioma also presents as a hypoechoic tumour, as in PM. Occasionally, PM may manifest as a confluent colour Doppler flow, mimicking haemangioma. However, infantile haemangioma often manifests in a homogeneous manner compared to PM and rarely displays calcification on grey-scale imaging. Calcification can be present in skin cysts on ultrasound. However, the calcifying type mainly present as scattered dots in the skin cysts. In addition, a hypoechoic rim is rarely present, while posterior acoustic enhancement is common in skin cysts.

The main method for PM management is surgical resection. However, surgery is usually not accepted for PM in young children because of the risk associated with surgery and systemic anaesthesia. Thus, ultra-high-frequency ultrasonography can be used to detect PM progression according to the calcifying type when a follow-up strategy is adopted. PM evolves into a regressive stage with age and can be resected with more safety at an older age. Moreover, preoperative evaluation of location, size, margin, and shape can be obtained by ultra-high-frequency ultrasonography.

In summary, PM is a heterogeneous, well-demarcated, hypoechoic tumour located between the deep dermis and subcutis on ultra-high-frequency ultrasonography. The most common features are calcification and a hypoechoic rim. Calcifying types can help in the staging of PM. Ultra-high-frequency ultrasound seems a useful tool for the diagnosis and evaluation of PM.

To our knowledge, this is the largest sample of PM used to explore ultra-high-frequency ultrasonographic characteristics based on histopathological stages. However, this study was limited by its retrospective nature and lack of vascularity analysis on colour Doppler ultrasonography. Further prospective studies with larger samples should be initiated to expatiate the results described herein.

## ETHICS STATEMENT

The studies involving human participants were reviewed and approved by Plastic Surgery Hospital, Chinese Academy of Medical Sciences and Beijing Children's Hospital, Capital Medical University. Written informed consent to participate in this study was provided by the participants' legal guardian/next of kin. Written informed consent was obtained from the individual(s), and minor(s)' legal guardian/next of kin, for the publication of any potentially identifiable images or data included in this article.

## AUTHOR CONTRIBUTIONS

LL and JX conceptualized and designed the study, drafted the initial manuscript, and reviewed and revised the manuscript. JX conceptualized and designed the study, coordinated and supervised data collection, conducted the initial analyses, drafted the initial manuscript, and critically reviewed the manuscript for important intellectual content. SW and JY designed the data collection instruments, collected data, conducted the initial analyses, and reviewed and revised the manuscript. All authors approved the final manuscript as submitted and agree to be accountable for all aspects of the work.

## REFERENCES


1. Julian CG, Bowers PW. A clinical review of 209 pilomatricomas. *J Am Acad Dermatol.* (1998) 39(2 Pt 1):191–5. doi: 10.1016/S0190-9622(98)70073-8
2. Malherbe A, Chenantis J. Note sur l'epitheliome calcifie des glandes sebacees. *Prog Med.* (1880) 8:826–8.
3. Hassanein AH, Alomari AI, Schmidt BA, Greene AK. Pilomatrixoma imitating infantile hemangioma. *J Craniofac Surg.* (2011) 22:734–6. doi: 10.1097/SCS.0b013e318207f29f

4. Kaddu S, Soyer HP, Hodl S, Kerl H. Morphological stages of pilomatricoma. *Am J Dermatopathol.* (1996) 18:333–8. doi: 10.1097/00000372-199608000-00001
5. Cevik HB, Erkan M, Kayahan S, Bulut G, Gumustas SA. A skin tumor from an orthopedic oncology perspective: Pilomatrixoma in extremities (11 years experience with 108 cases). *Dermatol Ther.* (2019) 32:e13004. doi: 10.1111/dth.13004
6. Jones CD, Ho W, Robertson BF, Gunn E, Morley S. Pilomatrixoma: a comprehensive review of the literature. *Am J Dermatopathol.* (2018) 40:631–41. doi: 10.1097/DAD.0000000000001118
7. Izzetti R, Vitali S, Aringhieri G, Nisi M, Oranges T, Dini V, et al. Ultra-high frequency ultrasound, a promising diagnostic technique: review of the literature and single-center experience. *Can Assoc Radiol J.* (2020). doi: 10.1177/0846537120940684. [Epub ahead of print].
8. Zaballos P, Llambrich A, Puig S, Malvehy J. Dermoscopic findings of pilomatricomas. *Dermatology.* (2008) 217:225–30. doi: 10.1159/000148248
9. Hughes J, Lam A, Rogers M. Use of ultrasonography in the diagnosis of childhood pilomatrixoma. *Pediatr Dermatol.* (1999) 16:341–4. doi: 10.1046/j.1525-1470.1999.00090.x
10. Lin SF, Xu SH, Xie ZL. Calcifying epithelioma of malherbe (Pilomatrixoma): clinical and sonographic features. *J Clin Ultrasound.* (2018) 46:3–7. doi: 10.1002/jcu.22517
11. Choo HJ, Lee SJ, Lee YH, Lee JH, Oh M, Kim MH, et al. Pilomatricomas: the diagnostic value of ultrasound. *Skeletal Radiol.* (2010) 39:243–50. doi: 10.1007/s00256-009-0678-x
12. Lim HW, Im SA, Lim GY, Park HJ, Lee H, Sung MS, et al. Pilomatricomas in children: imaging characteristics with pathologic correlation. *Pediatr Radiol.* (2007) 37:549–55. doi: 10.1007/s00247-007-0461-x
13. Marino MA, Ascenti G, Cardia R, Ieni A, Colonna MR. Pilomatrixoma of the right thigh: sonographic-pathologic correlation in a young man. *Radiol Case Rep.* (2020) 15:230–3. doi: 10.1016/j.radcr.2019.11.007
14. Ubals M, Castany A, Bassas P, Mollet J, Aparicio G, Garcia-Patos V. Utility of ultrasound in a rapidly growing cutaneous nodule in an infant. *J Pediatr.* (2017) 180:290–290e1. doi: 10.1016/j.jpeds.2016.09.038
15. Hwang JY, Lee SW, Lee SM. The common ultrasonographic features of pilomatricoma. *J Ultrasound Med.* (2005) 24:1397–402. doi: 10.7863/jum.2005.24.10.1397

12

# Nailfold Capillaroscopy with USB Digital Microscopy in Connective Tissue Diseases: A Comparative Study of 245 Patients and Healthy Controls

*Kumutnart Chanprapaph*[†]*, Wuttidej Fakprapai*[†]*, Preeyachat Limtong*[†] *and Poonkiat Suchonwanit*[*†]

*Division of Dermatology, Faculty of Medicine, Ramathibodi Hospital, Mahidol University, Bangkok, Thailand*

***Correspondence:**
*Poonkiat Suchonwanit*
*poonkiat@hotmail.com*

**Background:** Nailfold capillaroscopy (NFC) is a valuable tool to detect microcirculation abnormalities in connective tissue diseases (CTDs). However, whether the universal serial bus (USB) digital microscopy used as onychoscopy is as effective as the videocapillaroscopy in determining the diagnostic and prognostic values of CTDs remains to be determined.

**Objective:** This study aims to investigate NFC features of systemic lupus erythematosus (SLE), dermatomyositis (DM), and systemic sclerosis (SSc) patients and compare with normal controls as well as examine which feature could differentiate among CTDs. Furthermore, we aim to explore different capillaroscopic abnormalities and their association with disease activity.

**Methods:** Nailfold images were taken from patients and healthy controls using a USB digital microscopy. Patterns on the capillary morphology, diameter, architecture, and density were recorded and compared. We further determined the NFC findings in SLE, DM, and SSc and corresponded to their respective disease activity scoring system.

**Results:** A total of 245 participants, consisting of 54 SLE, 32 DM, and 51 SSc patients, as well as 108 controls, were enrolled. All capillaroscopic features, except for tortuous capillaries, were significantly more common in CTDs than healthy control (all $p < 0.05$). A multinomial logistic regression analysis revealed that bushy capillaries had significantly higher odds for both SLE and DM than SSc (OR: 4.10, 95% confidence interval (CI): 1.71–9.81, $p = 0.002$ and OR: 7.82, 95% CI, 2.86–21.38, $p < 0.001$, respectively). Elongated capillaries demonstrated significant odds for SLE compared with SSc (OR: 3.35, 95% CI: 1.005–11.20, $p = 0.049$), while prominent subpapillary plexus showed greater odds for SLE compared with both DM and SSc (OR: 2.75, 95% CI: 1.07–7.02, $p = 0.03$ and OR: 5.78, 95% CI: 2.29–14.58, $p < 0.001$, respectively). The presence of hemorrhage, enlarged capillaries, and the low-density index had significantly higher odds in favor of SSc than SLE. Bushy capillaries were the only pattern with a strong association for DM over SSc. The presence of enlarged capillaries indicated higher SLE severity, but no specific finding was related to DM or SSc skin scores.

**Conclusions:** Nailfold capillaroscopic examination using a digital microscope is a valuable method for the diagnosis of SLE, DM, and SSc. Several morphologic patterns can help differentiate among CTDs; however, the prognostic significance of this method requires further investigations.

**Keywords: capillaroscopy, dermoscopy, nailfold, systemic lupus erythematosus, dermatomyositis, systemic sclerosis**

## INTRODUCTION

Nailfold capillaroscopy (NFC) represents the best method to analyze microvascular abnormalities among connective tissue diseases (CTDs) since capillaroscopic changes of the nailfold have been well established in many CTDs. It is commonly used for differentiating primary from secondary Raynaud's phenomenon and for the diagnosis of scleroderma-spectrum disorders, including systemic sclerosis (SSc), dermatomyositis (DM), undifferentiated CTD, and mixed CTD (1). NFC changes can also be detected in other chronic autoimmune rheumatic diseases, namely systemic lupus erythematosus (SLE), Sjogren's syndrome, rheumatoid arthritis, and antiphospholipid syndrome (2–5).

SSc is a prototype of scleroderma-spectrum disorders which exhibits the typical scleroderma pattern through NFC assessments. Characteristic capillaroscopic changes of scleroderma contain enlarged capillaries, bushy capillaries, capillary hemorrhage, disorganization of the normal distribution of capillaries, and avascular area (6). At present, nailfold microvascular abnormalities are of great importance both at the time of diagnosis and during follow-up and have been established as a part of the most recent classification criteria for the diagnosis of SSc, the American College of Rheumatology and European League Against Rheumatism (ACR/EULAR) 2013 for SSc criteria (7).

Capillaroscopic alterations were described in patients with inflammatory myopathies, typically exhibiting scleroderma-capillary patterns. DM patients appear to have more frequent nailfold capillary abnormality than polymyositis. Giant capillaries and bushy capillaries with other characteristics in the scleroderma pattern were found in 74% of cases (8). Conversely, NFC changes in SLE have been documented to be less specific (2, 9). The most frequent capillaroscopic features of SLE are tortuous capillaries, elongated capillaries, and prominent subpapillary plexus (10, 11).

Although NFC is extremely useful for detecting various nailfold abnormalities, being the gold standard to discover microvascular changes in the nailfold, it requires a special equipment, the videocapillaroscopy, which is relatively expensive, time consuming, and not widely available in most healthcare settings. Videocapillaroscopy is the current gold standard for NFC assessment (12). Dermoscopy is an easily applicable, low-cost, noninvasive diagnostic technique generally used among dermatologists to evaluate inflammatory and pigmentary skin conditions. There are broadly two types of dermoscopy: (i) hand-held dermoscopy, allowing 10–20 times magnification and (ii) videodermoscopy, providing higher magnification up to 1,000 times (13). Hair and scalp dermoscopy, also known as trichoscopy, has become a standard evaluation for alopecia and other scalp disorders (14). Currently, trichoscopic features among CTDs have been well described and may indicate their diagnostic and prognostic values (15–19). Onychoscopy refers to the examination of the nail unit using dermoscopy. It has been further adapted for the assessment of nailfold vascular abnormalities. There is growing evidence suggesting that microvascular nailfold changes reflect the presence of certain autoantibodies and the disease activity in patients with CTDs (8, 11, 20–29). However, whether the NFC changes possess prognostic values in rheumatic disorders remains to be determined.

Currently, reports on nailfold capillaroscopic features using a digital microscope as an onychoscopy in CTDs are limited, and direct comparison among the most common rheumatologic disorders, namely, SLE, DM, and SSc are sparse. This study aimed to explore the differences among onychoscopic microvascular features in SLE, DM, SSc, and healthy controls. The secondary objective was to determine NFC findings and their association to the disease activity.

## MATERIALS AND METHODS

This cross-sectional, case-control study was approved by the Mahidol University Institutional Review Board (MURA 2019/263) and conducted at Ramathibodi Hospital, Bangkok, Thailand from February 2018 to February 2019. Informed consent to participate in the study was obtained from SLE, DM, and SSc patients, as well as healthy controls. SLE individuals who fulfilled the Systemic Lupus International Collaborating Clinics (SLICC) 2012 criteria and/or American College of Rheumatology (ACR) 1997 criteria (30), DM cases that met the Bohan and Peter criteria and/or the European League Against Rheumatism/American College of Rheumatology (EULAR/ACR) IIM criteria (31), and patients with SSc who satisfied the ACR/EULAR 2013 SSc criteria and/or the ACR 1980 criteria were recruited from the rheumatology and/or dermatology connective tissue disease clinics (7). The diagnosis and assessment of disease activity were made by a rheumatology-dermatology specialist. For healthy controls, healthcare personnel and patients who presented at the dermatology outpatient department for minor or cosmetic consultations, except for conditions involving the nails, and did not report signs and symptoms of CTD were recruited. Patients

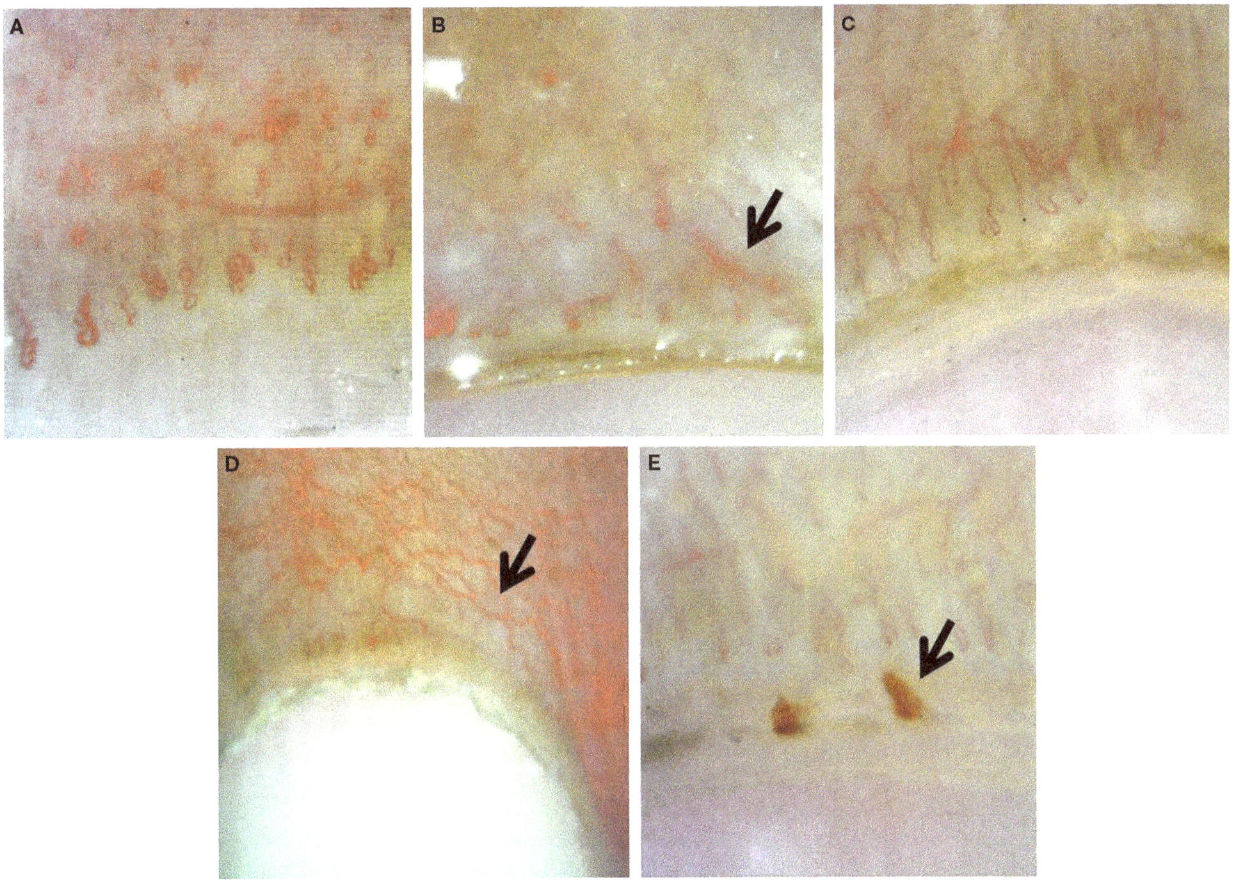


**FIGURE 1 |** Onychoscopic morphologic features: **(A)** tortuous capillaries, **(B)** bushy capillaries, **(C)** elongated capillaries, **(D)** prominent subpapillary plexus, and **(E)** capillary hemorrhage.

with other CTDs such as overlapping CTD, rheumatoid arthritis, Sjogren's syndrome, mixed CTD, and undifferentiated CTD were excluded from the study. Other exclusion criteria were patients who had traumatized finger and vascular occlusive diseases.

Nailfold examination was performed by a universal serial bus (USB) digital microscope with a polarizing light (Dinolite®; AnMo Electronics Corporation, Hsinchu, Taiwan) on both 4th and 5th fingers with × 200 magnification because their capillaries are the most visible. All examinations were operated by the same investigator. Patients were acclimatized for a minimum of 15–20 min before the examination at a room temperature (20–25°C). A drop of immersion oil was applied to the nailfold skin to improve resolution (32). Examination of the first distal row of capillaries was done to assess nailfold capillaroscopic features. Four consecutive images of each finger were captured. A blinded evaluation of images was conducted by an expert dermatologist.

Documented onychoscopic microvascular features consisted of morphology, diameter, architecture, and density of the nailfold capillaries. Morphologic parameters included tortuous capillaries (curled, crossed, or meandering capillaries; **Figure 1A**) (32), bushy capillaries (one capillary with three buddings; **Figure 1B**) (33), elongated capillaries (capillary loops longer than 300 $\mu$m; **Figure 1C**) (9, 34, 35), subpapillary plexus (vascular network at the base of the finger; **Figure 1D**) (34), and hemorrhages (extracapillary brown aggregations of erythrocytes and dived into punctate and confluent hemorrhages; **Figure 1E**) (9, 32, 35). The diameter index consisted of enlarged capillaries (capillaries with a diameter of arterial or venous limb wider than 20 $\mu$m; **Figure 2A**) (36), and giant capillaries (capillaries with a diameter wider than 50 $\mu$m; **Figure 2B**) (9, 32, 34). Architectural features included disorganized capillaries (irregular capillary pattern; **Figure 3A**) (34) and avascular area (distinct area in the nailfold where two or more adjacent capillaries are missing; **Figures 3B–D**) (34). Furthermore, the avascular area was quantitatively classified as grade 0 (no avascular area), grade 1 (mild or one or two avascular areas per millimeter), grade 2 (moderate or more than two avascular areas per millimeter), and grade 3 (severe or large and confluent avascular area) (35, 37). Capillary density was defined as the number of capillary loops in a 1-mm span of the distal row (9, 34, 37). We obtained capillary density by counting only the visible end row capillaries under a 90° angle. A capillary loop was considered a distal loop if the angle between the apex of that capillary and the apex of its two adjacent capillaries is >90° (**Figure 4**) (38). Any of the aforementioned

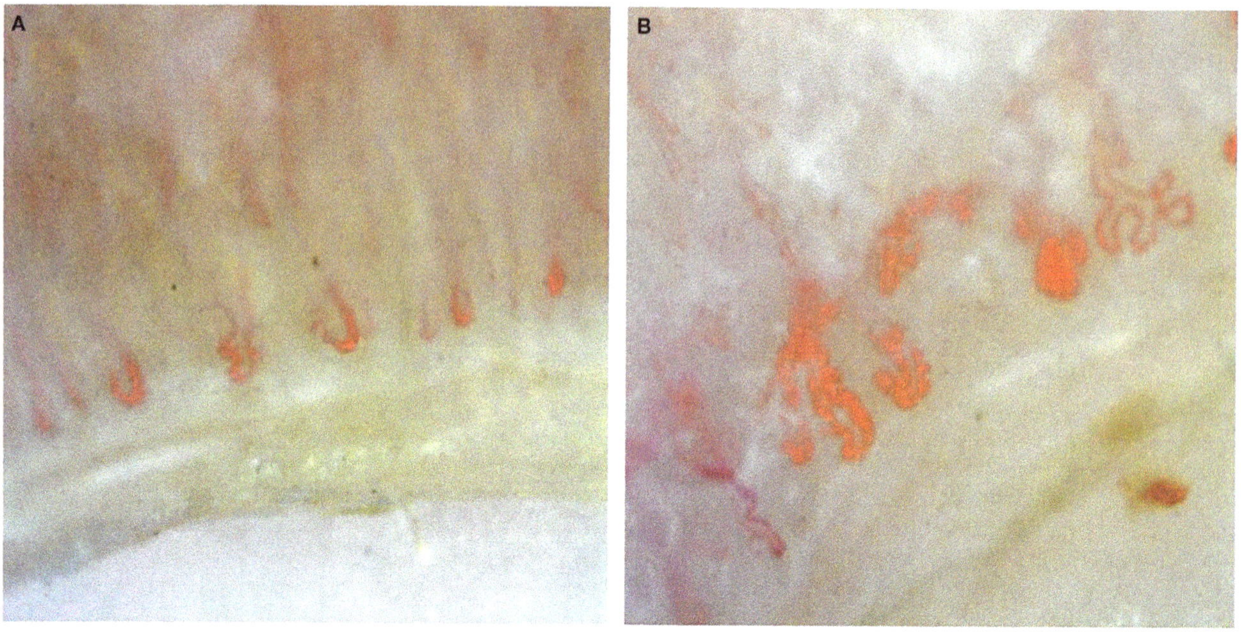

**FIGURE 2 |** Diameter index of onychoscopy: **(A)** enlarged capillaries and **(B)** giant capillaries.

features found at least in one finger was considered positive for capillary abnormality.

Nailfold capillaroscopic features among the three CTDs and controls were compared. Additionally, the correlation between onychoscopic microvascular changes and disease activity was additionally evaluated. The disease activity in SLE was assessed by using the Systemic Lupus Erythematosus Disease Activity Index 2000 (SLEDAI-2K) (39). We also evaluated the NFC changes in association to the skin scores of DM and SSC by using the Cutaneous Assessment tool for Myositis (CAT activity score) and modified Rodnan skin score, respectively (40, 41).

Data were analyzed using Stata 14.0 (Stata Corp LLC, College Station, TX). Results were expressed as mean ± standard deviation (SD) for continuous data and percentage for categorical data. Statistical analysis employed the chi-squared test or Fisher's exact test for categorical data and one-way ANOVA or Kruskal-Wallis test for continuous data. Multinomial logistic regression was used to determine the correlation among the three CTDs. A $p$-value of <0.05 was considered statistically significant. The magnitude of association was presented as odds ratio (OR) accounting for a 95% confidence interval (CI).

## RESULTS

Of 255 subjects included in the study, 10 were excluded due to the diagnosis of overlapping CTD ($n = 5$), inadequate data to assess disease severity ($n = 3$), and having traumatized fingers ($n = 2$). The remaining patients for SLE, DM, and SSc groups were 54, 32, and 51, respectively. For healthy controls, 108 subjects were enrolled. **Table 1** demonstrates demographic data in patients with SLE, DM, SSc, and healthy controls. The mean age of the SLE cases was younger than DM and SSc patients (34.9, 52.2, and 56.8, respectively). Female predominance was observed in patients with CTDs. All patients and healthy controls had Fitzpatrick skin type III-V and were of Southeast Asian ethnicity. Raynaud's phenomenon was reported in 5 (9.3%), 4 (12.5%), and 29 (56.9%) of SLE, DM, and SSc patients, respectively. Anti U1-ribonucleoprotein (U1RNP) antibody was present in 14/35 (40%) of SLE, 0/22 (0%) of DM, and 3/30 (10%) of SSc cases. Patients manifesting Raynaud's phenomenon and/or anti-U1RNP antibody were found in 15 (40.5%), 4 (16.7%), and 29 (69%) of SLE, DM, and SSc groups, respectively.

The comparison between onychoscopic microvascular features in patients with CTDs versus healthy controls revealed that all features, except for tortuous capillaries, were found more in CTDs with statistical significance (all $p < 0.05$) (**Table 2**). A comparison of NFC changes in SLE, DM, and SSc demonstrated that morphologic patterns consisting of bushy capillaries, subpapillary plexus, hemorrhage, and enlarged capillaries were significantly different among the three conditions. Bushy capillary pattern favored SLE and DM over SSc ($p < 0.001$), whereas elongated capillaries and subpapillary plexus were prominent features of SLE ($p = 0.003$ and $p < 0.001$, respectively). Hemorrhage and enlarged capillaries were also predominant in SSc ($p < 0.001$). The dilated capillaries and avascular areas were seen more in SSc patients, which was statistically greater than SLE and DM cases ($p = 0.01$ and $p = 0.004$, respectively). A quantitative analysis on the degree of avascular areas revealed that the majority of SLE cases had no or mild (72.2%), DM patients had mild to moderate (78.2%), while SSc cases had moderate to severe (64.7%) avascular areas (**Supplementary Table 1**).

A multinomial logistic regression analysis comparing nailfold capillaroscopic findings among the three CTDs is demonstrated

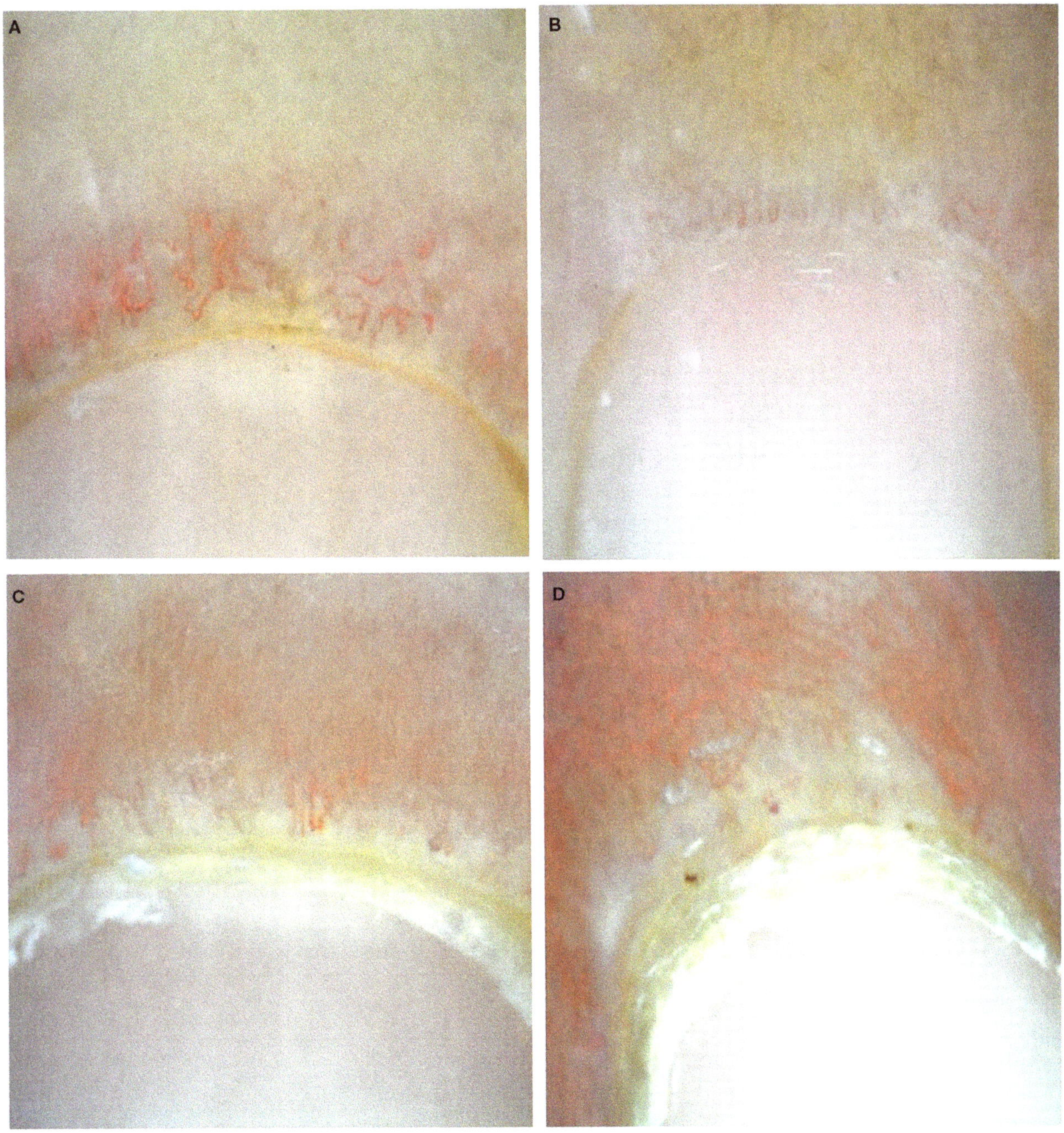


**FIGURE 3** | Onychoscopic architectural features: **(A)** disorganized capillaries, **(B)** avascular area grade 1, **(C)** grade 2, and **(D)** grade 3.

in **Table 3**. The results on morphologic pattern revealed that the presence of bushy capillaries had significantly higher odds for having both SLE and DM than SSc (OR: 4.10, 95% CI: 1.71–9.81; $p = 0.002$ and OR: 7.82, 95% CI: 2.86–21.38; $p < 0.001$, respectively). Elongated capillaries demonstrated significant odds for SLE compared with SSc (OR: 3.35, 95% CI: 1.005–11.20; $p = 0.049$), while prominent subpapillary plexus showed greater odds for SLE compared with both DM and SSc (OR: 2.75, 95% CI: 1.07–7.02; $p = 0.03$ and OR: 5.78, 95% CI: 2.29–14.58; $p < 0.001$, respectively). For other morphological and architectural patterns (i.e., hemorrhage, enlarged capillaries, and avascular area) as well as the low-density index, significantly higher odds were in favor of SSc than SLE. Bushy capillaries were the only pattern that showed a strong association for DM over SSc (OR: 7.82, 95% CI: 2.86–21.38; $p < 0.001$). We further performed quantitative analysis on the degree of avascular areas. The absence of avascular

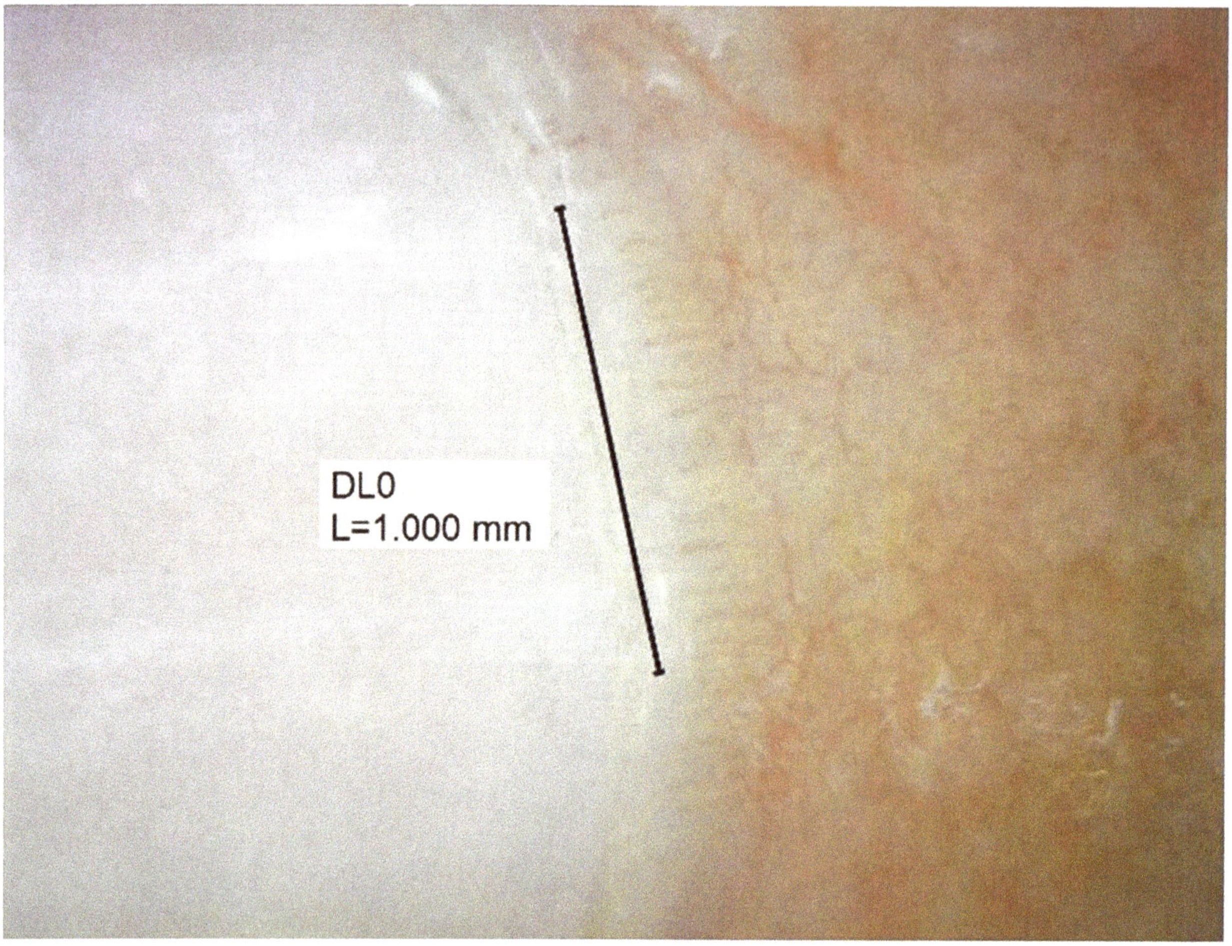


**FIGURE 4 |** Assessment of capillary density, counting the visible end row capillaries under a 90° angle.

**TABLE 1 |** Comparison of demographic data of patients with connective tissue diseases and healthy controls.

| Variable | SLE ($N$ = 54) | DM ($N$ = 32) | SSc ($N$ = 51) | Controls ($N$ = 108) |
|---|---|---|---|---|
| Mean age (year ± SD) | 34.9 ± 15.5 | 52.2 ± 16.9 | 56.8 ± 12.5 | 35.2 ± 10.4 |
| Sex | | | | |
| • Male | 6 (11.1%) | 8 (25%) | 9 (17%) | 41 (37.9%) |
| • Female | 48 (88.9%) | 24 (75%) | 42 (83%) | 67 (62.1%) |
| • F/M ratio | 8:1 | 3:1 | 4.6:1 | 1.6:1 |
| Mean disease duration (year ± SD) | 7.6 ± 8.9 | 3.8 ± 4.5 | 7.2 ± 6.0 | – |
| Fitzpatrick skin type | III–V | III–V | III–V | III–V |
| Southeast asian descent | 54 (100%) | 32 (100%) | 51 (100%) | 108 (100%) |

*DM, dermatomyositis; F, female; M, male; SD, standard deviation; SLE, systemic lupus erythematosus; SSc, systemic sclerosis.*

area revealed higher odds for SLE over SSc, while extensive avascular area (grades 2–3) had significantly greater odds for SSc and DM (**Supplementary Table 2**).

The correlation between NFC findings and disease activity of CTDs is shown in **Table 4**. The presence of enlarged capillaries was significantly associated with higher median

**TABLE 2 |** Comparison of onychoscopic features between connective tissue diseases and healthy controls.

| Onychoscopic features | SLE (*N* = 54) | DM (*N* = 32) | SSc (*N* = 51) | *p*-Value (among CTDs) | Controls (*N* = 108) | *p*-Value (CTDs vs. controls) |
|---|---|---|---|---|---|---|
| Tortous capillaries *N* (%) | 48 (88.8%) | 31 (96.8%) | 50 (98%) | 0.125 | 96 (88.8%) | 0.125 |
| Bushy capillaries *N* (%) | 27 (50%) | 21 (65.6%) | 10 (19.6%) | <0.001* | 4 (3.7%) | <0.001* |
| Elongated capillaries *N* (%) | 12 (22.2%) | 3 (9.3%) | 4 (7.8%) | 0.073 | 4 (3.7%) | 0.003* |
| Subpapillary plexus *N* (%) | 28 (51.8%) | 9 (28.1%) | 8 (15.6%) | <0.001* | 15 (13.8%) | <0.001* |
| Hemorrhage *N* (%) | 10 (18.5%) | 11 (34.4%) | 26 (50.9%) | 0.002* | 3 (2.7%) | <0.001* |
| Enlarged capillaries *N* (%) | 25 (46.2%) | 21 (65.6%) | 38 (74.5%) | 0.01* | 27 (25%) | <0.001* |
| Disorganized capillaries *N* (%) | 43 (79.6%) | 31 (96.8%) | 46 (90.1%) | 0.05 | 21 (19.4%) | <0.001* |
| Avascular areas *N* (%) | 41 (75.9%) | 30 (93.7%) | 49 (96%) | 0.004* | 10 (9.2%) | <0.001* |
| Density (mean ± SD) | 6.83 ± 1.95 | 5.31 ± 1.86 | 5.09 ± 1.69 | 0.592 | 7.43 ± 1.20 | <0.001* |

*CTDs, connective tissue diseases; DM, dermatomyositis; SD, standard deviation; SLE, systemic lupus erythematosus; SSc, systemic sclerosis. *Statistically significant.*

**TABLE 3 |** Multinomial logistic regression analysis of onychoscopic features in SLE, DM, and SSc patients.

| Onychoscopic features | SLE vs. DM | SLE vs. SSc | DM vs. SSc |
|---|---|---|---|
| Tortous capillaries | OR: 0.25 | OR: 0.16 | OR: 0.62 |
| | *p*-Value: 0.22 | *p*-Value: 0.095 | *p*-Value: 0.73 |
| | 95% CI: 0.02–2.24 | 95% CI: 0.01–1.37 | 95% CI: 0.03–10.27 |
| Bushy capillaries | OR: 0.52 | OR: 4.10 | OR: 7.82 |
| | *p*-Value: 0.16 | *p*-Value: 0.002* | *p*-Value: <0.001* |
| | 95% CI: 0.21–1.29 | 95% CI: 1.71–9.81 | 95% CI: 2.86–21.38 |
| Elongated capillaries | OR: 2.76 | OR: 3.35 | OR: 1.21 |
| | *p*-Value: 0.14 | *p*-value: 0.049* | *p*-Value: 0.80 |
| | 95% CI: 0.71–10.66 | 95% CI: 1.005–11.20 | 95% CI: 0.25–5.82 |
| Subpapillary plexus | OR: 2.75 | OR: 5.78 | OR: 2.10 |
| | *p*-Value: 0.03* | *p*-Value: <0.001* | *p*-Value: 0.17 |
| | 95% CI: 1.07–7.02 | 95% CI: 2.29–14.58 | 95% CI: 0.71–6.18 |
| Hemorrhage | OR: 0.43 | OR: 0.21 | OR: 0.50 |
| | *p*-Value: 0.10 | *p*-Value: 0.001* | *p*-Value: 0.14 |
| | 95% CI: 0.15–1.18 | 95% CI: 0.09–0.52 | 95% CI: 0.20–1.25 |
| Enlarged capillaries | OR: 0.45 | OR: 0.29 | OR: 0.65 |
| | *p*-Value: 0.08 | p-Value: 0.004* | *p*-Value: 0.38 |
| | 95% CI: 0.18–1.11 | 95% CI: 0.12–0.67 | 95% CI: 0.24–1.71 |
| Disorganized capillaries | OR: 0.12 | OR: 0.42 | OR: 3.36 |
| | *p*-Value: 0.053 | *p*-Value: 0.14 | *p*-Value: 0.27 |
| | 95% CI: 0.01–1.02 | 95% CI: 0.13–1.32 | 95% CI: 0.37–30.25 |
| Avascular areas | OR: 0.21 | OR: 0.12 | OR: 0.61 |
| | *p*-Value: 0.05 | *p*-Value: 0.009* | *p*-Value: 0.63 |
| | 95% CI: 0.04–1.00 | 95% CI: 0.02–0.60 | 95% CI: 0.08–4.57 |
| Density | OR: 1.21 | OR: 1.74 | OR: 0.22 |
| | *p*-Value: 0.09 | *p*-value: <0.001* | *p*-Value: 0.52 |
| | 95% CI: 0.91–2.42 | 95% CI: 1.12–2.35 | 95% CI: −0.48 to 0.93 |

*DM, dermatomyositis; OR, odds ratio; SLE, systemic lupus erythematosus; SSc, systemic sclerosis; 95% CI, 95% confidence interval.*
**Statistically significant.*

SLEDAI scores in SLE patients ($p = 0.01$). However, no specific feature was related to DM and SSc cutaneous changes using the CAT score and modified Rodnan skin score, respectively.

## DISCUSSION

Nailfold capillaroscopic examination using a USB digital microscopy has been demonstrated to provide high-quality

**TABLE 4** | Onychoscopic findings in relations to disease activity in SLE, DM, and SSc patients.

| Onychoscopic features | SLE | | | DM | | | SSc | | |
|---|---|---|---|---|---|---|---|---|---|
| | Median SLEDAI score in patients with the features (IQR) | Median SLEDAI score in patients without the features (IQR) | *p*-Value | Median CAT score in patients with the features (IQR) | Median CAT score in patients without the features (IQR) | *p*-Value | Median modified Rodnan score in patients with the features (IQR) | Median modified Rodnan score in patients without the features (IQR) | *p*-Value |
| Tortuous capillaries | 3.5 (0–8) | 10 (5–14) | 0.03* | 3 (2–5) | 0 (0–0) | 0.08 | 4 (1–12) | 10 (10) | 0.42 |
| Bushy capillaries | 4 (1–14) | 4 (0–6) | 0.18 | 3 (2–5) | 3 (2–5) | 0.82 | 7.5 (2–13) | 3 (1–10) | 0.27 |
| Elongated capillaries | 4 (1–11.5) | 4 (1–8) | 0.68 | 4 (2–5) | 3 (2–5) | 0.64 | 3 (0–10.5) | 5 (2–11) | 0.41 |
| Subpapillary plexus | 4 (0–9) | 4 (2–9) | 0.80 | 3 (2–5) | 3 (1–5) | 0.44 | 2 (0.5–7) | 6 (2–12.5) | 0.21 |
| Hemorrhage | 4.5 (2–10) | 4 (0.5–8.5) | 0.52 | 3 (2–5) | 4 (2–5) | 0.84 | 4 (1–8) | 6 (2–13) | 0.60 |
| Enlarged capillaries | 7 (2–14) | 2 (0–6) | 0.01* | 4 (2–5) | 2 (1–4) | 0.11 | 5 (2–12.5) | 4.5 (0.5–9) | 0.50 |
| Disorganized capillaries | 4 (1–11) | 2 (0–6) | 0.23 | 3 (2–5) | 0 (0–0) | 0.08 | 5 (1–11) | 6 (2–11.5) | 0.69 |
| Avascular areas | 4 (2–10) | 2 (0–6) | 0.07 | 3 (2–5) | 2 (0–4) | 0.34 | 6 (2–12) | 1 (0–2) | 0.15 |
| Decrease density | 4.5 (0–13) | 3 (1.5–6) | 0.24 | 3 (2–5) | 3 (1–4.5) | 0.62 | 5 (2–12) | 3.5 (0–7) | 0.43 |

*CAT, cutaneous assessment tool for myositis; DM, dermatomyositis; IQR, interquartile range; SLE, systemic lupus erythematosus; SLEDAI-2K, Systemic Lupus Erythematosus Disease Activity Index 2000; SSc, systemic sclerosis.*
**Statistically significant.*

images and comparable ability to differentiate between patients with SSc and healthy controls in previous studies with a small number of subjects (12, 42, 43). The method offers a cheaper and more readily available device comparing with videocapillaroscopy. Our study on a relatively high number of patients demonstrates the significant value of a USB digital microscope used as onychoscopy for the detection of nailfold capillary abnormalities among the three most common CTDs, namely SLE, DM, and SSc. To the best of our knowledge, this is the first study to compare NFC abnormalities among CTDs and the normal population with this method. Although information regarding the comparison of NFC features in patients with autoimmune CTDs vs. healthy controls has been previously reported in Caucasian and Japanese individuals (44, 45), there is no data in the Southeast Asian population. We confirm that numerous onychoscopic microvascular parameters in the morphologic indexes (i.e., bushy capillaries, elongated capillaries, subpapillary plexus, and hemorrhage), diameter patterns (i.e., enlarged capillaries), architectural forms (i.e., disorganized and avascular pattern), and decreased capillary density were distinct features for CTDs and rarely seen in normal individuals.

Previous reports have documented an increase in tortuosity as one of the important NFC findings in CTDs, particularly for SLE patients (9, 10). Our results have suggested otherwise, tortuous capillary morphology was a fairly common finding in healthy controls and should not be considered a valuable index to identify CTDs. The scleroderma pattern consists of two or more of the following features, enlarged capillaries, bushy capillaries, capillary hemorrhage, disorganized capillaries, and avascular area, presented in at least two nailfolds (6). These characteristic microvascular changes are well recognized for SSc. DM is considered a scleroderma-spectrum disorder; therefore, the scleroderma pattern is also commonly observed in DM patients (8, 46, 47). In the present study, we confirm that the majority (over 90%) of SSc and DM patients possessed NFC features of the scleroderma-type pattern. In multinomial logistic regression analysis, the scleroderma-type features on onychoscopy, namely, hemorrhage, enlarged capillary, and avascular area were not suggestive of SSc over DM or vice versa. However, only the bushy capillary morphology revealed significantly higher odds for DM (OR: 7.82, 95% CI: 2.86–21.38; $p < 0.001$). Therefore, we postulate that although DM is considered a scleroderma-spectrum disorder, possessing similar nailfold capillaroscopic features to SSc, bushy capillary formation is a valuable NFC finding that favored DM over SSc.

Evidence to date has shown that capillary nailfold changes in SLE patients present a smaller percentage of the scleroderma-type pattern and hold fewer specific characteristics (9, 10, 27–29, 39, 45, 48, 49). However, our results were discordant with previous reports. Of 51 SLE patients, 79.6%, 75.9%, 50%, 46.2%, and 18.5% had disorganized architecture, avascular areas, bushy capillaries, enlarged capillaries, and hemorrhage as their NFC findings, respectively. Therefore, using the aforementioned findings, over three-fourths of our SLE patients would fulfill the definition of the scleroderma pattern of NFC. In line with several previous reports, the higher prevalence of scleroderma-type pattern in SLE patients may be in part due to a relatively high number of SLE patients (40.5%) possessing Raynaud's phenomenon and/or anti-U1RNP antibody (50, 51). It would be informative to further explore whether or not scleroderma-type pattern on nail fold of SLE reflexes an SLE subset with subclinical features of SSc such as Raynaud's phenomenon. As our data showed that the scleroderma-type pattern may not invariably differentiate scleroderma-spectrum disorders from SLE, we suggest that individual microvascular nailfold changes and their severity should be considered rather than focusing on a specific pattern spectrum. SLE-type capillary nailfold pattern has been mentioned earlier consisting of tortuous, meandering capillaries, increase diameter, and prominent subpapillary plexus (9, 11, 28, 49). Our study results were concordant with the literature, but with regards to only the elongated capillary and prominent subpapillary plexus being more common in SLE. We also demonstrated that bushy capillary, elongated capillary, and prominent subpapillary plexus were patterns possessing significantly higher odds for SLE compared with SSc patients, while the prominent subpapillary plexus was the sole NFC finding that significantly favored SLE over DM. Moreover, in quantitative analysis for the degree of avascular areas, the absence of avascular area revealed significant odds for SLE over SSc, while extensive avascular areas favored both SSc and DM over SLE.

Microvascular changes play a central role in the pathophysiology of SLE, DM, and SSc. The similarities and dissimilarities on the NFC features may reflect their microvascular pathology. Endothelial injury is thought to be the initial vascular insult in SSc. Endothelial cell apoptosis, vasoconstriction, and vasculopathy are pronounced in SSc. A vast amount of tissue hypoxia in SSc patients may parallel the predominant nailfold avascular areas and the decrease capillary density seen on onychoscopy. Angiogenesis consequently occurs as compensation to chronic hypoxia, but the process is defective and dysregulated in SSc patients. An endothelial activation factor, namely vascular endothelial growth factor (VEGF), is highly expressed and has shown to be associated with decreased nailfold capillary density in patients with SSc (52).

VEGF is considered a key regulator of angiogenesis for SLE and DM as well. Kuryliszyn-Moskal et al. demonstrated that endothelial activation markers, namely VEGF, endothelin-1, E-selectin, and thrombomodulin were associated with increased capillaroscopic changes in SLE. Moreover, patients with moderate to severe capillaroscopic abnormalities (e.g., elongated, tortuous, meandering, ramified, and/or disarranged capillaries) showed higher levels of VEGF (23). In DM, microvascular injury is mediated by the humeral process with secondary vascular depletion, hypoxia, and myofiber necrosis. Subsequently, local angiogenesis occurs as compensation for vascular reduction. Angiogenic factors such as VEGF and angiogenin may play a role in the pathogenesis of DM and correspond to their onycoscopic changes (53). Therefore, similar to SSc, onychoscopic findings in DM may display both ischemia (e.g., avascular area and disorganized capillaries) and aberrant angiogenesis (e.g., enlarged capillaries and bushy capillaries). Nevertheless, further studies to determine the true pathomechanism and biomarkers that reflect the microvascular changes in CTDs are warranted.

The correlation of NFC alterations with the disease activity in SLE, DM, and SSc has been reported with variable results. In the present study, SLE patients with higher SLEDAI scores were associated with the presence of enlarged capillaries on onychoscopy than those without. Our results were in line with the literature showing higher disease activity defined by the SLEDAI, Systemic Lupus Activity Measures, and the European Consensus Activity Measures in SLE patients with NFC changes (11, 23, 27, 29). Documents on the microvascular nailfold abnormalities and disease activity in DM and SSc have been rather inconsistent. In DM and/or polymyositis, while several studies have shown a significant correlation between capillary damage with disease activity (e.g., myositis damage index, myositis disease activity assessment tools, and the global disease activity), many others have not (8, 54–59). Reports on the relationship between NFC and disease severity in SSc have been quite controversial, ranging from significant predictive association to no association. The significant heterogeneity reported are due to the differences in disease duration, specific organ complication (e.g., pulmonary vascular/parenchymal disease, myocardial dysfunction, and cutaneous sclerosis), scoring systems, and the parameter used in NFC (20, 60–64). In the present study, we found no correlation between nailfold capillaroscopic patterns with DM and SSc skin activity score, using the CAT score and modified Rodnan skin score, respectively. Further studies with validated disease severity/outcome parameters, analysis technique, and scoring system are much needed to determine the relationship between NFC features and the disease severity and organ-specific complications among CTDs.

The present study is subjected to several limitations. We did not determine NFC abnormalities of other chronic rheumatic disorders such as Sjogren's syndrome, rheumatoid arthritis, and antiphospholipid syndrome. Additional limitations were its cross-sectional, single-center study nature, with population restricted to Southeast Asians, and lack of prospective monitoring in order to evaluate alterations of NFC features and their relationship with disease activity over time. Our designated severity measures could not reflect the severity of disease in all aspects. Finally, being conducted in a tertiary care center means the study was prone to referral bias.

## CONCLUSION

Our study confirms that a USB digital microscope used as onychoscopy is a valuable tool to detect nailfold capillary changes in SLE, DM, and SSc patients. Several morphologic patterns and their severity can help differentiate among CTDs. Therefore, the device may serve as a relevant diagnostic instrument and could be implemented in clinical practice. However, determining the prognostic significance of onychoscopy requires a large cohort study with validating assessment on disease severity and organ-specific complication.

## ETHICS STATEMENT

The studies involving human participants were reviewed and approved by the Mahidol University Institutional Review Board for Ethics in Human Research. The patients/participants provided their written informed consent to participate in this study.

## AUTHOR CONTRIBUTIONS

PS: Conceptualization, writing-review and editing. PS, KC, and WF: methodology. PS and PL: validation. KC and WF: formal analysis PS, KC, WF, and PL: investigation. KC and WF: data curation and writing-original draft preparation. All authors have read and agreed to the published version of the manuscript.

## REFERENCES


1. Nagy Z, Czirják L. Nailfold digital capillaroscopy in 447 patients with connective tissue disease and Raynaud's disease. *J Eur Acad Dermatol Venereol.* (2004) 18:62–8. doi: 10.1111/j.1468-3083.2004.00853.x
2. Zhao T, Lin FA, Chen HP. Pattern of nailfold capillaroscopy in patients with systemic lupus erythematosus. *Arch Rheumatol.* (2020) 35:568–74. doi: 10.46497/ArchRheumatol.2020.7763
3. Corominas H, Ortiz-Santamaría V, Castellví I, Moreno M, Morlà R, Clavaguera T, et al. Nailfold capillaroscopic findings in primary Sjögren's syndrome with and without Raynaud's phenomenon and/or positive anti-SSA/Ro and anti-SSB/La antibodies. *Rheumatol Int.* (2016) 36:365–9. doi: 10.1007/s00296-015-3396-9
4. Pavlov-Dolijanovic S, Damjanov NS, Stojanovic RM, Vujasinovic Stupar NZ, Stanisavljevic DM. Scleroderma pattern of nailfold capillary changes as predictive value for the development of a connective tissue disease: a follow-up study of 3,029 patients with primary Raynaud's phenomenon. *Rheumatol Int.* (2012) 32:3039–45. doi: 10.1007/s00296-011-2109-2
5. Shenavandeh S, Habibi S, Habibi Y, Nazarinia M. Mechanic hands: clinical and capillaroscopy manifestations of patients with connective tissue diseases presented with and without mechanic hands. *Clin Rheumatol.* (2019) 38:2309–18. doi: 10.1007/s10067-018-04422-z
6. Chojnowski MM, Felis-Giemza A, Olesińska M. Capillaroscopy - a role in modern rheumatology. *Reumatologia.* (2016) 54:67–72. doi: 10.5114/reum.2016.60215
7. van den Hoogen F, Khanna D, Fransen J, Johnson SR, Baron M, Tyndall A, et al. 2013 classification criteria for systemic sclerosis: an American College of Rheumatology/European League against Rheumatism collaborative initiative. *Arthritis Rheum.* (2013) 65:2737–47. doi: 10.1002/art.38098
8. Mugii N, Hasegawa M, Matsushita T, Hamaguchi Y, Horie S, Yahata T, et al. Association between nail-fold capillary findings and disease activity in dermatomyositis. *Rheumatology (Oxford).* (2011) 50:1091–8. doi: 10.1093/rheumatology/keq430
9. Lambova SN, Müller-Ladner U. Capillaroscopic pattern in systemic lupus erythematosus and undifferentiated connective tissue disease: What we still have to learn? *Rheumatol Int.* (2013) 33:689–95. doi: 10.1007/s00296-012-2434-0
10. Cutolo M, Melsens K, Wijnant S, Ingegnoli F, Thevissen K, De Keyser F, et al. Nailfold capillaroscopy in systemic lupus erythematosus: A systematic review and critical appraisal. *Autoimmun Rev.* (2018) 17:344–52. doi: 10.1016/j.autrev.2017.11.025
11. Riccieri V, Spadaro A, Ceccarelli F, Scrivo R, Germano V, Valesini G. Nailfold capillaroscopy changes in systemic lupus erythematosus: correlations with disease activity and autoantibody profile. *Lupus.* (2005) 14:521–5. doi: 10.1191/0961203305lu2151oa
12. Berks M, Dinsdale G, Marjanovic E, Murray A, Taylor C, Herrick AL. Comparison between low cost USB nailfold capillaroscopy and videocapillaroscopy: a pilot study. *Rheumatology (Oxford).* (2020). doi: 10.1093/rheumatology/keaa723
13. Micali G, Lacarrubba F. Dermatoscopy: Instrumental Update. *Dermatol Clin.* (2018) 36:345–8. doi: 10.1016/j.det.2018.05.001
14. Sriphojanart T, Khunkhet S, Suchonwanit P, A. retrospective comparative study of the efficacy and safety of two regimens of diphenylcyclopropenone in the treatment of recalcitrant alopecia areata. *Dermatol Reports.* (2017) 9:7399. doi: 10.4081/dr.2017.7399
15. Chanprapaph K, Udompanich S, Visessiri Y, Ngamjanyaporn P, Suchonwanit P. Nonscarring alopecia in systemic lupus erythematosus: A cross-sectional study with trichoscopic, histopathologic, and immunopathologic analyses. *J Am Acad Dermatol.* (2019) 81:1319–29. doi: 10.1016/j.jaad.2019.05.053
16. Suchonwanit P, Udompanich S, Thadanipon K, Chanprapaph K. Trichoscopic signs in systemic lupus erythematosus: a comparative study with 109 patients and 305 healthy controls. *J Eur Acad Dermatol Venereol.* (2019) 33:774–80. doi: 10.1111/jdv.15421
17. Udompanich S, Chanprapaph K, Suchonwanit P. Hair and Scalp Changes in Cutaneous and Systemic Lupus Erythematosus. *Am J Clin Dermatol.* (2018) 19:679–94. doi: 10.1007/s40257-018-0363-8
18. Jasso-Olivares JC, Tosti A, Miteva M, Domínguez-Cherit J, Díaz-González JM. Clinical and Dermoscopic Features of the Scalp in 31 Patients with Dermatomyositis. *Skin Appendage Disord.* (2017) 3:119–24. doi: 10.1159/000464469
19. Kwiatkowska M, Rakowska A, Walecka I, Rudnicka L. The diagnostic value of trichoscopy in systemic sclerosis. *J Dermatol Case Rep.* (2016) 10:21–5. doi: 10.3315/jdcr.2016.1225
20. Herrick AL, Moore TL, Murray AK, Whidby N, Manning JB, Bhushan M, et al. Nail-fold capillary abnormalities are associated with anti-centromere antibody and severity of digital ischaemia. *Rheumatology (Oxford).* (2010) 49:1776–82. doi: 10.1093/rheumatology/keq139
21. Manfredi A, Sebastiani M, Cassone G, Pipitone N, Giuggioli D, Colaci M, et al. Nailfold capillaroscopic changes in dermatomyositis and polymyositis. *Clin Rheumatol.* (2015) 34:279–84. doi: 10.1007/s10067-014-2795-8
22. Souza EJ, Kayser C. [Nailfold capillaroscopy: relevance to the practice of rheumatology]. *Rev Bras Reumatol.* (2015) 55:264–71. doi: 10.1016/j.rbre.2014.09.005
23. Kuryliszyn-Moskal A, Ciolkiewicz M, Klimiuk PA, Sierakowski S. Clinical significance of nailfold capillaroscopy in systemic lupus erythematosus: correlation with endothelial cell activation markers and disease activity. *Scand J Rheumatol.* (2009) 38:38–45. doi: 10.1080/03009740802366050
24. Ingegnoli F. Capillaroscopy abnormalities in relation to disease activity in juvenile systemic lupus erythematosus. *Microvasc Res.* (2013) 87:92–4. doi: 10.1016/j.mvr.2013.02.004
25. Ciołkiewicz M, Kuryliszyn-Moskal A, Klimiuk PA. Analysis of correlations between selected endothelial cell activation markers, disease activity, and nailfold capillaroscopy microvascular changes in systemic lupus erythematosus patients. *Clin Rheumatol.* (2010) 29:175–80. doi: 10.1007/s10067-009-1308-7
26. Chanasumon N, Sriphojanart T, Suchonwanit P. Therapeutic potential of bimatoprost for the treatment of eyebrow hypotrichosis. *Drug Des Devel Ther.* (2018) 12:365–72. doi: 10.2147/DDDT.S156467
27. Shenavandeh S, Habibi S. Nailfold capillaroscopic changes in patients with systemic lupus erythematosus: correlations with disease activity, skin manifestation and nephritis. *Lupus.* (2017) 26:959–66. doi: 10.1177/0961203316686702
28. Tariq S, Tervaert JWC, Osman M. Nailfold Capillaroscopy in Systemic Lupus Erythematosus (SLE): a point-of-care tool that parallels disease activity and predicts future complications. *Curr Treat Options Rheumatol.* (2019) 5:336–45. doi: 10.1007/s40674-019-00133-x
29. Moneib HA, Salem SA, Aly DG, Khedr HT, Wafaey HA, Hassan HE. Assessment of serum vascular endothelial growth factor and nail fold capillaroscopy changes in systemic lupus erythematosus with and without cutaneous manifestations. *J Dermatol.* (2012) 39:52–7. doi: 10.1111/j.1346-8138.2011.01322.x
30. Petri M, Orbai AM, Alarcón GS, Gordon C, Merrill JT, Fortin PR, et al.

Derivation and validation of the Systemic Lupus International Collaborating Clinics classification criteria for systemic lupus erythematosus. *Arthritis Rheum.* (2012) 64:2677–86. doi: 10.1002/art.34473

31. Leclair V, Lundberg IE. New Myositis Classification Criteria-What We Have Learned Since Bohan and Peter. *Curr Rheumatol Rep.* (2018) 20:18. doi: 10.1007/s11926-018-0726-4
32. Cutolo M, Sulli A, Smith V. How to perform and interpret capillaroscopy. *Best Pract Res Clin Rheumatol.* (2013) 27:237–48. doi: 10.1016/j.berh.2013.03.001
33. von Bierbrauer A, Barth P, Willert J, Baerwald C, Mennel HD, Schmidt JA. Electron microscopy and capillaroscopically guided nailfold biopsy in connective tissue diseases: detection of ultrastructural changes of the microcirculatory vessels. *Br J Rheumatol.* (1998) 37:1272–8. doi: 10.1093/rheumatology/37.12.1272
34. Etehad Tavakol M, Fatemi A, Karbalaie A, Emrani Z, Erlandsson BE. Nailfold capillaroscopy in rheumatic diseases: which parameters should be evaluated? *Biomed Res Int.* (2015) 2015:974530. doi: 10.1155/2015/974530
35. Kabasakal Y, Elvins DM, Ring EF, McHugh NJ. Quantitative nailfold capillaroscopy findings in a population with connective tissue disease and in normal healthy controls. *Ann Rheum Dis.* (1996) 55:507–12. doi: 10.1136/ard.55.8.507
36. Lee P, Leung FY, Alderdice C, Armstrong SK. Nailfold capillary microscopy in the connective tissue diseases: a semiquantitative assessment. *J Rheumatol.* (1983) 10:930–8.
37. Ingegnoli F, Gualtierotti R, Lubatti C, Zahalkova L, Meani L, Boracchi P, et al. Feasibility of different capillaroscopic measures for identifying nailfold microvascular alterations. *Semin Arthritis Rheum.* (2009) 38:289–95. doi: 10.1016/j.semarthrit.2007.10.008
38. Emrani Z, Karbalaie A, Fatemi A, Etehadtavakol M, Erlandsson BE. Capillary density: An important parameter in nailfold capillaroscopy. *Microvasc Res.* (2017) 109:7–18. doi: 10.1016/j.mvr.2016.09.001
39. Mikdashi J, Nived O. Measuring disease activity in adults with systemic lupus erythematosus: the challenges of administrative burden and responsiveness to patient concerns in clinical research. *Arthritis Res Ther.* (2015) 17:183. doi: 10.1186/s13075-015-0702-6
40. Huber AM, Dugan EM, Lachenbruch PA, Feldman BM, Perez MD, Zemel LS, et al. The Cutaneous Assessment Tool: development and reliability in juvenile idiopathic inflammatory myopathy. *Rheumatology (Oxford).* (2007) 46:1606–11. doi: 10.1093/rheumatology/kem179
41. Khanna D, Furst DE, Clements PJ, Allanore Y, Baron M, Czirjak L, et al. Standardization of the modified Rodnan skin score for use in clinical trials of systemic sclerosis. *J Scleroderma Relat Disord.* (2017) 2:11–8. doi: 10.5301/jsrd.5000231
42. Bhakuni DS, Vasdev V, Garg MK, Narayanan K, Jain R, Mullick G. Nailfold capillaroscopy by digital microscope in an Indian population with systemic sclerosis. *Int J Rheum Dis.* (2012) 15:95–101. doi: 10.1111/j.1756-185X.2011.01699.x
43. Jakhar D, Grover C, Singal A. Nailfold capillaroscopy with USB dermatoscope: A cross-sectional study in healthy adults. *Indian J Dermatol Venereol Leprol.* (2020) 86:33–8. doi: 10.4103/ijdvl.IJDVL_240_18
44. Sekiyama JY, Camargo CZ, Eduardo L, Andrade C, Kayser C. Reliability of widefield nailfold capillaroscopy and video capillaroscopy in the assessment of patients with Raynaud's phenomenon. *Arthritis Care Res (Hoboken).* (2013) 65:1853–61. doi: 10.1002/acr.22054
45. Ohtsuka T. Dermoscopic detection of nail fold capillary abnormality in patients with systemic sclerosis. *J Dermatol.* (2012) 39:331–5. doi: 10.1111/j.1346-8138.2011.01357.x
46. HASEGAWA M. Dermoscopy findings of nail fold capillaries in connective tissue diseases. *J Dermatol.* (2011) 38:66–70. doi: 10.1111/j.1346-8138.2010.01092.x
47. Manfredi A, Sebastiani M, Cassone G, Pipitone N, Giuggioli D, Colaci M, et al. SAT0298 Nailfold capillaroscopic alterations in dermatomyositis and polymyositis. *Ann Rheum Dis.* (2014) 73:700–1. doi: 10.1136/annrheumdis-2014-eular.4305
48. Ingegnoli F, Zeni S, Meani L, Soldi A, Lurati A, Fantini F. Evaluation of nailfold videocapillaroscopic abnormalities in patients with systemic lupus erythematosus. *J Clin Rheumatol.* (2005) 11:295–8. doi: 10.1097/01.rhu.0000191193.93720.95
49. Wu PC, Huang MN, Kuo YM, Hsieh SC Yu CL. Clinical applicability of quantitative nailfold capillaroscopy in differential diagnosis of connective tissue diseases with Raynaud's phenomenon. *J Formos Med Assoc.* (2013) 112:482–8. doi: 10.1016/j.jfma.2012.02.029
50. Furtado RN, Pucinelli ML, Cristo VV, Andrade LE, Sato EI. Scleroderma-like nailfold capillaroscopic abnormalities are associated with anti-U1-RNP antibodies and Raynaud's phenomenon in SLE patients. *Lupus.* (2002) 11:35–41. doi: 10.1191/0961203302lu144oa
51. Chojer P, Mahajan BB. Nail fold dermoscopy in collagen vascular disorders: A cross-sectional study. *Indian J Dermatol Venereol Leprol.* (2019) 85:439. doi: 10.4103/ijdvl.IJDVL_495_18
52. Choi JJ, Min DJ, Cho ML, Min SY, Kim SJ, Lee SS, et al. Elevated vascular endothelial growth factor in systemic sclerosis. *J Rheumatol.* (2003) 30:1529–33.
53. Miossi R, de Souza FHC, Shinjo SK. Nailfold capillary changes in adult new-onset dermatomyositis: a prospective cross-sectional study. *Clin Rheumatol.* (2019) 38:2319–26. doi: 10.1007/s10067-019-04537-x
54. Ganczarczyk ML, Lee P, Armstrong SK. Nailfold capillary microscopy in polymyositis and dermatomyositis. *Arthritis Rheum.* (1988) 31:116–9. doi: 10.1002/art.1780310116
55. Brunner HI, Feldman BM, Bombardier C, Silverman ED. Sensitivity of the Systemic Lupus Erythematosus Disease Activity Index, British Isles Lupus Assessment Group Index, and Systemic Lupus Activity Measure in the evaluation of clinical change in childhood-onset systemic lupus erythematosus. *Arthritis Rheum.* (1999) 42:1354–60. doi: 10.1002/1529-0131(199907)42:7<1354::AID-ANR8>3.0.CO;2-4
56. Selva-O'Callaghan A, Fonollosa-Pla V, Trallero-Araguás E, Martínez-Gómez X, Simeon-Aznar CP, Labrador-Horrillo M, et al. Nailfold capillary microscopy in adults with inflammatory myopathy. *Semin Arthritis Rheum.* (2010) 39:398–404. doi: 10.1016/j.semarthrit.2008.09.003
57. Suchonwanit P, Hector CE, Bin Saif GA, McMichael AJ. Factors affecting the severity of central centrifugal cicatricial alopecia. *Int J Dermatol.* (2016) 55:e338–43. doi: 10.1111/ijd.13061
58. Schmeling H, Stephens S, Goia C, Manlhiot C, Schneider R, Luthra S, et al. Nailfold capillary density is importantly associated over time with muscle and skin disease activity in juvenile dermatomyositis. *Rheumatology (Oxford).* (2011) 50:885–93. doi: 10.1093/rheumatology/keq407
59. Shenavandeh S, Zarei Nezhad M. Association of nailfold capillary changes with disease activity, clinical and laboratory findings in patients with dermatomyositis. *Med J Islam Repub Iran.* (2015) 29:233.
60. Castellví I, Simeón-Aznar CP, Sarmiento M, Fortuna A, Mayos M, Geli C, et al. Association between nailfold capillaroscopy findings and pulmonary function tests in patients with systemic sclerosis. *J Rheumatol.* (2015) 42:222–7. doi: 10.3899/jrheum.140276
61. Smith V, Pizzorni C, De Keyser F, Decuman S, Van Praet JT, Deschepper E, et al. Reliability of the qualitative and semiquantitative nailfold videocapillaroscopy assessment in a systemic sclerosis cohort: a two-center study. *Ann Rheum Dis.* (2010) 69:1092–6. doi: 10.1136/ard.2009.115568
62. Greidinger EL, Gaine SP, Wise RA, Boling C, Housten-Harris T, Wigley FM. Primary pulmonary hypertension is not associated with scleroderma-like changes in nailfold capillaries. *Chest.* (2001) 120:796–800. doi: 10.1378/chest.120.3.796
63. Lovy M, MacCarter D, Steigerwald JC. Relationship between nailfold capillary abnormalities and organ involvement in systemic sclerosis. *Arthritis Rheum.* (1985) 28:496–501. doi: 10.1002/art.1780280505
64. Sato LT, Kayser C, Andrade LE. Nailfold capillaroscopy abnormalities correlate with cutaneous and visceral involvement in systemic sclerosis patients. *Acta Reumatol Port.* (2009) 34:219–27.

13

# A Novel Fuzzy Multilayer Perceptron (F-MLP) for the Detection of Irregularity in Skin Lesion Border Using Dermoscopic Images

*Abder-Rahman Ali [1*], Jingpeng Li [1], Summrina Kanwal [2], Guang Yang [3], Amir Hussain [4] and Sally Jane O'Shea [5]*

[1] Faculty of Natural Sciences, Computing Science and Mathematics, University of Stirling, Stirling, United Kingdom, [2] Department of Computing and Informatics, Saudi Electronic University, Al-Dammam, Saudi Arabia, [3] National Heart and Lung Institute, Imperial College London, London, United Kingdom, [4] Cognitive Big Data and Cybersecurity Research Lab, Edinburgh Napier University, Edinburgh, United Kingdom, [5] Mater Private Hospital, Cork, Ireland

***Correspondence:**
Abder-Rahman Ali
abder@cs.stir.ac.uk

Skin lesion border irregularity, which represents the B feature in the ABCD rule, is considered one of the most significant factors in melanoma diagnosis. Since signs that clinicians rely on in melanoma diagnosis involve subjective judgment including visual signs such as border irregularity, this deems it necessary to develop an objective approach to finding border irregularity. Increased research in neural networks has been carried out in recent years mainly driven by the advances of deep learning. Artificial neural networks (ANNs) or multilayer perceptrons have been shown to perform well in supervised learning tasks. However, such networks usually don't incorporate information pertaining the ambiguity of the inputs when training the network, which in turn could affect how the weights are being updated in the learning process and eventually degrading the performance of the network when applied on test data. In this paper, we propose a fuzzy multilayer perceptron (F-MLP) that takes the ambiguity of the inputs into consideration and subsequently reduces the effects of ambiguous inputs on the learning process. A new optimization function, the fuzzy gradient descent, has been proposed to reflect those changes. Moreover, a type-II fuzzy sigmoid activation function has also been proposed which enables finding the range of performance the fuzzy neural network is able to attain. The fuzzy neural network was used to predict the skin lesion border irregularity, where the lesion was firstly segmented from the skin, the lesion border extracted, border irregularity measured using a proposed measure vector, and using the extracted border irregularity measures to train the neural network. The proposed approach outperformed most of the state-of-the-art classification methods in general and its standard neural network counterpart in particular. However, the proposed fuzzy neural network was more time-consuming when training the network.

**Keywords: melanoma, irregularity, dermoscopy, multilayer perceptron, fuzzy logic**

## 1. INTRODUCTION

The increasing incidence of melanoma renders the attempts of the early detection of melanoma a continuing public health priority. Despite its aggressive infiltration of other body parts, melanoma is highly curable if diagnosed early and treated timely (1). Early detection is crucial since it contributes to a better survival; the 5-year survival rate for early stage invasive melanoma is 94%, compared to a 5-year survival rate of only 17% for melanomas that have spread to other parts of the body. There is a niche to develop an objective, bedside tool that could be used as an adjunct in the clinical assessment of skin lesions. Tracking tumor changes manually is also labor-intensive, especially for patients with multiple moles on their skin.

The ABCD rule (2) emerged in 1985 by a group of researchers at the New York University as a simple framework that physicians, novice dermatologists, and non-physicians could use to learn about the features of melanoma in its early curable stage, enhancing thereby the early detection of melanoma. The rule is more geared toward the public than the 7-point checklist which was designed for non-dermatological *medical* personnel. The approach has then been verified by the 1992 National Institutes of Health Consensus Conference Report on Early Melanoma, in addition to other studies published at the time (3–6), and is being advertised by the American Cancer Society as a method to help in seeking early medical evaluation of any suspicious pigmented lesions. The ABCD acronym refers to four parameters: (i) Asymmetry, (ii) Border irregularity, (iii) Color variegation, (iv) Diameter >6 mm. Such parameters provide simple means for appraisal of pigmented cutaneous lesions that may need to be further examined by a specialist, which might result on further work of dermoscopy or biopsy, or both. The rule is basically designed to be used on a daily life basis by both the layperson and the primary care physician (non-dermatologist) as a simple method to alert on the clinical features of melanoma, and is intended to help explain a subset of melanomas called *thin tumors* which could otherwise be confused with benign pigmented lesions.

One of the most significant factors in melanoma diagnosis is *border irregularity* (the B feature in the ABCD rule) (7). As opposed to benign pigmented lesions which tend to possess regular borders, melanoma lesions have irregular borders due to the uneven growth rate (8), the spread of melanocytes in various directions, and the regression of invasion and/or genetic instability of the lesion (9). In this paper we proposes a type-II fuzzy logic based multilayer perceptron that considers the ambiguity of neurons and attempts to reduce the effects of such ambiguous data on the network learning process. Such network will be used in detecting the skin lesion border irregularity and will be compared with its standard neural network counterpart. Detecting the other features (i.e., ACD) is explained in our other work (10).

Section 2 reviews related work, section 3 introduces the concepts of the perceptron, multilayer perceptron, and gradient descent, section 4 explains the notions of fuzzy sets and type-II fuzzy sets, fuzzy c-means clustering is explained in section 5, the proposed fuzzy multilayer perceptron (F-MLP) is described in section 6, sections 7–9 describe the skin lesion segmentation process, how we detect the skin lesion border, and how the border irregularity is measured, respectively, results are depicted in section 10, and the paper is concluded in section 11.

## 2. RELATED WORK

Although Artificial Neural Networks (ANNs) have been proved to work well with supervised learning tasks, they do not include information related to the ambiguity of the inputs. This issue can have a negative effect on how the weights are being updated in the learning process, and subsequently affecting the accuracy of the network results. The term *fuzzy neural network* was proposed in 1975 (11) when the authors attempted to extend the McCulloch-Pitts model of the neuron (12) in such a way that allows the activity of a neuron to be fuzzy rather than an all-or-none process. Different studies have then been published on combining fuzzy logic and neural networks. Keller and Hunt (13) proposed a fuzzy perceptron (the building block of fuzzy neural networks) to alleviate the major drawback with the crisp perceptron which is its inability to terminate when the data is not linearly separable. Goh et al. (14) developed an enhanced fuzzy perceptron that demonstrates higher stability and functionality compared to the fuzzy perceptron. A neural network classifier which uses the min-max hyperboxes as fuzzy sets aggregated into fuzzy set classes was introduced in Simpson (15), and was referred to as a fuzzy min-max classification neural network. As opposed to this supervised learning approach, an unsupervised learning pattern clustering sibling to this work, namely fuzzy min-max clustering neural network was proposed in Simpson (16). A fuzzy neural network based on the multilayer perceptron and capable of fuzzy classification of patterns has been proposed in Pal and Mitra (17) and Mitra et al. (18). Fuzzified neural networks, where fuzzy numbers are used for inputs, outputs, and/or connection weights have been proposed in Buckley and Hayashi (19), Ishibuchi et al. (20), Ishibuchi (21). Researchers attempted to enhance the fuzzy perceptron; Chen and Chang (22) proposed a fuzzy perceptron that addresses classification problems where it is capable of accepting two different kinds of input data: numerical data and fuzzy IF-THEN rules. Chen and Chen (23) proposed a fuzzy kernel perceptron where the fuzzy perceptron and the Mercer Kernels (24) are incorporated, such that input data is first mapped into a high-dimensional feature space and the fuzzy perceptron is then utilized in order to find a linear separating hyperplane in the high-dimensional feature space. A comprehensive review of proposed neurofuzzy systems in the periods 2002–2012 can be found in Samarjit et al. (25). Lixin Fan from Nokia Technologies wrote a detailed guide (26) that aims to bridge the gap between fuzzy logic and deep learning (64).

In this paper we propose a fuzzy multilayer perceptron (F-MLP) that uses a developed fuzzy gradient descent which incorporates the membership degrees of neurons (obtained using fuzzy c-means clustering) to reduce the effects of ambiguous neurons on the neural network learning process. Moreover, a proposed type-II fuzzy sigmoid activation function is used which allows to represent the range (lowest and highest) of performance the fuzzy neural network is able to achieve.

A radial search algorithm (27) was used to detect the skin lesion border in Golston et al. (28), where different sliding windows that represent the origin of a radii are automatically detected in the skin lesion. Sufficiently high jumps in luminance (also contain sufficiently sustained luminance) are searched for in the radii to form the candidate border points (29). Irregularity was eventually found using the *irregularity index*: $I = \frac{P^2}{4\pi A}$, where $P$ and $A$ are the perimeter (number of points on the detected border) and area (number of points on and within the border) of the closed boundary, respectively. Borders with an irregularity index greater than 1.8 were classified as being irregular. Sixty skin tumor images were labeled by a dermatologist as being regular or irregular (regular: 14, irregular: 46). 83.3% of the tumors were classified correctly (8/14 and 42/46 for regular and irregular borders, respectively).

Ng and Lee (30) used fractal dimensions (FDs) in measuring the irregularity of skin lesion borders. Four fractal dimension measures were found for each color image: direct FD, vertical smoothing FD, horizontal smoothing FD, and multi-fractal dimension of order two. Those FDs were also calculated on the blue band of the images. Four hundred and sixty eight melanocytic lesions (not hairy) have been segmented using a multi-stage method (31) and used to test the proposed approach. Results showed that the multi-fractal method performed the best. FDs were also used in Claridge et al. (32) and Ali et al. (33).

An approach which analyzes the structural irregularity of cutaneous melanocytic lesions was proposed in Lee et al. (34). The algorithm consists of two stages: (i) pre-processing: dark thick hair is removed by DullRazor (35) and the lesion border is extracted from the skin image, (ii) sigma-ratio: this is a measure derived from the scale-space filtering technique and used to analyze the structural shape of the lesion border. Results revealed that sigma-ratio is sensitive to structural indentations and protrusions (i.e., provides accurate estimation for the structure irregularity) as opposed to shape descriptors such as compactness index and fractal dimension which are more sensitive to texture irregularities than structure irregularities (36). The authors also proposed a new border irregularity measure in Lee and Atkins (36), Lee et al. (37), and Lee and Claridge (9), where all indentations and protrusions are firstly located along the lesion border and a new irregularity index is measured for each indentation and protrusion. Summing up all the individual indices provides an estimation on the overall border irregularity.

A new measure of border irregularity based on *conditional entropy* was proposed by Arbisala and Claridge (38), where it was observed that the entropy increases with the degree of irregularity. The results of the proposed measure were compared with the Indentation Irregularity Index (9) on 98 skin lesions (16 were melanoma) and showed to have a better discriminatory power; ROC curve 0.76 compared to 0.73 for the Indentation Irregularity Index.

Ma et al. (39) used *wavelet decomposition* to extract the skin lesion border structure to determine whether the lesion is naevus or melanoma. The discrete wavelet transform (DWT) was used to filter the 1D border into sub-bands down to level 9, where levels 6–9 (significant levels) have shown to contain information more relevant for classifying between melanoma and benign samples. Some statistical and geometrical feature descriptors of border irregularity were also extracted at each individual sub-band. Twenty-five measurements were formed by applying six features in four significant sub-bands and one feature in a single sub-band. A combination of features was eventually fed to a back-projection neural network. Using a small training set of 9 melanomas and 9 naevi, the best classifier was obtained when the best 13 features were used.

Jaworek-Korjakowska and Tadeusiewicz (40) used a simple method to measure border irregularity, in which a semi-quantitative evaluation method was used to divide the lesion into eight similar parts where the sharp abrupt cut-off in each part has a score of 1. A maximum score of 8 is obtained if the whole border is irregular, and a score 0 is obtained if the naevus is round with no ragged borders. Melanomas tend to have scores 4–8 (41). The approach was tested on 120 skin lesion cases with border irregularity <3 and 180 skin lesion cases with border irregularity >4, achieving a 79% accuracy.

Ali et al. (33) proposed a border irregularity measure that combines fractal dimension, zernike moments, and convexity, which are represented in a 27-value vector (zernike moments produced 25 values). Fractal dimension was found using the extracted border, and zernike moments and convexity were found using the segmented image. The extracted measures were then trained on a CNN (convolutional neural network) and Gaussian naive Bayes ensemble, which is then used for the automatic detection (i.e., classification) of skin lesion border irregularity on new images. The approach achieved outstanding results, obtaining an accuracy, sensitivity, specificity, and F-score of 93.6, 100, 92.5, and 96.1%, respectively. In this paper we use a similar skin lesion border irregularity measure, but use only fractal dimension and convexity.

## 3. PERCEPTRONS

The perceptron is normally used in supervised linear classification tasks in which a hyperplane would be tuned to fit a training dataset. This tuned hyperplane can then be used to classify new unknown samples. This is achieved by minimizing the hyperplane's error as it is applied on the training dataset through minimizing the *error function*: $\epsilon\,(w) = -\sum_{i \in M} t_i \mathbf{w}^T \mathbf{x}_i$, where $M$ is the set of misclassified samples, and $t_i \in \{-1, 1\}$ is the class of sample $\mathbf{x}_i$. If $\epsilon(\mathbf{w}) = 0$, this means that the hyperplane completely separates the classes. This minimization process is usually carried out in iterations such that after each iteration we move toward the minimum of $\epsilon(\mathbf{w})$. The $\mathbf{w}$ vector of iteration $k+1$ is obtained as the following weight updating step: $\mathbf{w}_{k+1} = \mathbf{w}_k + \Delta\mathbf{w}$ (weight update). Equation (1) shows the learning rule used in calculating the value for updating the weights at each increment:

$$\Delta \mathbf{w}_i = \eta \left( true_j - pred_j \right) x_i^j \quad (1)$$

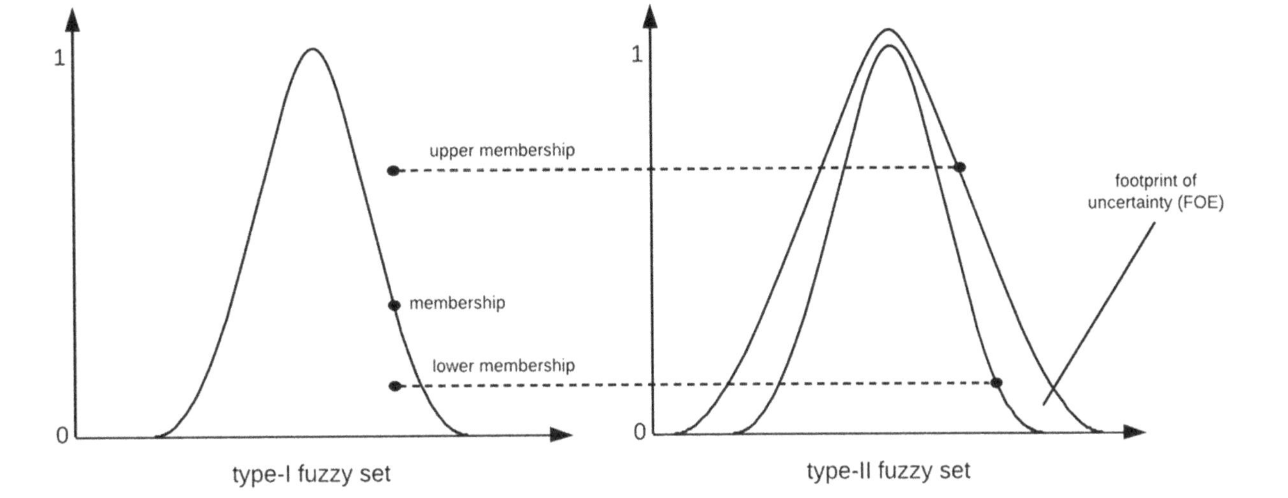


**FIGURE 1** | Creating a type-II fuzzy set.

where $\eta$ is the learning rate, $true_j$ is the true class label and $pred_j$ is the predicted class label.

The perceptron's learning process starts by initializing the weights to small random numbers [or 0]. For each training input sample the output value is calculated and the weights are updated until a minimum error is reached (i.e., backpropagation). The main drawback of perceptrons is that they are only able to converge when the two classes can be separated by a linear hyperplane.

A *multilayer perceptron* (also called Artificial Neural Network–ANN) is composed of neurons from the input layer, one or more hidden layers of neurons, and the output layer of neurons, where the input propagates through the network layer-by-layer in the forward direction where each layer of the network contains connections to the next layer. Such network is called a *feedforward* neural network and is typically used in supervised learning. The structure of the multilayer perceptron enables it to learn complex tasks by extracting more meaningful features from the input patterns. *Gradient descent* can be used to optimize model prediction by finding the local minimum of a function (i.e., minimize the network error), and is defined as follows:

$$\mathbf{w} = \mathbf{w} - \eta \times \frac{d}{d\mathbf{w}} F(\mathbf{w}) \tag{2}$$

where $\mathbf{w}$ are the weight values, $\eta$ is the learning rate, and $\frac{d}{dw}F(\mathbf{w})$ is the derivative of the objective function $F(\mathbf{w})$ representing the slope (gradient).

## 4. FUZZY SETS

Let $U = \{x_1, x_2, x_3, \ldots, x_n\}$ be the universe of discourse, a fuzzy set $A \in U$ is defined as the set of ordered pairs $\{(x_i, \mu_A(x_i))\}$, where $x_i \in U$, $\mu_A : U \to [0,1]$ is the membership function of $A$, and $\mu_A(x) \in [0,1]$ is the degree of membership of $x$ in $A$. Such fuzzy sets are called type-I fuzzy sets. However, this kind of fuzzy sets is unable to model different types of uncertainties since their membership functions are crisp. Membership functions of type-II fuzzy sets are on the other hand fuzzy and can model different types of uncertainties. A type-II fuzzy set $A'$ is characterized by a type-II membership function $\mu_{A'}(x, \mu)$, where $x \in U$ and $\mu \in [0,1]$, and is defined as:

$$A' = \{(x, \mu), \mu_{A'}(x, \mu) \,|\, \forall x \in U, \mu \in [0,1]\} \tag{3}$$

where $0 \leq \mu_{A'}(x, \mu) \leq 1$.

Type-II fuzzy sets can be simply formed by firstly defining a type-I fuzzy set and assigning lower and upper membership degrees to each element in order to construct the *footprint of uncertainty (FOU)*, that is, the interval between the lower and upper membership values (**Figure 1** depicts this concept). A type-II fuzzy set can be defined as (42):

$$A' = \{(x, \mu_U(x), x, \mu_L(x)) \,|\, \mu_L(x) \leq \mu(x) \leq \mu_U(x), \mu \in [0,1]\} \tag{4}$$

where $\mu_L$ and $\mu_U$ represent the *lower* and *upper* membership degrees of the initial membership function $\mu(x)$, respectively, defined as follows (42):

$$\mu_L(x) = [\mu(x)]^{\alpha} \tag{5}$$

$$\mu_U(x) = [\mu(x)]^{\frac{1}{\alpha}} \tag{6}$$

where $\alpha \in (1, \infty)$. In this paper, $\alpha = 2$ since $\alpha >> 2$ is not meaningful for image data (42).

## 5. FUZZY C-MEANS CLUSTERING

Let $X = \{x_1, \ldots, x_i, \ldots, x_n\}$ be the set of $n$ objects (i.e., pixels), $f(x_1, y_1), \ldots, f(x_i, y_j) : i \in [1, \ldots, m]; j \in [1, \ldots, n]$, and $V = \{v_1, \ldots, v_i, \ldots, v_c\}$ be the set of $c$ centroids in a $p$-dimensional

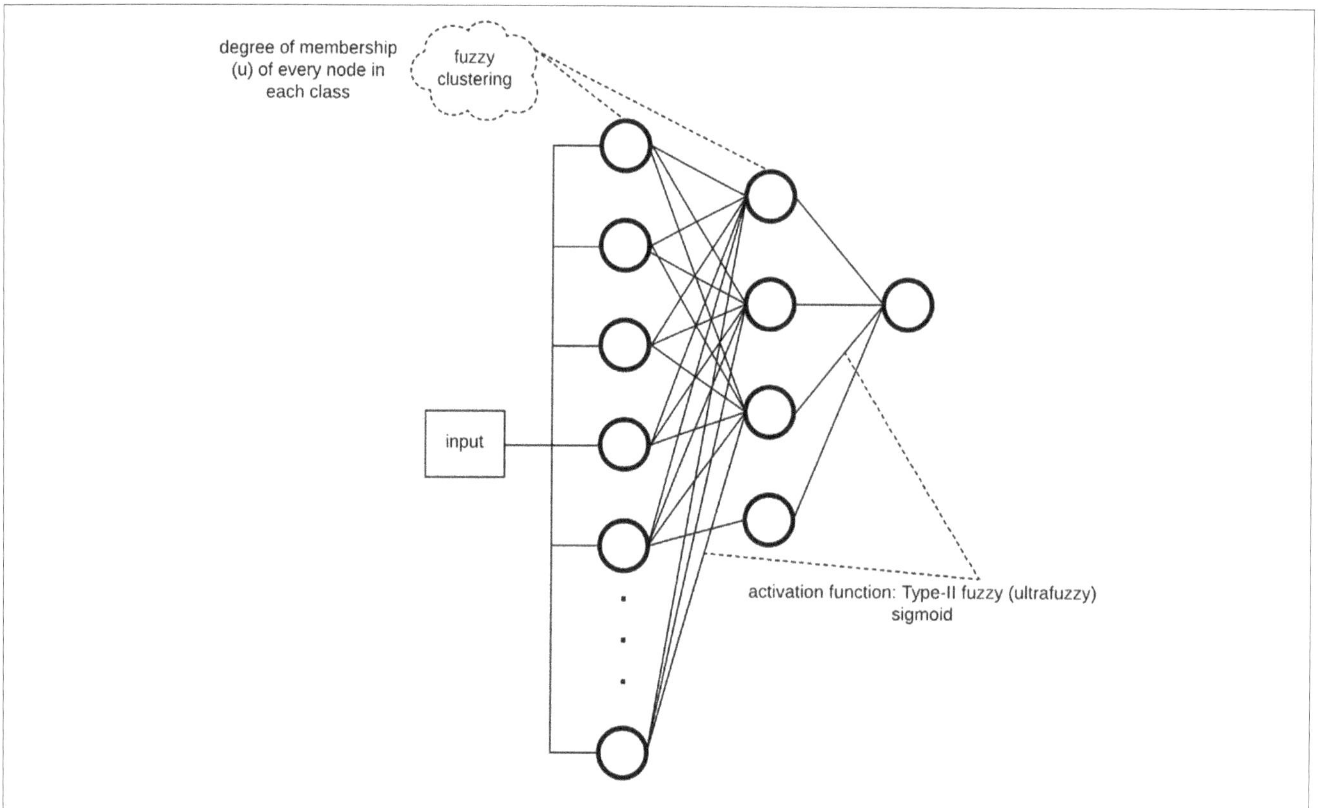


**FIGURE 2** | Proposed fuzzy multilayer perceptron (F-MLP) architecture.

feature space. In fuzzy c-means (FCM), $X$ is partitioned into $c$ clusters by minimizing the objective function $J$:

$$J = \sum_{j=1}^{n} \sum_{i=1}^{c} \left(u_{ij}\right)^m \left\|x_j - v_i\right\|^2 \tag{7}$$

where $1 \leq m \leq \infty$ is the *fuzzifier* (set to 2 in this paper), $v_i$ is the $i^{th}$ centroid corresponding to cluster $C_i$, $u_{ij} \in [0, 1]$ is the fuzzy membership of $x_j$ to cluster $C_i$, and $\|.\|$ is the distance norm, such that:

$$v_i = \frac{1}{n_i} \sum_{j=1}^{n} \left(u_{ij}\right)^m x_j \quad where \quad n_i = \sum_{j=1}^{n} \left(u_{ij}\right)^m \tag{8}$$

and,

$$u_{ij} = \frac{1}{\sum_{k=1}^{c} \left(\frac{d_{ij}}{d_{kj}}\right)^{\frac{2}{m-1}}} \quad where \quad d_{ij}{}^2 = \left\|x_j - v_i\right\|^2 \tag{9}$$

The process starts by randomly choosing $c$ objects that represent the centroids (means) of the $c$ clusters. Membership values $u_{ij}$ are calculated based on the relative distance (i.e., Euclidean distance) of the object $x_j$ to the centroids. The centroids $v_i$ of the clusters are calculated after the memberships of all objects have been found. If the centroids at the previous iteration are identical to the centroids generated at the current iteration the process terminates (43).

## 6. FUZZY MULTILAYER PERCEPTRON (F-MLP)

The proposed multilayer perceptron in this paper incorporates the membership degree of each input sample to the classes of interest (e.g., regular vs. irregular) in the learning process. Moreover, the gradient descent benefits from the membership values by reducing the effects of *ambiguous* features (i.e., features that have a membership degree of 0.5) when updating the weights (learning). Membership degrees are obtained by clustering each layer in the neural network (except the output layer) using fuzzy c-means. The proposed architecture is depicted in **Figure 2**.

A commonly used activation function in multilayer perceptrons is the *sigmoid* activation function (Equation 10). The sigmoid function is suitable for binary classification and provides continuous values in the range $[0, 1]$ that represent the probability of a class in the binary classification problem. As the sigmoid function introduces non-linearity in the hidden layers, it allows the neural network to learn more complex features (44).

$$sig\left(x\right) = \frac{1}{1 + e^{-x}} \tag{10}$$

Assuming that $\varphi$ is the fuzzy sigmoid activation function, the *type-II fuzzy sigmoid* activation function can be represented as:

$$\varphi_L\left(x\right) = \left[\frac{1}{1 + e^{-x}}\right]^\alpha \tag{11}$$

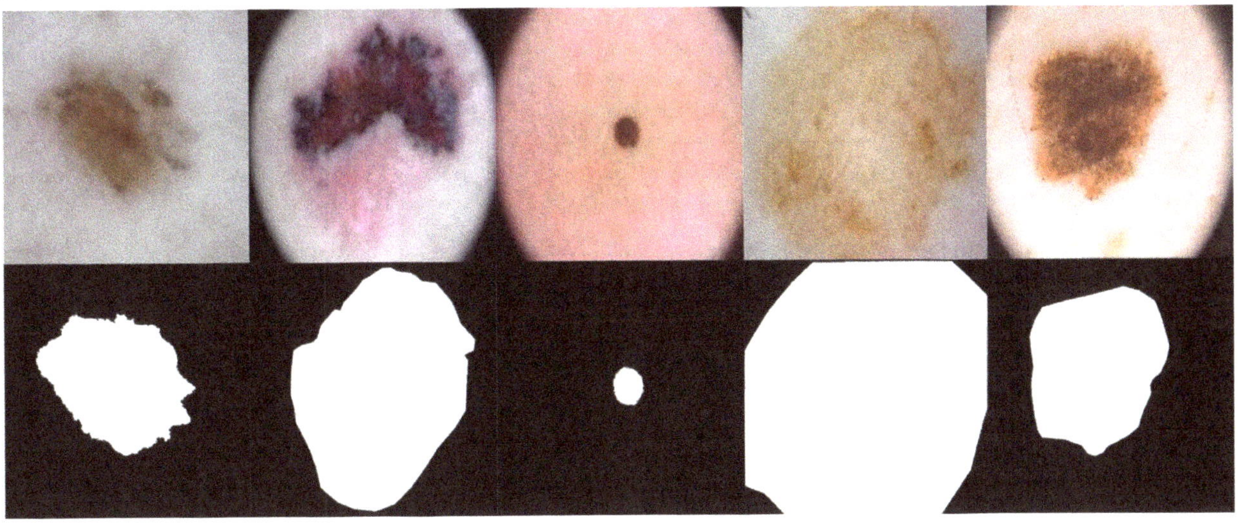

**FIGURE 3** | Samples of images used to train U-Net along with their groundtruth.

$$\varphi_U(x) = \left[\frac{1}{1+e^{-x}}\right]^{\frac{1}{\alpha}} \tag{12}$$

where $\varphi_L$ and $\varphi_U$ are the lower and upper sigmoid activation functions, respectively.

The proposed *fuzzy gradient descent* is defined as follows:

$$\mathbf{w} = \mathbf{w} - mean\left(|\mathbf{u}_1 - \mathbf{u}_2|^2\right) \times \eta \times \frac{d}{d\mathbf{w}}\varphi \tag{13}$$

where $\mathbf{w}$ are the weight values, $\mathbf{u}_1$ and $\mathbf{u}_2$ are the degrees of membership of each neuron to *class1* and *class2*, respectively; $\varphi$ is the type-II fuzzy sigmoid function, and *mean* is used to represent the square differences between the degrees of membership with a single value, which can be perceived as an *ambiguity* parameter. Notice that for ambiguous nodes $|\mathbf{u}_1 - \mathbf{u}_2|^2$ will evaluate to 0, thus having no effect on how weights are being updated. Incorporating degrees of membership in optimization will determine how input samples contribute to the learning process based on their ambiguity, such that more ambiguous features will have less effect on learning, and will rather be based on more non-ambiguous features The cost function used in our work is simply represented as the difference between the actual values and the predicted values. The F-MLP algorithm code has been open sourced and can be accessed via https://github.com/abderhasan/F-MLP.

## 7. SKIN LESION SEGMENTATION

To segment skin lesions (62) we use the U-Net architecture (45, 63), an end-to-end encoder-decoder network for semantic segmentation which was firstly used for medical image segmentation. U-Net has also been used for skin lesion segmentation in dermoscopic images (46, 47). The architecture consists of two sides: left (down) and right (up). The *down* part is the encoder part [follows the Convolutional Neural Network—CNN architecture (48)] where convolution blocks are applied followed by max-pooling in order to encode the input image into feature representations at multiple levels, provided that the number of feature channels are doubled at each downsampling step. In the *up* part, the feature map is upsampled and a convolution operation is applied, bringing the number of feature channels to half; a concatenation with the corresponding cropped feature map from the *down* part occurs, followed by two 3 × 3 convolutions which are also followed by two ReLU operations and one 2 × 2 max-pooling operation with stride 2 used for downsampling. Since border pixels are lost at each convolution, the cropping process is deemed essential. The higher resolution features from the *down* part are concatenated with the upsampled features in order to localize and learn representations better. The resulting architecture is one where the expansive path is symmetric to the concatenating path, yielding a U-shaped architecture. The network is composed of 23 convolutional layers in total and does not have any fully connected layers. The final layer of U-Net uses a 1 × 1 convolution to map each 64 feature vector to the desired number of classes. An *overlap-tile strategy* is used to predict the pixels of the border region where the missing context is extrapolated by mirroring the input image. The U-Net architecture was trained for 20 epochs on a Tesla P100 GPU on 1777 dermoscopy images (resized to 256 × 256 pixels) along with their corresponding groundtruth response masks from the "ISIC 2018: Skin Lesion Analysis Toward Melanoma Detection" grand challenge datasets (49, 50), and tested on 158 images from the same dataset (those images were not used in training U-Net). Training U-Net and testing it took 27.6 min and 25.9 s, respectively. **Figure 3** shows samples of the training dataset along with their groundtruth, and **Figure 4** shows samples of the segmentation results using U-Net (i.e., test dataset). The average Dice similarity achieved on the 158 images was 83.8%.

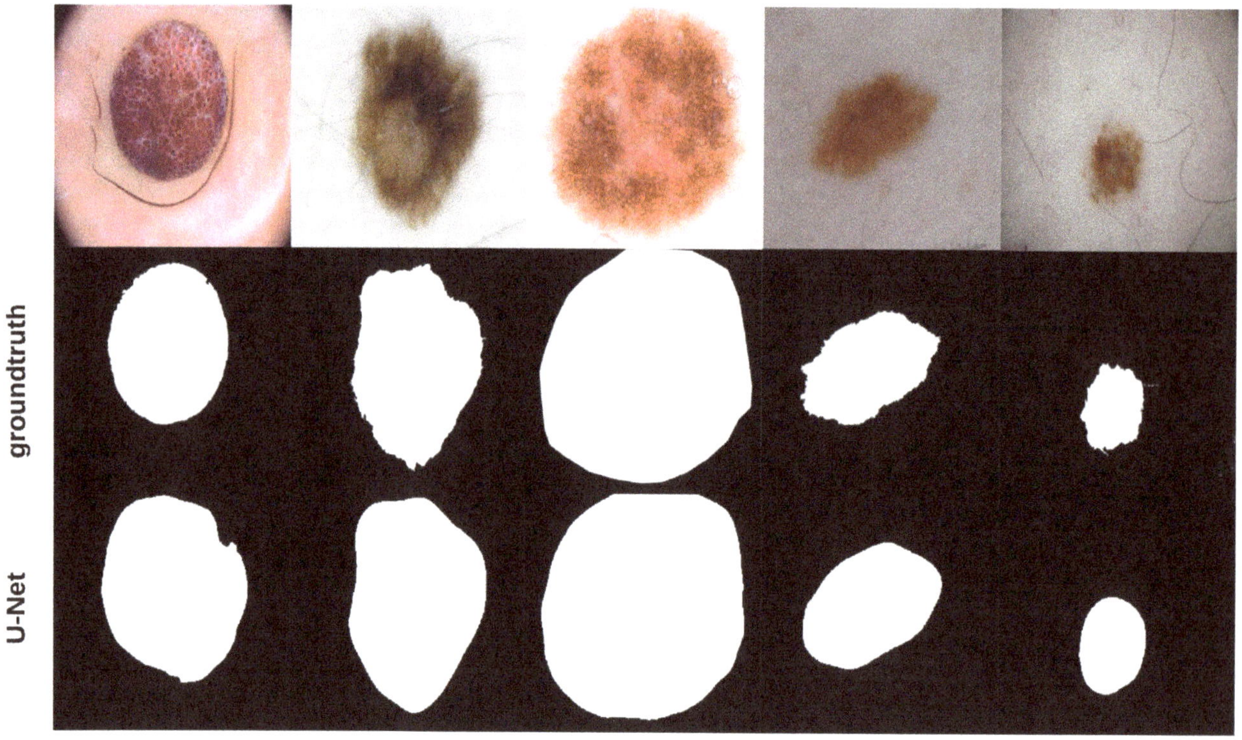


**FIGURE 4 |** Samples of images used to test U-Net, their groundtruth, and segmentation results.

## 8. SKIN LESION BORDER DETECTION

To detect the skin lesion border, we use the method we proposed in Ali et al. (46), namely *FuzzEdge*. Say that we have an image $G$ of size $M \times N$ pixels with $L$ gray levels: $G = [g(i,j)]_{M \times N}$, where $g(i,j) \in \{0, 1, \ldots, L-1\}$ refers to a pixel in the image. Let $X = [x(i,j)]_{M \times N}$ be the original input image, and $Y = [y(i,j)]_{M \times N}$ be the filtered output image; $y(i,j) = FuzzEdge(\underline{X}(i,j))$ represents the $(i,j)^{th}$ pixel of the filtered image $Y$, where $\underline{X}(i,j)$ is a $3 \times 3$ kernel centered at the input pixel $x(i,j)$ that will be affected by the filter, and $FuzzEdge(.)$ is the fuzzy filter function. Three fuzzy concepts (sets) are defined: *Bright*, *Dark*, and *Median*. Those concepts can be created using Algorithm.1.

The value associated with each pixel in the image is determined using the membership function (i.e., $f_{Median}$) of the corresponding fuzzy concept. FuzzEdge runs three standard deviation processes to determine the values of the filtered pixel (center pixel in the kernel) on each fuzzy concept, producing three values for each pixel: $y_{\bar{Bright}}(i,j)$, $y_{\bar{Dark}}(i,j)$, and $y_{\bar{Median}}(i,j)$. In the decision step of FuzzEdge, a standard deviation process similar to the above is applied on the pixels through a kernel, provided that the pixel values will be determined using a new membership function, that is, the fuzzy interval membership function. The final output of each filtered pixel is eventually determined by measuring the distance between $y_{\bar{Bright}}(i,j)$, $y_{\bar{Dark}}(i,j)$, and $y_{\bar{Median}}(i,j)$ to the fuzzy estimator, and taking the nearest pixel to the fuzzy estimator as the value of the filtered pixel in our kernel. **Figure 5** shows some samples of borders detected using FuzzEdge.

FuzzEdge code has been open sourced and can be accessed from: https://github.com/abderhasan/fuzzedge.

## 9. SKIN LESION BORDER IRREGULARITY

To measure skin lesion border irregularity, a measure that combines fractal dimension and convexity [similar to that proposed in our other work (33)] is used to form an *objective* quantitative measure of border irregularity, especially that many of the signs that the clinician relies on in diagnosis involve *subjective* judgment. This applies to visual signs such as border irregularity; it has been shown that both clinicians and patients find it hard in agreeing upon whether a naevus border is considered irregular or not (51). Such measure could thus aid in improving the diagnostic accuracy.

**Figure 6** depicts the process of extracting the skin lesion irregularity measure, which also shows that our measure will be represented as a vector of two values: convexity and fractal dimension, especially that those measures have been utilized in characterizing skin lesion border irregularity in literature.

Fractal dimension has been used in characterizing skin lesion border irregularity as in Claridge et al. (51), Ng and Lee (30), and (52). Fractal geometry (53) describes the space-filling capacity of irregular borders which is considered size independent and does not require any smoothing operations of irregular borders for measurement to be possible (54), meaning that structures don't

**Algorithm 1:** Fuzzy concept creation

**input** : grayscale image I
**output**: fuzzy set (concept)

1 For the fuzzy concepts *Bright*, *Dark*, and *Median*, specify the intervals of $[Bright_{begin}, Bright_{end}]$, $[Dark_{begin}, Dark_{end}]$, and $[Median_{begin}, Median_{end}]$, respectively.

2 Let $Bright_{begin} = (N_f - 1)\left[\frac{L-1}{N_f}\right]$, $Dark_{end} = \left[\frac{L-1}{N_f}\right]$, $Median_{begin} = Dark_{end} - left\_overlap$, and $Median_{end} = Bright_{begin} + right\_overlap$ /* $N_f$ *is the number of fuzzy concepts, and left_overlap and right_overlap determine the overlapping range of the fuzzy concepts (the overlap range was set to 0 in this paper)* */.

3 Set $Dark_{begin}$ to be the first $g_k$ from 0 to $Dark_{end}$.

4 Set $Bright_{end}$ to be the last $g_k$ from $Bright_{begin}$ to $L - 1$.

5 In interval $[Dark_{begin}, Dark_{end}]$, find a pixel $g_k$ with the maximum value of $p(g_k)$.

6 For the fuzzy concept *Dark*, create its membership function $f_{Dark}$ as follows: $m_{Dark} \leftarrow g_k$, $\alpha_{Dark} \leftarrow m_{Dark} - Dark_{begin}$, $\beta_{Dark} \leftarrow Dark_{end} - m_{Dark}$.

7 In interval $[Median_{begin}, Median_{end}]$, find a pixel $g_k$ with the maximum value of $p(g_k)$.

8 For the fuzzy concept *Median*, create its membership function $f_{Median}$ as follows: $m_{Median} \leftarrow g_k$, $\alpha_{Median} \leftarrow m_{Median} - Median_{begin}$, $\beta_{Median} \leftarrow Median_{end} - m_{Median}$.

9 In interval $[Bright, begin - Bright_{end}]$, find a pixel $g_k$ with the maximum value of $p(g_k)$.

10 For the fuzzy concept *Bright*, create its membership function $f_{Bright}$ as follows: $m_{Bright} \leftarrow g_k$, $\alpha_{Bright} \leftarrow m_{Bright} - Bright_{begin}$, $\beta_{Bright} \leftarrow Bright_{end} - m_{Bright}$.

need to possess a perfect geometric shape. Fractal dimension is a mathematical parameter that is able to quantify the irregularity of a skin lesion border via an objective observer-independent value, such that a higher fractal dimension refers to a higher degree of complexity of the analyzed pattern. A straight line in a 2-dimensional system has a fractal dimension of *one*, and more complicated lines (having fractal properties) will have larger dimensions (55). The fractal dimension is able to describe melanoma irregular borders that possess fractal properties more accurately than Euclidean measures (i.e., perimeter) (56). The *box-counting* method (57) is used to estimate the fractal dimension of the skin lesion border, and is defined as:

$$D = \lim_{e \to 0} \frac{\log N(e)}{\log\left(\frac{1}{e}\right)} \tag{14}$$

where $D = [1, 2]$ is the box-counting fractal dimension of the skin lesion border, $e > 0$ is the side (edge) length of the box, and $N$ is the smallest number of boxes of side length $e$ needed to completely cover the skin lesion border. The fractal dimension is the *slope* in the $\log N(e)/\log\left(\frac{1}{e}\right)$ graph. **Figure 7** demonstrates the box-counting method.

The straighter the skin lesion border the lower the value $D$, and vice versa. As melanoma borders tend to be irregular they are considered to be similar to fractals [i.e., Koch snowflake (58)] and are expected to have a higher fractal dimension than regular-boundary naevi. It was found in Cross et al. (54) that the fractal dimension of all lesions are greater than the topological dimension (i.e., one), indicating the existence of a fractal element in their structure.

Convexity, the ratio between the perimeter (the number of points/length of the boundary) of the convex hull of the skin lesion (the smallest convex polygon that surrounds all of the skin lesion pixels) and the skin lesion perimeter, can be used to characterize the skin lesion border shape and irregularity (37, 59, 60). Convex objects tend to have a convexity value of 1, as opposed to non-convex objects (i.e., irregular skin lesion borders) which tend to be less than 1. In other words, convexity shows the amount by which the object differs from the convex object.

## 10. RESULTS AND DISCUSSION

To prepare the training and testing data for F-MLP, 158 images segmented using U-Net were used, their skin lesion borders extracted using FuzzEdge, and the extracted borders sent to a dermatologist (Dr.Sally O'Shea) to label as *regular* or *irregular* borders (regular: 5, irregular: 153), which will eventually serve as our groundtruth (labels) for the training data. **Figure 8** shows some samples of regular and irregular borders along with their original and segmented images. However, due to the imbalance in data, an *augmentation* step (rotating, and flipping horizontally and vertically) has been carried out to increase the regular samples. Augmentation was carried out on the 5 regular bordered images, producing multiple versions of those images. The total number of images after augmentation was 310 images (regular: 157, irregular: 153).

**Table 1** shows the fractal dimension and convexity values for the images in **Figure 8**. It should be emphasized that fractal dimension is found for the edge images (i.e., FuzzEdge) and the convexity is found for the segmentation (i.e., U-Net) results of the image, as demonstrated in **Figure 6**. **Figure 9** shows box-and-whisker plots depicting the distribution of fractal dimension and convexity values for the regular and irregular skin lesions used in training and testing the neural networks.

The extracted skin lesion border irregularity measures were used to train and test a standard neural network and a type-II F-MLP. For both networks the number of neurons in the input layer is equal to the number of input features (2 features), the first hidden layer is composed of 4 neurons, the second hidden layer is composed of 2 neurons, the output layer is composed of 1 neuron which represents the final classification result, and the learning rate is 0.001. Experiments were run on a machine with an Intel Core i7 processor of speed 2.2 GHz and 16 GB memory.

After obtaining the *prediction probability* $\in [0, 1]$ of each test sample, a *threshold* is generated from the prediction probabilities

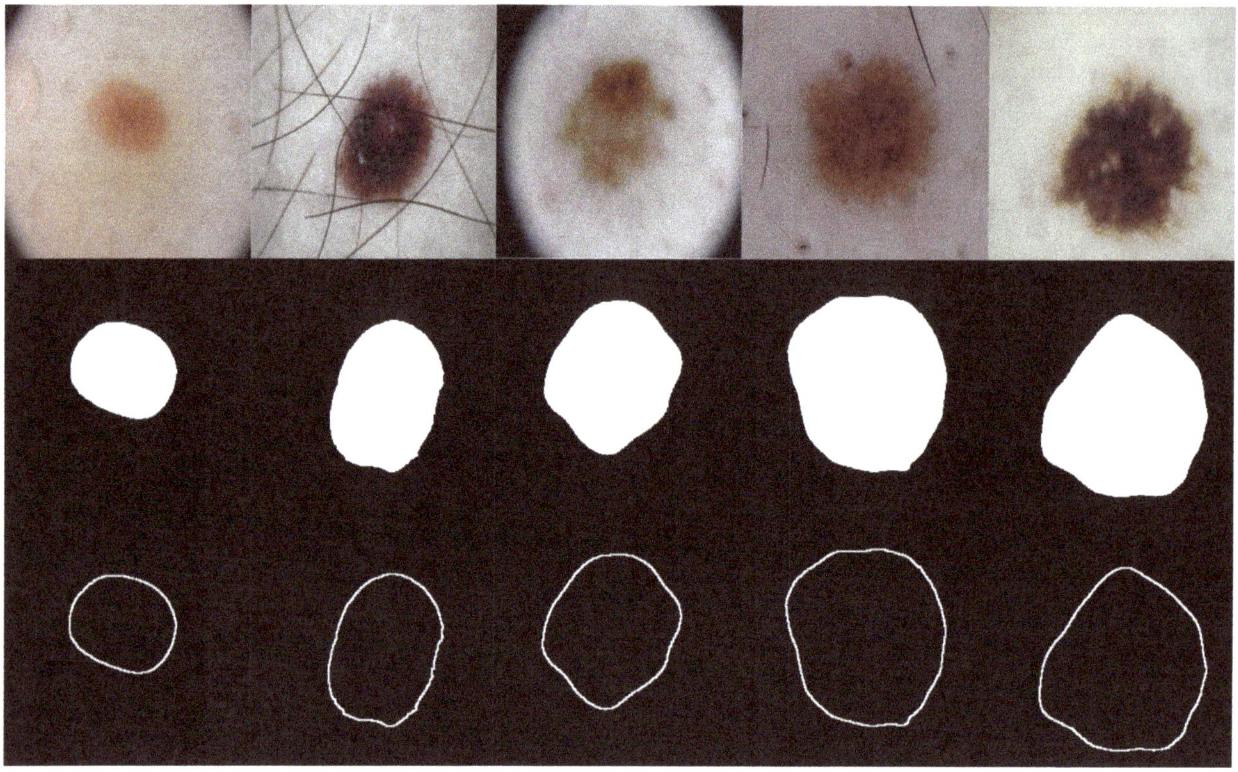

FIGURE 5 | Samples of test images, their segmentations using U-Net, and borders detected using FuzzEdge.

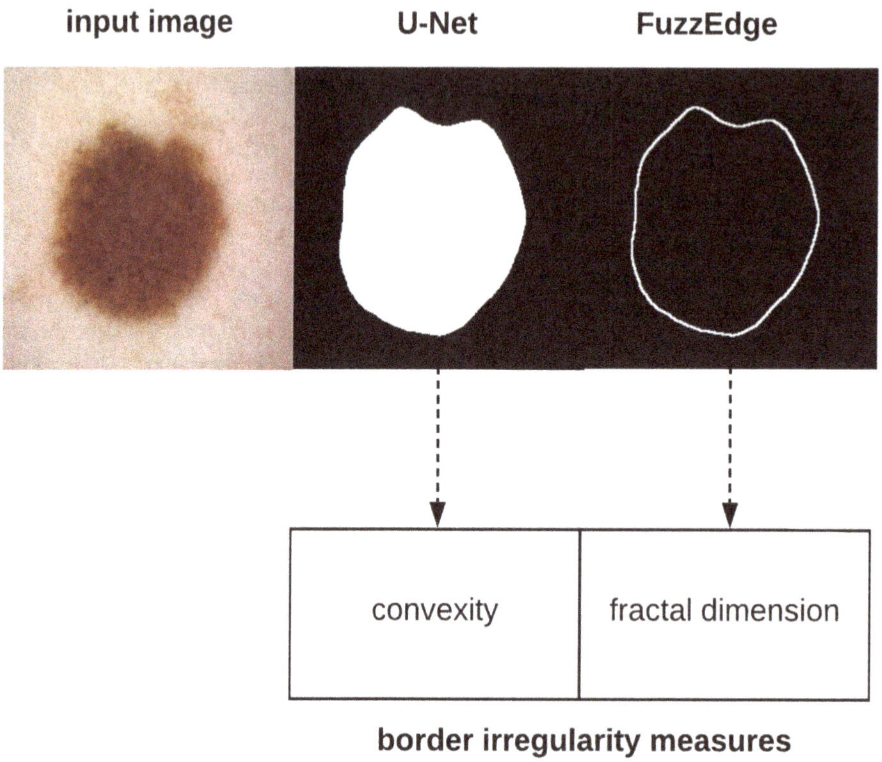


FIGURE 6 | Skin lesion border irregularity measures extraction.

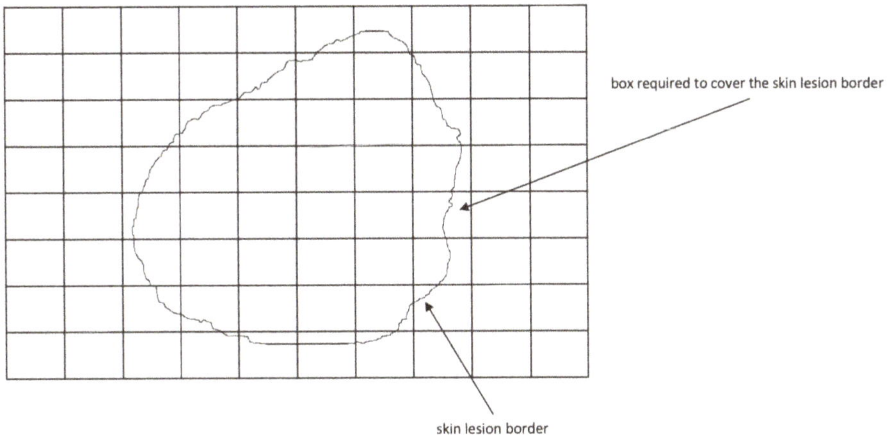


**FIGURE 7 |** Twenty-two boxes are required to cover the skin lesion border using the box-counting method.

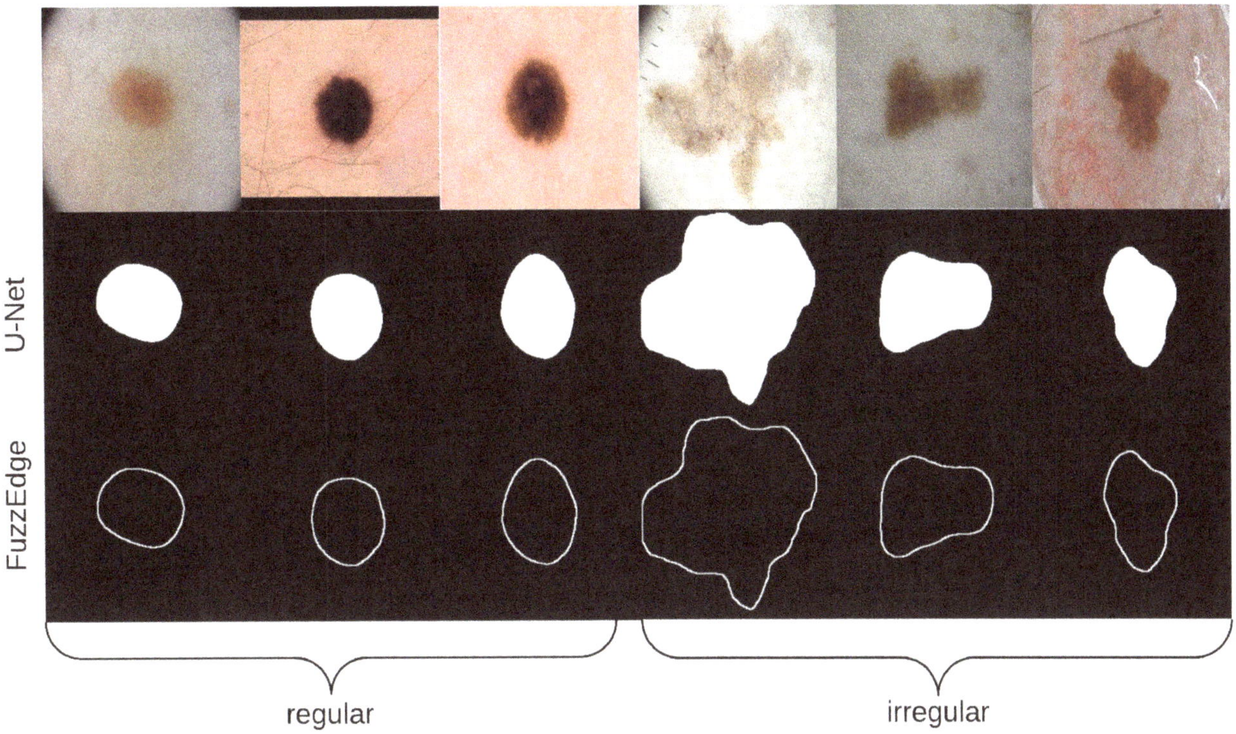


**FIGURE 8 |** Samples of regular and irregular borders labeled by the dermatologist.

to decide the final prediction (regular or irregular) according to Equation (15).

$$threshold = \frac{\sum_{i=1}^{n} p_i}{n} \tag{15}$$

where $n$ is the number of test samples, and $p_i$ is the prediction probability of test sample $i$. The final decision is obtained using Equation (16).

$$Decision = \begin{cases} regular, & p_i > threshold \\ irregular, & p_i \leq threshold \end{cases} \tag{16}$$

**Tables 2, 3** show the different training and testing split ratios used to evaluate the networks, number of iterations used in each network, time consumed (in seconds), and accuracy, for the standard neural network and F-MLP, respectively. The networks were run for only 1 iteration since more iterations didn't improve the accuracy.

Using two sigmoid activation functions reflects the type-II fuzzy set in that the error rates represent the range of performance that could be achieved using the fuzzy neural network (F-MLP), modeling thereby the potential uncertainty occurring within the input data. Two versions (lower and upper sigmoid) of F-MLP can be obtained, and the one with the best performance (maximum accuracy) can be used as shown in the following equation:

$$\lambda FMLP = \max\left(\lambda FMLP_{lower}, \lambda FMLP_{upper}\right) \quad (17)$$

where $\lambda FMLP$ is the accuracy of the fuzzy multilayer perceptron, $\lambda FMLP_{lower}$ is the accuracy of the fuzzy multilayer perceptron utilizing the lower sigmoid activation function, and $\lambda FMLP_{upper}$ represents the accuracy of the fuzzy multilayer perceptron utilizing the upper sigmoid activation function.

In comparing the standard neural network and F-MLP, we consider the 80:20 ratio as it results in better accuracy amongst the other ratios, evaluating to 91.9 and 95.2% for the standard neural network and F-MLP, respectively. **Tables 4, 5** depict the confusion matrices of the classification results, from which we derive the sensitivity and specificity values that evaluate to 100 and 82.8% for the standard neural network, respectively, and 100 and 89.7% for the F-MLP, respectively. **Figure 10** depicts the receiver operating characteristic (ROC) curves of the standard neural network and F-MLP.

To evaluate the proposed approach further, we compare it with other state-of-the-art classification methods as shown in **Table 6** which shows that F-MLP outperforms most of those methods.

Incorporating the membership degree in the gradient descent (Equation 13) helps in reducing the effects of ambiguous features/neurons when updating the weights, and thus increases the performance of learning (i.e., higher accuracy predictions). The proposed type-II F-MLP is able to perform better than its traditional neural network counterpart with fewer iterations.

**TABLE 1 |** Border irregularity measures for the images presented in **Figure 8**.

| Image | Fractal dimension | Convexity | Label |
|---|---|---|---|
| 1.r | 1.2527 | 0.9898 | 1 |
| 2.r | 1.2599 | 0.9890 | 1 |
| 3.r | 1.2875 | 0.9893 | 1 |
| 1.i | 1.4499 | 0.9031 | 0 |
| 2.i | 1.3056 | 0.9531 | 0 |
| 3.i | 1.3125 | 0.9586 | 0 |

*Images 1.r, 2.r, and 3.r from left to right refer to the first three images (regular), and images 1.i, 2.i, and 3.i refer to the last three images (irregular).*

**TABLE 2 |** Standard neural network evaluation on classifying regular and irregular borders using different training and testing split ratios.

| Ratio | Training | Testing | Training time | Testing time | Accuracy (%) |
|---|---|---|---|---|---|
| 80:20 | 248 | 62 | 0.02 | 0.007 | 91.9 |
| 70:30 | 217 | 93 | 0.02 | 0.008 | 91.4 |
| 60:40 | 186 | 124 | 0.01 | 0.007 | 87.9 |
| 50:50 | 155 | 155 | 0.02 | 0.009 | 79.4 |

**TABLE 3 |** F-MLP evaluation on classifying regular and irregular borders using different training and testing split ratios.

| Ratio | Training | Testing | Training time | Testing time | Lower sigmoid acc. (%) | Upper sigmoid acc. (%) |
|---|---|---|---|---|---|---|
| 80:20 | 248 | 62 | 0.58 | 0.01 | 95.2 | 90.3 |
| 70:30 | 217 | 93 | 0.8 | 0.07 | 91.4 | 89.2 |
| 60:40 | 186 | 124 | 0.6 | 0.08 | 90.3 | 87.9 |
| 50:50 | 155 | 155 | 0.7 | 0.08 | 83.9 | 75.5 |

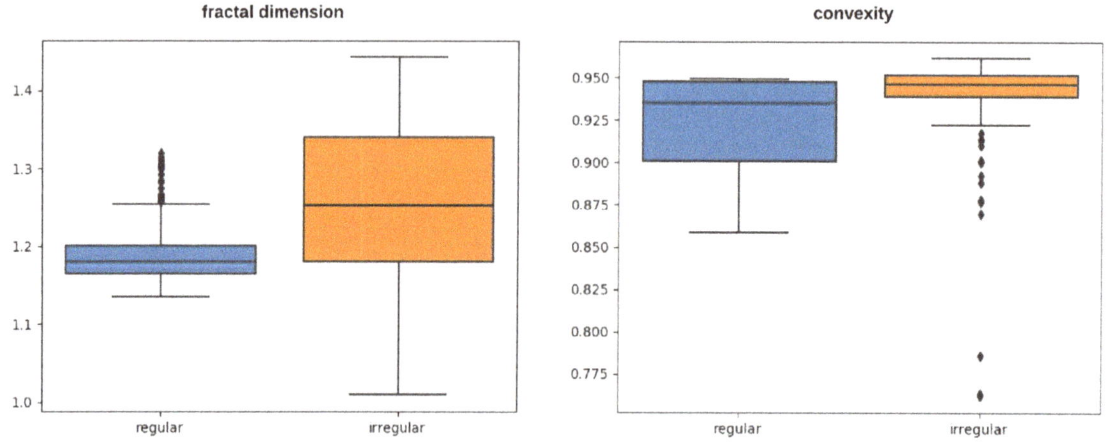


**FIGURE 9 |** Box-and-whisker plots representing the fractal dimension and convexity distributions of the skin lesions (regular and irregular) used in training and testing the neural network.

However, training F-MLP is more time-consuming than its traditional neural network counterpart.

## 11. CONCLUSION

An automatic approach for detecting the skin lesion border irregularity has been proposed. The approach starts by segmenting the skin lesion using U-Net, detecting the lesion border using FuzzEdge, extracting the irregularity measures (fractal dimension and convexity), training a F-MLP on the extracted measures, and predicting border irregularity on new images using the trained model. The proposed F-MLP utilizes type-II fuzzy sets and showed to provide better prediction accuracy than most of the state-of-the-art classification methods in general and its standard neural network counterpart in particular.

The proposed approach reflects three main contributions: (i) developing a fuzzy gradient descent that considers the membership degrees of neurons, minimizing thereby the effects of ambiguous neurons on the neural network learning process, (ii) proposing a type-II fuzzy sigmoid activation function which allows to represent the range (lowest and highest) of performance the fuzzy neural network is able to attain, where the fuzzy neural network with the highest performance (highest accuracy) could be utilized in the prediction process, (iii) proposing an irregularity measure that is represented as a vector of fractal dimension and convexity values. The

**TABLE 4 |** Standard neural network confusion matrix.

| | | Predicted | | |
|---|---|---|---|---|
| | | **Regular** | **Irregular** | **Total** |
| Actual | Regular | 33 | 0 | 33 |
| | Irregular | 5 | 24 | 29 |
| | Total | 38 | 24 | 62 |

**TABLE 5 |** F-MLP (lower sigmoid) confusion matrix.

| | | Predicted | | |
|---|---|---|---|---|
| | | **Regular** | **Irregular** | **Total** |
| Actual | Regular | 33 | 0 | 33 |
| | Irregular | 3 | 26 | 29 |
| | Total | 36 | 26 | 62 |

**TABLE 6 |** F-MLP evaluation on classifying regular and irregular borders using different training and testing split ratios.

| Method | TP | TN | FP | FN | Accuracy (%) |
|---|---|---|---|---|---|
| F-MLP (lower sigmoid) | 33 | 26 | 3 | 0 | 95.2 |
| Stochastic gradient descent | 33 | 26 | 3 | 0 | 95.2 |
| Random forests | 32 | 28 | 1 | 1 | 96.8 |
| Logistic regression | 32 | 22 | 7 | 1 | 87.1 |
| K-nearest neighbors | 32 | 26 | 3 | 1 | 93.5 |
| Gaussian naive bayes | 32 | 22 | 7 | 1 | 87.1 |
| Support vector machine | 28 | 23 | 11 | 0 | 87.1 |
| Decision tree | 32 | 26 | 3 | 1 | 93.5 |

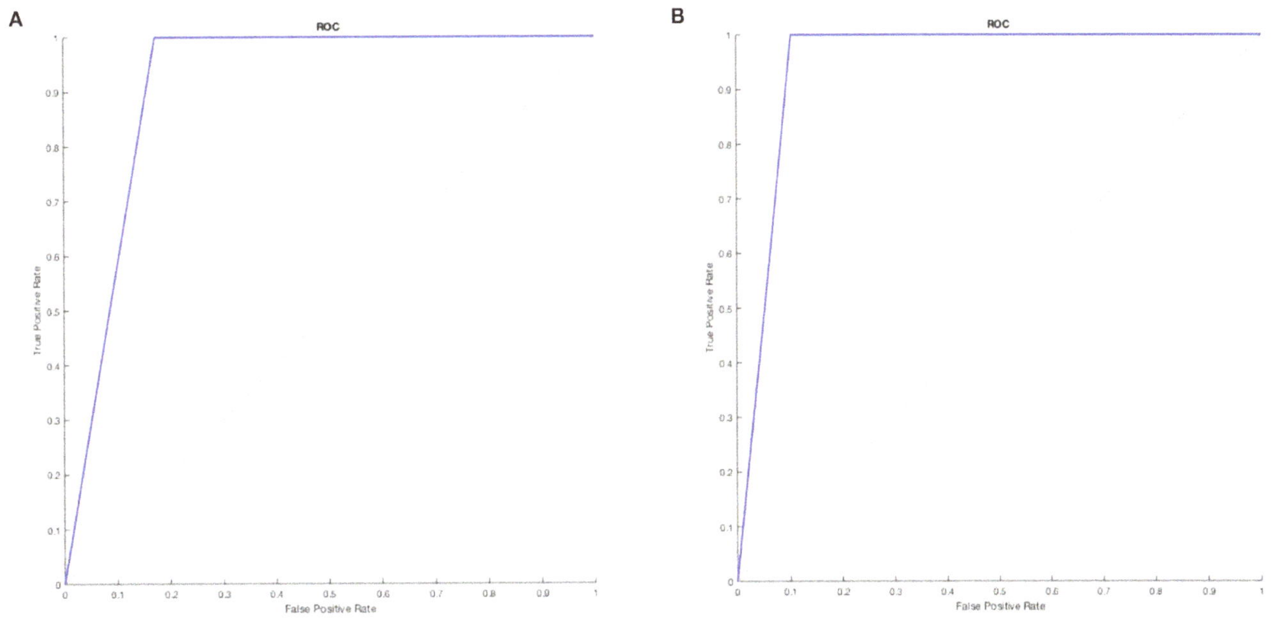


**FIGURE 10 | (A)** Standard neural network ROC curve **(B)** F-MLP (lower sigmoid) ROC curve.

approach is however more time-consuming when training the neural network.

The process of assigning regular and irregular labels to the skin lesion borders in the F-MLP training phase is considered laborious and might involve a larger team to be able to label thousands of lesion borders, a task that could eventually improve the prediction accuracy.

This work leads us to what we call fuzzy deep learning, in which we hypothesize that it would improve the traditional deep learning approaches currently used in literature. We are aiming to investigate further the combination of fuzzy logic and CNNs. There could be different approaches to fuzzifying the CNN such as using fuzzy arithmetic instead of the currently used convolution arithmetic (61) for instance. This will be demonstrated further in a future study.

As future work, we would also like to investigate introducing more metrics in the skin lesion border irregularity measure vector to increase the robustness of such measure. Moreover, we would like to apply the method on problems incorporating more than two classes, and on skin lesion images taken using a mobile phone camera (i.e., less quality) as opposed to dermoscopic images.

## AUTHOR CONTRIBUTIONS

A-RA was the main author of the paper, designed and implemented the method, and drafted the paper. JL was the main author's Ph.D. supervisor and provided deep analytical thoughts, suggestions, comments, and feedback that improved the paper dramatically. GY and SK provided comments and feedback on the paper and raised some questions about the proposed method. AH provided comments and feedback on the paper and raised some questions about the proposed method and how to improve it. SO'S acted as the dermatologist who annotated our skin lesion border images which were used as a ground truth throughout our experiments. All authors contributed to the article and approved the submitted version.

## ACKNOWLEDGMENTS

The work was supported by Natural Science Foundation of China (Grant No. 71571076).

## REFERENCES

1. Hintz-Madsen M. *A Probabilistic Framework for Classification of Dermatoscopic Images.* Technical University of Denmark (1998).
2. Friedman R, Rigel D, Kopf A. Early detection of malignant melanoma: the role of physician examination and self-examination of the skin. *Cancer J Clin.* (1985) 35:130–51. doi: 10.3322/canjclin.35.3.130
3. McGovern T, Litaker M. Clinical predictors of malignant pigmented lesions: a comparison of the Glasgow seven point check list and the American Cancer Society's ABCDs of pigmented lesions. *J Dermatol Surg Oneal.* (1992) 18:22–6. doi: 10.1111/j.1524-4725.1992.tb03296.x
4. Barnhill R, Roush G, Ernstoff ea MS. Interclinician agreement on the recognition of selected gross morphologic features of pigmented lesions. *J Dermatol Surg Oneal.* (1992) 26(2 Pt 1):185–90. doi: 10.1016/0190-9622(92)70023-9
5. Cascinelli N, Ferrario M, Tonelli ea T. A possible new tool for the clinical diagnosis of melanoma: the computer. *J Am Acad Oermatol.* (1987) 16:361–7. doi: 10.1016/S0190-9622(87)70050-4
6. White R, Rigel O, Friedman R. Computer applications in the diagnosis and prognosis of malignant melanoma. *Dermatol Clin.* (1991) 9:695–702. doi: 10.1016/S0733-8635(18)30374-7
7. Keefe M, Dick DC, Wakeel R. A study of the value of the seven-point checklist in distinguishing benign pigmented lesions from melanoma. *Clin Exp Dermatol.* (1990) 15:167–71. doi: 10.1111/j.1365-2230.1990.tb02064.x
8. Dellavalle R. *United States Skin Disease Needs Assessment, An Issue of Dermatologic Slinics - E-Book.* Philadelphia, PA: Elsevier Health Sciences (2012).
9. Lee T, Claridge E. Predictive power of irregular border shapes for malignant melanomas. *Skin Res Technol.* (2005) 11:1–8. doi: 10.1111/j.1600-0846.2005.00076.x
10. Ali A-R, Li J, O'Shea SJ. Towards the automatic detection of skin lesion shape asymmetry, color variegation and diameter in dermoscopic images. *PLoS ONE.* (2020) 15:e0234352. doi: 10.1371/journal.pone.0234352
11. Lee S, Lee E. Fuzzy neural networks. *Math Biosci.* (1975) 23:151–77. doi: 10.1016/0025-5564(75)90125-X
12. McCulloch W, Pitts W. A logical calculus of the ideas immanent in nervous activity. *Bull Math Biophys.* (1943) 5:115–33. doi: 10.1007/BF02478259
13. Keller J, Hunt D. Incorporating fuzzy membership functions into the perceptron algorithm. *IEEE Trans. Pattern Anal. Mach. Intell.* (1985) I:693–9. doi: 10.1109/TPAMI.1985.4767725
14. Goh T, Wang P, Lui H. Learning algorithm for enhanced fuzzy perceptron. *Proc IJCNN.* (1992) 2:435–40.
15. Simpson P. Fuzzy min–max neural networks–part I: classification. *IEEE Trans Neural Netw.* (1992) 3:776–86. doi: 10.1109/72.159066
16. Simpson P. Fuzzy min-max neural networks–part 2: clustering. *IEEE Trans Fuzzy Syst.* (1993) 1:32–45. doi: 10.1109/TFUZZ.1993.390282
17. Pal S, Mitra S. Multilayer perception, fuzzy sets and classification. *IEEE Trans Neural Netw.* (1992) 3:683–96. doi: 10.1109/72.159058
18. Mitra S, Pal SK, Kundu MK. Fingerprint classification using fuzzy multilayer perceptron. *Neural Comput Appl.* (1994) 2:227–33. doi: 10.1007/BF01414811
19. Buckley J, Hayashi Y. Fuzzy neural networks: a survey. *Fuzzy Sets Syst.* (1994) 66:1–13. doi: 10.1016/0165-0114(94)90297-6
20. Ishibuchi H, Kwon K, Tanaka H. A learning algorithm of fuzzy neural networks with triangular fuzzy weights. *Fuzzy Sets Syst.* (1995) 71:277–93. doi: 10.1016/0165-0114(94)00281-B
21. Ishibuchi H. Development of fuzzy neural networks. In: *Fuzzy Modeling: Paradigms and Practices.* Norwell, MA: Kluwer. (1996) p. 185–202.
22. Chen J, Chang D. Fuzzy perceptron neural networks for classifiers with numerical data and linguistic rules as inputs. *IEEE Trans Fuzzy Syst.* (2000) 8:730–45. doi: 10.1109/91.890331
23. Chen J, Chen C. Fuzzy kernel perceptron. *IEEE Trans Neural Netw.* (2002) 13:1364–73. doi: 10.1109/TNN.2002.804311
24. Vapnik V. *The Nature of Statistical Learning Theory.* New York, NY: Springer-Verlag (1995).
25. Samarjit K, Dasb S, Ghoshb PK. Applications of neuro fuzzy systems: a brief review and future outline. *Appl Soft Comput.* (2014) 15:243–59. doi: 10.1016/j.asoc.2013.10.014
26. Fan L. Revisit fuzzy neural network: bridging the gap between fuzzy logic and deep learning. *arXiv [preprint].* arXiv:17110265.. (2018).

27. Golston J, Moss R, W S. Boundary detection in skin tumor images: an overall approach and a radial search algorithm. *Pattern Recogn.* (1990) 23:1235–47. doi: 10.1016/0031-3203(90)90119-6
28. Golston J, Stoecker R W Moss, Dhillon I. Automatic detection of irregular borders in melanoma and other skin tumors. *Comput Med Imaging Graph.* (1992) 16:199–203. doi: 10.1016/0895-6111(92)90074-J
29. Leondes CT. *General Anatomy.* Amsterdam: CRC Press (1997).
30. Ng V, Lee T. Measuring border irregularities of skin lesions using fractal dimensions. In: *SPIE Photonics China, Electronic Imaging and Multimedia Systems.* Beijing (1996). p. 64–72.
31. Lee T, Ng V, McLean D, Coidman A, Gallagher R, Sale J. A multi-stage segmentation method for images of skin lesions. In: *Proceedings of IEEE Pacific Rim Conference on Commnnicaions, Compulers, and Signal Processing.* Victoria, BC (1995). p. 602–5.
32. Claridge E, Smith J, Hall P. Evaluation of border irregularity in pigmented skin lesions against a consensus of expert clinicians. In: Berry E, Hogg D, Mardia K, Smith M, editors. *Proceedings of Medical Image Understanding and Analysis (MIUA98).* Leeds: BMVA (1998). p. 85–8.
33. Ali A, Li J, Yang G, O'Shea SJ, Trappenberg T. A machine learning approach to automatic detection of irregularity in skin lesion border using dermoscopic images. *PeerJ Comput Sci.* (2020).
34. Lee T, Atkins M, Gallagher R, MacAulay C, Coldman A, McLean D. Describing the structural shape of melanocytic lesions. In: Hanson KM, editor. *Proceedings of SPIE.* San Diego, CA (1999). p. 1170–9.
35. Lee T, Ng V, Gallagher R, Coldman A, McLean D. DullRazor: a software approach to hair removal from images. *Comput Biol Med.* (1997) 27:533–43. doi: 10.1016/S0010-4825(97)00020-6
36. Lee T, Atkins M. A new approach to measure border irregularity for melanocytic lesions. *SPIE J.* (2000) 668–75. doi: 10.1117/12.387728
37. Lee T, McLean D, Stella M. Irregularity index: a new border irregularity measure for cutaneous melanocytic lesions. *Med Image Anal.* (2003) 7:47–64. doi: 10.1016/S1361-8415(02)00090-7
38. Aribisala B, Claridge E. A border irregularity measure using a modified conditional entropy method as a malignant melanoma predictor. In: *International Conference Image Analysis and Recognition.* Toronto, ON (2005). p. 914–21.
39. Ma L, Qin B, Xu W, Zhu L. Multi-scale descriptors for contour irregularity of skin lesion using wavelet decomposition. In: *Proceedings of the 3rd International Conference on Biomedical Engineering and Informatics.* Toronto, ON (2010) p. 414–8.
40. Jaworek-Korjakowska J, Tadeusiewicz R. Determination of border irregularity in dermoscopic color images of pigmented skin lesions. *Conf Proc IEEE Eng Med Biol Soc.* (2015) 2015:2665–8. doi: 10.1109/EMBC.2014.6945107
41. Argenziano G, et al. *Interactive Atlas of Dermoscopy.* Milan: Edra Medical Publishing and New Media (2000).
42. Tizhoosh H. Image thresholding using type II fuzzy sets. *Pattern Recogn.* (2005) 38:2363–72. doi: 10.1016/j.patcog.2005.02.014
43. Maji P, Pal S. Maximum class separability for rough-fuzzy c-means based brain MR image segmentation. *T Rough Sets.* (2008) 9:114–34. doi: 10.1007/978-3-540-89876-4_7
44. Pattanayak S. *Pro Deep Learning With tensorFlow: A Mathematical Approach to Advanced Artificial Intelligence in Python, 1st Edition.* Bangalore: Apress (2017).
45. Ronneberger O, Fischer P, Brox T. U-net: Convolutional networks for biomedical image segmentation. In: *MICCAI.* Munich (2015).
46. Ali A, Li J, O'Shea S, Yang G, Trappenberg T, Ye X. A deep learning based approach to skin lesion border extraction with a novel edge detector in dermoscopy images. In: *The International Joint Conference on Neural Networks - IEEE IJCNN.* Budapest (2019).
47. Ali A, Li J, O'Shea S, Trappenberg T. Supervised versus unsupervised deep learning based methods for skin lesion segmentation in dermoscopy images. In: *Canadian Conference on Artificial Intelligence.* (2019) At Kingston, ON. p. 373–9.
48. Krizhevsky A, Sutskever I, Hinton G. Imagenet classification with deep convolutional neural networks. In: *NIPS.* Nevada (2012).
49. Codella N, Gutman D, Emre Celebi M, Helba B, Marchetti M, Dusza S, et al. Skin lesion analysis toward melanoma detection: A challenge at the 2017 international symposium on biomedical imaging (ISBI), Hosted by the International Skin Imaging Collaboration (ISIC). *arXiv:171005006.* (2017). doi: 10.1109/ISBI.2018.8363547
50. Tschandl P, Rosendahl C, Kittler H. The HAM10000 dataset, a large collection of multi-source dermatoscopic images of common pigmented skin lesions. *arXiv preprint arXiv:180310417.* (2018). doi: 10.1038/sdata.2018.161
51. Claridge E, Hall P, Keefe J, Allen P. Shape analysis for classification of malignant melanoma. *J Biomed Eng.* (1992) 14:229–34. doi: 10.1016/0141-5425(92)90057-R
52. Piantanelli A, Maponi P, Scalise L, Serresi S, Cialabrini A, Basso A. Fractal characterisation of boundary irregularity in skin pigmented lesions. *Med Biol Eng Comput.* (2005) 43:436–42. doi: 10.1007/BF02344723
53. Mandelbrot B. *The Fractal Geometry of Nature.* W. H. Freeman and Co. (1982).
54. Cross S, McDonagh A, Stephenson T, Cotton D, Underwood J. Fractal and integer-dimensional geometric analysis of pigmented skin lesions. *Am J Dermatopathol.* (1995) 17:374–8. doi: 10.1097/00000372-199508000-00012
55. Falconer K. *The Fractal Geometry of Nature.* Chicester: John Wiley (1990).
56. Cross S, Cotton D. The fractal dimension may be a useful morphometric discriminant in histopathology. *J Pathol.* (1992) 166:409–11. doi: 10.1002/path.1711660414
57. Feder J. Fractals. *J Pathol.* (1992) 166:409–11.
58. Li JM, Lü L, Lai MO, Ralph B. *Image-Based Fractal Description of Microstructures.* New York, NY: Springer Science & Business Media (2003).
59. Rosin PL. Classification of pathological shapes using convexity measures. *Pattern Recogn Lett.* (2009) 30:570–8. doi: 10.1016/j.patrec.2008.12.001
60. Do T, Hoang T, Pomponiu V, Zhou Y, Chen Z, Cheung N, et al. Accessible melanoma detection using smartphones and mobile image analysis. *IEEE Trans Multimed.* (2018) 20:2849–64. doi: 10.1109/TMM.2018.2814346
61. Vincent D, Francesco V. A guide to convolution arithmetic for deep learning. *arXiv [preprint].* arXiv:160307285. (2016). 179–88.
62. Zhang L, Yang G, Ye X. Automatic skin lesion segmentation by coupling deep fully convolutional networks and shallow network with textons. *J. Med. Imaging.* (2019) 6:024001. doi: 10.1117/1.JMI.6.2.024001
63. Jiang H, Huang K, Zhang R, Hussain A. Style-neutralized pattern classification based on adversarially trained upgraded U-Net. *Cogn. Comput.* (2019). doi: 10.1007/s12559-019-09660-0
64. Huang K, Hussain A, Wang Q-F, Zhang R. *Deep Learning: Fundamentals, Theory and Applications, vol.2.* Cham: Springer Nature (2019). doi: 10.1007/978-3-030-06073-2

# 14

# IMPROVE 1.0: Individual Monitoring of Psoriasis Activity by Regular Online App Questionnaires and Outpatient Visits

*Natalie Garzorz-Stark* [1,2*†], *Sarah Beicht* [1†], *Veronika Baghin* [1], *Sebastian P. Stark* [1], *Tilo Biedermann* [1] *and Felix Lauffer* [1]

[1] *Department of Dermatology and Allergy, Technical University of Munich, Munich, Germany,* [2] *Division of Dermatology and Venereology, Department of Medicine Solna, Center for Molecular Medicine, Karolinska Institutet, Stockholm, Sweden*

***Correspondence:***
*Natalie Garzorz-Stark*
*natalie.garzorz@tum.de*

† *These authors have contributed equally to this work*

Smartphone apps gain more and more importance in supporting management of chronic diseases. Psoriasis is a highly prevalent, lifelong chronic inflammatory skin disease with a high impact on patient's quality of life. Disease management includes regular topical and systemic treatment of skin lesions as well as co-treatment of metabolic and psychologic disorders. In this study, we investigated the potential of a new smartphone app (IMPROVE 1.0) for individual monitoring of disease activity and disease influencing factors. Twelve out of 50 psoriasis patients asked for study participation performed self-assessment of psoriasis severity, life quality, and stress scores using the app over a period of 1 year. Every 2 months, study participants were carefully examined by a dermatologist in order to control the quality of app-reported data. We found that psoriasis severity and life quality values as entered in the app closely correlate to physician's examination. Furthermore, we detected strong correlations of disease activity with life quality and psoriasis serum biomarker. Temporal relations between psoriasis aggravation and previous changes of lifestyle factors, such as increased stress levels, were observed in individual patients, indicating a high potential for preventive interventions in future psoriasis apps. The vast majority of study participants evaluated IMPROVE 1.0 app positively and wish to include the app into their daily life. Hence, we demonstrate that smartphone apps are a useful tool to raise self-awareness for the dimensions of complex diseases and fully integrate psoriasis patients into individual disease management. These data are important to develop more advanced digital tools supporting the management of chronic diseases in the future.

**Keywords: smartphone, application, psoriasis, inflammatory skin disease, personalized medicine**

## INTRODUCTION

Smartphone apps play an increasingly important part in daily life. They are easily accessible, are handy, and facilitate access to information, communication, or management of routine tasks such as banking. As health care systems are limited by financial restrictions and personal capacities, smartphone apps might more and more support or take over routine physician's work. Several digital health tools have been developed over the last decade (1). While a plethora of smartphone apps are created for patient education and mainly deliver information in a more convenient way (2, 3), the major restriction of more advanced apps is the lack of objective measurement tools to perform long-term disease monitoring. Therefore, many apps are linked to a conventional medical device in order to assess, for example, blood pressure, blood glucose, or overall healthy lifestyle in a prospective way (4, 5). However, to establish an app in a larger cohort of patients, all essential tools must be executable by the patients themselves without any further technical devices. For this purpose, inflammatory skin diseases (ISD) are an ideal disease model, as disease activity is usually assessed by morphological scores, such as the psoriasis area and severity index (PASI).

Psoriasis is one of the most common ISD, which affects up to 3% of the general population in western countries (6). Patient's life quality if critically diminished by visible and stigmatizing plaques of inflamed skin, itch, scaling, and comorbidities (7, 8). In the latter case, the metabolic syndrome, addictive diseases, and psychological disorders are the major causes of morbidity and mortality (7). However, obesity or distress can—vice versa—also impair psoriasis severity (9). Therefore, psoriasis patients need a disease management considering individual disease and lifestyle factors (10)—a comprehensive approach that might profit from digital support by a smartphone app. However, it is so far unknown if patients are capable to reliably judge psoriasis severity and reflect about comorbidities using an app and if they appreciate a digital tool for their individual disease management.

To test whether apps are useful to monitor psoriasis disease activity, we created a new app (IMPROVE 1.0) and asked psoriasis patients to regularly enter self-PASI, life quality, and stress questionnaires as well as lifestyle factors over a period of 12 months. In a prospective study, we compared data collected by the app with physician's examination, with disease scoring performed by dermatologists and biomarkers. Furthermore, we collected patients' feedback on utility and helpfulness of IMPROVE 1.0 in order to gain further insight into the potential of a psoriasis app in clinical practice.

# METHODS

## Study Cohort

Fifty adult patients (age $\geq$ 18 years) with histologically confirmed diagnosis of psoriasis regularly seen at our outpatient clinic who used a smartphone and had experience with smartphone apps were asked to participate in the study. Reasons for not participating were lack of time and/or no smartphone with Android system (app only programmed for Android system) at patient's disposal. Thirteen of these patients were enrolled, and 12 of the enrolled patients completed the 48-week study. One patient did not continue the study after the first outpatient visit for personal reasons. Patients were given an introduction of the app and every 2 weeks $\pm$ 1 week; they filled in the smartphone app questionnaire assessing disease severity and lifestyle factors (see below). Lifestyle factors and their potentially aggravating effect on psoriasis were explained at the beginning of the study to each patient but no intervention with regard to lifestyle factors was initiated. Every 8 $\pm$ 2 weeks, patients were examined by a physician during an outpatient visit. Moreover, blood samples were taken at each visit and analyzed for serum markers and blood count (see **Figure 1A**). At the end of the study, patients completed a final evaluation questionnaire on the app and the study. The study was approved by the Ethics Committee of the Faculty of Medicine of the Technical University of Munich (63/16S) and written informed consent was obtained from the patients.

## Smartphone App Improve 1.0

The app was programmed using Eclipse for androids, an IDE for developers creating Android applications (http://www.eclipse.org). The app was sent to the patient *via* e-mail and downloaded by the patient. An introduction to the app was given by the study team. The app consisted of the DLQI questionnaire to measure the quality of life (11), the PSS questionnaire to measure the perception of stress (12), and of questions on their lifestyle (consumption of alcohol, cigarettes, and fast food; frequency of doing sports; body weight; and sleep), which were assessed on a verbal rating scale that was converted to a numeric rating scale for analysis (0–4, except for the amount of cigarettes 0–5). Besides, the patients assessed the severity of psoriasis according to the simplified PASI (SPASI) (13). The area of involvement (area score) was assessed on a 0–6 scale [0: no lesions, 1: $\leq$10 palms of the hand (PTH), 2: $\leq$30 PTH, 3: $\leq$50 PTH, 4: $\leq$70 PTH, 5: $\leq$90 PTH, and 6: complete body affected]. The average redness (R), thickness (T), and scaliness (S) of the lesions were assessed using a verbal rating scale that was converted to a numeric rating scale for analysis (0–4 scale). To facilitate this assessment, each scale point was visualized by a representative picture of the severity (see **Figure 1B**). SPASI was calculated as follows: SPASI = Area score $\times$ (R + T + S).

## Blood Parameters

Blood counts (leukocytes, lymphocytes, neutrophils, eosinophils, basophils, and monocytes) and serum proteins (Cortisol, C3, C4, IgA, CRP, HbA1c, cholesterol, triglycerides, and LDL) were assessed by clinical routine laboratory. ELISA for human squamous cell carcinoma antigen 2 (SCCA2; PeproTech, Germany) and Beta-defensin-2 protein (HBD2; MyBioSource, CA, USA) were performed according to the manufacturer's instructions.

## Statistical Analysis

Statistical analysis was performed using GraphPad Prism 7.00 Software (GraphPad Software, La Jolla, CA). Two-tailed paired sample test was used to compare variables of two different time points (beginning vs. end of the study) or of two different evaluators (mean PASI or DLQI as assessed by the physician vs. mean SPASI or DLQI as assessed by the patient *via* app) within individuals. Variables were correlated using Pearson correlation. Average Pearson coefficients across patients were obtained by transforming each correlation coefficient using Fisher's $z$, calculation of the mean of the $z$ values, and back-transformation of the mean $z$ value to the mean correlation coefficient. Parameters of outpatient visits were correlated with parameters assessed by the app if data of both visits and app were

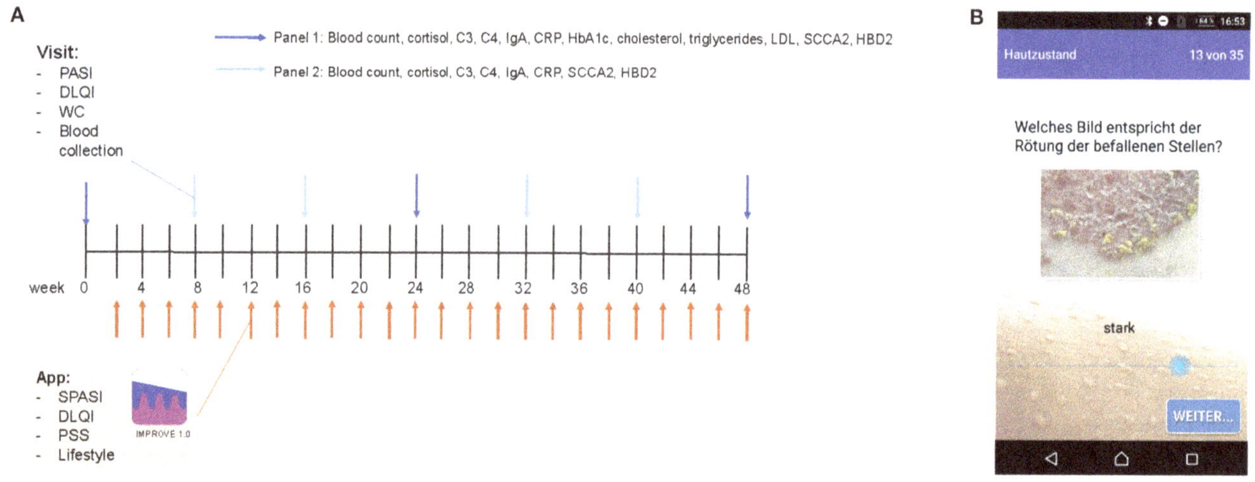


**FIGURE 1 |** Study design and app. PASI, DLQI, and waist circumference (WC) of psoriasis patients were assessed every 8 weeks. Besides, blood was taken and examined for blood counts and serum parameters (Panel 1 at visits 2, 3, 5, and 6 and Panel 2 at visits 1, 4, and 7) **(A)**. Biweekly, patients filled out an app questionnaire including SPASI, DLQI, PSS, and questions on lifestyle factors. Assessment of disease severity was supported visually by example pictures of psoriasis for redness, thickness, and scaling (here exemplarily shown for redness) **(B)**.

available from the same week. Correlation matrix was built using the agglomerative clustering tool within the scikit-learn package of Python 0.23.2 (https://scikit-learn.org/stable/). Mean values are shown with standard error of the mean (SEM).

## RESULTS

### Design of the Study and Characterization of the Study Cohort

Twelve psoriasis patients completed the 48-week study consisting of biweekly online smartphone app questionnaires and clinical outpatient visits every 8 weeks including clinical examination and blood tests (see **Figures 1A,B**). Details on the study cohort are listed in **Table 1**. Within the study cohort, the mean age of patients was 43.25 ± 4.11 years and 67.7% of the participants were male. Mean age of onset of psoriasis was 20.92 ± 3.77 years, and PASI at the time of the individual start with the study (week 0) was 7.37 ± 1.79. Fifty percent of participants were smoker, mean BMI at week 0 was 28.38 ± 1.68, and 8 out of 12 patients suffered from comorbidities such as type 2 diabetes and obesity.

### App-Reported PASI and DLQI Correlate Closely to Physician's Objective Assessment

To assess if patients' reported disease activity would be in line with the physician's objective scoring of disease activity, curves for both SPASI as reported *via* app and PASI as determined by the physician during the outpatient visits were plotted together and are exemplarily shown for two patients (**Figures 2A,B**). Indeed, both curves showed a similar course (**Figures 2A,B**; other patients, **Supplementary Figure 1**) and mean PASI and SPASI did not significantly differ ($p = 0.2409$): Eight out of the 12 patients evaluated their PASI lower as the physician did, as shown by the mean over all PASI and SPASI values, respectively, over the course of the study (**Figure 2C**). However, SPASI and PASI values over all patients showed significant correlation ($r = 0.75$, $p < 0.0001$, **Figure 2D**). We next sought to compare DLQI as determined *via* app ($DLQI_{app}$) with DLQI values given by the patient during the outpatient visit ($DLQI_{visit}$). Also, here, both curves showed high accordance (**Figures E,F**; other patients, **Supplementary Figure 2**) and DLQI determined during visits and *via* app did not significantly differ ($p = 0.27$): 7 out of 12 patients reported lower quality of life *via* app than during outpatient visits as shown by the mean of all $DLQI_{app}$ and $DLQI_{visit}$ values, respectively, during the study (**Figure 2G**). Also, for DLQI, high correlation of $DLQI_{app}$ and $DLQI_{visit}$ over all patients could be found ($r = 0.997$, $p < 0.0001$, **Figure 2E**).

### DLQI and HBD2 Correlate With Disease Activity, While Stress Shows Individual Temporal Correlation With PASI

To next assess factors correlating with PASI and SPASI on individual patient level but also across patients, we correlated PASI with serum parameters and $DLQI_{visit}$. Besides, SPASI was correlated with $DLQI_{app}$, BMI, stress, and lifestyle factors (see **Figures 3A,B**). Across all patients, PASI (SPASI) showed a mean correlation coefficient of 0.65 (0.64) with $DLQI_{visit}$ ($DLQI_{app}$). Moreover, human beta defensin 2 (HBD2), a previously described serum marker for psoriasis disease severity, showed the highest correlation coefficient among all measured blood parameters with disease activity ($r = 0.56$), which objectively confirmed correct assessment of PASI and SPASI in our cohort. Percentage of basophil granulocytes and levels of HbA1c showed a trend toward negative correlation with PASI.

**TABLE 1** | Clinical characteristics of the patients included in the study.

| Patient (no.) | Sex | Age | Psoriasis therapy (week of study: 0–48) | Comorbidities | Age of onset of psoriasis | Course of disease | Smoker | PASI at week 0 | BMI at week 0 |
|---|---|---|---|---|---|---|---|---|---|
| 1 | M | 33 | Secukinumab (0–56) | Overweight | 20 | Stable with no symptom-free intervals | No | 0.5 | 28.4 |
| 2 | F | 54 | Methotrexate (0–23), none (23–37), topical glucocorticosteroids (37–48) | Type 2 diabetes, obesity, COPD, hypothyroidism, myocardial infarction at age 49 | 20 | Progression | No (until age 49) | 18 | 38.3 |
| 3 | M | 26 | Ustekinumab (0–47) | | 0 | Progression | No | 10.7 | 25.9 |
| 4 | F | 42 | Secukinumab (0–42), ixekizumab (42–48) | Obesity | 20 | Stable with no symptom-free intervals | No | 3.6 | 29.7 |
| 5 | F | 27 | Methotrexate (36–48), topical glucocorticosteroids (0–48) | Atopic dermatitis, allergic rhinoconjunctivitis | 9 | Progression | Yes | 0.9 | 23.9 |
| 6 | M | 36 | Fumaric acid (0–31), methotrexate (31–48) | Allergic rhinoconjunctivitis, migraine, arterial hypertension, overweight | 33 | Progression | No | 12.6 | 29.8 |
| 7 | M | 32 | Fumaric acid (0–4), topical glucocorticosteroids (0–52) | | 31 | Progression | Yes | 10.2 | 22.8 |
| 8 | F | 56 | Topical glucocorticosteroids (0–4) | | 4 | No symptoms age 12–35, thereafter progression | No | 16 | 20.9 |
| 9 | M | 57 | Secukinumab (0–44) | Obesity, prediabetes | 36 | Stable with symptom-free interval at age 52–57 years | Yes | 1 | 30.7 |
| 10 | M | 45 | Methotrexate (0–18 and 31–48) | Obesity, prediabetes | 43 | Progression | Yes | 6.8 | 38.5 |
| 11 | M | 73 | Fumaric acid (0–4), apremilast (4–23), secukinumab (23–48) | Type 2 diabetes, obesity | 21 | Stable with symptom-free interval at age 21–56 years | Yes | 1.2 | 30 |
| 12 | M | 38 | Apremilast (0–48) | | 14 | Stable with no symptom-free intervals | Yes | 6.9 | 21.67 |

Interestingly, none of the lifestyle factors such as sleep, smoking, and consumption of fruits or vegetables correlated with SPASI across all patients. Instead, correlations on individual patient level between PASI and assessed parameters could be found (**Figures 3A,B** and **Supplementary Figures 3A,B**): For example, in patient 2, waist circumference (WC) and BMI significantly correlated with PASI and SPASI, respectively, whereas in patients 5 and 8, inflammatory activity is reflected on serum level by positive correlations between PASI and levels of leukocytes and neutrophils in the blood. In patient 3, e.g., amount of night sleep negatively correlated with SPASI. As stress has been discussed as a potential aggravator of psoriasis disease activity (14, 15), we next sought to investigate the influence of stress on PASI, SPASI, cortisol levels, and DLQI. Exemplarily shown for patient 12, a significant correlation between SPASI and $DLQI_{app}$ ($r = 0.91, p < 0.0001$) and also for PASI and $DLQI_{visit}$ ($r = 0.85, p < 0.015$) was found. No correlation of PASI with cortisol levels was observed; however, a trend for weak correlation with stress as measured by the PSS ($r = 0.39, p = 0.077$, **Figure 3C**) was observed, indicating that decrease of stress levels was timely accompanied by decrease in disease activity. In patient 10, however, one may come up with the hypothesis that rising cortisol and PSS levels preceded the increase of PASI (**Figure 3D**). Indeed, when shifting cortisol and PSS curves 20 weeks ahead, correlation values between SPASI and PSS increased from $r = 0.3$ and $p = 0.07$ to $r = 0.7$ and $p = 0.0004$ (**Figure 3E**). Increase in cortisol and PSS may also follow increasing PASI, as exemplified in patient 2 (**Figure 3F**): Indeed, when shifting both cortisol and PSS curves 10 weeks back, correlation values, though not at significant level, become positive for PSS and SPASI (PASI and cortisol) from $r = -0.34$ and $p = 0.23$ to $r = 0.23$ and $p = 0.6$ (from $r = -0.54, p = 0.2146$ to $r = 0.72, p = 0.1671$) (**Figure 3G**). Interestingly, PSS did not correlate with DLQI ($r = 0.12$) and cortisol levels ($r = -0.31$) across all patients (see **Supplementary Figure 3C**).

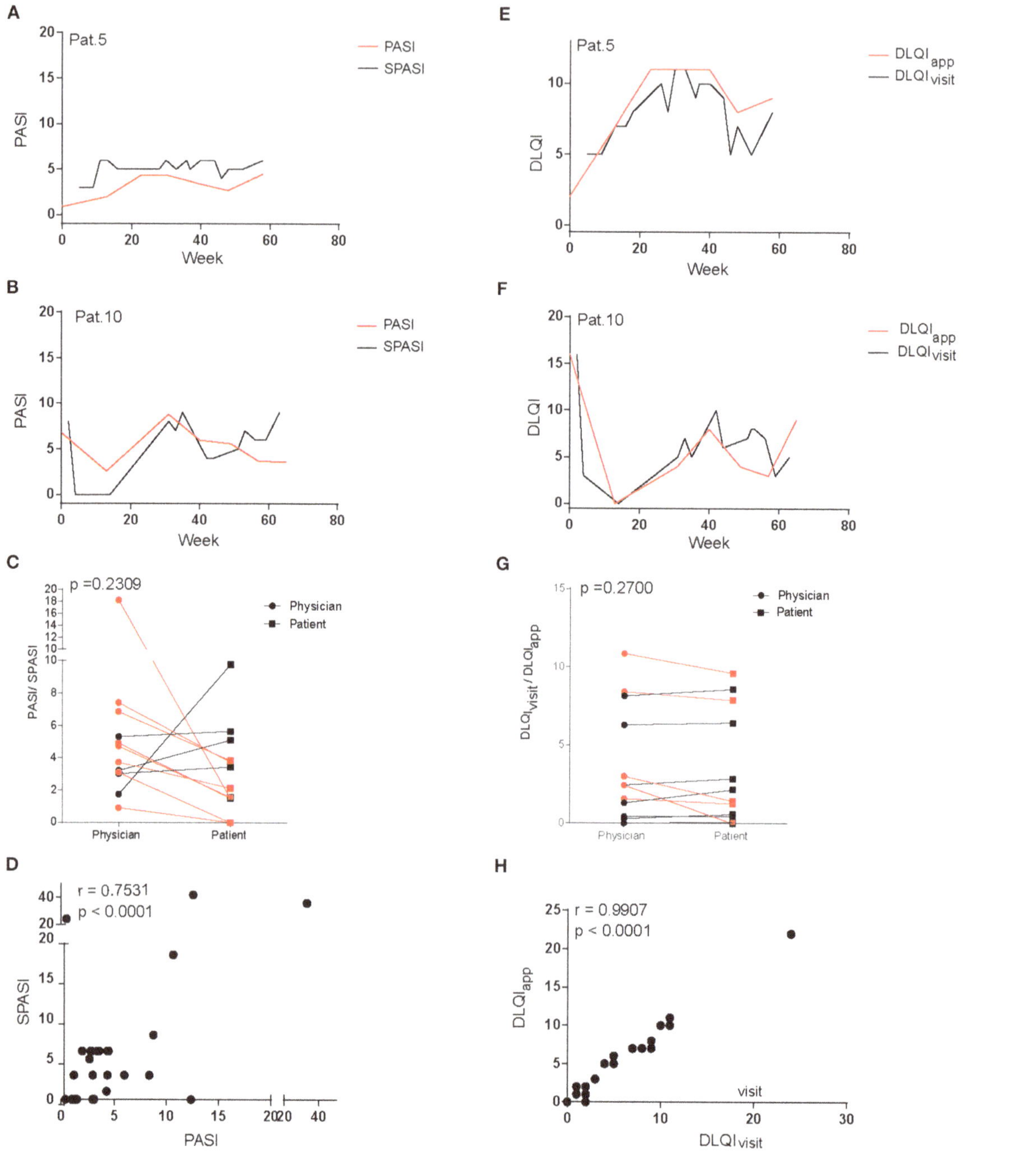


**FIGURE 2 |** Comparison of dermatology life quality index and disease severity assessed at outpatient visits and *via* app questionnaire. Curves of PASI and SPASI take a similar course as exemplarily shown for patients 5 **(A)** and 10 **(B)**. Comparison of mean PASI values as measured by physicians and mean SPASI values as measured by patients during the course of the study show no difference on patient level **(C)**. SPASI and PASI across patients show high correlation **(D)**. Also, curves of $DLQI_{app}$ and $DLQI_{visit}$ take a similar course in patients 5 **(E)** and 10 **(F)**. Mean $DLQI_{visit}$ values as stated during outpatient visits and mean $DLQI_{app}$ values as determined via app during the course of the study do not differ on patient level **(G)**. $DLQI_{app}$ and $DLQI_{visit}$ across patients show high correlation **(H)**.

## Patients Reported Benefits of the Smartphone App

At the end of the study, patients were asked to evaluate the study regarding the skin condition, the study design and the app. More than 80% of the participants considered the study to have had a beneficial effect on their skin lesions (**Figure 4**); in particular, the individual care was highly appreciated. Indeed, PASI significantly decreased across all patients (7.37 ± 1.78 at the beginning of the study vs. 2.58 ± 0.45 at the end of the study, $p = 0.0249$, **Supplementary Figure 4A**). Only 3 out of 12 patients dealt more intensively with the disease by filling out the app questionnaire. This is reflected by the fact that none

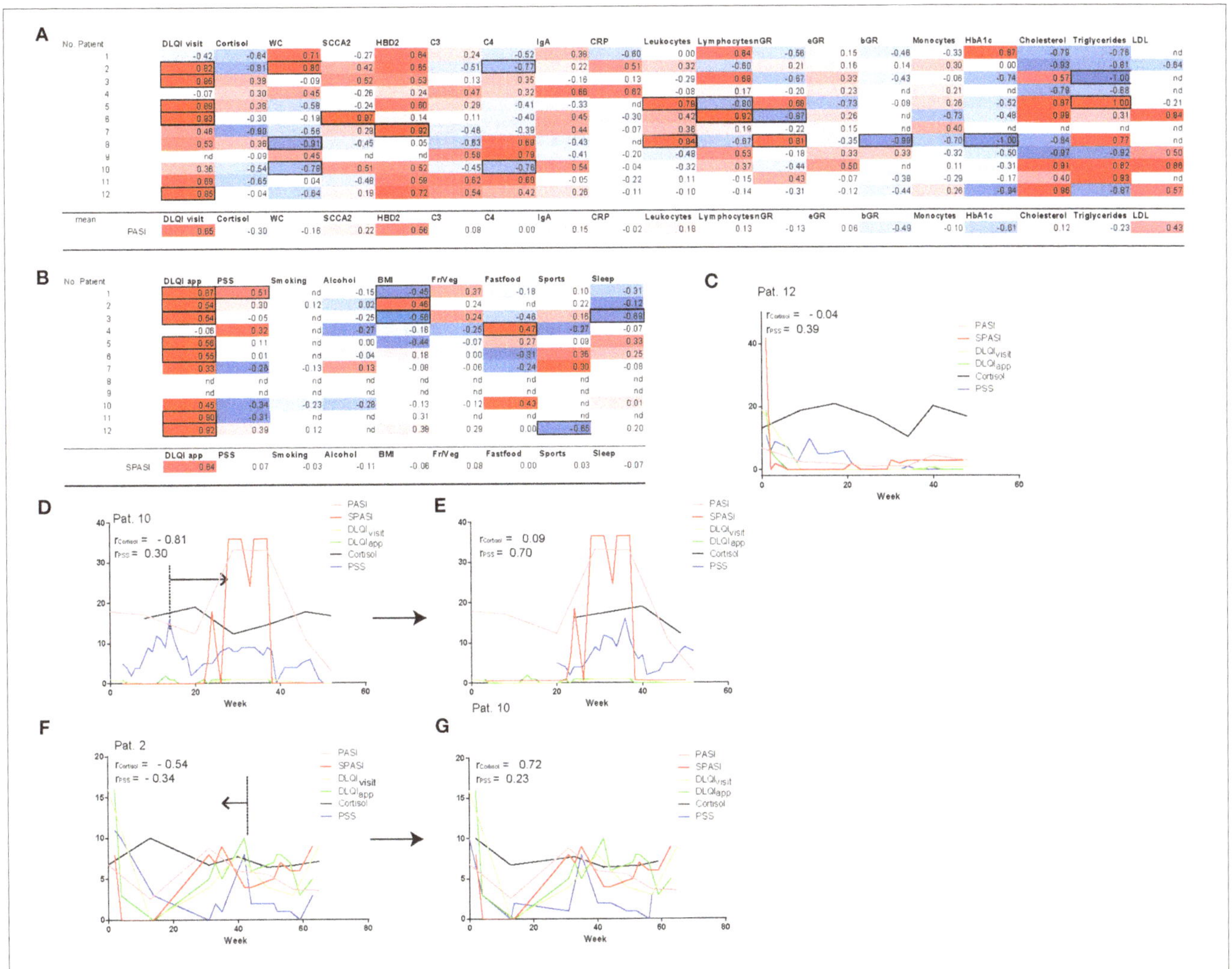


**FIGURE 3 |** Correlation of disease severity with parameters assessed at outpatient visits and *via* app. PASI shows correlation with $DLQI_{visit}$ and HBD2 **(A)**, SPASI with $DLQI_{app}$ **(B)**. Significance of parameters ($p < 0.01$) on patient level are shown in black frames. Besides, mean correlation coefficients of all patients are shown for each parameter with PASI/SPASI. Nd = no correlation could be calculated. Fr/Veg = consumption of fruits and vegetables. Curves of cortisol, PSS, $DLQI_{visit}$, $DLQI_{app}$, PASI, and SPASI are exemplarily shown in patient 12 **(C)**, patient 10 **(D,E)**, and patient 2 **(F,G)** and reveal temporal correlation of stress and PASI. In patients 10 and 2, curves of PSS and cortisol are timely shifted **(E,G)** to reveal PSS and cortisol as factors temporally preceding **(D)** or succeeding **(F)** increase of PASI. nGR, neutrophils, eGR, eosinophils; bGR, basophils; Fr/Veg, consumption of fruits and vegetables.

of the lifestyle factors (BMI, sports, consumption of fruits and vegetables, alcohol, and smoking) showed significant differences at the beginning of the study as compared to the end of the study (**Supplementary Figures 4B–F**). In contrast, consumption of fast food even increased ($p = 0.0281$). Fifty percent of patients would appreciate an updated version of the app supplemented with a lifestyle manager to achieve individual lifestyle goals.

## DISCUSSION

In this study, we investigated the potential of a new smartphone app for assessment of psoriasis severity, life quality, and lifestyle factors. We found that patient reported disease severity (SPASI) using the app closely resembles PASI scoring performed by a dermatologist. Furthermore, we demonstrate that both PASI and SPASI significantly correlate to life quality (DLQI) and the well-established serum biomarker HBD2 (16). More than 80% of study participants gave a positive evaluation of the smartphone app, and mean PASI values significantly decreased during the entire course of the study.

Psoriasis is a lifelong inflammatory disease, which requires a comprehensive therapeutic concept. Patients need to be treated by several medical disciplines, for example, dermatologists primarily evaluating skin lesions or general physicians caring about metabolic disorders. Often, interdisciplinary communication, if any, relies on written reports and intuitively every physician involved mainly focuses on his own specialty, a situation that can be ineffective and time-consuming for both patients and physicians. Often, there is an active–passive relationship between health care professionals and patients, with patients being in a passive and inanimate role (17). Here, a smartphone app used by the patients would help to bring the patient back into the center of disease management as it was already shown for, e.g., neurological disorders (18). Regular

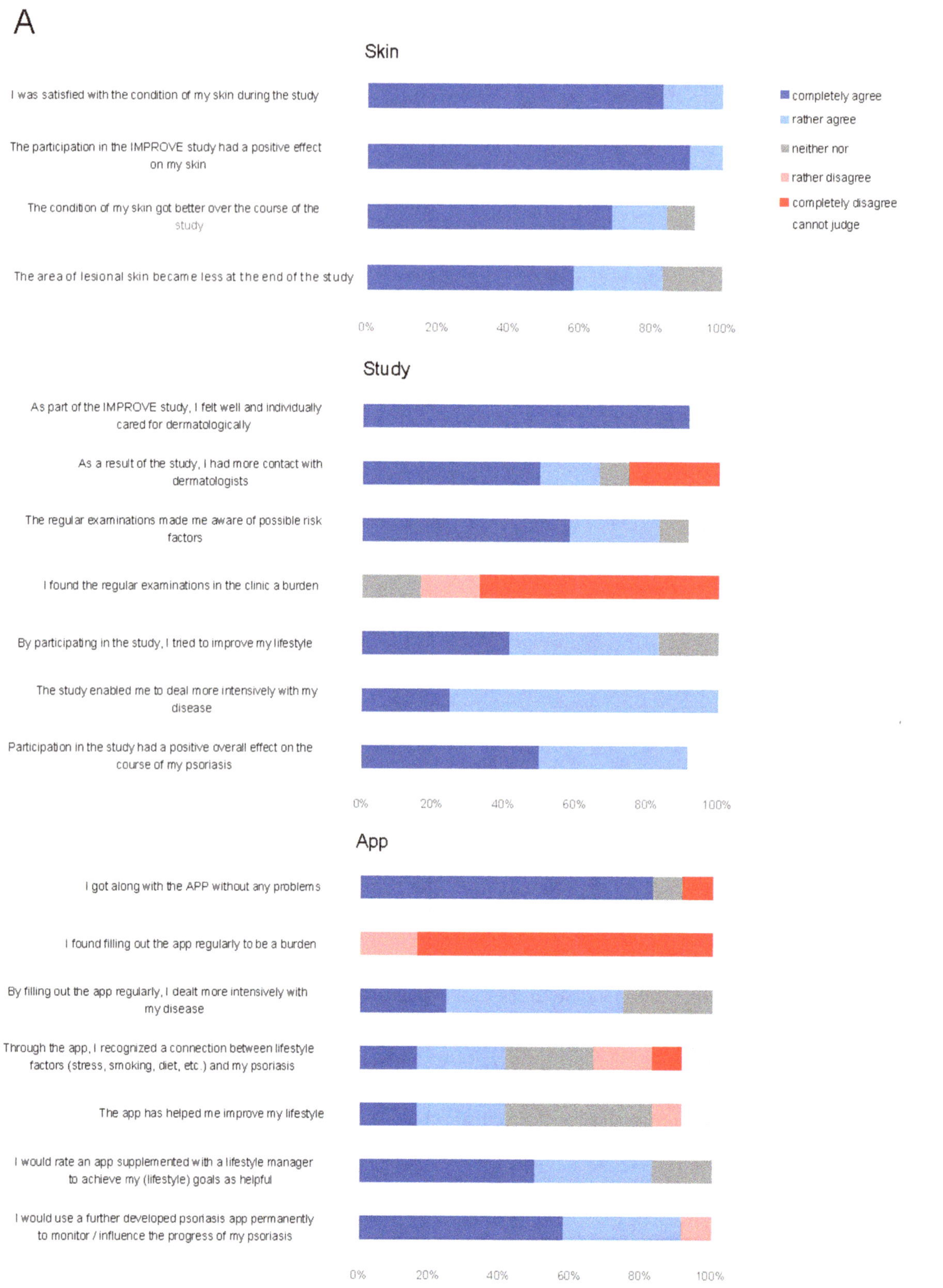


**FIGURE 4 |** Final questionnaire at the end of the study on skin, study design, and app. Shown are patients' responses in percent on a verbal rating scale.

assessment of the disease activity by the patients and easy display of disease course and disease-related factors *via* the app would clearly facilitate doctor–patient communication. Saving time of a detailed medical history allows more time for individual medical consultation. Furthermore, a structured evaluation of all disease-related factors in a smartphone app raises awareness and reflection about disease dimensions for health care professionals of different disciplines and patients.

Several apps supporting patients with chronic diseases or cancer have already been developed (19–21). In case of psoriasis in two randomized controlled trials, Sevendsen et al. demonstrated that a smartphone app improved patients' adherence to topical treatment and Spencer et al. showed that psoriasis patients learned more about their disease when using an app than a control group without digital support (22, 23). In contrast to these studies, IMPROVE 1.0 aims at not only facing one aspect of psoriasis, but on monitoring all disease-related factors. We did not choose a randomized, placebo-controlled study design, as the primary aim of the study was to compare data reliability between app and physician's examination in the same cohort of patients. Here, we could prove that data collected by the app, such as SPASI, correlate well to physician's scoring. Based on these findings, the next step of development will be to integrate more app functions. While PASI values decreased significantly during the study period, there was no change of lifestyle factors in our cohort, since no intervention for modulation of possibly aggravating lifestyle factors was initiated. However, we observed in individual patients that a change in BMI or stress level during the 12-month observation period was followed by an increase of PASI, indicating that our app can detect lifestyle changes preceding a shift in PASI. Thus, a valuable feature of an updated app version (IMPROVE 2.0) would be an implementation of an "alert system" drawing patient's attention to increasing stress levels or weight gain to optimize both psoriasis treatment and lifestyle to prevent an acute flare. Given that IMPROVE 2.0 is able to not only monitor psoriasis severity but also serve as an individualized feedback system for each patient, positive effects on psoriasis and overall healthy way of life can be expected and investigated by future randomized, controlled trials.

Our study has some limitations. First, we investigated only a limited cohort of patients in a proof-of-concept approach. Due to the small study cohort, a more advanced data analysis including robust statistical tests for significance of factors influencing future PASI changes was not possible. Second, IMPROVE 1.0 was only compatible to Android smartphones and many psoriasis patients were unwilling to participate due to technical difficulties in handling a smartphone app in general. Though both might lead to a selection bias, these observations are important to estimate psoriasis patients' willingness to use digital tools in real life and demonstrate that an app can only support a subgroup of patients with technical affinity. Furthermore, improvement of PASI scores during study participation must be interpreted with caution as they might be influenced by frequent physician consultation based on the study design. Despite these limitations, the strength of our study is that patients were followed up closely in a prospective manner over a period of 12 months. By comparing app performance to the current gold standard, namely, dermatologist's examination and collecting patient's feedback, this study proves that smartphone apps can be an important future component of a comprehensive therapeutic approach.

In summary, we demonstrated that a smartphone app is a valuable and reliable tool to assess disease activity, life quality, and potential influencing factors in psoriasis patients. This tool can markedly improve doctor–patient communication, facilitate interdisciplinary collaboration, and, most importantly, assign the patients an active role in disease management. Of note, we assessed temporal interrelations between PASI increase and lifestyle factors in individual patients. This points toward a high value of automated feedback loops—for example, by virtual disease managers helping patients to control individual risk factors—to improve disease activity in a future IMPROVE 2.0 app. These data are essential for the future implementation of digital tools in clinical routine care of complex, inflammatory diseases.

## ETHICS STATEMENT

The studies involving human participants were reviewed and approved by the Ethics Committee of the Faculty of Medicine of the Technical University of Munich (63/16S). The patients/participants provided their written informed consent to participate in this study.

## AUTHOR CONTRIBUTIONS

NG-S and FL designed the study and wrote the paper. NG-S, SB, VB, and FL generated the data. NG-S and SB analyzed the data. SS programmed the app. TB revised the manuscript. All authors contributed to the article and approved the submitted version.

## ACKNOWLEDGMENTS

The authors thank Jana Sänger for excellent technical assistance.

## REFERENCES

1. King ALS, Padua MK, Goncalves LL, Santana de Souza Martins A, Nardi AE. Smartphone use by health professionals: a review. *Digit Health.* (2020) 6:2055207620966860. doi: 10.1177/2055207620966860
2. Wilson R, Cochrane D, Mihailidis A, Small J. Mobile apps to support caregiver-resident communication in long-term care: systematic search and content analysis. *JMIR Aging.* (2020) 3:e17136. doi: 10.2196/17136
3. Staiger PK, O'Donnell R, Liknaitzky P, Bush R, Milward J. Mobile apps to reduce tobacco, alcohol, and illicit drug use: systematic review of the first decade. *J Med Internet Res.* (2020) 22:e17156. doi: 10.2196/17156

4. Dörr M, Weber S, Birkemeyer R, Leonardi L, Winterhalder C, Raichle CJ, et al. iPhone app compared with standard blood pressure measurement -The iPARR trial: the iPARR trial. *Am Heart J.* (2021) 233:102–8. doi: 10.1016/j.ahj.2020.12.003
5. Kriventsov S, Lindsey A, Hayeri A. The diabits app for smartphone-assisted predictive monitoring of glycemia in patients with diabetes: retrospective observational study. *JMIR Diabetes.* (2020) 5:e18660. doi: 10.2196/18660
6. Boehncke WH, Schon MP. Psoriasis. *Lancet.* (2015) 386:983–94. doi: 10.1016/S0140-6736(14)61909-7
7. Dalgard FJ, Gieler U, Tomas-Aragones L, Lien L, Poot F, Jemec GB, et al. The psychological burden of skin diseases: a cross-sectional multicenter study among dermatological out-patients in 13 European countries. *J Invest Dermatol.* (2015) 135:984–91. doi: 10.1038/jid.2014.530
8. Zink A, Herrmann M, Fischer T, Lauffer F, Garzorz-Stark N, Bohner A, et al. Addiction: an underestimated problem in psoriasis health care. Journal of the European Academy of Dermatology and Venereology. *JEADV.* (2017) 31:1308-15. doi: 10.1111/jdv.14204
9. Kamiya K, Kishimoto M, Sugai J, Komine M, Ohtsuki M. Risk factors for the development of psoriasis. *Int J Mol Sci.* (2019) 20:4347. doi: 10.3390/ijms20184347
10. Nast A, Erdmann R, Pathirana D, Rzany B. Translating psoriasis treatment guidelines into clinical practice—the need for educational interventions and strategies for broad dissemination. *J Eval Clin Pract.* (2008) 14:803–6. doi: 10.1111/j.1365-2753.2008.00971.x
11. Finlay AY, Khan GK. Dermatology life quality index (DLQI)-a simple practical measure for routine clinical use. *Clin Exp Dermatol.* (1994) 19:210–6. doi: 10.1111/j.1365-2230.1994.tb01167.x
12. Cohen S, Kamarck T, Mermelstein R. A global measure of perceived stress. *J Health Soc Behav.* (1983) 24:385–96. doi: 10.2307/2136404
13. Louden BA, Pearce DJ, Lang W, Feldman SR. A simplified psoriasis area severity index (SPASI) for rating psoriasis severity in clinic patients. *Dermatol Online J.* (2004) 10:7.
14. Mueller SM, Itin PH, Navarini AA, Goldust M, Brandt O, Griffiths CEM, et al. The relationship between PASI and DLQI with itch, stress, and depression: do we need additional decision-making tools in psoriasis? *Dermatolo Ther.* (2020) 33:e13276. doi: 10.1111/dth.13276
15. Kwan Z, Bong YB, Tan LL, Lim SX, Yong ASW, Ch'ng CC, et al. Determinants of quality of life and psychological status in adults with psoriasis. *Arch Dermatol Res.* (2018) 310:443–51. doi: 10.1007/s00403-018-1832-x
16. Jansen PA, Rodijk-Olthuis D, Hollox EJ, Kamsteeg M, Tjabringa GS, de Jongh GJ, et al. Beta-defensin-2 protein is a serum biomarker for disease activity in psoriasis and reaches biologically relevant concentrations in lesional skin. *PLoS ONE.* (2009) 4:e4725. doi: 10.1371/journal.pone.0004725
17. Chipidza FE, Wallwork RS, Stern TA. Impact of the doctor-patient relationship. *Prim Care Companion CNS Disord.* (2015) 17. doi: 10.4088/PCC.15f01840
18. Winberg C, Kylberg M, Pettersson C, Harnett T, Hedvall PO, Mattsson T, et al. Feeling controlled or being in control? Apps for self-management among older people with neurological disability. *Disabil Rehabil Assist Technol.* (2019) 1–6. doi: 10.1080/17483107.2019.1685017. [Epub ahead of print].
19. Yin H, Wardenaar KJ, Wang Y, Wang N, Chen W, Zhang Y, et al. Mobile mental health apps in china: systematic app store search. *J Med Internet Res.* (2020) 22:e14915. doi: 10.2196/14915
20. Kong FW, Horsham C, Ngoo A, Soyer HP, Janda M. Review of smartphone mobile applications for skin cancer detection: what are the changes in availability, functionality, and costs to users over time? *Int J Dermatol.* (2020) 60:289–308. doi: 10.1111/ijd.15132
21. Harada N, Harada S, Ito J, Atsuta R, Hori S, Takahashi K. Mobile Health App for Japanese Adult Patients With Asthma: clinical Observational Study. *J Med Internet Res.* (2020) 22:e19006. doi: 10.2196/19006
22. Hawkins SD, Barilla S, Feldman SR. Web app based patient education in psoriasis—a randomized controlled trial. *Dermatol Online J.* (2017) 23:13030/qt26d525z5.
23. Svendsen MT, Andersen F, Andersen KH, Pottegard A, Johannessen H, Moller S, et al. A smartphone application supporting patients with psoriasis improves adherence to topical treatment: a randomized controlled trial. *Br J Dermatol.* (2018) 179:1062–71. doi: 10.1111/bjd.16667

# 15

# The Role of DICOM in Artificial Intelligence for Skin Disease

**_Liam J. Caffery_**[1,2]**_*, Veronica Rotemberg_**[3]**_, Jochen Weber_**[3]**_, H. Peter Soyer_**[2,4]**_,_**
**_Josep Malvehy_**[5] **_and David Clunie_**[6]

*[1] Centre for Online, Centre for Health Services Research, The University of Queensland, Brisbane, QLD, Australia, [2] Dermatology Research Centre, The University of Queensland Diamantina Institute, The University of Queensland, Brisbane, QLD, Australia, [3] Dermatology Service, Department of Medicine, Memorial Sloan Kettering Cancer Center, New York, NY, United States, [4] Department of Dermatology, Princess Alexandra Hospital, Brisbane, QLD, Australia, [5] Department of Dermatology, Institut d'Investigacions Biomèdiques August Pi i Sunyer, Hospital Clinic of Barcelona, University of Barcelona, Barcelona, Spain, [6] PixelMed Publishing, Bangor, PA, United States*

***Correspondence:**
*Liam J. Caffery*
*l.caffery@uq.edu.au*

There is optimism that artificial intelligence (AI) will result in positive clinical outcomes, which is driving research and investment in the use of AI for skin disease. At present, AI for skin disease is embedded in research and development and not practiced widely in clinical dermatology. Clinical dermatology is also undergoing a technological transformation in terms of the development and adoption of standards that optimizes the quality use of imaging. Digital Imaging and Communications in Medicine (DICOM) is the international standard for medical imaging. DICOM is a continually evolving standard. There is considerable effort being invested in developing dermatology-specific extensions to the DICOM standard. The ability to encode relevant metadata and afford interoperability with the digital health ecosystem (e.g., image repositories, electronic medical records) has driven the initial impetus in the adoption of DICOM for dermatology. DICOM has a dedicated working group whose role is to develop a mechanism to support AI workflows and encode AI artifacts. DICOM can improve AI workflows by encoding derived objects (e.g., secondary images, visual explainability maps, AI algorithm output) and the efficient curation of multi-institutional datasets for machine learning training, testing, and validation. This can be achieved using DICOM mechanisms such as standardized image formats and metadata, metadata-based image retrieval, and de-identification protocols. DICOM can address several important technological and workflow challenges for the implementation of AI. However, many other technological, ethical, regulatory, medicolegal, and workforce barriers will need to be addressed before DICOM and AI can be used effectively in dermatology.

**Keywords: dermatology, artificial intelligence, DICOM, standards, imaging**

## INTRODUCTION

The Digital Imaging and Communications in Medicine (DICOM) standard (1) is a comprehensive, international standard for medical imaging. DICOM defines a standard medical image file format and a metadata model and network services for the storage, transmission, and query and retrieval of objects. DICOM has also specified other network services to improve the efficiency of medical imaging workflows.

The most common DICOM data object is an image file. A DICOM image file consists of metadata and the pixel data of the image melded into a single file. The pixel data may be encoded using the Joint Photographic Expert Group format or other standard compression methods. The metadata model is standardized by object type, meaning there are different metadata models for, say, a magnetic resonance image, and a photographic image. The metadata model is described in an Information Object Definition (IOD). An IOD consists of an amalgamation of modules, where each module is a collection of patient, study, equipment, and image metadata attributes.

Although DICOM is ubiquitous in some medical image-producing specialties (e.g., radiology, cardiology, and radiation therapy), to date, the use of DICOM for dermatological imaging has been limited. There is, however, a growing realization that the adoption of DICOM for dermatological imaging is advantageous compared with other methods of image management (2). Clinical imaging for dermatology can be encoded using the existing, visible light photography IOD. Dermatology-specific IODs for dermoscopy have been developed and included in the DICOM standard. Future work items proposal will be for total body photography and reflectance confocal microscopy (3).

One of the primary motivations for adopting DICOM for dermatology imaging has been interoperability with digital health ecosystems such as electronic medical records, picture archiving and communication systems (PACS), and enterprise imaging repositories. In addition to these interoperability benefits, DICOM adoption is also likely to facilitate the use of artificial intelligence (AI) in clinical dermatology.

The application of AI for dermatology most often uses an image as input into a machine learning algorithm and results in the algorithm outputting a diagnostic or risk prediction of a disease condition. This use of AI is a form of image classification, and convolutional neural networks (CNNs) are becoming the most promising of AI algorithms for dermatology image classification (4). Melanoma diagnosis is a common application of dermatology image classifiers for which several reader studies have found that under experimental conditions, the diagnostic performance of AI can match that of an experienced dermatologist (5–7). Similar results have been reported for psoriasis (8) and onychomycosis (9).

DICOM is an evolving medical imaging standard with continual additions to the standard in the form of supplements and corrections. The increasing interest in AI image classifiers in medical imaging is, in turn, catalyzing the inclusion of AI-specific content in the DICOM standard. The DICOM Standards Committee has a dedicated AI working group (WG 23). The role of this working group is to develop a DICOM mechanism to support AI workflows and encode AI artifacts (10). This paper aims to discuss the role of DICOM in the AI in the context of dermatological imaging and review the current status of AI-specific content in the DICOM standard.

## DERIVED OBJECTS

Preprocessing and post-processing of images for prediction analysis by machine learning create derived image objects such as resized or down-sampled images, segmentation images, visual explanation (e.g., saliency maps) images, and the algorithm's output. Research has shown that the output of an AI model influences the clinical decision of even experienced dermatologists (7, 11). Hence, derived objects should form part of the patient's medical record if AI is used in clinical practice to meet the health-care provider's regulatory and legal obligation to retain medical records. In addition to regulatory and legal requirements to store derived objects, there are also ethical aspects. The Joint European and North American Multi-society Statement on the Ethics of AI in radiology (12) recommended that the output of AI algorithms need to be stored in an auditable format to permit the investigation of errors and the monitoring over time to ensure there is no degradation of performance.

In practical terms, encoding the derived objects as DICOM objects with the appropriate identifying and descriptive metadata would allow them to be stored alongside the original image files in the health-care organization PACS or enterprise imaging repositories and visualized in conjunction with the clinical images.

Further, the use of DICOM is likely to improve image acquisition and image review workflows. AI has been shown to substantially reduce the amount of time radiologists spend on image review without compromising diagnostic accuracy (13–15). The same potential exists in dermatology, and the greatest efficiency gains are likely to be achieved for dermatologists reviewing total skin imaging studies. In hospitals, medical imaging infrastructure, including acquisition devices and image repositories, nearly all use DICOM as the underlying communication protocol. Speaking a common language can improve the efficiency of workflows, for example, automatic population of patient demographics at acquisition or the automated storage of images to an image repository. Implementing AI as a standalone product, as opposed to being integrated within the medical imaging ecosystems, may negate the diagnostic efficiencies afforded by using AI.

Original images often need to be resized to a fixed image size before inputting into a CNN. In some instances, we have seen dermoscopic images resized to a fixed resolution of 224 × 224 pixels (7). However, other datasets have reported using a fixed resolution of 448 × 448 pixels (16) or 1,024 × 1,024 pixels (17). Choosing the fixed resolution is a trade-off be computational efficiency and predictive accuracy (18). Therefore, storing the resized or down-sampled images can document the input into the CNN in an auditable and reproducible format.

Visual explanation maps assign each feature in an image a level of importance that the feature contributes to AI algorithm output. An example of two common visual explanation methods is Shapley additive explanation (SHAP) (19), and Gradient-Weighted Class Activation Mapping (Grad-CAM) (20). Examples of these visual explanations are shown in **Figures 1**, **2**. Visual explanation maps can be used by clinicians to help them understand how the AI algorithm came to its output and to assess

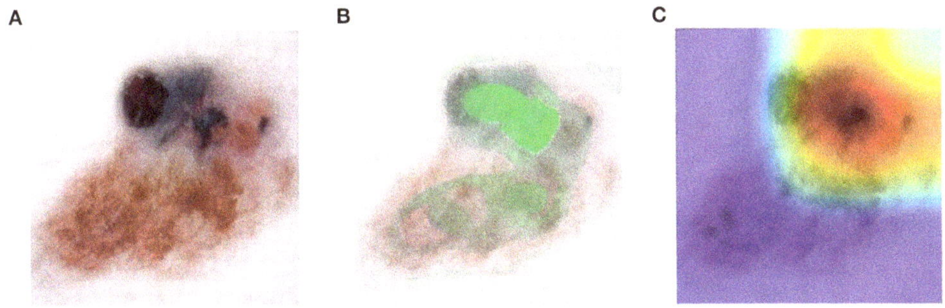


**FIGURE 1 |** Visual explanation images where AI algorithm correctly classified the skin lesion as melanoma **(A)** original image **(B)** SHAP visual explanation where green indicates the most important area of contribution to the AI result and red indicates the least important area; and **(C)** Grad-CAM visual explanation image where red is the most important area of contribution to AI result and blue is the least important part of the image to AI result. Image courtesy of Sally Shrapnel.

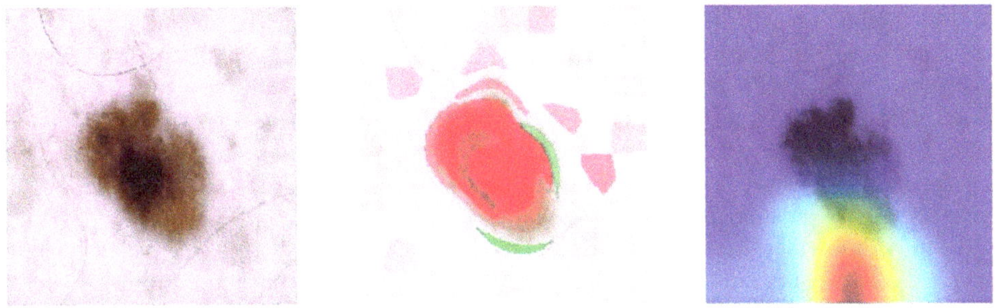

**FIGURE 2 |** Visual explanation images where the AI algorithm incorrectly classified the skin lesion as benign. Note the pigmented lesion was not considered an important feature by either SHAP or Grad-CAM. Image courtesy of Sally Shrapnel.

the quality of the output (21). Therefore, visual explanation maps can provide insight into potential sources of bias in AI algorithms (22). For example, if an AI algorithm predicted a high probability of melanoma but the visual explanation maps showed that the area of pigmentation in the lesion was not of high importance in determining this, then the clinician may be suspicious of the accuracy of the prediction (see **Figure 2**).

Resized or down-sampled images can be encoded as DICOM photographic or secondary capture objects. DICOM segmentation objects can be used to encode both binary and fractional segmentation images as multi-frame images. The multiple frames include the referenced image instance and segmentation image instances (**Figure 3**). Visual explanation images can be encoded as parametric map objects. A current proposal is to be able to link segmentation objects and parametric map objects to DICOM Structured Reports (SR) for the measurement objects (23). DICOM is also trialing the use of Javascript Object Notation (JSON) for encoding the output of AI algorithms (e.g., risk prediction of skin disease) in DICOM SR format (24). The goal of this trial is to harmonize with the machine learning community where JSON is the preferred format for algorithm output. Additionally, JSON encoding will achieve encoding of ground truth diagnosis that can be used to train, test, and validate future machine learning algorithms.

## METADATA

The current use of CNNs for image classification has relied on image data as the only input. However, clinicians also rely on metadata as part of the diagnostic process (4). To emulate this, there have been several studies that have assessed the inclusion of metadata along with images as input into machine learning algorithms. One study found metadata resulted in a small improvement (1–2%) in sensitivity. Improvements were most noticeable in smaller, lower-performing models (25), which may indicate that the metadata compensates for fewer pixel data. A further study found the sensitivity and specificity improved from 82.1 to 95.2% and 86.1 to 91.0%, respectively (26). Both of these studies relied on simple metadata (age, sex, and lesion site). When lesion characteristics of bleeding, pain, and itchiness were added to age and the anatomical site as input, the accuracy of the algorithm improved by around 7% (27).

As previously noted, the DICOM file format (28) is an amalgamation of metadata with the pixel data of the image. The metadata is stored in the DICOM file header. The standardized metadata includes identifying and descriptive patient metadata (e.g., age, sex) and study metadata (e.g., lesion site). Most DICOM viewers allow the metadata encoded in the DICOM file header to be viewed in text format.

**FIGURE 3** | Segmentation images **(a)** referenced instance **(b)** binary segmentation instance **(c)** fractional segmentation instance.

The DICOM supplement for dermoscopy has proposed the use of a skin cancer acquisition context. An acquisition context is a method of embedding descriptors of clinical metadata in the DICOM header using codes from standard lexicons [such as SNOMED CT (29)] for both concepts and values (30). The proposed skin cancer acquisition context includes rich clinical metadata such as a personal and familial history of melanoma, *in situ* melanoma, and other skin cancers; Fitzpatrick skin type; the degree of ultraviolet damage; atypical mole syndrome; and other relevant genetic conditions. Furthermore, the skin cancer acquisition context also includes lesion-level metadata such as history of growth, itch, erythema, and other relevant patient-observed changes. As DICOM is extensible, there is the ability to define acquisition contexts for different skin disease classes (e.g., inflammatory disease). There is the potential that using rich metadata stored in the acquisition context as an AI algorithm input will improve the performance of machine learning algorithms, perhaps more so than simple metadata. However, at this time it remains untested. The use of metadata is an area for further research, as it has been shown that not all metadata improve the performance of skin lesion image classifiers, and that selective metadata selection will likely be necessary (31).

## DATASETS

One of the main limitations of deep learning is the input data used to train the system (32). AI models trained and validated from the same dataset risk overfitting, which is a phenomenon of "knowing the training data too well (33)." Overfitting results in the predictive output of an AI model only being reliable for the population on which the AI model was trained. To overcome this limitation, external validation or cross-validation is necessary and can be achieved by training the AI model on datasets amalgamated from multiple clinical sources, including different populations and ethnicities. Having images from these disparate sources in a standardized format facilitates the amalgamation of datasets and reduces the cost and effort of dataset curation. The lack of deployment of imaging and metadata standards in dermatology has inhibited the development of large image collections suitable for machine learning (34). DICOM is a universally recognized standard for medical imaging and would be ideal as a standardized image encoding to address this challenge.

The use of metadata-based retrieval (30), using queries based on DICOM metadata attributes, could also facilitate the creation of machine learning datasets with high levels of granularity. For example, to develop an AI algorithm specific to polarized light dermoscopy, one could assemble an appropriate dataset using query (based on DICOM attributes for the dermoscopy image type and polarization) and retrieve images from the repository where they are stored.

The amalgamation of datasets does increase the risk of unauthorized access to patient-identifiable information. DICOM's de-identification profiles (35), which are used to address privacy issues for multi-center clinical trials, can be directly applied to the amalgamation of machine learning datasets. The DICOM Attribute Confidentiality Profiles contain a comprehensive list of attributes that potentially provide identifying information and should be removed to protect the patient's privacy. Adopting an established de-identification profile has many advantages, including avoidance of repeating the same complex technical and legal consideration for de-identification, being less error-prone for participating sites to deploy, and implying a level of rigor that would potentially satisfy ethics committees.

Excluding images from datasets where the DICOM attribute Recognizable Visual Features (0028, 0302) is set is a further way to enhance the privacy of a dataset for machine learning. The Recognizable Visual Features flag is most often set when the subject's face is included in an image. In the forthcoming DICOM supplement for dermoscopy, this attribute is set if the images contain the patient's fingerprints.

## DISCUSSION AND CONCLUSION

The increasing use of imaging in dermatology is being driven by many factors, including diagnostic imaging (as opposed to documentary imaging) such as teledermatology, sequential dermoscopic imaging, and melanoma screening using total body photography (36). The ability of DICOM to encode relevant metadata and afford interoperability with the digital health ecosystem has driven the initial interest in the adoption of DICOM for dermatology (2). DICOM can improve AI workflows by encoding derived objects (e.g., secondary images, visual explainability maps, AI algorithm output) and the efficient curation of multi-institutional datasets for machine learning training, testing, and validation. This can be achieved using DICOM mechanisms such as standardized image formats and metadata, metadata-based image retrieval, and de-identification protocols.

Currently, the use of DICOM to manage dermatological imaging is not widespread. Further, the use of DICOM to support AI workflows in dermatology is likely more limited still. There has, however, been a successful proof-of-concept trial using DICOM to encode datasets for AI of skin disease (37). DICOM adoption by dermatology may be more challenging than for other medical specialties. Clinical photographs captured on a mobile device constitute most imaging in dermatology. This type of imaging lacks standardization (38). Cameras used for clinical photography in dermatology are often commercial-off-the-shelf products as opposed to dedicated medical devices, hence, unlikely to support DICOM. As opposed to other medical specialties where formal diagnostic reports are produced, dermatology images can be simply viewed, which lessens the importance of integration with PACS. There is a lot of enthusiasm for AI in dermatology (32). More widespread understanding of the role that DICOM has in facilitating the adoption of AI in dermatology may strongly influence the dermatology community to adopt DICOM.

AI workflows for dermatology would require some interoperable actors on a medical imaging network. A potential workflow would be that images are acquired and stored in an image archive using typical DICOM image acquisition and storage workflows. Images could be automatically routed from the archive to an AI evidence creator actor (e.g., CNN). The evidence creator may undertake image post-processing to produce resized or down-sampled images and/or segmentation objects. These images would be encoded as DICOM objects and be automatically stored in the image archive. The AI evidence creator would analyze the image of the skin and create evidence documents (e.g., DICOM SR) containing the risk prediction of skin disease and potentially visual explainability maps. Again, these derived objects would be encoded as DICOM objects and automatically stored in the image archive using DICOM network services. All derived objects created by the AI evidence creator would use the same study identifier as the original images to facilitate linkage. A dermatologist or other clinician could use a DICOM viewer to subsequently query and retrieve an imaging study and display the original images and derived objects (e.g., a structured report containing algorithm output and/or visual explainability maps) that would help with image interpretation. DICOM-facilitated interoperability between AI actors and other devices in a medical imaging network is likely to facilitate workflow efficiencies. In addition to the transmission of images and results, interoperability is likely to play a key role in the continual adaptive learning of machine learning algorithms (39). Interoperability will also allow health-care organizations to use "best-of-breed" AI actors rather than being locked into an existing vendor's product.

The use of DICOM for the management of dermatological images will not guarantee effective clinical use of AI in dermatology. DICOM can address several important technological and workflow challenges for the implementation of AI. However, many other technological, ethical, regulatory, medicolegal, and workforce barriers will need to be addressed before DICOM and AI can be used effectively in dermatology.

## AUTHOR CONTRIBUTIONS

All authors contributed equally to the preparation of this perspective piece.

## REFERENCES

1. National Electrical Manufacturers Association. *About DICOM: Overview*. National Electrical Manufacturers Association (2020). Available online at: https://www.dicomstandard.org/current (accessed September 01, 2020).
2. Caffery LJ, Clunie D, Curiel-Lewandrowski C, Malvehy J, Soyer HP, Halpern AC. Transforming dermatologic imaging for the digital era: metadata and standards. *J Digit Imaging*. (2018) 31:568–77. doi: 10.1007/s10278-017-0045-8
3. DICOM Standards Committee. *Supplement 221: Dermoscopy (Letter Ballot)*. (2020). Available online at: ftp://medical.nema.org/MEDICAL/Dicom/Supps/LB/sup221_lb_dermoscopy.pdf (accessed October 01, 2020).
4. Wada M, Ge Z, Gilmore SJ, Mar VJ. Use of artificial intelligence in skin cancer diagnosis and management. *Med J Aust*. (2020) 213:256–9.e1. doi: 10.5694/mja2.50759
5. Esteva A, Kuprel B, Novoa RA, Ko J, Swetter SM, Blau HM, et al. Dermatologist-level classification of skin cancer with deep neural networks. *Nature*. (2017) 542:115–8. doi: 10.1038/nature21056
6. Haenssle HA, Fink C, Schneiderbauer R, Toberer F, Buhl T, Blum A, et al. Man against machine: diagnostic performance of a deep learning convolutional neural network for dermoscopic melanoma recognition in comparison to 58 dermatologists. *Ann Oncol*. (2018) 29:1836–42. doi: 10.1093/annonc/mdy166
7. Tschandl P, Rinner C, Apalla Z, Argenziano G, Codella N, Halpern A, et al. Human-computer collaboration for skin cancer recognition. *Nat Med*. (2020) 26:1229–34. doi: 10.1038/s41591-020-0942-0
8. Zhao S, Xie B, Li Y, Zhao X, Kuang Y, Su J, et al. Smart identification of psoriasis by images using convolutional neural networks: a case study in China. *J Eur Acad Dermatol Venereol*. (2020) 34:518–24. doi: 10.1111/jdv.15965
9. Han SS, Park GH, Lim W, Kim MS, Na JI, Park I, et al. Deep neural networks show an equivalent and often superior performance to dermatologists in onychomycosis diagnosis: automatic construction of onychomycosis datasets by region-based convolutional deep neural network. *PLoS ONE*. (2018) 13:e0191493. doi: 10.1371/journal.pone.0191493
10. National Electrical Manufactuerres Association. *AI and DICOM*. (2020). Available online at: https://www.dicomstandard.org/ai (accessed October 01, 2020).
11. Haenssle HA, Fink C, Toberer F, Winkler J, Stolz W, Deinlein T, et al. Man against machine reloaded: performance of a market-approved convolutional neural network in classifying a broad spectrum of skin lesions in comparison with 96 dermatologists working under less artificial conditions. *Ann Oncol*. (2020) 31:137–43. doi: 10.1016/j.annonc.2019.10.013
12. Geis JR, Brady AP, Wu CC, Spencer J, Ranschaert E, Jaremko JL, et al.

Ethics of artificial intelligence in radiology: summary of the joint European and North American multisociety statement. *Radiology*. (2019) 293:436–40. doi: 10.1148/radiol.2019191586

13. Booz C, Yel I, Wichmann JL, Boettger S, Al Kamali A, Albrecht MH, et al. Artificial intelligence in bone age assessment: accuracy and efficiency of a novel fully automated algorithm compared to the greulich-pyle method. *Eur Radiol Exp*. (2020) 4:6. doi: 10.1186/s41747-019-0139-9
14. Conant EF, Toledano AY, Periaswamy S, Fotin SV, Go J, Boatsman JE, et al. Improving accuracy and efficiency with concurrent use of artificial intelligence for digital breast tomosynthesis. *Radiol Artif Intell*. (2019) 1:e180096. doi: 10.1148/ryai.2019180096
15. Pesapane F, Codari M, Sardanelli F. Artificial intelligence in medical imaging: threat or opportunity? radiologists again at the forefront of innovation in medicine. *Eur Radiol Exp*. (2018) 2:35. doi: 10.1186/s41747-018-0061-6
16. Mahbod A, Tschandl P, Langs G, Ecker R, Ellinger I. The effects of skin lesion segmentation on the performance of dermatoscopic image classification. *Comput Methods Programs Biomed*. (2020) 197:105725. doi: 10.1016/j.cmpb.2020.105725
17. Combalia M, Codella NC, Rotemberg V, Helba B, Vilaplana V, Reiter O, et al. BCN20000: dermoscopic lesions in the wild. *arXiv*. (2019). *arXiv* 1908.02288v2.
18. Hashemi M. Enlarging smaller images before inputting into convolutional neural network: zero-padding vs. interpolation. *J Big Data*. (2019) 6:98. doi: 10.1186/s40537-019-0263-7
19. Lundberg SM and Lee S-I. A unified approach to interpreting model predictions. In: von Luxburg U, Guyon I, editors. *Proceedings of the 31st International Conference on Neural Information Processing Systems*. Long Beach, CA: Curran Associates Inc., (2017). p. 4765–74.
20. Selvaraju RR, Cogswell M, Das A, Vedantam R, Parikh D, Batra D. Grad-CAM: visual explanations from deep networks via gradient-based localization. *Int J Comput Vision*. (2020) 128:336–59. doi: 10.1007/s11263-019-0 1228-7
21. Holzinger A, Langs G, Denk H, Zatloukal K, Muller H. Causability and explainability of artificial intelligence in medicine. *Wiley Interdiscip Rev Data Min Knowl Discov*. (2019) 9:e1312. doi: 10.1002/widm.1312
22. Young K, Booth G, Simpson B, Dutton R, Shrapnel S. Deep neural network or dermatologist? In: Suzuki K, Reyes M, Syeda-Mahmood T, et al. editors. *Interpretability of Machine Intelligence in Medical Image Computing and Multimodal Learning for Clinical Decision Support: Proceedings of the Second International Workshop on Interpretability of Machine Intelligence in Medical Image Computing, iMIMIC 2019, and the 9th International Workshop on Multimodal Learning for Clinical Decision Support, ML-CDS 2019, held in conjunction with the 22nd International Conference on Medical Imaging and Computer-Assisted Intervention, MICCAI 2019*. Shenzhen: Springer International Publishing (2019). p. 48–55.
23. DICOM Standards Committee. *CP-1867 Add codes for visual Explanation maps*. (2020). Available online at: https://dicom.nema.org/Dicom/News/September2019/docs/cpack103/cp1867.pdf (accessed October 01, 2020).
24. DICOM Standards Commiteee. *Supplement 219: JSON Representation of DICOM Structured Reports*. (2020). Available online at: ftp://medical.nema.org/medical/dicom/supps/Frozen/sup219_fz_14_JSONSR.pdf (accessed October 01, 2020)
25. Gessert N, Nielsen M, Shaikh M, Werner R, Schlaefer A. Skin lesion classification using ensembles of multi-resolution efficientnets with meta data. *MethodsX*. (2020) 7:100864. doi: 10.1016/j.mex.2020.100864
26. Liu Z, Sun J, Smith M, Smith L, Warr R. Incorporating clinical metadata with digital image features for automated identification of cutaneous melanoma. *Br J Dermatol*. (2013) 169: 1034–40. doi: 10.1111/bjd.12550
27. Pacheco AGC, Krohling RA. The impact of patient clinical information on automated skin cancer detection. *Comput Biol Med*. (2020) 116:103545. doi: 10.1016/j.compbiomed.2019.103545
28. National Electrical Manufacturers Association. *Digital Imaging and Communications in Medicine (DICOM) Standard PS3.10 - Media Storage and File Format for Media Interchange*. (2020). Available online at: https://dicom.nema.org/medical/dicom/current/output/pdf/part10.pdf (accessed October 01, 2020).
29. Donnelly K. SNOMED-CT: the advanced terminology and coding system for eHealth. *Stud Health Technol Inform*. (2006) 121:279–90.
30. Bidgood WD Jr, Bray B, Brown N, Mori AR, Spackman KA, Golichowski A, et al. Image acquisition context: procedure description attributes for clinically relevant indexing and selective retrieval of biomedical images. *J Am Med Inform Assoc*. (1999) 6:61–75. doi: 10.1136/jamia.1999.0060061
31. Li W, Zhuang J, Wang R, Zhang J, Zheng W. Fusing metadata and dermoscopy images for skin disease diagnosis. In: *2020 IEEE 17th International Symposium on Biomedical Imaging (ISBI)*. (2020). p. 1996–2000.
32. Du-Harpur X, Watt FM, Luscombe NM, Lynch MD. What is AI? Applications of artificial intelligence to dermatology. *Br J Dermatol*. (2020) 183:423–30. doi: 10.1111/bjd.18880
33. Chan S, Reddy V, Myers B, Thibodeaux Q, Brownstone N, Liao W. Machine learning in dermatology: current applications, opportunities, and limitations. *Dermatol Ther*. (2020) 10:365–86. doi: 10.1007/s13555-020-00372-0
34. Curiel-Lewandrowski C, Novoa RA, Berry E, Celebi ME, Codella N, Giuste F, et al. *Artificial Intelligence Approach in Melanoma. Melanoma*. New York, NY: Springer (2019). p. 1–31.
35. National Electrical Manufacturers Association Digital Imaging and Communications in Medicine (DICOM). *Standard PS3.15 - Security and System Management Profiles - E.1 Attribute Confidentiality Profiles - De-identifier*. (2020). Available online at: https://dicom.nema.org/medical/dicom/current/output/chtml/part15/chapter_E.html#sect_E.1.1 (accessed October 01, 2020)
36. Rayner JE, Laino AM, Nufer KL, Adams L, Raphael AP, Menzies SW, et al. Clinical perspective of 3D total body photography for early detection and screening of Melanoma. *Front Med*. (2018) 5:152. doi: 10.3389/fmed.2018.00152
37. Rotemberg V, Kurtansky N, Betz-Stablein B, Caffery L, Chousakos E, Codella N, et al. A patient-centric dataset of images and metadata for identifying melanomas using clinical context. *arXiv*. (2020). *arXiv* 2008.07360v1.
38. Quigley EA, Tokay BA, Jewell ST, Marchetti MA, Halpern AC. Technology and technique standards for camera-acquired digital dermatologic images: a systematic review. *JAMA Dermatol*. (2015) 151:883–90. doi: 10.1001/jamadermatol.2015.33
39. Dikici E, Bigelow M, Prevedello L, White R, Erdal B. Integrating AI into radiology workflow: levels of research, production, and feedback maturity. *J Med Imaging*. (2020) 7:016502. doi: 10.1117/1.JMI.7.1.016502

# 16

# Automatic Segmentation of Epidermis and Hair Follicles in Optical Coherence Tomography Images of Normal Skin by Convolutional Neural Networks

*Rocío del Amor [1*], Sandra Morales [1], Adrián Colomer [1], Mette Mogensen [2], Mikkel Jensen [3], Niels M. Israelsen [3], Ole Bang [3] and Valery Naranjo [1]*

[1] Instituto de Investigación e Innovación en Bioingeniería, I3B, Universitat Politècnica de València, Valencia, Spain,
[2] Department of Dermatology, Bispebjerg Hospital, University of Copenhagen, Copenhagen, Denmark,
[3] DTU Fotonik, Department of Photonics Engineering, Technical University of Denmark, Kongens Lyngby, Denmark

***Correspondence:**
Rocío del Amor
madeam2@upv.es

Optical coherence tomography (OCT) is a well-established bedside imaging modality that allows analysis of skin structures in a non-invasive way. Automated OCT analysis of skin layers is of great relevance to study dermatological diseases. In this paper, an approach to detect the epidermal layer along with the follicular structures in healthy human OCT images is presented. To the best of the authors' knowledge, the approach presented in this paper is the only epidermis detection algorithm that segments the pilosebaceous unit, which is of importance in the progression of several skin disorders such as folliculitis, acne, lupus erythematosus, and basal cell carcinoma. The proposed approach is composed of two main stages. The first stage is a Convolutional Neural Network based on U-Net architecture. The second stage is a robust post-processing composed by a Savitzky-Golay filter and Fourier Domain Filtering to fully define the borders belonging to the hair follicles. After validation, an average Dice of 0.83 $\pm$ 0.06 and a thickness error of 10.25 $\mu m$ is obtained on 270 human skin OCT images. Based on these results, the proposed method outperforms other state-of-the-art methods for epidermis segmentation. It demonstrates that the proposed image segmentation method successfully detects the epidermal region in a fully automatic way in addition to defining the follicular skin structures as main novelty.

**Keywords: skin OCT, follicular structures, layer segmentation, epidermis, convolutional neural networks, pilosebaceous unit**

## 1. INTRODUCTION

Optical coherence tomography (OCT) is a well-established imaging modality used to capture various aspects of biological tissues (1). OCT has been routinely used in ophthalmology due to the ease of light in penetrating ocular structures (2). In addition, as OCT is a non-invasive technique and therefore, does not require direct contact with the eye, it allows the *in-vivo* study of internal ocular structures such as the retina without performing any perforation.

Less established is the use of the OCT for the analysis of other biological tissues such as the skin due to the limited resolution and penetration of the light waves within this structure (3). **Figure 1** shows the skin structure mainly composed of epidermis and dermis layers. However, during the last decade, this technique has gained great relevance for the study of the skin layers because of the last advances in optical, fiber, and laser technology (4).

Although skin biopsies are currently the gold standard for the diagnosis of a large number of dermatological diseases, this technique is invasive, time-consuming and can cause side effects that make disease monitoring difficult (2, 3). Therefore, the analysis of the main skin structures through non-invasive techniques such as OCT provides a useful non-traumatic alternative to the biopsy.

As well as other quantitative analyses of skin OCTs, the calculation of the epidermal layer thickness, which is important for the diagnosis of several skin disorders, often requires manual segmentation that is very time-consuming and suffers from inter and intra-observer variability. This fact has motivated the development of semi- and fully automated epidermis segmentation methods from OCT images (5–9). Li et al. defined the segmentation of the epidermis in three steps: preprocessing weighted by least squares, detection of the surface of the skin based on graphics, and local integral projection for the detection of the DEJ. The proposed method was evaluated with a dataset composed of five volumes belonging to healthy skin of the arm, obtaining an average overlap ratio of 0.744 (5). Taghavikhalilbad et al. proposed a semi-automated method to detect the location of the DEJ on 115 B-Scan OCT skin images taken from different body parts, obtaining a root-mean-square error between 8 and 14 $\mu m$. The proposed method was based on a graphical representation of an attenuation coefficient map through a uniform-cost search method. In addition, for border thinning, a fuzzy-based nonlinear smoothing technique was used (6). Note that the aforementioned works were based on classical image processing techniques. In fact, despite the existence of state-of-the-art methods for segmentation of different skin structures, only few are based on deep learning algorithms (8, 9). Calderon-Delgado et al. proposed a fully convolutional network (FCN) to segment 1756 human skin OCT images into dermis, dermal-epidermal junction, epidermis, glycerol, and glass, obtaining an average accuracy of 88, 91, 90, and 96%, respectively. Note that the main limitation of this work is that complex structures, such as hair follicles, were not segmented (8). Kepp et al. presented a deep learning algorithm based on the U-net architecture which was modified with densely connected convolutions to segment mouse skin OCT volumes. They divided the skin into five classes: (epi-)dermis layer, subcutaneous fat layer, fascia and muscle layer, tattoos and background. They applied their algorithms to 72 B-scans of the mice inguinal region and achieved an average Dice similarity coefficient of 0.86 over all segmented skin structures (9). Note that this work did not differentiate between the epidermis and the dermis region.

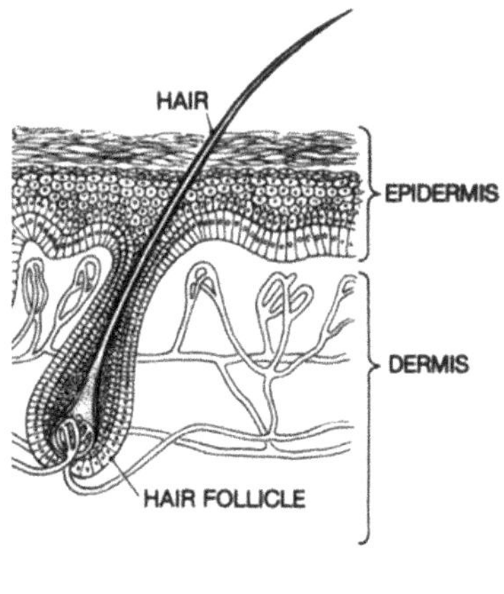


**FIGURE 1** | Main parts of skin: epidermal and dermal layers and follicular structures.

After a thorough search of the relevant literature, it was found that no previous studies have been focused on the segmentation of the epidermis layer along with the follicular structures in human skin OCT images. Note that the epidermis detection is of importance in several clinical dermatology applications such as the epidermal thickness determination in healthy versus unhealthy skin (6). In addition, the identification and measurement of pilosebaceous unit and the size and condition of hair follicles can be useful in monitoring several diseases such as lupus erythematosus, folliculitis, alopecia areata, and basal cell carcinomas (BCCs) (10). However, before interpreting pathological processes and identifying skin pathologies using OCT, the healthy skin appearance has to be studied to establish morphological features of normal skin (4, 11). For all of the above, in this paper, a method to detect the epidermis layer with the hair follicles in healthy human skin OCT images is proposed.

## 2. MATERIALS AND METHODS

### 2.1. Skin Database

The human skin OCT database used in this paper is composed of a total of 270 images from nine healthy humans with ages between 28 and 72 years old (**Table 1**). The research protocol was approved by the Ethics Committee of the Capital Region of Denmark: no. H-16039077. The skin images were acquired from the cheek of the subjects using a UHR-OCT (ultrahigh-resolution) system developed by the Technical University of Denmark (DTU) (3). Compared with a commercial OCT system, which has a lateral resolution around between 10 and 15 $\mu$m and axial resolution of 5-10 $\mu$m, the used UHR-OCT system achieves 6 and 2.2 $\mu$m for lateral and axial resolution, respectively. Therefore, the UHR-OCT system is able to improve the definition of some structures of the skin images such as follicular structures that are of great importance to detect some skin disorders (3). In terms of image size, the number of image pixels varies from one patient to another (**Table 1**). In order to be segmented through deep learning techniques, it is required that all images have the same dimension. For this reason, a rescaling of all images to the minimal dimension was performed, in this case, to $526 \times 975$ pixels.

**TABLE 1** | Content of the skin OCT database.

| Patients | Images | Dimensions |
|---|---|---|
| Patient 01 | 30 | 601 × 975 |
| Patient 02 | 30 | 601 × 975 |
| Patient 03 | 30 | 601 × 975 |
| Patient 04 | 30 | 526 × 975 |
| Patient 05 | 30 | 601 × 975 |
| Patient 06 | 30 | 601 × 995 |
| Patient 07 | 30 | 601 × 995 |
| Patient 08 | 30 | 551 × 995 |
| Patient 09 | 30 | 601 × 995 |

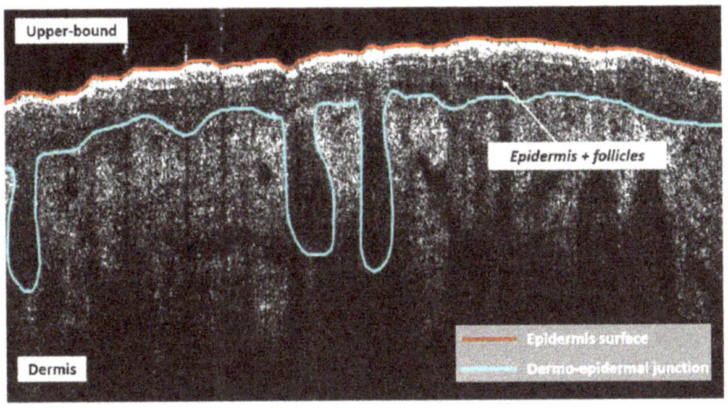


**FIGURE 2** | Ground truth of skin layer boundaries.

As was mentioned before, the goal of the method presented in this paper is to segment the epidermis regions as well as the follicular structures, which can be identified in the skin OCT images as variations of the dermo-epidermal junction. These structures were manually segmented by an expert for training and validation purposes (**Figure 2**). The complete database, including original images and the ground truth, is available as **Supplementary Material**.

## 2.2. Segmentation Algorithm

In this paper, we present an automatic algorithm able to segment the epidermis regions in OCT volumes from human skin. This algorithm consists of an encoder-decoder fully convolutional network combined with a robust post-processing[1].

### 2.2.1. Fully Convolutional Network (FCN)

Skin layers segmentation can be interpreted as a classification problem. The aim is to assign each pixel of an OCT image, into its label $l$ in the label space $L = \{l\} = \{1, ..., \lambda\}$. In this work $\lambda = 3$, being $\lambda$ the number of classes (i.e., upper bound, epidermis+follicles, dermis). Note that these layers are shown between the boundaries exposed in **Figure 3**. The encoder-decoder architecture proposed to address the segmentation task can be observed in **Figure 3**. The input to the whole algorithm is the original image along with its corresponding ground-truth mask, whereas the outputs are the obtained probability maps, one per class. The architecture components and the training and testing processes will be exposed below.

- ***Encoder-decoder block***

Each encoder block is composed of four layers, in sequence: convolution layer, batch normalization layer, ReLU activation layer and max-pooling layer. The convolutional layer is composed of 64 rectangular kernels of $7 \times 3$ and zero padding to preserve the spatial dimensions. The batch normalization technique is applied to improve the convergence speed and the performance of the neural network. ReLu activation introduces non-linearities and max-pooling condenses the feature information reducing the spatial dimensions. The pooling indexes of this operation are transferred to the corresponding unpooling layer in the decoder block. In conclusion, the main objective of the encoder part is the extraction of relevant features from the images.

Each decoder block consists of five layers, in sequence: unpooling layer, concatenation layer, convolution layer, batch normalization, and ReLU activation function. The unpooling layer upsamples the feature maps from the previous decoder block to a double resolution by using the achieved pooling indexes to the matched encoder block. After this step, a concatenation of the upsampled feature maps with the corresponding output feature maps is performed. Finally, convolutional layer, batch normalization, and ReLu are applied to the concatenated feature map. The main objective of this part is to collect the characteristics extracted by the encoder to build the output image as accurately as possible and with the same spatial dimension as the input image.

The final decoder block consists of a convolutional layer with $1 \times 1$ kernel and the softmax activation function. This part is responsible to associate each pixel to one of the three possible classes (upper bound, epidermis+follicles, dermis).

- ***Training process***

**Data partitioning.** According to section 2.1, the used dataset is composed of 270 images coming from nine different subjects. To avoid biased results due to a specific partition of the skin OCT images database into training and test subsets and to obtain the segmentation of all images, an external $K$-fold cross-validation technique was carried out. Specifically, $K = 9$ partitions were created, one per patient. Consequently, in the training process, $K - 1$ different folds in each external iteration were used, while the remaining partition was utilized to test the model performance. In addition, an internal leave-one-out cross-validation was carried out, using the images from one different training fold in each internal iteration as a validation set (**Figure 4**).

**Data conditioning.** Because the images used for training have large dimensions, a patch-wise learning methodology was applied in order to avoid memory problems. In this case, patches of size $526 \times 75$ were used, with a total of 2,730 patches for training and 390 patches for validation. Furthermore, we

[1]Request for materials should be addressed to RA (email: madeam2@upv.es).

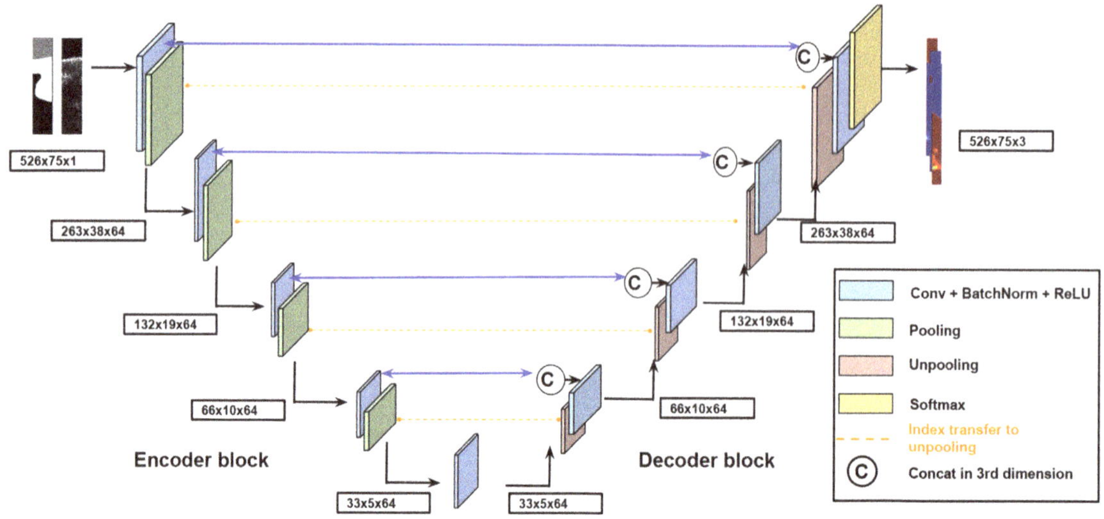


**FIGURE 3 |** Encoder-decoder architecture proposed to address the segmentation task.

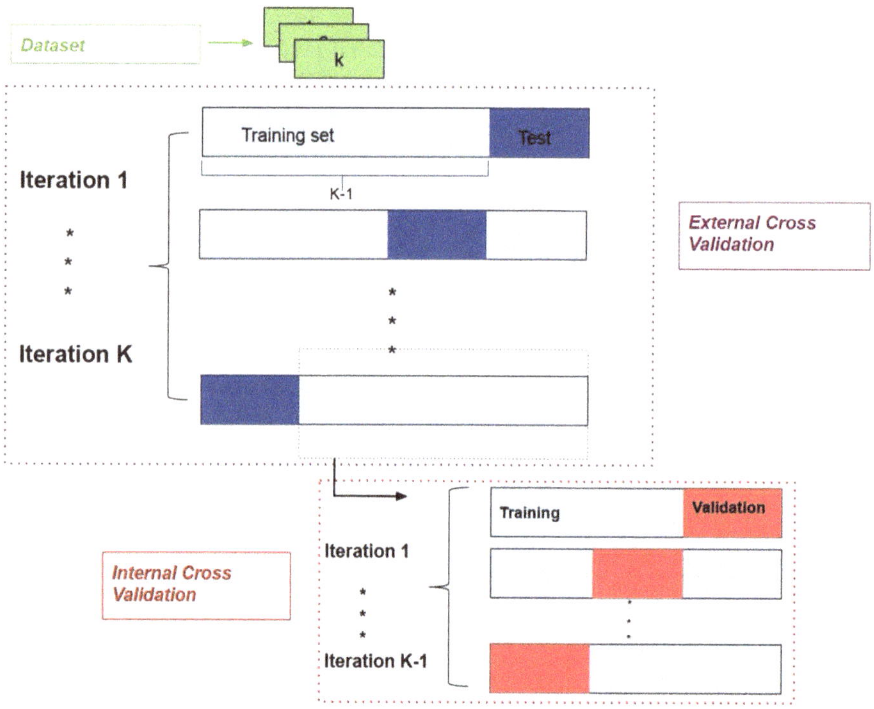


**FIGURE 4 |** *K*-fold cross-validation technique used to data partitioning.

augmented the sliced data by introducing random geometric transformations such as rotations, horizontal flips, croppings, and translations that permit avoiding the overfitting. In the testing stage, memory requirements were more permissive allowing to predict a test sample into two slices of $526 \times 512$ with a Titan V GPU.

**Loss function.** The proposed network was trained by optimizing the Soft-Dice loss function. This function evaluates spatial overlap between the algorithm prediction and the ground truth. Since the Soft-Dice loss is a value ranging between 0 and 1, the aim is to maximize this function during the training stage.

The used Soft-Dice loss function can be defined as follows:

$$\zeta_{dice} = 1 - \frac{2\sum_{x\in\Omega} p_l(x)g_l(x)}{\sum_{x\in\Omega} p_l^2(x) + \sum_{x\in\Omega} g_l^2(x)} \quad (1)$$

where $p_l(x)$ is the predicted multiclass segmentation and $g_l(x)$ is the ground truth.

**Hyper-parameter configuration.** The proposed network was learned through the stochastic gradient descent (SGD) optimizer. Using this optimizer, each epoch of training was composed of a set of $N$ iterations $N = \frac{n^o\ training\ samples}{Batch\ Size}$, in which the gradient was calculated only for a batch of training data. In this case, $Batch\ Size = 4$ and $N = 683$ per epoch. A momentum value of 0.97 was used and the learning rate was initially established to 0.001 and reduced by one order after every 20 epochs. The training stage was composed of 60 epochs and the model that minimizes the validation loss was chosen as the best one.

- ***Testing process***

After training the different models, the images belonging to each patient partition ($K = 9$) were predicted. As was mentioned, an external and internal cross-validation technique was used, obtaining a set of $K \times (K-1)$ models. Therefore, for the final prediction of each test subset belonging to each patient $P_i$ ($i = 1, 2, \ldots, K$), $(K-1)$ models were used:

$$P_i = \frac{1}{K-1}\sum_{j=1}^{K} T_j \quad \forall j \neq i \quad (2)$$

where $T_j$ is the test subset prediction of each model created with different validation subsets ($j = 1, 2, \ldots, K$) with $j \neq i$. The final prediction had a depth equal to the number of classes, so the maximum value in the depth direction was calculated, obtaining for each pixel the class with the highest probability.

### 2.2.2. Post-processing

After testing all skin OCT images of the database (**Figure 5A**) with the trained models, segmentation maps as those shown in **Figure 5B** were obtained. As it can be observed in **Figure 5C**, the proposed network was not able to obtain the characteristic smoothed borders of the follicular structures due to the lack of a pronounced gradient of intensity in its contours. Thus, a post-processing on the obtained segmentation maps was carried out. The implemented post-proccssing was composed of two main stages that are explained below.

- ***Savitzky-Golay filter***

Hair follicles can be considered invaginations of the epidermis into the dermis. The first step to perform a correct definition of the hair follicles consisted in obtaining the contours of those structures. To achieve this purpose, it was necessary to detect the baseline of the dermo-epidermal signal to discriminate between the part belonging to the epidermis to that belonging to the hair follicles. So that, the Savitzky-Golay (SG) filter was used.

The Savitzky-Golay filter is considered a type of finite response digital filter (FIR) based on the polynomial adjustment of a set of points by means of least squares (12). If a symmetric window of size $N$ and centered on point $x_0$ of a vector $\mathbf{x}$ of size $N = 2M + 1$ is considered, the points contained in this window are symmetric on each side of $x_0$ as follows:

$$\mathbf{x} = [x_{-M}, \ldots, x_{-1}, x_0, x_1, \ldots, x_M]^T \quad (3)$$

The $N$ samples contained in $\mathbf{x}$ can be adjusted by a polynomial of order $d$ with ($0 \leq d \leq M$), following the next equation:

$$\hat{x}_m = c_0 + c_1 m + \ldots + c_d m^d \quad -M \leq m \leq M \quad (4)$$

where $\hat{x}_m$ represents the $m_{th}$ sample of the smoothing data. The coefficients $c_i$ are real and must be determined in an optimal way, minimizing the least-squares adjustment errors.

$$e = \sum_{m=-M}^{M} (x_m - \hat{x}_m)^2 = \sum_{m=-M}^{M} (x_m - (c_0 + c_1 m + \ldots + c_d m^d))^2 \quad (5)$$

To obtain the value of these coefficients and therefore the smoothing values, $d + 1$ polynomial base vectors represented by $\mathbf{s}_i$ ($i = 0, 1, \ldots, d$) are defined:

$$\mathbf{s}_i(m) = m^i \quad -M \leq m \leq M \quad (6)$$

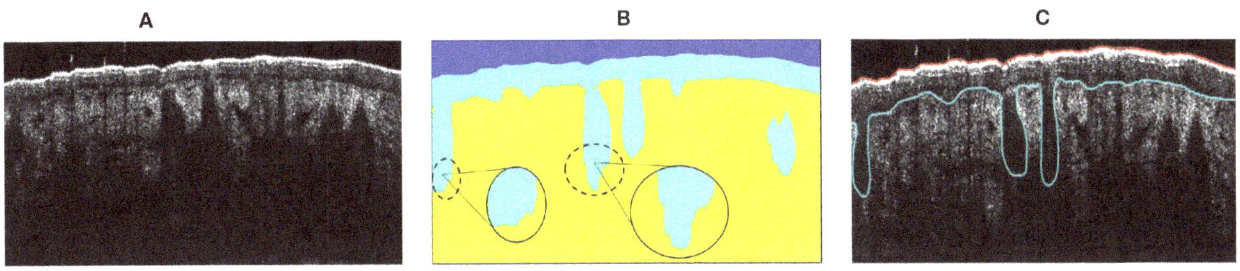


**FIGURE 5 | (A)** Original OCT image. **(B)** Segmentation maps obtained before post-processing. **(C)** Ground truth image.

The corresponding **S** matrix ($N \times (d+1)$) is established as $\mathbf{S} = [\mathbf{s_0}, \mathbf{s_1}, \ldots, \mathbf{s}_d]$ and the smoothing values can be organized in a vector as follows:

$$\hat{\mathbf{x}} = \mathbf{B}\mathbf{x} = \sum_{i=0}^{d} c_i \mathbf{s}_i \tag{7}$$

where **B** is established as $\mathbf{B} = [\mathbf{b}_{-M}, \ldots, \mathbf{b}_0, \ldots, \mathbf{b}_M]$.

The value $y_0 = \hat{x_0}$ is given in terms of the center of the filter $\mathbf{b}_0$ according to the following equation:

$$y_0 = \mathbf{b}_0^T \mathbf{x} = \sum_{m=-M}^{M} b_0(m) x_m \tag{8}$$

In addition, the N-dimensional vector **x** can be shifted of $n$ instants of time as follows:

$$\mathbf{x} = [x_{n-M}, \ldots, x_{n-1}, x_n, x_{n+1}, \ldots, x_{n+M}]^T \tag{9}$$

Therefore, the response of the SG filter with $N$ length to smooth a $x(n)$ signal in a steady-state period can be represented by:

$$y(n) = \sum_{m=-M}^{M} b_0(-m) x(n-m) \tag{10}$$

Note that in input-on and input-off transients periods (at the beginning and the end of the signal), the window goes beyond the limits of the signal and becomes undefined. To handle this problem, in input-on transients periods where $n = 0, \ldots, M-1$:

$$y(n) = \sum_{m=0}^{2M} b_{M-n}(m-M) x(m) \tag{11}$$

and in input-off transients periods where $n = L-M, \ldots, L-1$, being $L$ the length of the whole signal:

$$y(n) = \sum_{m=0}^{2M} b_{-M-n+(L-1)}(m-M) x(L-1-2M+m) \tag{12}$$

The larger the size of the chosen window, the smaller the variance of the error at the filter output. However, if the window is too large, the filter output will be biased compared to the real signal, so the output signal will be very smoothed.

Since the purpose of applying this method was to obtain the baseline of the dermo-epidermal junction, a polynomial order $d = 1$ and a large window size of 449 pixels were established to obtain the signal as smooth as possible. Note that both the polynomial order and the window size were obtained empirically. The results after the application of this filter can be observed in **Figure 6A**.

As it is shown in **Figure 6A**, the obtained baseline of the dermo-epidermal junction (green line) was not completely adjusted at the outset of the three follicular structures content in this image. Therefore, a baseline correction was carried out:

$$bl_c(x) = bl(x) - dif(x) \tag{13}$$

where $dif(x) = max(s_{dej}(x)) - max(bl(x))$ with $s_{dej}(x)$ is the signal of dermo-epidermal junction and $bl(x)$ the baseline obtained after the application of Savitzky-Golay filter. In **Figure 6B**, the corrected baseline is shown. As it can be observed, the baseline is now more precisely adjusted to obtain the full follicular structures.

The hair follicles are structures located below the baseline of the dermis-epidermis junction obtained. However, after the SG application, not all structures below the obtained baseline are hair follicles. To obtain only the follicular structures, a morphological area opening was performed (13). This operation removes the connected components with an area smaller than a parameter $\alpha$. In this case, $\alpha = 0.3 \times \max(\mathbf{A_c})$, with $\mathbf{A_c}$ being the area of the components below the obtained baseline.

After the application of the Savitzky-Golay filter, the upper epidermis region, **Figure 7B**, and the follicular structures, **Figure 7C**, were obtained removing any structure that not accomplishes the condition to be a hair follicle as that located on the right side of **Figure 7A**. These follicular structures are the input to the following post-processing stage.

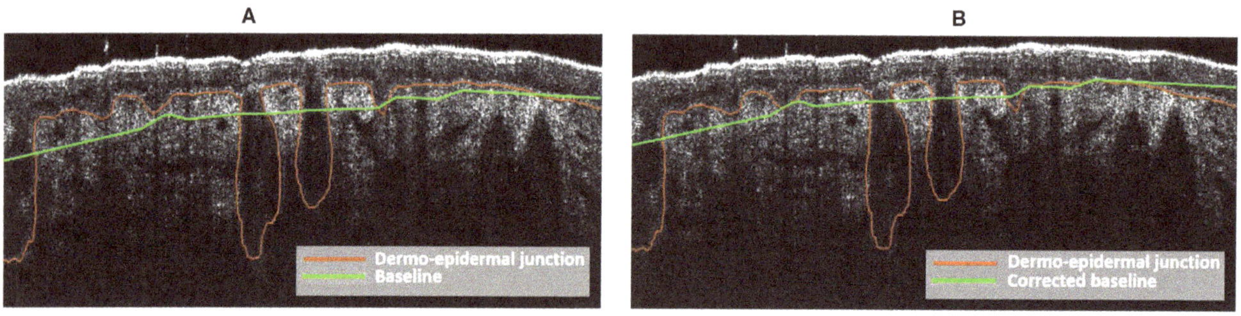


**FIGURE 6** | Baseline of the dermo-epidermis junction. **(A)** Baseline obtained after the application of Savitzky and Golay filter. **(B)** Baseline obtained after the correction process.

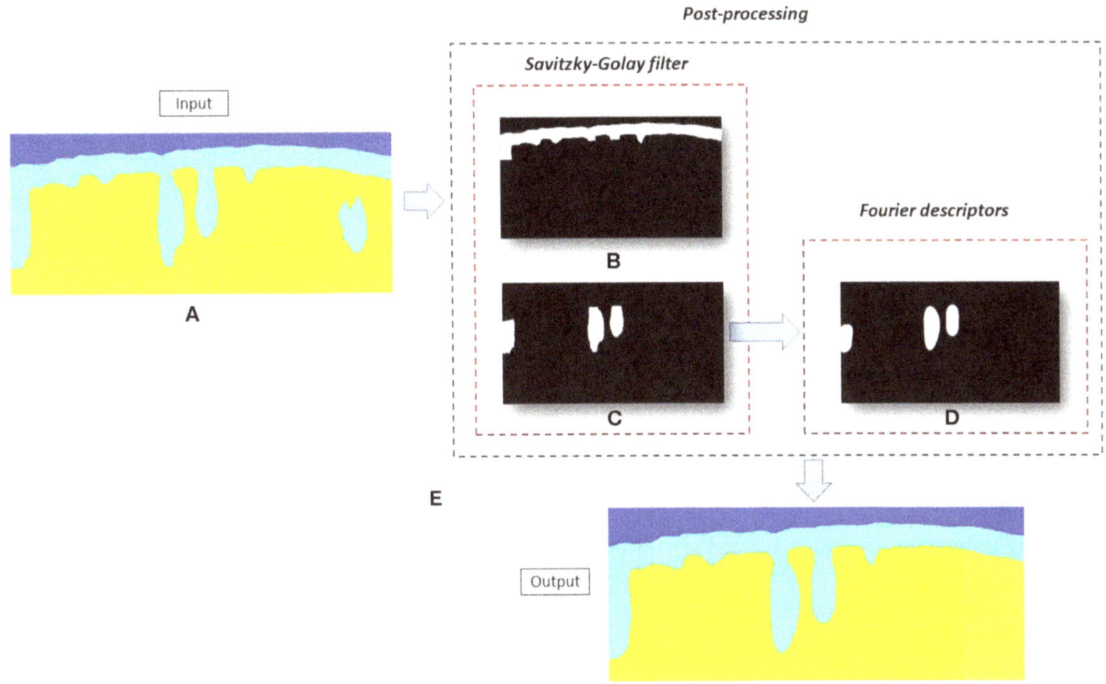


**FIGURE 7** | Post-processing. **(A)** Segmentation maps obtained by the fully convolutional network. **(B)** Upper epidermis without follicular structures. **(C)** Follicular structures obtained after the Savitzky-Golay filter. **(D)** Follicular structures softened after the Fourier Domain Filtering application. **(E)** Segmentation maps obtained after post-processing.

- ***Fourier Domain Filtering***

After applying the Savitzky-Golay filter to obtain the baseline of the dermo-epidermal junction signal and therefore, detect each follicular structure, a Fourier Domain Filtering is applied to soften their contours. Fourier Domain Filtering is a useful mathematical tool to describe the shape of objects defined by a closed contour line. The first step in the application of the Fourier transform is to obtain the coordinates $(x, y)$ of the object contour to be analyzed. The application of the Fourier method requires that the contour was discretized in equispaced coordinates and that the number of contour points $N$ was a power of two and belongs to the complex plane:

$$s[n] = x[n] + jy[n] \tag{14}$$

where $x[n]$ and $y[n]$ are the coordinates of the points of the resampled contour, in this case, the follicular contour.

After obtaining the points of the contour in the complex plane, the Fourier transform is calculated as:

$$S[k] = \sum_{n=0}^{N-1} s[n]e^{-j\frac{2\pi kn}{N}} \tag{15}$$

where $k = (0, \dots N-1)$. After this step, the contour of the object, that in this case is each follicular structure, is transformed into a frequency vector. Since the Fourier transform has inverse, the outline of each object can be reconstructed from its Fourier descriptors. The reconstruction is carried out by applying this equation:

$$s[n] = \frac{1}{N}\sum_{n=0}^{P-1} S[k]e^{j\frac{2\pi kn}{P}} \tag{16}$$

being $P \leq N$. Note that the first descriptors that make up the object, which correspond to the low frequencies, represent the general shape of the contour. However, the latest descriptors, which correspond to high frequencies, represent the finest details. In this case, the roughness of the contour of the hair follicles. Therefore, if the number of descriptors used in the object reconstruction process, $P$ decreases, the contour of the object is softened. As the aim of the application of the Fourier Domain Filtering method is the smoothing of the hair follicles and the bandwidth of this signal was approximately 0.06, a frequency cut off ($f_c$) around 0.007 was used. This means that all descriptors with a frequency greater than $f_c$ were removed. Note that the $f_c$ value was heuristically determined. The number of total descriptors used to define the final object can be calculated with the following equation $P = f_cN$, being $N$ equal to the number of total descriptors, about 57 in this case. Therefore, the number of descriptors used to define the hair follicles was $P = 4$. The follicular structures softened after the Fourier Domain Filtering stage are shown in **Figure 7D**.

Final segmentation maps were obtained by combining the upper epidermis (**Figure 7B**) with the smoothed follicular

**TABLE 2** | Dice's and Jaccard's metrics (mean and standard deviation) comparing the results of the proposed method before and after post-processing (PP) with the ground truth.

| Layers | Dice | | Jaccard | |
|---|---|---|---|---|
| | Before PP | After PP | Before PP | After PP |
| Epidermis + follicles | $0.81 \pm 0.06$ | **$0.83 \pm 0.06$** | $0.69 \pm 0.09$ | **$0.71 \pm 0.09$** |
| Dermis | $0.95 \pm 0.01$ | **$0.96 \pm 0.01$** | $0.92 \pm 0.02$ | **$0.93 \pm 0.02$** |

structures (**Figure 7D**). As it can be observed, in **Figure 7E**, all follicles irregularities have been removed. This allows a better shape definition of the follicular structures, more similar to the manually segmented by experts.

## 3. RESULTS

First, six quantitative measures were computed: Dice's and Jaccard's coefficients, the relative success rate for the number of detected follicles per patient, epidermal thickness, root-mean-square and mean absolute error of the epidermal thickness. Dice's and Jaccard's metrics were calculated for both, the epidermis with hair follicles and the dermis since the layer below the dermo-epidermal junction belongs to the dermis. In addition, these metrics were obtained before and after the post-processing stage to demonstrate the utility of the post-processing in the results of the proposed method (**Table 2**). As **Table 2** demonstrates the improvement of segmentation by including post processing (bold values), from this point, the remaining metrics will be computed on the segmentation results after post-processing.

The relative success rate (RSR) for the number of the detected follicles was calculated with the following equation:

$$RSR = 1 - \frac{|F_{GT} - F_P|}{F_{GT}} \tag{17}$$

where $F_{GT}$ and $F_P$ are the number of follicles detected by the ground truth and by the proposed method, respectively (**Table 3**). To obtain the follicular structures, the Savizky-Golay filter was used. After the application of the SG filter and the morphological area opening explained in section 2.2.2, the follicular structures of the ground truth and the proposed method were obtained per patient. After that, the connected components were automatically counted.

For the epidermal thickness (ET), the average distance between the dermo-epidermal junction (DEJ) and the epidermis surface is considered. The dermo-epidermis junction without hair follicles was calculated for this measure because, according to experts' knowledge, it is better to consider the thin region of the epidermis for the diagnosis of disorders associated with loss of epidermal thickness (11, 14). The hair follicles were manually removed from the GT by experts. The averaged values as well as standard deviation of ET for each healthy subject are reported and compared with the values of the ground truth (**Table 4**). The three lowest values of RSME and MAE are shown in bold.

**TABLE 3** | Number of detected follicles comparing the results of the proposed method with the ground truth (GT).

| Patients | $F_{GT}$ | $F_P$ | RSR |
|---|---|---|---|
| Patient 01 | 5 | 5 | 1.00 |
| Patient 02 | 3 | 4 | 0.67 |
| Patient 03 | 5 | 6 | 0.80 |
| Patient 04 | 4 | 5 | 0.75 |
| Patient 05 | 5 | 5 | 1.00 |
| Patient 06 | 7 | 7 | 1.00 |
| Patient 07 | 3 | 3 | 1.00 |
| Patient 08 | 4 | 6 | 0.50 |
| Patient 09 | 4 | 4 | 1.00 |
| Mean total | | | 0.86 |

**TABLE 4** | Epidermis thickness (ET) comparing the results of the proposed method with the ground truth (GT).

| Patients | GT-based ET ($\mu$m) | Proposed-method-based ET ($\mu$m) | RMSE ($\mu$m) | MAE ($\mu$m) |
|---|---|---|---|---|
| Patient 01 | 56.06±2.05 | $65.02 \pm 0.76$ | 9.13 | 8.95 |
| Patient 02 | 49.20±1.50 | $58.19 \pm 1.77$ | 9.28 | 8.98 |
| Patient 03 | $78.90 \pm 3.83$ | $62.50 \pm 2.75$ | **8.90** | **8.68** |
| Patient 04 | $82.47 \pm 2.63$ | $87.00 \pm 1.90$ | **5.75** | **4.62** |
| Patient 05 | $71.30 \pm 3.83$ | $83.65 \pm 3.02$ | 13.29 | 12.9 |
| Patient 06 | $71.43 \pm 2.40$ | $77.90 \pm 1.99$ | **7.30** | **6.61** |
| Patient 07 | $92.12 \pm 3.37$ | $106.00 \pm 1.20$ | 14.40 | 13.87 |
| Patient 08 | $76.12 \pm 1.67$ | $85.42 \pm 0.76$ | 9.70 | 9.29 |
| Patient 09 | 85.16± 2.94 | $98.69 \pm 1.18$ | 14.10 | 13.52 |
| Mean total | $73.60 \pm 2.69$ | $80.50 \pm 1.70$ | 10.20 | 9.76 |

The root-mean-square error (RMSE) and the mean absolute error (MAE) were calculated with the following equations:

$$RMSE = \sqrt{\frac{\sum_{k=1}^{N}(G[k] - P[k])^2}{N}} \tag{18}$$

$$MAE = \frac{1}{N}\sum_{k=1}^{N}|G[k] - P[k]| \tag{19}$$

where in both metrics $G$ and $P$ are the ET obtained by experts and the prediction of the proposed method, respectively, and $N$ is the number of OCT images.

Secondly, for qualitative evaluation, **Figure 8** shows three examples of representative segmentation results obtained by the proposed method.

## 4. DISCUSSION

In this work, we presented an automatic algorithm for the segmentation of the epidermis along with the follicular structures in healthy patients. As no previous studies have been based on the detection of follicular structures, the results of Dice's

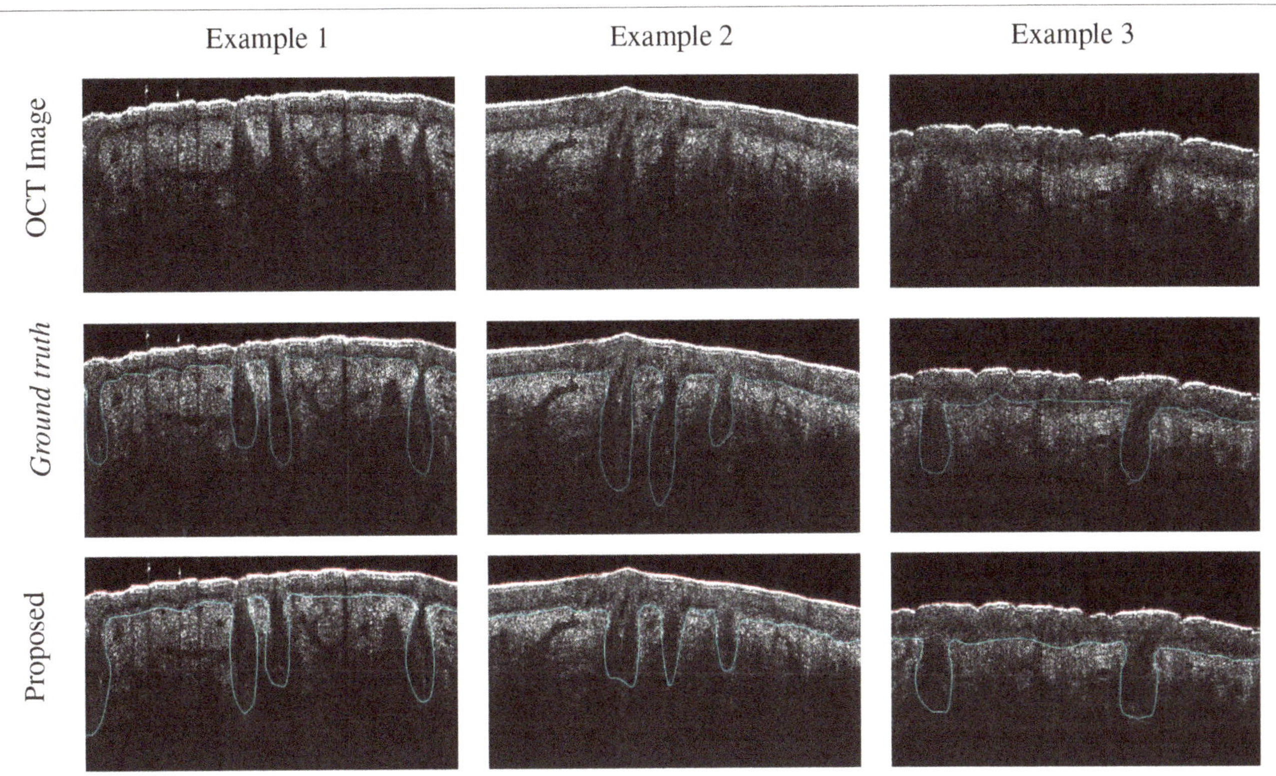


**FIGURE 8 |** Segmentation results (including post-processing) on three representative examples of human skin OCT images. Color code: skin surface (red), dermo-epidermal junction along with hair follicles (blue).

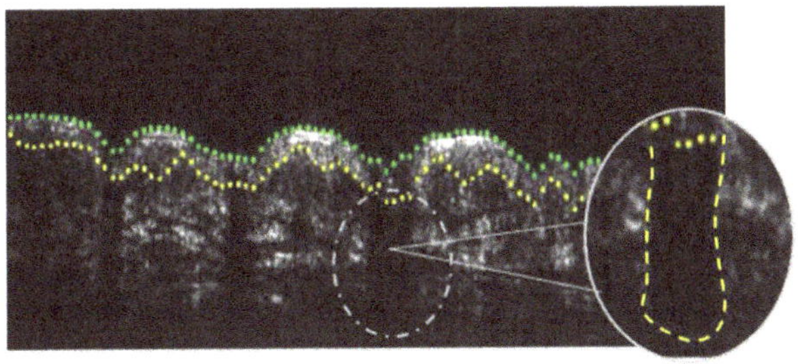

**FIGURE 9 |** Segmentation of follicular structures in another state-of-the-art work. Note that the method misdetect the hair follicles. The area where follicles should be detected is marked and zoomed in with the correct segmentation. Image directly extracted from Li et al. (5).

and Jaccard's coefficients obtained in this study cannot be extrapolated and reliably compared with those existing in the state of the art. However, there are some studies focused only on the segmentation of the epidermal layer (5). It satisfactory segments the epidermis but fails in the detection of the hair follicles (**Figure 9**). In particular, the method presented by Li et al. (5) obtains a Dice's coefficient of 0.74 in the segmentation of the epidermis layer in contrast to the 0.83 obtained by the proposed method that segments the epidermis along with follicular structures, which adds considerable difficulty.

Regarding the amount of follicles detected per patient, the proposed method achieves a mean relative success rate of 0.86, which demonstrates that the proposed algorithm successfully detects the follicles structures from patients with different ages.

With respect to the measurement of epidermal thickness, only the epidermis region was considered because hair follicles were not considered relevant enough in this case. Compared to the RSME error provided by another semi-automatic method of the state of the art, the proposed method achieves an error of 10.2, while (6) obtains an error between 8 and 14 $\mu$m. Note that this is an indirect comparison since the epidermal thickness was calculated on two different databases focused on different body parts and acquired with different OCT devices. However, in addition to be a fully automatic method, the error presented by the developed algorithm is among the lowest errors obtained by the semi-automatic method which were body-part dependent (6). Note that no publicly available skin OCT segmentation method that can be tested on our images to perform a direct comparison was found because most methods designed for this goal are not open access.

As commented in section 1, the detection of follicular structures is of importance in some skin disorders. For example, basal cell carcinoma, the most prevalent cancer in Caucasians human, is related to hair follicles. In fact, several studies confirm that BCCs arise from basal cells specifically of the hair follicles (15, 16). Therefore, in this case, the obtaining of the hair follicles in the OCT images would be useful to study the changes in follicular volume and size produced by cancerous effects. The follicular structures are also the main target in a subtype of cutaneous lupus erythematosus (LE) called chronic discoid LE (CDLE), which results in an irreversible hair loss due to the recruitment of the cells to the bulge region of the hair follicles coupled with the collapse of immune privilege ultimately (17).

Acne is another disorder related to alterations in hair follicles that is easily detected in OCT images (18). Several studies demonstrate that the dynamics of the acne skin are characterized by the increase in the number of dysmorphic pilosebaceous units and the hyperkeratinization of the acroinfundibulum of the pilosebaceous duct before the occurrence of inflammatory events around the follicle. Furthermore, superficial inflammation of the hair follicles in the epidermis is also produced when folliculitis occurs (19). The OCT images show an ill-defined border of the follicular structures in this type of disorder (20).

Due to the fact that the algorithm presented in this work allows to detect hair follicles and distinguish them from the epidermis in an automatic way, it could be of interest to the analysis of diseases such as those mentioned above. The detection of hair follicles carried out by the proposed algorithm could be used to detect a significant decrease in the number of follicles of a patient during a period of time. In addition, the obtaining each follicular structure would also facilitate a further automatic analysis and comparison of its shape and area with a reference pattern which is useful in diseases that cause a significant change in the follicular structures.

## 5. CONCLUSION

OCT analysis in human skin is of great relevance because, compared to other invasive techniques such as biopsies, the OCT allows to capture the most important skin structures without perforation. This fact is especially important for the follow-up of dermatological treatments or the detection of skin tumors. However, before analyzing pathological images, it is necessary to study images from healthy patients to establish reference markers to be compared. In that context, this paper proposes an approach to segment the epidermal layer along with follicular structures in healthy human OCT images. The proposed algorithm is composed of two main stages. The first stage is a CNN based on U-Net architecture. The second stage is a robust post-processing based on a Savitzky-Golay filter and Fourier Domain Filtering. The Savitzky-Golay filter is used to obtain the baseline of DEJ junction and detect the hair follicles. The Fourier Domain Filtering is used over the hair follicles to smooth their contour. To the best of the authors' knowledge, this approach is the only epidermis detection algorithm that segments the follicular structures, which are of importance in the progress of several skin disorders. So, the introduction of the proposed method into clinical practice would accelerate the process of segmentation some important skin structures, allowing the early diagnosis of several skin disorders in a near future. With the aim of facilitating further comparisons and avoid having to use different databases to evaluate the goodness of the segmentation method, the dataset used in this work along with their ground truth (expert-reviewed segmentation) were made publicly as **Supplementary Material**.

From a technical perspective, the future lines of work will focus on adapting the network architecture, if it is necessary, to segment pathological images of different disorders. In this way, a distinction between healthy and pathological images would be carried out.

## ETHICS STATEMENT

The studies involving human participants were reviewed and approved by the Ethics Committee of the Capital Region of Denmark: no. H-16039077. The patients/participants provided their written informed consent to participate in this study.

## AUTHOR CONTRIBUTIONS

RA is the corresponding author. She is the specialist researcher in image processing and the main author of this work. AC is the specialist researcher in deep learning. He guided RA to investigate deep learning techniques and develop the proposed algorithm. SM supervised and reviewed the manuscript carefully and she gave helpful tips to RA for the manuscript writing. MM is the dermatology specialist and brought her expertise about the skin and provided interesting comments. MJ is a specialist in OCT image refinement and has been in charge of the shadow compensation algorithm and contributed to the numerical dispersion compensation. Both methods were applied for refinement of the UHR OCT images in terms of improved contrast and improved resolution. NI is the specialist researcher in OCT and he constructed the UHR-OCT system and provided the UHR-OCT images. Additionally, he helped in defining the results provided for the proposed algorithm. OB is the specialist researcher in charge of UHR-OCT system development. He provided the used database. VN is the lead researcher, she defined the goal of this work, and participated in the revision of the final manuscript providing interesting comments and ideas.

## ACKNOWLEDGMENTS

We gratefully acknowledge the support of NVIDIA Corporation with the donation of the Titan V GPU used for this research. NVIDIA Corporation had no role in study design, data collection and analysis, decision to publish or preparation of the manuscript.

## REFERENCES


1. Kafieh R, Rabbani H, Abramoff M, Sonka M. Intra-retinal layer segmentation of optical coherence tomography using diffusion map. In: *2013 IEEE International Conference on Acoustics, Speech and Signal Processing* (Vancouver, BC). (2013). p. 1080–4. doi: 10.1109/ICASSP.2013.6637816
2. Hussain AA, Themstrup L, Mogensen M, Jemec GB. Optical coherence tomography imaging of the skin. In: Humbert P, Fanian F, Maibach HI, Agache P, editor. *Agache's Measuring the Skin: Non-invasive Investigations, Physiology, Normal Constants* (Cham: Springer). (2017) p. 493–502. doi: 10.1007/978-3-319-32383-1_53
3. Israelsen NM, Maria M, Mogensen M, Bojesen S, Jensen M, Haedersdal M, et al. The value of ultrahigh resolution OCT in dermatology-delineating the dermo-epidermal junction, capillaries in the dermal papillae and vellus hairs. *Biomed Opt Exp.* (2018) 9:2240–65. doi: 10.1364/BOE.9.002240
4. Park ES. Skin-layer analysis using optical coherence tomography (OCT). *Med Lasers.* (2014) 3:1–4. doi: 10.25289/ML.2014.3.1.1
5. Li A, Cheng J, Yow A, Wall C, Wong D, Tey HL, et al. Epidermal segmentation in high-definition optical coherence tomography. In: *2015 37th Annual International Conference of the IEEE Engineering in Medicine and Biology Society (EMBC)* (Milan). (2015). p. 3045–8.
6. Taghavikhalilbad A, Adabi S, Clayton A, Soltanizadeh H, Mehregan D, Avanaki MR. Semi-automated localization of dermal epidermal junction in optical coherence tomography images of skin. *Appl Opt.* (2017) 56:3116–21. doi: 10.1364/AO.56.003116
7. Srivastava R, Yow AP, Cheng J, Wong DW, Tey HL. Three-dimensional graph-based skin layer segmentation in optical coherence tomography images for roughness estimation. *Biomed Opt Exp.* (2018) 9:3590–606. doi: 10.1364/BOE.9.003590
8. Calderon-Delgado M, Tjiu JW, Lin MY, Huang SL. High resolution human skin image segmentation by means of fully convolutional neural networks. In: *2018 International Conference on Numerical Simulation of Optoelectronic Devices (NUSOD)* (Hong Kong). (2018). p. 31–2. doi: 10.1109/NUSOD.2018.8570241
9. Kepp T, Droigk C, Casper M, Evers M, Hüttmann G, Salma N, et al. Segmentation of mouse skin layers in optical coherence tomography image data using deep convolutional neural networks. *Biomed Opt Exp.* (2019) 10:3484–96. doi: 10.1364/BOE.10.003484
10. Mogensen M, Bojesen S, Israelsen NM, Maria M, Jensen M, Podoleanu A, et al. Two optical coherence tomography systems detect topical gold nanoshells in hair follicles, sweat ducts and measure epidermis. *J Biophoton.* (2018) 11:e201700348. doi: 10.1002/jbio.201700348
11. Mogensen M, Morsy HA, Thrane L, Jemec GB. Morphology and epidermal thickness of normal skin imaged by optical coherence tomography. *Dermatology.* (2008) 217:14–20. doi: 10.1159/000118508
12. Savitzky A, Golay MJ. Smoothing and differentiation of data by simplified least squares procedures. *Anal Chem.* (1964) 36:1627–39. doi: 10.1021/ac60214a047
13. Heijmans HJ. Connected morphological operators for binary images. *Comput Vis Image Understand.* (1999) 73:99–120. doi: 10.1006/cviu.1998.0703
14. Mogensen M, Nürnberg B, Forman JL, Thomsen JB, Thrane L, Jemec G. *In vivo* thickness measurement of basal cell carcinoma and actinic keratosis with optical coherence tomography and 20-MHz ultrasound. *Br J Dermatol.* (2009) 160:1026–33. doi: 10.1111/j.1365-2133.2008.09003.x
15. Wang GY, Wang J, Mancianti ML, Epstein EH Jr. Basal cell carcinomas arise from hair follicle stem cells in Ptch1+/- mice. *Cancer Cell.* (2011) 19:114–24. doi: 10.1016/j.ccr.2010.11.007
16. Peterson SC, Eberl M, Vagnozzi AN, Belkadi A, Veniaminova NA, Verhaegen ME, et al. Basal cell carcinoma preferentially arises from stem cells within hair follicle and mechanosensory niches. *Cell Stem Cell.* (2015) 16:400–12. doi: 10.1016/j.stem.2015.02.006
17. Berekméri A, Tiganescu A, Alase A, Vital EM, Stacey M, Wittmann M. Non-invasive approaches for the diagnosis of autoimmune/autoinflammatory skin diseases-a focus on psoriasis and lupus erythematosus. *Front Immunol.* (2019) 10:1931. doi: 10.3389/fimmu.2019.01931
18. Fuchs CS, Ortner VK, Mogensen M, Philipsen PA, Haedersdal M. Transfollicular delivery of gold microparticles in healthy skin and acne vulgaris, assessed by *in vivo* reflectance confocal microscopy and optical coherence tomography. *Lasers Surg Med.* (2019) 51:430–8. doi: 10.1002/lsm.23076
19. Durdu M, Ilkit M. First step in the differential diagnosis of folliculitis: cytology. *Crit Rev Microbiol.* (2013) 39:9–25. doi: 10.3109/1040841X.2012.682051
20. Andersen AJB, Fuchs C, Ardigo M, Haedersdal M, Mogensen M. *In vivo* characterization of pustules in Malassezia Folliculitis by reflectance confocal microscopy and optical coherence tomography. A case series study. *Skin Res. Technol.* (2018) 24:535–41. doi: 10.1111/srt.12463

# 17

# Dermoscopy Features of Acquired Perforating Dermatosis Among 39 Patients

*Wenju Wang[1†], Yansen Liao[2†], Lixin Fu[1], Bei Kan[1], Xiaodong Peng[2*] and Yonghong Lu[1*]*

*[1] Department of Dermatovenereology, Chengdu Second People's Hospital, Chengdu, China, [2] Department of Oncology, Chengdu Second People's Hospital, Chengdu, China*

***Correspondence:**
*Xiaodong Peng*
*3260172243@qq.com*
*Yonghong Lu*
*1255395583@qq.com*

*† These authors have contributed equally to this work*

In this report, we concluded there are four dermoscopic features of APD including a yellow-brown homogeneous structureless area in the center of the lesion, dotted and linear vessels distribution radially and a dam shape uplift at the periphery, as well as a white irregular ring surrounding the lesion. There are three features, including the yellow-brown homogeneous structureless area in the center of the lesion, the dotted and linear vessels distribution radially and the white irregular ring surrounding the lesion were correspond to the report of Emma Ormerod et al.These features are also similar to those previously discribed in three separated reports of seven cases with APD. In our report, we found a new dermoscopic features: the dam shape uplift at the periphery. These finding may be contributed to improve the rate of clinical diagnosis of APD.

**Keywords: dermoscopy, acquired perforating dermatosis, characteristic, new dermoscopic features, clinical diagnosis**

Acquired perforating dermatosis (APD) is a penetrating skin disease characterized by the excretion of denatured collagen from the epidermis. The most common clinical symptom of APD is pruritus. The lesions are distributed widely and characterized by umbilicated papules and plaques with central crusted ulceration (1). The histopathological presentation of APD often shows local epidermal erosion and loss, homogenized denaturation of dermal superficial fibers, and denaturated fiber bundles penetrating the epidermis (2, 3).MASSON's trichrome and elastic fiber stain showed collagen fibers penetrating the epidermis in the dermis. APD is a rare disorder and the clinical presentation can vary from patient to patient, and it is difficult to differentiate clinically from prurigo nodularis, solar dermatitis, or other diseases. The real diagnosis is often missed or delayed.

Dermoscopy is a non-invasive technique that is used to aid the diagnosis of skin tumors and other inflammatory dermatoses (4, 5) In our clinical work, we found the APD is characteristic under dermoscopy. To the best of our knowledge, the dermoscopic features of APD have been described in three previous case reports (6–8). Here we analyze and report the dermoscopic feature in a series of 39 patients with APD.

We identified 39 patients (19 male and 20 female) with a diagnosis of APD in our department over the past 4 years. The age of these patients ranged from 18 to 65 years, the average age was 48.5 years. All of the patients were diagnosed by clinical (**Figure 1**) and histopathological examination (**Figure 2**).

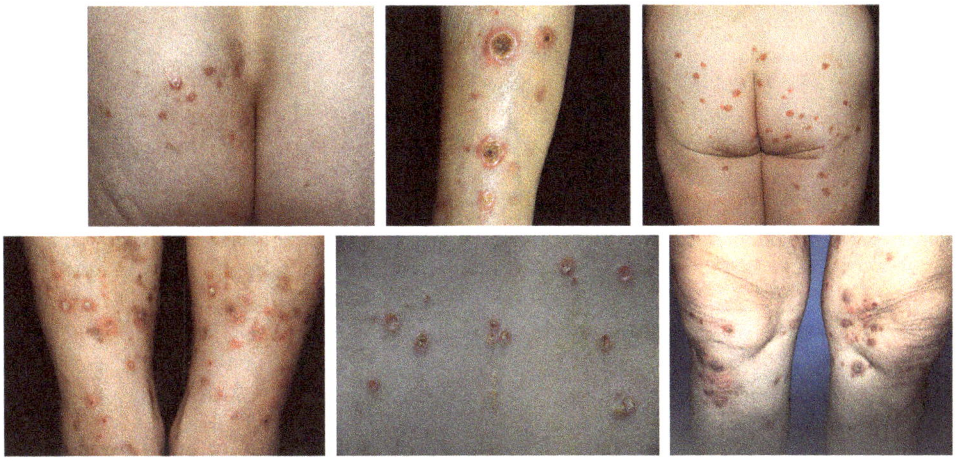

FIGURE 1 | The clinical presentation of an APD patient. Skin lesions were widely distributed all over the trunk and limbs, the main manifestations were keratinized purplish-red papules or ulcers, about rice to bean size. The center of most papules was navel concave, the surface was a yellow adhesive exfoliated scab shell surrounded by a purplish-red halo. The edge of the ulcer was levee shaped and palpated with moderate hardness.

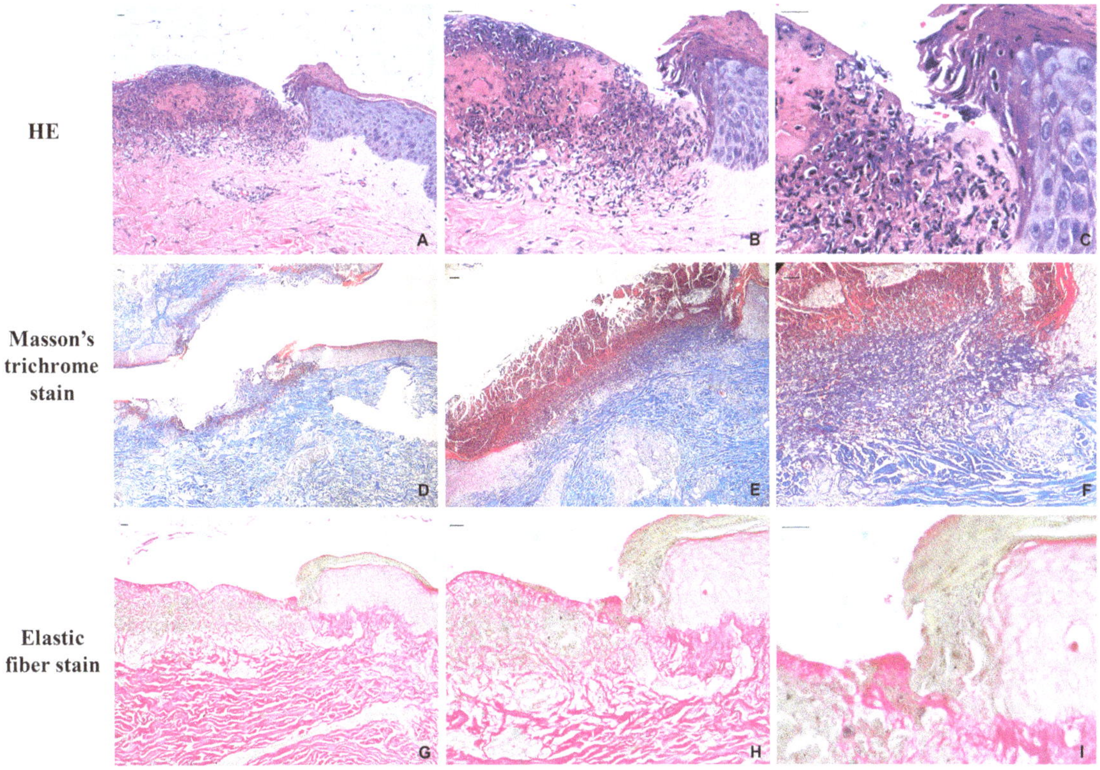


FIGURE 2 | Histopathological features at initial presentation. **(A)** the HE staining of APD patients (10x); **(B)** the HE staining of APD patients (200x); **(C)** the HE staining of APD patients (400x); **(D)** Masson trichrome staining (40x); **(E)** Masson trichrome staining (100x); **(F)** Masson trichrome staining (200x); **(G)** elastic fiber staining (100x); **(H)** elastic fiber staining (200x); **(I)** elastic fiber staining (400x). Scale bars, 200 μm.

We analyzed the dermoscopy pictures of all 39 patients (**Table 1**). Dermoscopic images revealed that there are nine features: (1) a yellow-brown homogeneous structureless area in the center of the lesion were found in 38 of the 39 cases, the accrue rate was about 97.43% (**Figure 3A**); (2) dotted and linear vessel distribution radially were found in 38 of the 39 cases, the accrue rate was about 97.43% (**Figure 3B**); (3) a dam shape uplift at the periphery of the lesion was found in 37 of the 39 cases, the accrue rate was about 94.87% (**Figure 3C**); (4) a white irregular halo surrounding the lesion was found in 34 of the

39 cases, the accrue rate was about 87.18% (**Figure 3D**); (5) a thin scale ring surrounding the lesion was found in 21 of the 39 cases, the accrue rate was about 53.84% (**Figure 3E**); (6) a pink background in the lesion were found in 16 of the 39 cases, the accrue rate was about 41.02% (**Figure 3F**); (7) we found an an orange background in the lesion in 12 of the 39 cases, the accrue rate was about 30.77% (**Figure 3G**); (8) we found a red background in the lesion in 11 of the 39 cases, the accrue rate is about 28.20% (**Figure 3H**); (9) a pigment structure surrounding the lesion were found in 3 of the 39 cases, the accrue rate is about 7.69% (**Figure 3I**).

**TABLE 1** | Dermoscopic features observed in 39 ARPC patients with relative frequencies.

| Dermoscopic features | *N* (Total 39) | Rate (%) |
|---|---|---|
| yellow-brown homogeneous structureless area in the center | 38 | 97.43 |
| dotted and linear vessels distribution radially | 38 | 97.43 |
| adam shape uplift at the periphery | 37 | 94.87 |
| white irregular halo surrounding the lesion | 34 | 87.18 |
| thin scale ring surrounding the lesion | 21 | 53.84 |
| pink background | 16 | 41.02 |
| orange background | 12 | 30.77 |
| red background | 11 | 28.20 |
| pigment structure surrounding the lesion | 3 | 7.69 |

Dermatoscopic images reveal that the first four clear and consistent features corresponded to the histopathology changes of APD. The yellow-brown homogeneous structureless area in the center of the lesion was found to correspond to the collagen bundle that penetrates the epidermis vertically. The dotted and linear vessel distribution radially in the lesion was found to correspond to the perivascular inflammatory cells. The dam shape uplift at the periphery was found to correspond to the thickening of stratum spinosum and the form of cup-shaped depression of the epidermis by extruded collagen. This white irregular ring surrounding the lesion indicates pigment loss. The first three features also corresponded to a report of Emma Ormerod et al. (6). As described above, the dermoscopic features may be an aid in diagnosing APD and improve the rate of clinical diagnosis.

At present, there is no special treatment method for APD. Common treatment methods are to treat the primary disease to eliminate inducement. In this report, all patients were treated with oral antihistamines, topical glucocorticoid, and retinoic acid ointment combined with NB-UVB irradiation, and the efficacy was satisfactory. In conclusion, we found there are four common dermoscopic features of APD including a yellow-brown homogeneous structureless area in the center of the lesion, dotted

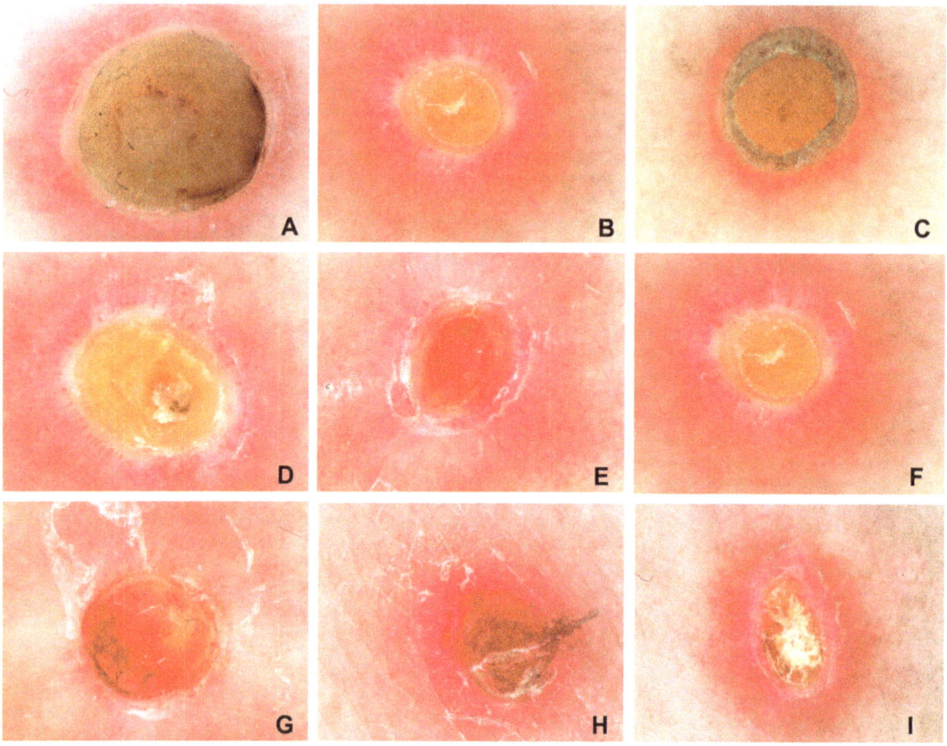


**FIGURE 3** | The common dermatoscopic features of the typical lesions from the 39 patients. **(A)** the yellow-brown homogeneous structureless area in the center of the lesion; **(B)** dotted and linear vessels distribution radially; **(C)** a dam shape uplift at the periphery of the lesion; **(D)** the white irregular halo surrounding the lesion; **(E)** a thin scale ring surrounding the lesion; **(F)** pink background; **(G)** orange background; **(H)** red background; **(I)** pigment structure surrounding the lesion. **(A–D)** the four common dermoscopic features of APD.

and linear vessel distribution radially, and a dam shape uplift at the periphery, as well as a white irregular ring surrounding the lesion. There are three features, including the yellow-brown homogeneous structureless area in the center of the lesion, the dotted and linear vessel distribution radially, and a white irregular ring surrounding the lesion, which corresponds with the findings of Emma Ormerod et al. (6). These features are also similar to those previously described in three separate reports relating to seven cases of APD. In our report, we found a new dermoscopic feature: the dam shape uplift at the periphery. These findings could improve the rate of clinical diagnosis of APD.

According to our understanding, the kind of penetrating dermatosis, such as penetrating folliculitis, Kyrle disease, and elastosis perforans, have common features under the pathology, including parakeratosis keratotic plug or elastic fiber through the epidermis. We also summarized the differences in dermoscopic features between prurigo and APD. The dermoscopic features of prurigo show pale brown solitary raised papules with sticky white scabs, irregular white unstructured areas, and spotty, linear vascular foci. Different from the dermoscopic features of APD, there is no yellow-brown homogeneous structureless area in the center, no dam shape uplift at the periphery of the lesion, a white irregular halo surrounding the lesion, and the vascular arrangement is irregular. Therefore, hypothesize that the four dermoscopic features of APD described above are common dermoscopic features of penetrating collagen disease. The question of whether these four features can be defined simply as APD, requires further confirmation and study.

## ETHICS STATEMENT

Human research was approved by the Ethics Committee of Chengdu Second People's Hospital. The authors certify that they have obtained all appropriate patient consent forms and patients provided consent, confirming that their clinical information could be reported in journal articles.

## AUTHOR CONTRIBUTIONS

All authors listed have made a substantial, direct and intellectual contribution to the work, and approved it for publication.

## REFERENCES

1. Millard PR, Young E, Harrison DE, Wojnarowska F. Reactive perforating collagenosis: light, ultrastructural and immunohisto-logical studies. *Histopathology.* (1986) 10:1047–56. doi: 10.1111/j.1365-2559.1986.tb02541.x
2. Kim SW, Kim MS, Lee JH, Son SJ, Park KY, Li K, et al. A clinicopathologic study of thirty cases of acquired perforating dermatosis in Korea. *Ann Dermatol.* (2014) 26:162–71. doi: 10.5021/ad.2014.26.2.162
3. Cerio R, Calnan CD, Wilson-Jones E. A clinic-pathological study of reactive perforating collagenosis: report of 10 cases. *Br J Dermatol.* (1987) 117:16–7. doi: 10.1111/j.1365-2133.1987.tb11997.x
4. Argenziano G, Soyer HP, Chimenti S, Talamini R, Corona R, Sera F, et al. Dermoscopy of pigmented skin lesions: results of a consensus meeting via the internet. *J Am Acad Dermatol.* (2003) 48:679–93. doi: 10.1067/mjd.2003.281
5. Goncharova Y, Attia EA, Souid K, Protzenko O, Koktishev I. Dermoscopic features of clinically inflammatory dermatoses and their correlation with histopathologic reaction patterns. *Arch Dermatol Res.* (2015) 307:23–30. doi: 10.1007/s00403-014-1513-3
6. Ormerod E, Atwan A, Intzedy L, Stone N. Dermoscopy features of acquired reactive perforating collagenosis: a case series. *Dermatol Pract Concept.* (2018) 8:303–5. doi: 10.5826/dpc.0804a11
7. Kittisak P, Tanaka M. Dermoscopic findings in a case of reactive perforating collagenosis. *Dermatol Pract Concept.* (2015) 5:75–7. doi: 10.5826/dpc.0502a13
8. Ramirez-Fort MK, Khan F, Rosendahl CO, Mercer SE, Shin-Chang H, Levitt JO. Acquired perforating dermatosis: a clinical and der-matoscopic correlation. *Dermatol Online J.* (2013) 19:18958.

# 18

# Convolutional Neural Network for Skin Lesion Classification: Understanding the Fundamentals Through Hands-On Learning

*Marta Cullell-Dalmau [1], Sergio Noé [1], Marta Otero-Viñas [2], Ivan Meić [1,3] and Carlo Manzo [1*]*

*[1] The QuBI Lab, Facultat de Ciències i Tecnologia, Universitat de Vic – Universitat Central de Catalunya, Vic, Spain, [2] Tissue Repair and Regeneration Laboratory, Facultat de Ciències i Tecnologia, Universitat de Vic – Universitat Central de Catalunya, Vic, Spain, [3] University of Zagreb, Zagreb, Croatia*

***Correspondence:**
*Carlo Manzo*
*carlo.manzo@uvic.cat*

Deep learning architectures for the classification of images have shown outstanding results in a variety of disciplines, including dermatology. The expectations generated by deep learning for, e.g., image-based diagnosis have created the need for non-experts to become familiar with the working principles of these algorithms. In our opinion, getting hands-on experience with these tools through a simplified but accurate model can facilitate their understanding in an intuitive way. The visualization of the results of the operations performed by deep learning algorithms on dermatological images can help students to grasp concepts like convolution, even without an advanced mathematical background. In addition, the possibility to tune hyperparameters and even to tweak computer code further empower the reach of an intuitive comprehension of these processes, without requiring advanced computational and theoretical skills. This is nowadays possible thanks to recent advances that have helped to lower technical and technological barriers associated with the use of these tools, making them accessible to a broader community. Therefore, we propose a hands-on pedagogical activity that dissects the procedures to train a convolutional neural network on a dataset containing images of skin lesions associated with different skin cancer categories. The activity is available open-source and its execution does not require the installation of software. We further provide a step-by-step description of the algorithm and of its functions, following the development of the building blocks of the computer code, guiding the reader through the execution of a realistic example, including the visualization and the evaluation of the results.

**Keywords: convolutional neural networks, skin lesion analysis, classification, melanoma, deep learning**

## INTRODUCTION: BACKGROUND AND RATIONALE FOR THE EDUCATIONAL ACTIVITY INNOVATION

Over the last two decades, convolutional neural networks (CNNs) (1) have become established as an invaluable tool for biomedical image classification and have been proposed as an instrument for clinical diagnosis in disciplines such as radiology, histology, ophthalmology, and dermatology (2).

The rapid spread of CNNs and other deep learning techniques, has created the need for non-experts to become familiar with these complex tools and understand their principles of operation. There is a broad literature of introductory articles offering basic reviews on CNNs principles and applications. However, on the practical side, tutorials to start working with CNNs often require a familiarity with terms and concepts that could discourage readers without a solid background in mathematics and/or computer programming to obtain a further understanding of these techniques.

In this scenario, we aim to close this gap by offering a hands-on activity based on the step-by-step execution of a computer code involving all the procedures carried out when implementing a CNN classification, along with their description. Similar educational activities have been recently proposed for other research fields (3). The activity guides the student through two complete examples based on images of skin lesions, starting from the pre-processing of the dataset, and leading through the steps of data augmentation, the choice of the network architecture and its fine-tuning, until the final evaluation of the results.

In our opinion, this hands-on activity can help students to obtain an intuitive understanding of the operations performed by the CNN building blocks, e.g., by visualizing the effect of image convolution with a specific kernel, the feature map generated at specific network layers, or even by performing the network training and exploring the effect of different hyperparameters on the results. The activity can be performed at different levels of difficulty, depending on the user expertise in programming. At the basic level of execution, the students can interactively play with the different sections just by changing input parameters from simple form fields and can run the program by pushing the play button, without even visualizing the code. At the intermediate/advanced levels, students can unfold cells to show, read and (possibly) modify portions of the code. In both cases, the use of the Google Colab and GitHub platforms allows to run the activity in the cloud from any internet browser, without any software installation, strongly simplifying configuration requirements and enabling the capability to use hardware accelerators.

## PEDAGOGICAL FRAMEWORK AND LEARNING ENVIRONMENT

We aimed at developing a hands-on activity mainly directed to students (medical school, biomedical engineering), but with the potential of being of interest also for clinicians and other professionals willing to get acquainted with deep learning and CNNs. Four major developments make such a learning-by-doing experience nowadays possible, even for non-experts. First, the creation of specific software libraries, which have reduced the complexity and length of the code necessary to implement these networks, thus allowing their use to operators with a basic knowledge of computer programming. Secondly, the distribution of pre-trained classical CNN under license for reuse has enabled the possibility to perform transfer learning further simplifying the coding and speeding up the training. Third, the free availability of cloud computing on virtual machines with graphics (GPUs) and tensor processing units (TPUs), which has played an important role in speeding up training procedures. The last development of note is the accessibility of databases containing labeled images for training.

Along these lines, for the proposed activity we use Keras (4), an open-source framework developed by Francois Chollet. Several open-source frameworks are nowadays available for deep learning such as PyTorch or Caffe. However, Keras is recommended for beginners since it is relatively easy to use and has a high-level API that permits to build complex models by writing a few lines of code. In addition, Keras has several models of the best performing architecture (Alexnet, ResNet, VGGNet, Inception, etc.) pre-trained on large datasets (e.g., the one used for the ImageNet Large Scale Visual Recognition Challenge (ILSVRC, http://image-net.org) containing millions of photographs from 1,000 categories) that have thus achieved very general classification capabilities. These trained networks can be "reconverted" to the classification of different target images in few simple steps and their learnable parameters (weights and biases) are fine-tuned to provide high classification accuracy, through a procedure called transfer learning.

The code for the activity is provided on the Google Colaboratory platform (Colab, https://colab.research.google.com/notebooks/intro.ipynb). Colab is a free cloud service that enable coding in Python and program execution in a web browser, in a highly interactive fashion. In addition, it requires a minimum number of configuration steps, offers free access to GPUs and TPUs, and allows sharing of contents in a straightforward manner. The notebooks and metadata necessary for the activity are shared on GitHub (www.github.com), a free hosting service for software development and version control.

Deep learning requires a massive amount of information in the form of labeled images. Several repositories contain high-quality images associated to dermatology, available as research tools in clinical training and computer science. For example, the archive of the International Skin Imaging Collaboration (ISIC, https://isic-archive.com/), or the Edinburgh Dermofit Library (https://licensing.edinburgh-innovations.ed.ac.uk/i/software/dermofit-image-library.html) host images of skin lesions, labeled according to their diagnoses. For the activity, we use images from the dataset that has been recently made available for the training of methods competing for the ISIC 2019 challenge (https://challenge2019.isic-archive.com), a competition aimed at supporting research toward automated melanoma detection. The full dataset contains 25,331 images of skin lesions associated to 8 different diagnostic categories (melanoma, melanocytic nevus, basal cell carcinoma, actinic keratosis, benign keratosis, dermatofibroma, vascular lesion, and squamous cell carcinoma) and can be accessed by registering to the ISIC website.

## DESCRIPTION OF THE HANDS-ON ACTIVITY

The files to perform the activity are stored on the GitHub public repository https://github.com/qubilab/CNN-for-skin-lesion-classification. The two links, associated to examples of a binary (benign/malignant) and a multiclass (melanoma/melanocytic nevus/basal cell carcinoma/actinic keratosis/benign keratosis/dermatofibroma/vascular lesion/squamous cell carcinoma) classification of images of skin lesions, automatically redirect to the respective Colab notebooks.

For the basic use of the notebook, no configuration is needed. For applications requiring hardware accelerators (e.g., training or fine-tuning), GPU or TPU can be enabled by picking the required accelerator from the menu that appears by selecting Runtime/Change runtime type.

For a better pedagogical support, the notebook is organized in consecutive sections, each with a brief explanation of the task performed, that guide the user steps-by-step along the activity. To execute the code in a cell, it is sufficient to select it with a click and then either press the play button within the cell box or use the keyboard shortcut "Command/Ctrl+Enter." For more advanced applications, the visualization of input form fields or code is achieved by unfolding the cell content, by clicking on the little arrowhead at the left of the cell, thus enabling the necessary editing.

## Image Pre-processing and CNN Basics

The first cell "0. Imports" gives access to the code provided in other modules and libraries and defines some basic functions. Once this operation has been performed, we enter into the core of the activity. In fact, since most of the deep learning approaches are data-driven, a major focus must be set on the dataset and its organization. The cell "1. Loading and organizing the dataset" loads the labeled images on the Colab cloud space and arrange them into folders (**Figure 1A**). The first block of this section requires the input of user credential to login on the ISIC archive and the selection of the number of images per category. The photographs will then be organized into folders according to their category and further randomly split into training, validation, and test sets. A variable percentage of images (10–30%) can be used for the final testing, whereas the others are split between training (70–80%) and validation. The folder tree can be visualized in the left frame of Colab, by selecting "Files." In the example, we use percentages of 65, 20, and 15% of the total number of images for training, validation and test, respectively. These percentages can be changed by the user through the form fields of block 1.3.

The cell "2. Understanding images and convolution" allows the user to visualize an image from a selected folder, together with its decomposition into layers according to RGB color model and the representation of the pixel intensity value. To provide an intuitive understanding of the principle of CNN, the activity shows different convolution kernels and their pixel values. The convolution of the image with these kernels is further provided. An introductory description of the convolution and of the hyperparameters of a convolutional layer can be found in our previous article (5).

Often, the limited amount of data available for training might produce the memorization of specific details of the training images, leading to overfitting and the inability of the model to generalize. In this case, it is recommendable to perform a procedure called data augmentation. The augmentation generates modified images by applying random transformations, such as rotation, shift, scaling, and reflection, to existing data (**Figure 1B**). Typically, the computer function used for augmentation also takes care of resizing the images to the input size required by the network. These steps can be visualized on a random image by executing the cell "3. Data augmentation."

## CNN Selection

Once the data have been obtained and properly organized, the following step entails the choice of the classification network. In principle, users could build their own network by assembling it layer-by-layer. Application program interfaces allow one to create a CNN from scratch relatively easily. However, this is generally not recommended for beginners, since it requires some background knowledge, a good dose of intuition, and some trial and error. Moreover, unless one is facing a new and very specific image classification task, a personalized CNN is often not needed: many popular deep learning architectures are released under a permissive license for reuse. Even in the case that it is essential to build a custom model, classic networks might still serve as an inspiration, a scaffold, or as a block of the new model. Nowadays, several networks offering outstanding performance for image classification are available, therefore choosing the most suitable CNN for one's application is not straightforward. Since these CNNs have been originally built for applications on different datasets, the selection should be based on their performance on the target dataset and thus requires their evaluation and comparison (6).

## ResNet-50

We use the CNN ResNet-50 (7). ResNet architectures were developed by the Microsoft Research team (7) and are available in several versions with different number of layers, such as 50, 101, 152 (https://github.com/KaimingHe/deep-residual-networks). Notably, the ResNet-152 won the 1st places in all the sections of the ILSVRC and COCO (http://cocodataset.org/#detection-2015) competitions in 2015. Pre-trained ResNet architectures have been frequently used for the classification of skin lesions, even by several participants to ISIC challenges (8–12).

A schematic representation of the architecture and functions of ResNet-50 is shown in **Figure 2**. **Figure 2A** shows examples of feature maps obtained at specific layers. Moreover, the code of the hands-on activity displays the feature map for any selected layer of the CNN (cell "8.5 Visualize features generated at a specific layer"). **Figure 2B** contains a scheme of the layers and the connections of the network. **Figure 2C** shows the effect of the application of specific operations (convolution, batch normalization, activation and maxpooling) on an image.

As shown in **Figure 2A** and in cell "2. Understanding images and convolution," an image is a collection of two-dimensional matrices (channels) which elements (pixels) have numeric values representing the brightness in each channel. Color images are composed of multiple channels (e.g., 3 for the RGB representation) whereas grayscale images only have one. The application of the network over an input image, produces its progressive transformation into a larger number of features with smaller lateral dimensions. Eventually, the features are combined to obtain a set of scalar values with the same dimension of the

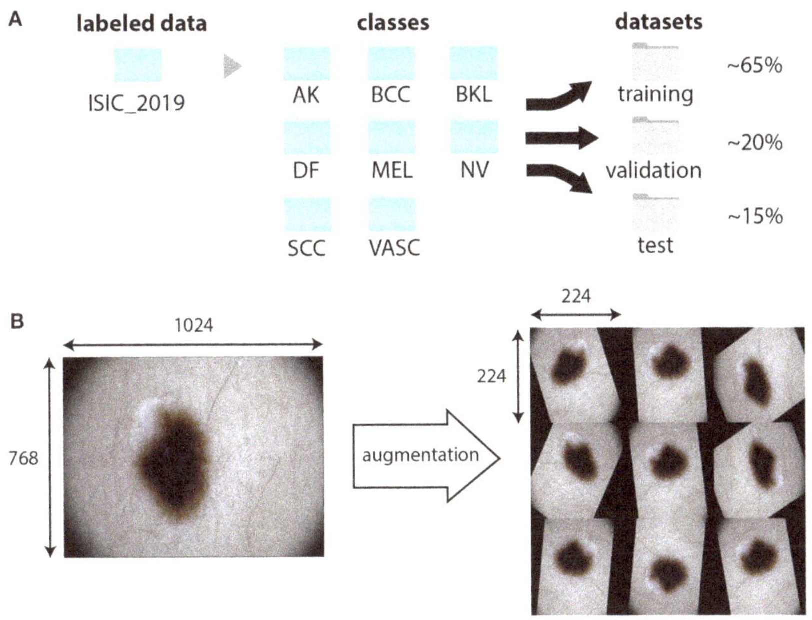


**FIGURE 1 |** Data pre-processing and augmentation. **(A)** Example of the organization of the training dataset ISIC 2019. Images are first divided into folders associated to the different categories. A specific function split them randomly into training, validation and test datasets. **(B)** An original image from the training dataset ISIC 2019 (class NV) and possible outputs of the application of the augmentation procedure, consisting in combinations of random shift, rotation, and reflection. The data augmentation function resizes the images to fit the input size of the network (224 × 224 × 3).

output categories. This is achieved through the repetition of mathematical operations performed by the layers and depending on a large number of learnable parameters.

The input is first processed by a convolutional layer. Convolution is a mathematical operation involving the input image and a kernel, typically a matrix with smaller lateral dimensions with respect to the input. During CNN training, kernels are randomly generated and each kernel produces a different feature. Convolution is performed by sequentially shifting the kernel along the input image by a fixed number of pixels, called stride. At each step, the sum of the element-by-element multiplication between overlapping pixels returns the pixel value of the convolutional feature. In cell "2. Understanding images and convolution" the output provided by different kernels can be interactively explored. It must be pointed out that a stride larger than one can be used to obtain features with reduced lateral size with respect to the input.

The first convolutional layer of the ResNet-50 uses 64 kernels of 7 × 7 pixels$^2$ with a stride of 2 pixels and thus produces 64 features with half the lateral size of the input image (**Figure 2**). The features are regularized through a batch normalization layer (**Figure 2C**), that performs the standardization of the input, corresponding to the subtraction of the mean of the batch and the division by the standard deviation. The convolutional and batch normalization layers are generally followed by an activation function that performs a non-linear transformation of the feature map, providing the input for the next convolutional layer. Non-linear functions (like sigmoid or hyperbolic tangent) are used as activation functions for their similarity to the behavior of real neurons, i.e., the transformation of a continuous input into a digital output. The most widely used function is the rectified linear unit (ReLU). The ReLU performs a simple calculation: it returns the same value provided by the input if the input is positive. However, if the input value is negative or null, it returns zero. Inputs that are converted to zero constitute non-activated neurons. In this way, not all neurons are firing simultaneously. The sparse activation and the simpler mathematical operation guarantee a higher computational efficiency for ReLU as compared with other non-linear functions.

The batch normalization and the activation layers preserve the lateral size of features obtained at the output of the convolution layer. However, it is often recommendable to create a lower resolution version (downsampling) of the output image to reduce the number of parameters and account for variations in the position of features in the input image. A common approach is to use a pooling layer, which substitutes adjacent subregions of specific size with the sum, average or maximum values of the corresponding pixels. The ResNet-50 uses a maxpooling layer (**Figure 2C**) to downsample images by taking the maximum of the input over 3 × 3 regions.

Combinations of these layers are applied along the network, progressively reducing the lateral size from 224 × 224 to 7 × 7 and increasing the depth of the feature map from 3 (the RGB layers of the input image) to 2048. At this point, a group of three layers flattens the feature map, i.e., transforms it into a score vector with the same length as the number of categories. The values of elements of this vector correspond to the probability that the input image belongs to each category (**Figure 2B**) and

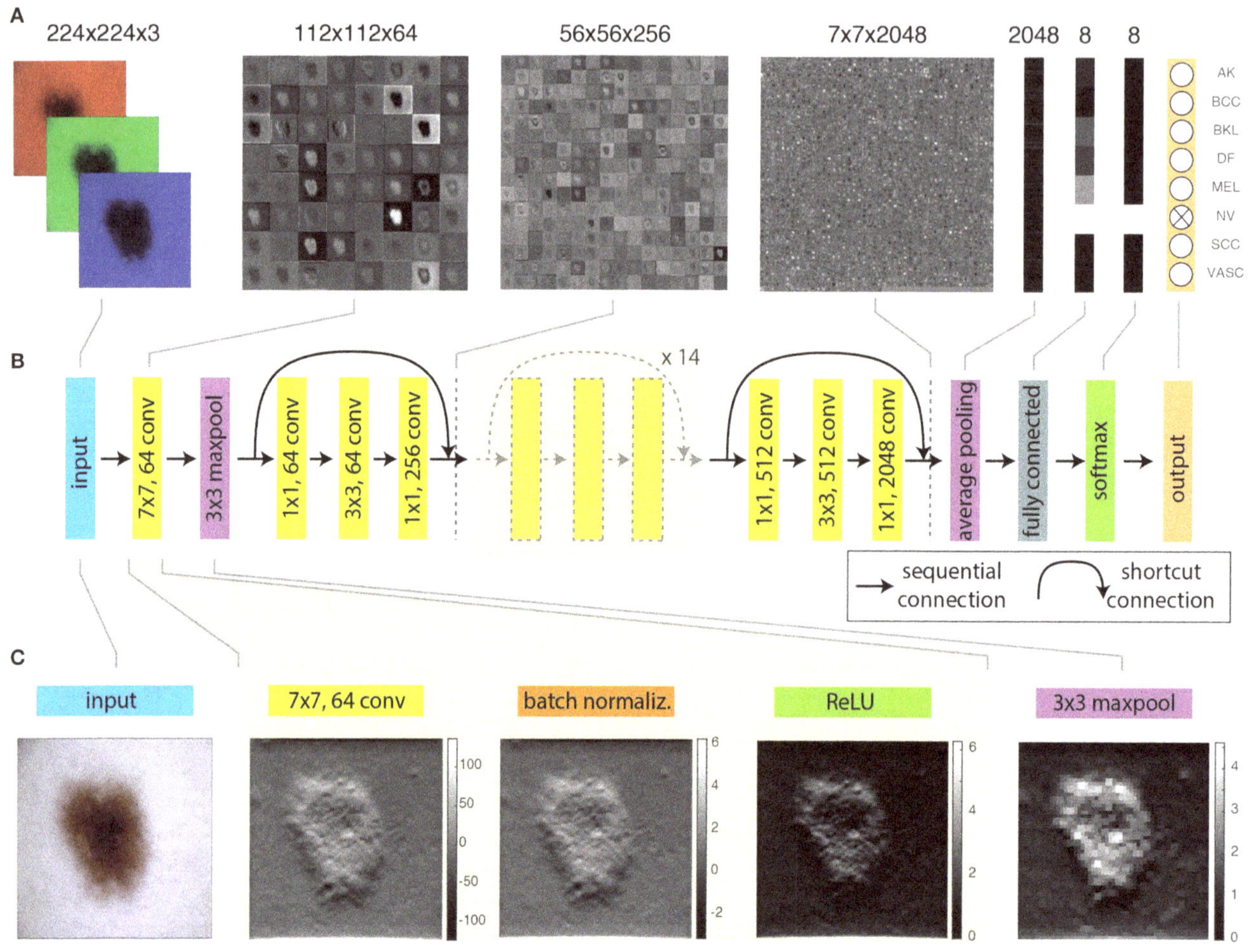


**FIGURE 2 |** Schematic and operations of a ResNet-50. **(A)** Feature maps obtained at different layers of a trained ResNet-50, from the input RGB image, to the 8-element probability vector predicting the image class. **(B)** Schematic illustration of representative layers of the network. **(C)** Effect of convolution, batch normalization, activation, and maxpooling on 1 of the 64 features produced by the first convolutional layer from the input image.

the maximum of this vector will correspond to the category assigned to the input image by the CNN. The first layer of the group performs a downsampling through average pooling, a pooling operation returning the mean of the region of the image considered. By using an average pooling over 7 × 7 regions, each of the 2048 features is thus reduced to a single value given by the average of all the pixels in the 7 × 7 map (**Figure 2A**).

The further reduction of the number of elements of the vector to a size equal to the number of categories is obtained through the fully connected layer. Each output value of this layer has a complete connection with all the 2048 inputs, as it is obtained as their weighted sum. The very last layer normalizes these values into the probabilities to belong to each labeled category. Usually, this task is performed through a softmax function that generalizes binary logistic regression to the case of a multiclass problem.

## Training

Once the dataset is ready and the CNN has been chosen, it is possible to start the actual training of the network. During this procedure, values of the learnable parameters are randomly changed, and the corresponding features are calculated to provide a tentative classification of the images in the training set. The performance of the network is evaluated by the calculation of a metric (loss function) that quantifies the similarity between the prediction and the ground-truth. Parameters are iteratively adjusted to optimize the loss function and thus increase correct predictions.

However, as mentioned earlier, we need to distinguish between two different situations. The first refers to the case in which the network needs to be fully trained. In this case, the values of all the parameters of the network need to be learned from scratch. This procedure requires very large datasets, often not available for medical applications. However, the use of a classical network further enables the possibility of performing transfer learning: besides using the same architecture as a classical network, one can also take advantage of parameters learned by the previous training of the CNN on a different, larger dataset. In transfer learning, the parameters obtained from the training of the model over a large dataset are only fine-tuned to adapt the network for the classification of a different target dataset. In this way, one can skip the time-consuming training steps but still take advantage of the features learned from the training over many photographs. As reported in (6), the top-performing methods submitted for ISIC challenges 2016, 2017, and 2018 used CNNs pre-trained on the ImageNet database. In cells 4–6, we perform these steps using the ResNet-50 pre-trained on the ImageNet dataset.

The ResNet-50 is designed for the ImageNet challenge and thus its output is composed of 1,000 categories. To use the ResNet-50 to classify skin lesion images among a different number of classes, it is first necessary to replace the last layers by ones providing an output over the desired number (2 or 8) of categories (**Figure 2B**). This procedure is performed in the section "4. The CNN: ResNet-50."

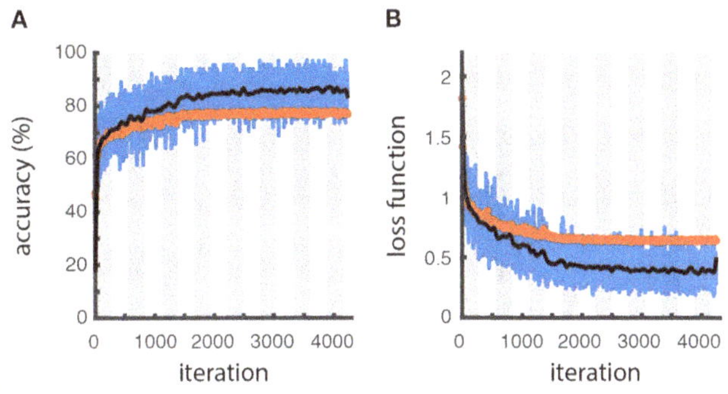


**FIGURE 3 |** Learning curves. Accuracy **(A)** and loss function **(B)** as a function of the number of iterations for the training batch (blue line for raw data, black line for filtered data) and validation sets (red symbols), as obtained through the optimization procedure. The white and gray areas delimit different epochs. The slightly higher accuracy and lower loss values obtained for the training dataset respect to the validation one reveals a slight overfitting.

## Hyperparameters

The CNN will learn weights and biases by minimizing the loss function over the training set using a method called stochastic gradient descent. However, due to the large size of the dataset and the limited memory, it is not possible to feed all the images simultaneously to the CNN. Therefore, training images are generally passed to the CNN in smaller groups called batches (cell 4.1). The optimum batch size must be set by trial and error in order to provide the fastest convergence. As a rule of thumb, small but not too small batch sizes (e.g., 32, 64, 128) are preferred, since they show higher accuracy than very large batches (13). The number of iterations necessary for the network to "see" the entire training dataset constitutes an epoch.

Another relevant hyperparameter is the global learning rate (cell 5.1), a number between 0 and 1 determining the step size used to update the weights at each iteration. The learning rate sets the speed at which the model is adjusted to the data. A low learning rate applies small changes to the weights at each update, thus requires more epochs of training. Although a high learning rate produces faster changes, if too high it might not converge to an optimal model. The correct learning rate should be empirically chosen to obtain convergence in a reasonable amount of time. Typically, the learning rate is not fixed but is progressively reduced during the optimization. Large rates are first used to quickly obtain values of the weights corresponding to a loss function close to its minimum. At that point, smaller rates further adjust the weights to better approximate the exact minimum of the loss function (cell 5.2). In addition, since in CNN the features provided by the early layers are more generic, whereas those belonging to the last layers are dataset specific, one can introduce non-uniform learning rates and either "freeze" the early layers or train the new layers at a faster rate with respect to the others (cell 5.1 and 5.3). Besides, several other hyperparameters need to be set in relation to the optimization procedure. In the activity, we adopt a procedure and use hyperparameters similar as those described in (11).

## Optimization

The algorithm is now ready to start the optimization process, a procedure involving the minimization of a loss function that measure the distance between the predicted and the ground-truth classification. For classification tasks, the cross-entropy function is the usual choice (cell 5.4). The optimization will run until some convergence condition is met. This condition is set by the user based either on the value of accuracy/error calculated on the validation set, or on a maximum number of validations without improving the loss value (cell 5.2).

The actual training is performed in section "6. Fine-tuning the model." The learning process can be visually monitored by displaying the trend of learning curves calculated from both the training and validation datasets as a function of algorithm iterations, to have an idea about how well the model is, respectively, learning and generalizing (defined in cell 5.5). Typically, plots of learning curves associated to optimization (e.g., cross-entropy loss) and performance (e.g., accuracy) are simultaneously created for both datasets (**Figures 3A,B**). The comparison of learning curves obtained for training and validation datasets is a valuable diagnostic method for the model behavior. A training loss showing a continuous decrease with a validation loss showing a minimum, in general correspond to an overfitting model. A good fit is usually associated with training and validation losses decreasing simultaneously toward closely spaced horizontal asymptotes (4). However, a higher accuracy (lower loss) of the training set with respect to the validation can still indicate some degree of overfitting, as obtained for the example shown in **Figures 3A,B**.

Since the training can sometimes run for quite a long time, in section "7. Load a trained network" we also provide a previously-trained model with weights. By loading this model, the user can perform the remaining part of the activity without having to wait for the completion of the training procedure.

## Performance Evaluation

Once the learning phase is complete, the network can be finally applied to predict the class of the images contained in the test dataset, that were not used for the training. Since the ground-truth of these images is known, they can be used to calculate

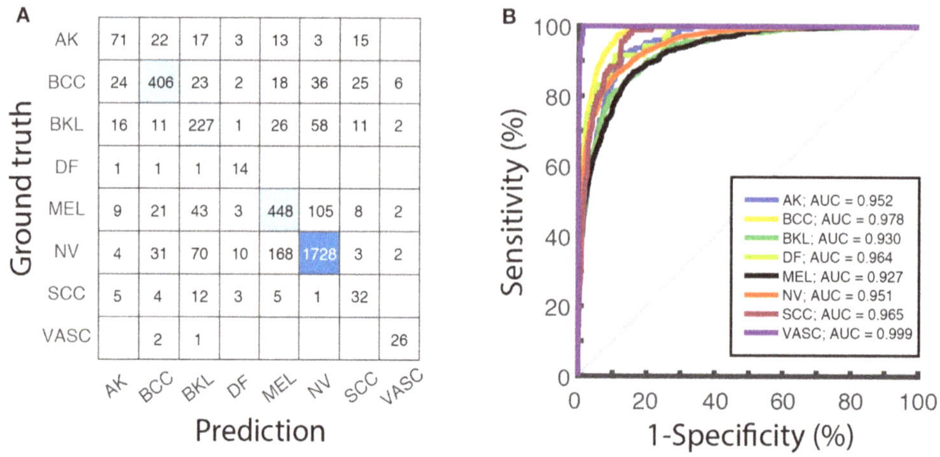


| | AK | BCC | BKL | DF | MEL | NV | SCC | VASC |
|---|---|---|---|---|---|---|---|---|
| AK | 71 | 22 | 17 | 3 | 13 | 3 | 15 | |
| BCC | 24 | 406 | 23 | 2 | 18 | 36 | 25 | 6 |
| BKL | 16 | 11 | 227 | 1 | 26 | 58 | 11 | 2 |
| DF | 1 | 1 | 1 | 14 | | | | |
| MEL | 9 | 21 | 43 | 3 | 448 | 105 | 8 | 2 |
| NV | 4 | 31 | 70 | 10 | 168 | 1728 | 3 | 2 |
| SCC | 5 | 4 | 12 | 3 | 5 | 1 | 32 | |
| VASC | | 2 | 1 | | | | | 26 |

**FIGURE 4 |** Model evaluation over the test dataset. **(A)** Confusion matrix displaying the number of images of the test dataset associated to each category by the ResNet-50 network. **(B)** ROC curves obtained on the same dataset and the corresponding values of the AUC for each class.

metrics to assess the performance of the classifier (section "8. Performance assessment"). Besides the overall accuracy, the confusion matrix, reporting the number of correct and incorrect predictions over all the classes, (**Figure 4A**) visually summarize classification and mis-classification performance of the model. The evaluation of the model performance further includes the plot of the receiver operating characteristic (ROC) curves and the calculation of the area under the curve (AUC) for each category (**Figure 4B**), obtained as detailed in (5).

## DISCUSSION AND CONCLUSIONS

We have developed a hands-on activity based on the interactive computer code and a detailed description of the steps needed to implement and fine-tune a CNN to perform the classification of dermatological images, together with an intuitive explanation, suitable for non-experts, of the functions performed by the main blocks of the network. The description is based on two practical examples, consisting of the fine-tuning of a pre-trained ResNet-50 network on a public dataset, containing images of skin lesions corresponding to different diagnoses. The use of *ad hoc* toolboxes and libraries largely simplifies the coding and makes it accessible to beginners.

In our opinion, the hands-on example, together with the description provided in this article, can act as a tool for students interested in obtaining a first understanding of the inner working of a CNN. However, the same activity can also be offered to provide a tutorial for beginners' initiation to computer programming for building and optimizing CNNs. In the first case, the code can be simply executed with the default parameters to visualize the output of each cell. The visualization of the results provides an intuitive understanding of CNN principles. As an example, plotting the feature maps obtained at consecutive layers allows comparing the changes introduced on the features by pooling, batch normalization and activation layers. In the second case, the user can further explore how modifications of the dataset and the change of hyperparameters affect the network's performance. Examples in this sense might involve the comparison of performance upon the change of learning rates (or even the freezing) of specific layers.

The use of an interactive hands-on activity reproducing a novel approach in its complexity might be a powerful strategy to approach the development of problem-solving and analytical skills, possibly through group work in the classroom. In addition, we believe that making this technology more accessible for non-expert will contribute to further strengthen the collaboration between dermatologists and computer scientists, toward the joint effort of improving image-based medical diagnosis.

## AUTHOR CONTRIBUTIONS

CM and MC-D contributed to conception and design of the study. SN, IM, and CM wrote the code and performed analyses. MC-D wrote the first draft of the manuscript. CM wrote the final version of the manuscript. CM and MO-V supervised the research. All authors contributed to manuscript revision, read, and approved the submitted version.

## FUNDING

CM gratefully acknowledges funding from FEDER/Ministerio de Ciencia, Innovación y Universidades – Agencia Estatal de Investigación through the Ramón y Cajal program 2015 (Grant No. RYC-2015-17896), and the Programa Estatal de I+D+i Orientada a los Retos de la Sociedad (Grant No. BFU2017-85693-R); from the Generalitat de Catalunya (AGAUR Grant No. 2017SGR940). CM also acknowledges the support of NVIDIA Corporation with the donation of the Titan Xp GPU. MO-V gratefully acknowledges funding from the PO FEDER of Catalonia 2014-2020 (project PECT Osona Transformació Social, Ref. 001-P-000382) and the Spanish Ministry of Science, Innovation, and Universities through the Instituto de Salud Carlos III-FEDER program (FIS PI19/01379). IM acknowledges the support of the Erasmus+ program of the European Union.

## REFERENCES


1. LeCun Y, Haffner P, Bottou L, Bengio Y. Object recognition with gradient-based learning. In: *Shape, Contour and Grouping in Computer Vision Lecture Notes in Computer Science, vol 1681*. Berlin; Heidelberg: Springer (1999). p. 319–45. doi: 10.1007/3-540-46805-6_19
2. Litjens G, Kooi T, Bejnordi BE, Setio AAA, Ciompi F, Ghafoorian M, et al. A survey on deep learning in medical image analysis. *Med Image Anal.* (2017) 42:60–88. doi: 10.1016/j.media.2017.07.005
3. Erickson BJ. Magician's corner: how to start learning about deep learning. *Radiol Artif Intell.* (2019) 1:e190072. doi: 10.1148/ryai.2019190072
4. Chollet F. *Deep Learning with Python*. Shelter Island: Manning Publications Company (2018).
5. Cullell-Dalmau M, Otero-Viñas M, Manzo C. Research techniques made simple: deep learning for the classification of dermatological images. *J Invest Dermatol.* (2020) 140:507–14.e1. doi: 10.1016/j.jid.2019.12.029
6. Perez F, Avila S, Valle E. Solo or ensemble? Choosing a CNN architecture for melanoma classification. In: *Proceedings of the IEEE Conference on Computer Vision and Pattern Recognition Workshops*. Long Beach, CA (2019).
7. He K, Zhang X, Ren S, Sun J. Deep residual learning for image recognition. *Proc IEEE Comput Soc Conf Comput Vis Pattern Recognit.* (2016) 2016-Decem:770–8. doi: 10.1109/CVPR.2016.90
8. Gutman D, Codella NCF, Celebi E, Helba B, Marchetti M, Mishra N, et al. Skin lesion analysis toward melanoma detection. *In: A Challenge at the International Symposium on Biomedical Imaging (ISBI) 2016, hosted by the International Skin Imaging Collaboration (ISIC)* (2016). Available online at: https://arxiv.org/abs/1605.01397
9. Marchetti MA, Codella NCF, Dusza SW, Gutman DA, Helba B, Kalloo A, et al. Results of the 2016 international skin imaging collaboration international symposium on biomedical imaging challenge: comparison of the accuracy of computer algorithms to dermatologists for the diagnosis of melanoma from dermoscopic images. *J Am Acad Dermatol.* (2018) 78:270–7.e1. doi: 10.1016/j.jaad.2017.08.016
10. Codella NCF, Gutman D, Celebi ME, Helba B, Marchetti MA, Dusza SW, et al. Skin lesion analysis toward melanoma detection: a challenge at the 2017 International symposium on biomedical imaging (ISBI), hosted by the international skin imaging collaboration (ISIC). In: *2018 IEEE 15th International Symposium on Biomedical Imaging (ISBI 2018)*. New York, NY: IEEE (2018). p. 168–72.
11. Han SS, Kim MS, Lim W, Park GH, Park I, Chang SE. Classification of the clinical images for benign and malignant cutaneous tumors using a deep learning algorithm. *J Invest Dermatol.* (2018) 138:1529–38. doi: 10.1016/j.jid.2018.01.028
12. Codella N, Rotemberg V, Tschandl P, Celebi ME, Dusza S, Gutman D, et al. Skin lesion analysis toward melanoma detection 2018. In: *A Challenge Hosted by the International Skin Imaging Collaboration (ISIC)*. Washington, DC (2019).
13. Mishkin D, Sergievskiy N, Matas J. Systematic evaluation of convolution neural network advances on the Imagenet. *Comput Vis Image Underst.* (2017) 161:11–9. doi: 10.1016/j.cviu.2017.05.007

# 19

# Artificial Intelligence Applications in Dermatology: Where do we Stand?

*Arieh Gomolin [1], Elena Netchiporouk [1], Robert Gniadecki [2*] and Ivan V. Litvinov [1*]*

*[1] Division of Dermatology, McGill University Health Centre, Montreal, QC, Canada, [2] Division of Dermatology, University of Alberta, Edmonton, AB, Canada*

***Correspondence:**
*Robert Gniadecki*
*r.gniadecki@ualberta.ca*
*Ivan V. Litvinov*
*ivan.litvinov@mcgill.ca*

Artificial intelligence (AI) has become a progressively prevalent Research Topic in medicine and is increasingly being applied to dermatology. There is a need to understand this technology's progress to help guide and shape the future for medical care providers and recipients. We reviewed the literature to evaluate the types of publications on the subject, the specific dermatological topics addressed by AI, and the most challenging barriers to its implementation. A substantial number of original articles and commentaries have been published to date and only few detailed reviews exist. Most AI applications focus on differentiating between benign and malignant skin lesions, however; others exist pertaining to ulcers, inflammatory skin diseases, allergen exposure, dermatopathology, and gene expression profiling. Applications commonly analyze and classify images, however, other tools such as risk assessment calculators are becoming increasingly available. Although many applications are technologically feasible, important implementation barriers have been identified including systematic biases, difficulty of standardization, interpretability, and acceptance by physicians and patients alike. This review provides insight into future research needs and possibilities. There is a strong need for clinical investigation in dermatology providing evidence of success overcoming the identified barriers. With these research goals in mind, an appropriate role for AI in dermatology may be achieved in not so distant future.

**Keywords: artificial intelligence, barriers, contact allergens, dermatology, melanoma, nevi, psoriasis, machine learning**

## INTRODUCTION

Dermatology is a field with the growing interplay of digitalization, telehealth, and informatics (1). The increasing presence of artificial intelligence (AI) worldwide, has led to numerous attempts to leverage this technology for dermatological applications (2). In a recent international survey of 1,271 dermatologists, 85.1% of responders were aware of AI as an emerging topic in their field yet only 23.8% had good or excellent knowledge on the subject (3). Moreover, 77.3% agreed that AI will improve dermatologic care and 79.8% thought that AI should be a part of medical training. Informing stakeholders on the current stance of AI is thus necessary to promote what dermatologists themselves believe to be a growing, beneficial and potentially obligatory aspect of the field. To date, many publications exist on specific AI topics in dermatology but few provide a basic overview and address the wide landscape. In this article, we summarize the status of the literature on AI in dermatology using three sections. First, we highlight the types of articles published on this subject. We then focus on dermatologic diseases targeted by AI, and finally, we spotlight the identified barriers impeding AI implementation.

# TYPES OF ARTICLES PUBLISHED

## Original Research

The overwhelming majority of articles published to date are original research articles. These describe the design of AI applications that can perform dermatology-related tasks. For example, articles have studied tools that can segment a psoriasis lesion or differentiate between benign and malignant skin lesions (4, 5). Although these AI tools have not yet been implemented clinically, these papers describe their technological feasibility and identify the potential clinical relevance should they be further validated. Most of these studies are authored by engineering researchers with few dermatologists as co-authors. Although the number is increasing, relatively few papers involve significant dermatologist collaboration in conceiving, designing and interpreting the studies. To overcome known barriers to clinical implementation, partnership with dermatologists is key. Zakhem et al. highlight in their recent review of melanoma screening applications, that when dermatologists were involved in the study design, the AI applications leveraged significantly larger patient datasets that were more representative of true clinical scenarios (6). Another important form of collaboration is conducting prospective clinical trials and very few of these exist (7). One landmark study was conducted by Dreiseitl et al. (8). In their protocol, patients with undiagnosed pigmented lesions presented to a dermatology clinic and were assessed separately by both non-expert physicians using an AI device and by expert dermatologists. The study design therefore resembled a realistic clinical practice scenario. The results indicated inferiority of the automated system, and unfortunately, no similar studies have been published to date. Whether the lack of similar studies is a publication bias or a literature gap remains unclear.

## Reviews

A small number of systematic reviews exist at this time. Most of these cover the potential use of AI in differentiating between benign and malignant skin lesions. For example, studies have reviewed the specificities and sensitivities of AI tools for melanoma screening (9). To the best of our knowledge, only one systematic review has been published on dermatological applications of AI in general, not limited to neoplastic lesions (10).

## Commentaries

An extensive amount of commentaries exist on the topic of AI in dermatology. These papers either highlight the potential impact of AI or stress the challenges of its implementation (11, 12).

# DERMATOLOGICAL APPLICATIONS OF AI

## Keratinocyte Carcinomas and Melanoma

There is an abundant and growing body of research demonstrating the preliminary success of AI applications at distinguishing between benign nevi *vs.* melanoma (5, 13–34). The main principle behind these applications is that dermatoscopic or non-dermatoscopic images of lesions can be broken down into individual pixels for analysis. A representative example by Jafari et al. describes an application that examines images pixel by pixel and extracts 60 features from each to predict disease classification (24). These applications are typically validated by comparing their ability to correctly diagnose lesions to the ability of certified dermatologists (32). One review of photo recognition applications by Safran et al. included 48 melanoma-screening tools and demonstrated a mean sensitivity of 87.60% and a mean specificity of 83.54% (9). Interest toward this topic has grown to the extent that an international skin imaging competition was founded in 2016 and has been occurring annually since (32, 35). Although these applications have become more robust, prospective clinical trials are rare and known implementation barriers are continuously debated.

An increasing number of original studies have also begun classifying non-melanoma skin cancers (also known as keratinocyte carcinomas) vs. benign and pre-malignant lesions (36–44). For example, Spyridonos et al. developed an AI model that could differentiate between actinic keratosis and normal skin with a specificity of 89.8% and a sensitivity of 91.7% (37). Altogether, most of the research on the topic of skin cancer demonstrates technological feasibility combined with the growing evidence supporting clinical utility. What remains to be demonstrated is whether such tools can be implemented and relied upon in daily clinical practice.

AI has also been used beyond photo recognition. Rather than processing image pixels, applications can also process numerical values in various sequences and extract trends. For example, Tan et al. described an application that predicted the complexity of micrographic Mohs surgery based on variables assessed at the initial evaluation visit such as tumor size and patient age (43). They were able to create a preliminary model that could theoretically be used to triage patients and prioritize Mohs referrals. Although most of the research on AI and skin cancer is based on photo recognition algorithms, other opportunities exist.

## Ulcer Assessment

There is a growing body of research on diabetic and pressure ulcer applications (45–48). Thus, far most studies demonstrate methods for improving wound assessments using image recognition (45).

Articles have described applications capable of measuring precise wound boundaries, and differentiating between the types of tissue involved (45–47, 49). For example, Dhane et al. demonstrated an AI application's ability to segment the area of ill-defined ulcers with a sensitivity of 87.3% and specificity of 95.7% (47). Mukerjee et al. demonstrated an AI application's ability to classify granulation, slough and necrotic tissue with 87.61% accuracy (46). Risk prediction tools also exist. Alderden et al. described a tool that leverages data in the electronic health records of admitted patients, to predict their tendency to develop pressure ulcers (50). Altogether, these applications have preliminarily been shown to be technologically feasible, they have not yet been validated extensively in clinically trials.

## Psoriasis and Other Inflammatory Skin Diseases

Several original research articles exist on AI applications for inflammatory dermatoses. Most of these studies thus far have focused on improving psoriasis classification methods using image recognition (4, 51, 52). A representative example is a study conducted by Shrivasta et al., which compared the ability of several applications at classifying the severity of psoriasis lesions. The systems described achieved average sensitivities between 93.81 and 99.76% and average specificities between 97 and 99.99% (4).

Emam et al. described a psoriasis application beyond image recognition. They demonstrated a system's ability to predict psoriasis patient responses to biologic therapy using parameters gauged at an initial visit such as patient's weight and age of onset of psoriasis (53). They were able to create a preliminary model that could theoretically be used to optimize therapy for patients.

Beyond psoriasis, applications have been described classifying acne, lichen planus, pityriasis lichenoides and dermatomyositis (10, 54–58). Seite et al. developed a smartphone AI tool that grades and classifies types of acne lesions (e.g., comedonal, inflammatory, post inflammatory hyperpigmentation, etc.) (59). Huang et al. developed a multi disease classifier that could analyse 34 attributes (e.g., erythema, scaling, definite borders, etc.) and differentiate several papulosquamous diseases such as psoriasis, seborheic dermatitis, lichen planus, pityriasis, and chronic dermatitis (58).

Although most of these experiments relied on images of skin, one application assessed muscle ultrasound images and differentiated between normal muscle, dermatomyosisits, polymyositis, and inclusion body myositis with accuracies between 76.2 and 86.6% (60). Altogether, the theoretical utility of these applications for inflammatory diseases is significant, both further technological validation and clinical experimentation are needed.

## Predicting Skin Sensitization Substances

Research is also accumulating on using AI to minimize exposure to skin-sensitizing substances (61–65). A representative example by Zang et al. described an application capable of analyzing physiochemical properties of substances (e.g., melting point) and determining whether the substance could be a sensitizer or not (65). This application yielded an accuracy of 81% when the substances were studied in a human cohort. Wilm et al. reviewed current advances in skin sensitization testing and highlighted several other examples, where AI has provided a method to reduce animal testing (66). While this use of AI can have an impact on a population wide level, significant technological and clinical validation studies are necessary.

## Novel Applications in Pathology and Gene Expression Profiling

Applications have been described that can automate histology image processing and classification (67–71). For example, Arevalo et al. described a system that analyzes histopathological images and can classify basal cell carcinoma with 98.1% accuracy (67). Olsen et al. described a system that diagnosed dermal nevi and seborrheic keratosis with high accuracies and may serve as a future method to increase the efficiency of analyzing these prevalent benign tumors (72). Algorithms have also been described that can identify predictive genes and biomarkers for diseases (73–83). A representative example by Reimann et al., described an AI model capable of diagnosing psoriasis vulgaris based on the expression level of 4 genes with 96.4% accuracy (78). In another study assessing genetic differences in psoriasis genotypes, Patrick et al. used a combination of statistical learning and machine learning to identify new loci and predict the tendency of cutaneous psoriasis patients to develop psoriatic arthritis symptoms (84). While these investigations are in an early phase, the potential for their impact can be significant.

# IDENTIFIED BARRIERS

## Choice of Predictive Model

AI algorithms are continually being developed and each has advantages and challenges. Beam et al. discussed the relationship of AI compared to more classic statistical models (85). They detail how predictive technologies can be viewed on a machine-learning spectrum. Statistical models are lower on the spectrum because humans impose assumptions and guide many aspects of the algorithm. True machine learning is highest on the spectrum because the algorithms evolve without human involvement. A systematic review by Christodoulou et al. found no objective advantage of machine learning compared to longitudinal regression for binary clinical prediction (86). However, the review does summarize various theoretical reasons why machine learning may be superior to longitudinal regression in certain instances such as processing data with a strong signal to noise ratio (e.g., handwriting) or with a significant number of predictor subcategories (e.g., images) (86). There are therefore many unanswered questions regarding whether advanced forms of AI are actually needed or if more primitive technologies can accomplish the same tasks.

## Generalizability

One of the main limitations to AI is that the decisions made by these technologies are ultimately a reflection of the input data used to train the system (87). This theoretically implies that applications can only be used reliably in populations they were trained to assess. If applications are trained in one population and tested in another, the results are technically not generalizable and are subject to systematic biases such as overfitting. For example, Han et al. experimented with a skin cancer detection algorithm and concluded that overall performance could be improved if trained with a wide variety of data from multiple ethnic populations (36). However, simply using more data does not necessarily solve this problem. For example, Navarrete-Dechent et al. took Han et al.'s established an AI algorithm that was trained with a relatively diverse set of data and tested it in a unique database of Caucasian Americans from the southern United States. They found that the performance was suboptimal compared to how it was reported originally (88). The issue of generalizability is thus not simple to solve and may require either unique or extended data depending on the composition of the population being tested. This tendency for systematic bias has numerous implications for dermatology given the various demographic factors that affect making a diagnosis such as age, gender, race, and ethnicity to name a few.

### Standardization

Even if the application is trained using data from the correct population, images of new lesions need to be comparable. What angle should the image be taken at? What lighting should the room have? What should the background be? Are there pen markings? These are factors that can affect decision-making by AI. For example, a study by Winkler et al. showed that surgical markings significantly interfered with the ability of a system to correctly diagnose dermatoscopic images of melanoma and increased the false positive rate (89). Artificial intelligence relies on standardization and there are numerous non-standardized aspects to dermatology unlike in other specialties (e.g., radiology) (90). Although databases are intentionally large to account for variability, factors such as these create an infinite possibility for divergence.

### Data Requirements

One large barrier is the prerequisite for copious quantities of data of appropriate quality to power AI algorithms (91). A growing effort in the United States has been to solve this barrier using DataDerm, the American Academy of Dermatology's electronic health record system. Worldwide collaboration is likely required to achieve the ideal scenario where all of the necessary data categories are represented.

### Interpretability

Artificial intelligence algorithms are formed, re-evaluated and constantly changing without human input. This is why the technology has often been termed a "black box" technology (92). Although AI is therefore flexible and can theoretically accomplish more than humans and human-guided statistical algorithms, many aspects and certainly the logic behind the decision-making is often not interpretable. When a certified dermatologist conducts a personalized assessment and arrives at a conclusion, that conclusion can be rationalized and explained based on existing clinical evidence. At this time, decisions made by AI cannot be interpreted in this way. This is a strong limitation which influences whether society and regulatory bodies will accept it in the daily practice of medicine.

### Acceptance

A proper history followed by a physical examination in a well-lit examining room, while assessing for texture and eliciting specific signs for a given lesion (e.g., Darier, dimple, buttonhole signs, etc.) complemented by additional investigations/imaging or a biopsy is a standard way to establish a diagnosis in dermatology. Furthermore, it is accepted that while some diagnoses are clinical, others rest solely on histologic findings or a combination of clinical and histologic results correlation. This holistic approach cannot be fully replaced by computer programs and this is felt to be one of the most important barriers to implementing AI (93). Many patients also want to see and partner with a physician who is vested in helping them and may not be satisfied with isolated computerized tools (12).

### Liability

There is also the issue of liability (94). If AI is relied upon and an adverse outcome ensues, is the dermatologist responsible? With this in mind, a common belief is that AI will only become a guidance tool and not an absolute diagnostic tool.

### Next Steps

To address these barriers, several broad recommendations have been made to date. One clear need is for prospective clinical trials. If the question is whether AI can improve a dermatologic clinical encounter then studies that revolve around the clinical encounter are crucial (7). Dermatologist collaboration has also been highlighted as essential (6). Systems need to be trained with the full spectrum of human populations and clinical presentations that challenge dermatologists in clinical practice (88). Systems can also benefit from receiving inputs on other metrics available to physicians such as anatomic location, duration of the lesion and images of unaffected skin (88). Standardization practices also need to be implemented for photographing new lesions. Finally, given the lack of interpretability of many AI applications, we hypothesize that improving the lay descriptions of the algorithms and study designs can lead to improved acceptance by physicians and society at large. This would also aid regulatory decision makers who will need to adopt stances on liability.

## CONCLUSION

AI is being increasingly studied in dermatology. Although most applications involve analyzing and classifying images, there are other tools such as risk assessment calculators. The most progress thus far has taken place in the field of melanoma diagnosis, followed by ulcer and psoriasis assessment tools, then followed by numerous less frequently studied applications. However, critical barriers and literature gaps exist that significantly limit AI's applicability to clinical practice at this time. For the less common applications, technological papers and commentaries are needed to improve capabilities and provoke interest. For the more saturated topics, there is a larger need for clinical trials providing evidence of clinical efficacy, while successfully overcoming the identified barriers. With these research goals in mind, an appropriate role for AI in dermatology may be achieved.

## AUTHOR CONTRIBUTIONS

AG, EN, RG, and IL performed the literature review and wrote the paper. RG and IL supervised the project.

## REFERENCES

1. El-Azhary RA. The inevitability of change. *Clin Dermatol.* (2019) 37:4–11. doi: 10.1016/j.clindermatol.2018.09.003
2. Jiang F, Jiang Y, Zhi H, Dong Y, Li H, Ma S, et al. Artificial intelligence in healthcare: past, present and future. *Stroke Vasc Neurol.* (2017) 2:230–43. doi: 10.1136/svn-2017-000101

3. Polesie S, Gillstedt M, Kittler H, Lallas A, Tschandl P, Zalaudek I, et al. Attitudes towards artificial intelligence within dermatology: an international online survey. *Br J Dermatol.* (2020). doi: 10.1111/bjd.18875. [Epub ahead of print].
4. Shrivastava VK, Londhe ND, Sonawane RS, Suri JS. A novel and robust Bayesian approach for segmentation of psoriasis lesions and its risk stratification. *Comp Methods Programs Biomed.* (2017) 150:9–22. doi: 10.1016/j.cmpb.2017.07.011
5. Xie F, Fan H, Li Y, Jiang Z, Meng R, Bovik A. Melanoma classification on dermoscopy images using a neural network ensemble model. *IEEE Trans Med Imaging.* (2017) 36:849–58. doi: 10.1109/TMI.2016.2633551
6. Zakhem GA, Fakhoury JW, Motosko CC, Ho RS. Characterizing the role of dermatologists in developing AI for assessment of skin cancer: a systematic review. *J Am Acad Dermatol.* (2020). doi: 10.1016/j.jaad.2020.01.028. [Epub ahead of print].
7. Dick V, Sinz C, Mittlbock M, Kittler H, Tschandl P. Accuracy of computer-aided diagnosis of melanoma: a meta-analysis. *JAMA Dermatol.* (2019) 155:1291–9. doi: 10.1001/jamadermatol.2019.1375
8. Dreiseitl S, Binder M, Hable K, Kittler H. Computer versus human diagnosis of melanoma: evaluation of the feasibility of an automated diagnostic system in a prospective clinical trial. *Melan Res.* (2009) 19:180–4. doi: 10.1097/CMR.0b013e32832a1e41
9. Safran T, Viezel-Mathieu A, Corban J, Kanevsky A, Thibaudeau S, Kanevsky J. Machine learning and melanoma: the future of screening. *J Am Acad Dermatol.* (2018) 78:620–1. doi: 10.1016/j.jaad.2017.09.055
10. Thomsen K, Iversen L, Titlestad TL, Winther O. Systematic review of machine learning for diagnosis and prognosis in dermatology. *J Dermatol Treat.* (2019) 1–15. doi: 10.1080/09546634.2019.1682500
11. Krittanawong C. The rise of artificial intelligence and the uncertain future for physicians. *Eur J Internal Med.* (2018) 48:e13–e4. doi: 10.1016/j.ejim.2017.06.017
12. Lallas A, Argenziano G. Artificial intelligence and melanoma diagnosis: ignoring human nature may lead to false predictions. *Dermatol Pract Concept.* (2018) 8:249–51. doi: 10.5826/dpc.0804a01
13. Yu C, Yang S, Kim W, Jung J, Chung KY, Lee SW, et al. Acral melanoma detection using a convolutional neural network for dermoscopy images. *PLoS ONE.* (2018) 13:e0193321. doi: 10.1371/journal.pone.0193321
14. Pour MP, Seker H, Ling S. Automated lesion segmentation and dermoscopic feature segmentation for skin cancer analysis. *Conf Proc.* (2017) 2017:640–3. doi: 10.1109/EMBC.2017.8036906
15. Jafari MH, Samavi S, Karimi N, Soroushmehr SM, Ward K, Najarian K. Automatic detection of melanoma using broad extraction of features from digital images. *Conf Proc.* (2016) 2016:1357–60. doi: 10.1109/EMBC.2016.7590959
16. Sabouri P, GholamHosseini H, Larsson T, Collins J. A cascade classifier for diagnosis of melanoma in clinical images. *Conf Proc.* (2014) 2014:6748–51. doi: 10.1109/EMBC.2014.6945177
17. Abedini M, von Cavallar S, Chakravorty R, Davis M, Garnavi R. A cloud-based infrastructure for feedback-driven training and image recognition. *Stud Health Technol Inform.* (2015) 216:691–5. doi: 10.3233/978-1-61499-564-7-691
18. Sabbaghi S, Aldeen M, Garnavi R. A deep bag-of-features model for the classification of melanomas in dermoscopy images. *Conf Proc.* (2016) 2016:1369–72. doi: 10.1109/EMBC.2016.7590962
19. Esteva A, Kuprel B, Novoa RA, Ko J, Swetter SM, Blau HM, et al. Dermatologist-level classification of skin cancer with deep neural networks. *Nature.* (2017) 542:115–8. doi: 10.1038/nature21056
20. Bi L, Kim J, Ahn E, Kumar A, Fulham M, Feng D. Dermoscopic image segmentation via multistage fully convolutional networks. *IEEE Trans Bio-Med Eng.* (2017) 64:2065–74. doi: 10.1109/TBME.2017.2712771
21. Riaz F, Hassan A, Javed MY, Tavares Coimbra M. Detecting melanoma in dermoscopy images using scale adaptive local binary patterns. *Conf Proc.* (2014) 2014:6758–61. doi: 10.1109/EMBC.2014.6945179
22. Garcia Arroyo JL, Garcia Zapirain B. Detection of pigment network in dermoscopy images using supervised machine learning and structural analysis. *Comp Biol Med.* (2014) 44:144–57. doi: 10.1016/j.compbiomed.2013.11.002
23. Liu Z, Sun J, Smith L, Smith M, Warr R. Distribution quantification on dermoscopy images for computer-assisted diagnosis of cutaneous melanomas. *Med Biol Eng Comp.* (2012) 50:503–13. doi: 10.1007/s11517-012-0895-7
24. Jafari MH, Nasr-Esfahani E, Karimi N, Soroushmehr SMR, Samavi S, Najarian K. Extraction of skin lesions from non-dermoscopic images for surgical excision of melanoma. *Int J Comp Assist Radiol Surg.* (2017) 12:1021–30. doi: 10.1007/s11548-017-1567-8
25. Shimizu K, Iyatomi H, Celebi ME, Norton KA, Tanaka M. Four-class classification of skin lesions with task decomposition strategy. *IEEE Trans Bio-Med Eng.* (2015) 62:274–83. doi: 10.1109/TBME.2014.2348323
26. Lingala M, Stanley RJ, Rader RK, Hagerty J, Rabinovitz HS, Oliviero M, et al. Fuzzy logic color detection: blue areas in melanoma dermoscopy images. *Comput Med Imaging Graph.* (2014) 38:403–10. doi: 10.1016/j.compmedimag.2014.03.007
27. Nasr-Esfahani E, Samavi S, Karimi N, Soroushmehr SM, Jafari MH, Ward K, et al. Melanoma detection by analysis of clinical images using convolutional neural network. *Conf Proc.* (2016) 2016:1373–6. doi: 10.1109/EMBC.2016.7590963
28. Souza S, Abe JM. Nevus and melanoma paraconsistent classification. *Studies Health Technol Inform.* (2014) 207:244–50. doi: 10.1007/978-3-319-19722-7_9
29. Premaladha J, Ravichandran KS. Novel approaches for diagnosing melanoma skin lesions through supervised and deep learning algorithms. *J Med Syst.* (2016) 40:96. doi: 10.1007/s10916-016-0460-2
30. Tschandl P, Kittler H, Argenziano G. A pretrained neural network shows similar diagnostic accuracy to medical students in categorizing dermatoscopic images after comparable training conditions. *Br J Dermatol.* (2017) 177:867–9. doi: 10.1111/bjd.15695
31. Kaur R, Albano PP, Cole JG, Hagerty J, LeAnder RW, Moss RH, et al. Real-time supervised detection of pink areas in dermoscopic images of melanoma: importance of color shades, texture and location. *Skin Res Technol.* (2015) 21:466–73. doi: 10.1111/srt.12216
32. Marchetti MA, Codella NCF, Dusza SW, Gutman DA, Helba B, Kalloo A, et al. Results of the 2016 international skin imaging collaboration international symposium on biomedical imaging challenge: comparison of the accuracy of computer algorithms to dermatologists for the diagnosis of melanoma from dermoscopic images. *J Am Acad Dermatol.* (2018) 78:270–7.e1. doi: 10.1016/j.jaad.2017.08.016
33. Li Y, Shen L. Skin lesion analysis towards melanoma detection using deep learning network. *Sensors.* (2018) 18:E556. doi: 10.3390/s18020556
34. Afifi S, GholamHosseini H, Sinha R. SVM classifier on chip for melanoma detection. *Conf Proc.* (2017) 2017:270–4. doi: 10.1109/EMBC.2017.8036814
35. Marchetti MA, Liopyris K, Dusza SW, Codella NCF, Gutman DA, Helba B, et al. Computer algorithms show potential for improving dermatologists' accuracy to diagnose cutaneous melanoma: results of the international skin imaging collaboration 2017. *J Am Acad Dermatol.* (2020) 82:622–7. doi: 10.1016/j.jaad.2019.07.016
36. Han SS, Kim MS, Lim W, Park GH, Park I, Chang SE. Classification of the clinical images for benign and malignant cutaneous tumors using a deep learning algorithm. *J Invest Dermatol.* (2018) 138:1529–38. doi: 10.1016/j.jid.2018.01.028
37. Spyridonos P, Gaitanis G, Likas A, Bassukas ID. Automatic discrimination of actinic keratoses from clinical photographs. *Comput Biol Med.* (2017) 88:50–9. doi: 10.1016/j.compbiomed.2017.07.001
38. Kefel S, Pelin Kefel S, LeAnder RW, Kaur R, Kasmi R, Mishra NK, et al. Adaptable texture-based segmentation by variance and intensity for automatic detection of semitranslucent and pink blush areas in basal cell carcinoma. *Skin Res Technol.* (2016) 22:412–22. doi: 10.1111/srt.12281
39. Cheng B, Joe Stanley R, Stoecker WV, Stricklin SM, Hinton KA, Nguyen TK, et al. Analysis of clinical and dermoscopic features for basal cell carcinoma neural network classification. *Skin Res Technol.* (2013) 19:e217–22. doi: 10.1111/j.1600-0846.2012.00630.x
40. Cheng B, Joe Stanley R, Stoecker WV, Osterwise CT, Stricklin SM, Hinton KA, et al. Automatic dirt trail analysis in dermoscopy images. *Skin Res Technol.* (2013) 19:e20–6. doi: 10.1111/j.1600-0846.2011.00602.x
41. Odeh SM, Baareh AK. A comparison of classification methods as diagnostic system: a case study on skin lesions. *Comp Methods Programs Biomed.* (2016) 137:311–9. doi: 10.1016/j.cmpb.2016.09.012

42. Chang WY, Huang A, Yang CY, Lee CH, Chen YC, Wu TY, et al. Computer-aided diagnosis of skin lesions using conventional digital photography: a reliability and feasibility study. *PLoS ONE.* (2013) 8:e76212. doi: 10.1371/journal.pone.0076212
43. Tan E, Lin F, Sheck L, Salmon P, Ng S. A practical decision-tree model to predict complexity of reconstructive surgery after periocular basal cell carcinoma excision. *JEADV.* (2017) 31:717–23. doi: 10.1111/jdv.14012
44. Guvenc P, LeAnder RW, Kefel S, Stoecker WV, Rader RK, Hinton KA, et al. Sector expansion and elliptical modeling of blue-gray ovoids for basal cell carcinoma discrimination in dermoscopy images. *Skin Res Technol.* (2013) 19:e532–6. doi: 10.1111/srt.12006
45. Wang L, Pedersen PC, Agu E, Strong DM, Tulu B. Area determination of diabetic foot ulcer images using a cascaded two-stage SVM-based classification. *IEEE Trans Bio-Med Eng.* (2017) 64:2098–109. doi: 10.1109/TBME.2016.2632522
46. Mukherjee R, Manohar DD, Das DK, Achar A, Mitra A, Chakraborty C. Automated tissue classification framework for reproducible chronic wound assessment. *BioMed Res Int.* (2014) 2014:851582. doi: 10.1155/2014/851582
47. Manohar Dhane D, Maity M, Mungle T, Bar C, Achar A, Kolekar M, et al. Fuzzy spectral clustering for automated delineation of chronic wound region using digital images. *Comp Biol Med.* (2017) 89:551–60. doi: 10.1016/j.compbiomed.2017.04.004
48. de Franciscis S, Fregola S, Gallo A, Argiro G, Barbetta A, Buffone G, et al. PredyCLU: a prediction system for chronic leg ulcers based on fuzzy logic; part I - exploring the venous side. *Int Wound J.* (2016) 13:1349–53. doi: 10.1111/iwj.12529
49. Garcia-Zapirain B, Elmogy M, El-Baz A, Elmaghraby AS. Classification of pressure ulcer tissues with 3D convolutional neural network. *Med Biol Eng Comp.* (2018) 56:2245–58. doi: 10.1007/s11517-018-1835-y
50. Alderden J, Pepper GA, Wilson A, Whitney JD, Richardson S, Butcher R, et al. Predicting pressure injury in critical care patients: a machine-learning model. *Am J Crit Care.* (2018) 27:461–8. doi: 10.4037/ajcc2018525
51. Lu J, Kazmierczak E, Manton JH, Sinclair R. Automatic segmentation of scaling in 2-D psoriasis skin images. *IEEE Trans Med Imaging.* (2013) 32:719–30. doi: 10.1109/TMI.2012.2236349
52. Shrivastava VK, Londhe ND, Sonawane RS, Suri JS. Computer-aided diagnosis of psoriasis skin images with HOS, texture and color features: a first comparative study of its kind. *Comp Methods Programs Biomed.* (2016) 126:98–109. doi: 10.1016/j.cmpb.2015.11.013
53. Emam SDA, Thomsen SF, Greiner R, Gniadecki R. Predicting the long-term outcomes of biologics in psoriasis patients using machine learning. *Br J Dermatol.* (2019) doi: 10.1111/bjd.18741. [Epub ahead of print].
54. Min S, Kong HJ, Yoon C, Kim HC, Suh DH. Development and evaluation of an automatic acne lesion detection program using digital image processing. *Skin Res Technol.* (2013) 19:e423–32. doi: 10.1111/j.1600-0846.2012.00660.x
55. Daliri MR. Feature selection using binary particle swarm optimization and support vector machines for medical diagnosis. *Biomed Tech Biomed Eng.* (2012) 57:395–402. doi: 10.1515/bmt-2012-0009
56. Begic Fazlic L, Avdagic K, Omanovic S. GA-ANFIS expert system prototype for prediction of dermatological diseases. *Studies Health Technol Inform.* (2015) 210:622–6. doi: 10.3233/978-1-61499-512-8-622
57. Khan J, Malik AS, Kamel N, Dass SC, Affandi AM. Segmentation of acne lesion using fuzzy C-means technique with intelligent selection of the desired cluster. *Conf Proc.* (2015) 2015:3077–80. doi: 10.1109/EMBC.2015.7319042
58. Huang ML, Hung YH, Lee WM, Li RK, Jiang BR. SVM-RFE based feature selection and Taguchi parameters optimization for multiclass SVM classifier. *Scient World J.* (2014) 2014:795624. doi: 10.1155/2014/795624
59. Seite S, Khammari A, Benzaquen M, Moyal D, Dreno B. Development and accuracy of an artificial intelligence algorithm for acne grading from smartphone photographs. *Exp Dermatol.* (2019) 28:1252–7. doi: 10.1111/exd.14022
60. Burlina P, Billings S, Joshi N, Albayda J. Automated diagnosis of myositis from muscle ultrasound: exploring the use of machine learning and deep learning methods. *PLoS ONE.* (2017) 12:e0184059. doi: 10.1371/journal.pone.0184059
61. Forreryd A, Zeller KS, Lindberg T, Johansson H, Lindstedt M. From genome-wide arrays to tailor-made biomarker readout - Progress towards routine analysis of skin sensitizing chemicals with GARD. *Toxicol vitro.* (2016) 37:178–88. doi: 10.1016/j.tiv.2016.09.013
62. Johansson H, Rydnert F, Kuhnl J, Schepky A, Borrebaeck C, Lindstedt M. Genomic allergen rapid detection in-house validation–a proof of concept. *Toxicol Sci.* (2014) 139:362–70. doi: 10.1093/toxsci/kfu046
63. Strickland J, Zang Q, Paris M, Lehmann DM, Allen D, Choksi N, et al. Multivariate models for prediction of human skin sensitization hazard. *J Appl Toxicol.* (2017) 37:347–60. doi: 10.1002/jat.3366
64. Tsujita-Inoue K, Hirota M, Ashikaga T, Atobe T, Kouzuki H, Aiba S. Skin sensitization risk assessment model using artificial neural network analysis of data from multiple *in vitro* assays. *Toxicol in vitro.* (2014) 28:626–39. doi: 10.1016/j.tiv.2014.01.003
65. Zang Q, Paris M, Lehmann DM, Bell S, Kleinstreuer N, Allen D, et al. Prediction of skin sensitization potency using machine learning approaches. *J Appl Toxicol.* (2017) 37:792–805. doi: 10.1002/jat.3424
66. Wilm A, Kuhnl J, Kirchmair J. Computational approaches for skin sensitization prediction. *Crit Rev Toxicol.* (2018) 48:738–60. doi: 10.1080/10408444.2018.1528207
67. Arevalo J, Cruz-Roa A, Arias V, Romero E, Gonzalez FA. An unsupervised feature learning framework for basal cell carcinoma image analysis. *Artif Intell Med.* (2015) 64:131–45. doi: 10.1016/j.artmed.2015.04.004
68. Cruz-Roa AA, Arevalo Ovalle JE, Madabhushi A, Gonzalez Osorio FA. A deep learning architecture for image representation, visual interpretability and automated basal-cell carcinoma cancer detection. *Med Image Comp Comp Assist Interv.* (2013) 16(Pt 2):403–10. doi: 10.1007/978-3-642-40763-5_50
69. Masood A, Al-Jumaily A. Differential evolution based advised SVM for histopathalogical image analysis for skin cancer detection. *Conf Proc.* (2015) 2015:781–4. doi: 10.1109/EMBC.2015.7318478
70. Zhang G, Yin J, Li Z, Su X, Li G, Zhang H. Automated skin biopsy histopathological image annotation using multi-instance representation and learning. *BMC Med Genomics.* (2013) 6 (Suppl. 3):S10. doi: 10.1186/1755-8794-6-S3-S10
71. Zhang G, Yin J, Su X, Huang Y, Lao Y, Liang Z, et al. Augmenting multi-instance multilabel learning with sparse bayesian models for skin biopsy image analysis. *BioMed Res Int.* (2014) 2014:305629. doi: 10.1155/2014/305629
72. Olsen TG, Jackson BH, Feeser TA, Kent MN, Moad JC, Krishnamurthy S, et al. Diagnostic performance of deep learning algorithms applied to three common diagnoses in dermatopathology. *J Pathol Inform.* (2018) 9:32. doi: 10.4103/jpi.jpi_31_18
73. Ghosh D, Ding L, Sivaprasad U, Geh E, Biagini Myers J, Bernstein JA, et al. Multiple transcriptome data analysis reveals biologically relevant atopic dermatitis signature genes and pathways. *PLoS ONE.* (2015) 10:e0144316. doi: 10.1371/journal.pone.0144316
74. Mays AC, Chou J, Craddock AL, Miller L, Browne JD. Gene variability between perineural-positive and perineural-negative squamous cell skin cancers. *Antican Res.* (2016) 36:4007–11. doi: 10.4172/2472-128X.1000133
75. Son YA, Yucebas SC. A novel SVM-ID3 hybrid feature selection method to build a disease model for melanoma using integrated genotyping and phenotype data from dbGaP. *Studies Health Technol Inform.* (2014) 205:501–5. doi: 10.3233/978-1-61499-432-9-501
76. Wei D. A multigene support vector machine predictor for metastasis of cutaneous melanoma. *Mol Med Rep.* (2018) 17:2907–14. doi: 10.3892/mmr.2017.8219
77. Yang S, Xu J, Zeng X. A six-long non-coding RNA signature predicts prognosis in melanoma patients. *Int J Oncol.* (2018) 52:1178–88. doi: 10.3892/ijo.2018.4268
78. Reimann E, Lattekivi F, Keermann M, Abram K, Koks S, Kingo K, et al. Multicomponent biomarker approach improves the accuracy of diagnostic biomarkers for psoriasis vulgaris. *Acta Derm Venereol.* (2019) 99:1258–65. doi: 10.2340/00015555-3337
79. Lefrancois P, Tetzlaff MT, Moreau L, Watters AK, Netchiporouk E, Provost N, et al. TruSeq-based gene expression analysis of formalin-fixed paraffin-embedded (FFPE) cutaneous T-cell lymphoma samples: subgroup analysis results and elucidation of biases from FFPE sample processing on the TruSeq Platform. *Front Med.* (2017) 4:153. doi: 10.3389/fmed.2017.00153
80. Lefrançois P, Xie P, Wang L, Tetzlaff MT, Moreau L, Watters AK, et al. Gene expression profiling and immune cell-type deconvolution highlight robust disease progression and survival markers in multiple

cohorts of CTCL patients. *OncoImmunology.* (2018) 7:e1467856. doi: 10.1080/2162402X.2018.1467856
81. Litvinov IV, Cordeiro B, Huang Y, Zargham H, Pehr K, Dore MA, et al. Ectopic expression of cancer-testis antigens in cutaneous T-cell lymphoma patients. *Clin Cancer Res.* (2014) 20:3799–808. doi: 10.1158/1078-0432.CCR-14-0307
82. Litvinov IV, Netchiporouk E, Cordeiro B, Dore MA, Moreau L, Pehr K, et al. The use of transcriptional profiling to improve personalized diagnosis and management of cutaneous T-cell lymphoma (CTCL). *Clin Cancer Res.* (2015) 21:2820–9. doi: 10.1158/1078-0432.CCR-14-3322
83. Litvinov IV, Tetzlaff MT, Thibault P, Gangar P, Moreau L, Watters AK, et al. Gene expression analysis in Cutaneous T-Cell Lymphomas (CTCL) highlights disease heterogeneity and potential diagnostic and prognostic indicators. *Oncoimmunology.* (2017) 6:e1306618. doi: 10.1080/2162402X.2017.1306618
84. Patrick MT, Stuart PE, Raja K, Gudjonsson JE, Tejasvi T, Yang J, et al. Genetic signature to provide robust risk assessment of psoriatic arthritis development in psoriasis patients. *Nat Commun.* (2018) 9:4178. doi: 10.1038/s41467-018-06672-6
85. Beam AL, Kohane IS. Big data and machine learning in health care. *JAMA.* (2018) 319:1317–8. doi: 10.1001/jama.2017.18391
86. Christodoulou E, Ma J, Collins GS, Steyerberg EW, Verbakel JY, Van Calster B. A systematic review shows no performance benefit of machine learning over logistic regression for clinical prediction models. *J Clin Epidemiol.* (2019) 110:12–22. doi: 10.1016/j.jclinepi.2019.02.004
87. Du-Harpur X, Watt FM, Luscombe NM, Lynch MD. What is AI? Applications of artificial intelligence to dermatology. *Br J Dermatol.* (2020) doi: 10.1111/bjd.18880. [Epub ahead of print].
88. Navarrete-Dechent C, Dusza SW, Liopyris K, Marghoob AA, Halpern AC, Marchetti MA. Automated dermatological diagnosis: hype or reality? *J Invest Dermatol.* (2018) 138:2277–9. doi: 10.1016/j.jid.2018.04.040
89. Winkler JK, Fink C, Toberer F, Enk A, Deinlein T, Hofmann-Wellenhof R, et al. Association between surgical skin markings in dermoscopic images and diagnostic performance of a deep learning convolutional neural network for melanoma recognition. *JAMA Dermatol.* (2019) 155:1135–41. doi: 10.1001/jamadermatol.2019.1735
90. Narla A, Kuprel B, Sarin K, Novoa R, Ko J. Automated classification of skin lesions: from pixels to practice. *J Invest Dermatol.* (2018) 138:2108–10. doi: 10.1016/j.jid.2018.06.175
91. Park AJ, Ko JM, Swerlick RA. Crowdsourcing dermatology: dataderm, big data analytics, and machine learning technology. *J Am Acad Dermatol.* (2018) 78:643–4. doi: 10.1016/j.jaad.2017.08.053
92. Wang F, Kaushal R, Khullar D. Should health care demand interpretable artificial intelligence or accept "black box" medicine? *Ann Internal Med.* (2019). doi: 10.7326/M19-2548. [Epub ahead of print].
93. Lim BCW, Flaherty G. Artificial intelligence in dermatology: are we there yet? *Br J Dermatol.* (2019) 181:190–1. doi: 10.1111/bjd.17899
94. Mattessich S, Tassavor M, Swetter SM, Grant-Kels JM. How I learned to stop worrying and love machine learning. *Clin Dermatol.* (2018) 36:777–8. doi: 10.1016/j.clindermatol.2018.06.003

20

# A Deep Learning Based Framework for Diagnosing Multiple Skin Diseases in a Clinical Environment

*Chen-Yu Zhu* [1†], *Yu-Kun Wang* [1†], *Hai-Peng Chen* [2], *Kun-Lun Gao* [2], *Chang Shu* [1], *Jun-Cheng Wang* [1], *Li-Feng Yan* [2], *Yi-Guang Yang* [3], *Feng-Ying Xie* [3] *and Jie Liu* [1*]

[1] *Department of Dermatology, State Key Laboratory of Complex Severe and Rare Diseases, Peking Union Medical College Hospital, Chinese Academy of Medical Sciences and Peking Union Medical College, Beijing, China,* [2] *DeepWise AI Lab, Beijing, China,* [3] *Image Processing Center, School of Astronautics, Beihang University, Beijing, China*

***Correspondence:**
*Jie Liu*
*liujie04672@pumch.cn*

† *These authors have contributed equally to this work*

**Background:** Numerous studies have attempted to apply artificial intelligence (AI) in the dermatological field, mainly on the classification and segmentation of various dermatoses. However, researches under real clinical settings are scarce.

**Objectives:** This study was aimed to construct a novel framework based on deep learning trained by a dataset that represented the real clinical environment in a tertiary class hospital in China, for better adaptation of the AI application in clinical practice among Asian patients.

**Methods:** Our dataset was composed of 13,603 dermatologist-labeled dermoscopic images, containing 14 categories of diseases, namely lichen planus (LP), rosacea (Rosa), viral warts (VW), acne vulgaris (AV), keloid and hypertrophic scar (KAHS), eczema and dermatitis (EAD), dermatofibroma (DF), seborrheic dermatitis (SD), seborrheic keratosis (SK), melanocytic nevus (MN), hemangioma (Hem), psoriasis (Pso), port wine stain (PWS), and basal cell carcinoma (BCC). In this study, we applied Google's EfficientNet-b4 with pre-trained weights on ImageNet as the backbone of our CNN architecture. The final fully-connected classification layer was replaced with 14 output neurons. We added seven auxiliary classifiers to each of the intermediate layer groups. The modified model was retrained with our dataset and implemented using Pytorch. We constructed saliency maps to visualize our network's attention area of input images for its prediction. To explore the visual characteristics of different clinical classes, we also examined the internal image features learned by the proposed framework using t-SNE (t-distributed Stochastic Neighbor Embedding).

**Results:** Test results showed that the proposed framework achieved a high level of classification performance with an overall accuracy of 0.948, a sensitivity of 0.934 and a specificity of 0.950. We also compared the performance of our algorithm with three most widely used CNN models which showed our model outperformed existing models with the highest area under curve (AUC) of 0.985. We further compared this model with 280 board-certificated dermatologists, and results showed a comparable performance level in an 8-class diagnostic task.

**Conclusions:** The proposed framework retrained by the dataset that represented the real clinical environment in our department could accurately classify most common dermatoses that we encountered during outpatient practice including infectious and inflammatory dermatoses, benign and malignant cutaneous tumors.

**Keywords: artificial intelligence, deep learning, convolutional neural networks, dermatology, skin diseases, skin imaging, dermoscopy**

## INTRODUCTION

Dermatology is a branch of clinical medicine of which the diagnosis and treatment monitor greatly rely on the morphology of various cutaneous lesions. The traditional diagnostic process of dermatoses is thus based on the integration of patients' medical history, clinical manifestation, dermoscopic images and sometimes histopathological evaluation by the dermatologists. However, the training of becoming an experienced dermatologist is time-consuming. Furthermore, cutaneous diseases are vast in type and can be very similar in appearance under human eyes, leading to the difficulties in accurate and effective diagnosis. Recent advances on artificial intelligence (AI), particularly convolutional neural networks (CNN) based deep learning algorithms, have made it possible to learn the most predictive features of diseases directly from medical images given a large dataset of labeled examples (1, 2). Esteva et al. proposed a dermatologist level classification of skin cancer via fine-tuning a pre-trained Inception-v3 network (3). Menegola et al. also conducted experiments comparing training from scratch with fine-tuning of pre-trained networks on images with skin lesions (4). Their work showed that fine-tuning of pre-trained networks worked better than training from scratch. Numerous researches based on AI using dermoscopic and non-dermoscopic images have attempted to apply this technology in the dermatological field, including segmentation and classification of melanocytic tumors, keratinocyte tumors, ulcers, psoriasis and other inflammatory dermatoses (5–11). Some of the AI models showed astonishing diagnostic capacity that could reach or even surpass a dermatologist level (3, 7, 12, 13). Therefore, currently those computer-aided diagnostic model applications are tied with great hope and promise in screening and helping to diagnose cutaneous diseases.

Although these studies have achieved acceptable accuracy in specific diseases with different models trained by various databases, researches under real clinical settings are scarce. Additionally, previous studies applying AI models in real clinical settings showed relatively poorer performance outcomes comparing with that using their own experimental datasets (14, 15). In clinical practice, the most frequently encountered diseases are not limited to the kinds mentioned above, especially in Asian countries like China where the incidence of melanoma is relatively lower. Therefore, for better adaption of the AI application in dermatological field, we investigated the imaging database of the Department of Dermatology, Peking Union Medical College Hospital, and extracted the imaging data of the 14 most frequently encountered dermatoses to form a dataset that represented the real clinical environment of our clinics. The disease categories included melanocytic nevus (MN), seborrheic keratosis (SK), dermatofibroma (DF), keloid and hypertrophic scar (KAHS), basal cell carcinoma (BCC), hemangioma (Hem), port wine stain (PWS), eczema/dermatitis (EAD), psoriasis (Pso), seborrheic dermatitis (SD), rosacea (Rosa), acne vulgaris (AV), lichen planus (LP), and viral warts (VW). We used this dataset to construct a novel framework based on deep learning, aiming to verifying the classification performance of this proposed framework under a more practical and representative circumstance, and further compare its diagnostic accuracy with certificated dermatologists in China.

This novel CNN model we proposed here was on the basis of the EfficientNet-b4 CNN algorithm. We utilized multiple auxiliary prediction modules among different intermediate layers to accumulate discriminative information from different levels of features. The proposed CNN model was trained on 13,603 clinical images from 2,538 patient cases, and had been evaluated on expert-confirmed clinical images grouped into 14 different dermatologist-labeled diagnoses mentioned above. According to the experiment, it outperformed common convolutional networks and was competitive with dermatologists in real-world diagnosis.

## MATERIALS AND METHODS

### Ethical Approval

We conducted this research according to the ethical tenets of the *Declaration of Helsinki*. And this study was approved by the Medical Ethics Committee of Peking Union Medical College Hospital (NO. JS-2003). Informed written consents were obtained from all the included adult patients or the guardians of juvenile patients.

### Datasets

Our dataset was collected and formed from the imaging database of the Department of Dermatology, Peking Union Medical College Hospital in China from October 2016 to April 2020. All the included patients were Asian with Fitzpatrick skin type III or IV, and their dermoscopic images were consecutively acquired using a digital dermoscopy system (MoleMax HD 1.0 dermoscope, Digital Image Systems, Vienna, Austria) by the same technician to ensure the quality and standardization of the images. Generally, multiple dermoscopic images were captured of a single lesion in different angles or in subsequent follow-up presentations. The annotation process was performed by 2 dermatologists with more than 5-years experience according to the patients' medical history, clinical manifestations and dermoscopic features independently. All the patients with BCC and few ambiguous cases with benign conditions were confirmed by histopathological investigations. Whenever there was a disagreement between the annotators, consensus was reached through discussion or consultant with a third dermatological expert. Cases with unclear or incomplete medical history, whose images were poorly focused, and lesions located on the nail or mucosa areas were excluded. The final dataset for the development of the model and the demographic characteristics of the included patients were shown in **Table 1**.

## CNN and Deep Learning Algorithm

Instead of training a new model from scratch, we applied a fine-tuning strategy directly on pre-trained models via a multi-step retraining strategy with our dataset. In this strategy, we gradually unfroze the layer weights in steps with the first few layers being unfrozen last. In these steps, we reduced learning rates progressively from 1e-3 to 1e-5 and kept other parameters unchanged. As shown in **Figure 1**, we applied Google's EfficientNet-b4 (16) with pre-trained weights on the 2015 ImageNet dataset (17) with 1,000 object categories as the backbone of the proposed deep learning framework. The final fully-connected classification layer was replaced with 14 output neurons of our classifier. We also add seven auxiliary classifiers at the end of each intermediate layer (18) to make the model learn classification information from different level of features as shown in **Figure 2**.

Our deep learning network was implemented using Pytorch. Initially, a global learning rate 0.001 was used and it decayed to 0.0001 at epoch 25. We used a mini-batch gradient descent with a momentum 0.9 as the model parameters optimizer. In training, each image was resized to 380*380 pixels in RGB channels, the optimized input size of EfficientNet-b4. For each epoch, each image would be rotated from $-30^\circ$ to $30^\circ$ randomly, together with 50% probabilities for vertical and horizontal flipping. Color constancy method was also applied to eliminate the color deviation.

The raw output of our classifiers (seven auxiliary classifiers plus 1 final classifier) was summarized by 14 classification neurons. And then an argmax operation was used to find the most likely classification of the input image. The formula is as follows:

$$\text{classification} = \text{argmax}\left(\sum_{i=1}^{\text{Classifiers\_number}} \text{output}_i\right)$$

where $\text{output}_i$ is the classification vector with dimension (1, 14) and the sum of eight classification vectors is an element-wise summation.

## Saliency Maps

As illustrated in **Figure 3**, to facilitate triaging referrals and focusing one's clinical examination, we also created a heatmap via gradient-weighted class activation mapping (Grad-CAM) algorithm (20), which can produce visual explanations for CNN based deep learning models. Grad-CAM uses the gradient information flowing into the last convolutional layer to understand the importance of each neuron for a decision of interest thereby highlighting the important regions in the image for prediction. In our case, we used gradients of 14 classification neurons which flowed into the final convolutional layer to produce a coarse localization map highlighting the important regions in the image for predicting the label. It can be noticed that our network has the capability of focusing on the skin area affected by the disease and neglecting the background pixels and healthy skin around the lesions.

## Comparison Between the Proposed CNN Model and Previous Reported Methods

To both quantitatively and qualitatively demonstrate the effectiveness of the proposed deep learning framework, we compared the performance of our algorithm with previous reported methods, namely Inception-v3 (19), ResNet-101 (21), and the original EfficientNet-b4 (16) using our test set.

## Comparison Between our CNN Model and Dermatologists

We also compared the proposed framework with 280 board-certified dermatologists who previously participated in at least 72-h systemic dermoscopic training on diagnosing clinical cases, using an independent test set that consisted of 200 cases with a clinical image and a dermoscopic image. These cases were composed by eight categories of diseases, namely MN, SK, BCC, EAD, SD, Pso, VW and Rosa, with 25 cases each (also demonstrated in **Table 1**). For this reader study, every dermatologist was asked for the most likely diagnosis of each case from eight choices of included diseases. This questionnaire reflects the actual in-clinic task that dermatologists will decide whether or not to request further examinations or biopsies. For a fair comparison, the proposed deep learning framework also output the top-1 diagnosis with probabilities/confidence scores of the same 8 categories. However, clinical images were not provided to our CNN model. The outcome was considered "Correct" when the diagnosis made by the proposed deep learning framework or a dermatologist was the real diagnosis for the corresponding case.

## Statistical Analysis

In the reader study, Kappa coefficients were used to assess the consistency between dermatologists (or CNN) and the reference standard on the classification of each disease. Kappa coefficient $>0.75$ indicates good consistency, 0.40–0.75 indicates moderate consistency, and $<0.40$ indicates poor consistency. Adjusted Z-tests were used to assess differences in Kappa coefficients between dermatologists and CNN. We also calculated the Kappa coefficients of the dermatologists (as standard) and included CNNs. Results were considered statistically significant at the $P <$ 0.05 level. All analyses were carried out using Scikit-learn 0.22.2 and Numpy 1.16.4.

**TABLE 1** | Dataset overview.

| Characteristics | Development set | | Test set of the reader study | |
|---|---|---|---|---|
| | Images | Patients | Images | Patients |
| Numbers included in study (*n*) | 13,603 | 2,538 | 200 | 200 |
| Mean age (years), mean ± SD (range) | - | 57.38 ± 16.81 | - | 43.55 ± 19.68 |
| Female, *n* (%) | - | 1,532 (60.36) | - | 123 (61.50) |
| Lichen planus, *n* (%) | 804 (5.91) | 126 (4.96) | - | - |
| Rosacea, *n* (%) | 597 (4.39) | 80 (3.15) | 25 (12.5) | 25 (12.5) |
| Viral warts, *n* (%) | 1,110(8.16) | 298 (11.74) | 25 (12.5) | 25 (12.5) |
| Acne vulgaris, *n* (%) | 2,023(14.87) | 277 (10.91) | - | - |
| Keloid and hypertrophic scar, *n* (%) | 438 (3.22) | 96 (3.78) | - | - |
| Eczema/dermatitis, *n* (%) | 2,440 (17.94) | 419 (16.51) | 25 (12.5) | 25 (12.5) |
| Dermatofibroma, *n* (%) | 343 (2.52) | 116 (4.57) | - | - |
| Seborrheic dermatitis, *n* (%) | 767 (5.64) | 124 (4.89) | 25 (12.5) | 25 (12.5) |
| Seborrheic keratosis, *n* (%) | 553 (4.07) | 143 (5.63) | 25 (12.5) | 25 (12.5) |
| Melanocytic nevus, *n* (%) | 1,214 (8.92) | 345 (13.59) | 25 (12.5) | 25 (12.5) |
| Hemangioma, *n* (%) | 200 (14.70) | 61 (2.40) | - | - |
| Psoriasis, *n* (%) | 1,707 (12.55) | 234 (9.22) | 25 (12.5) | 25 (12.5) |
| Port wine stain, *n* (%) | 920 (6.76) | 112 (4.41) | - | - |
| Basal cell carcinoma, *n* (%) | 487 (3.58) | 107 (4.22) | 25 (12.5) | 25 (12.5) |

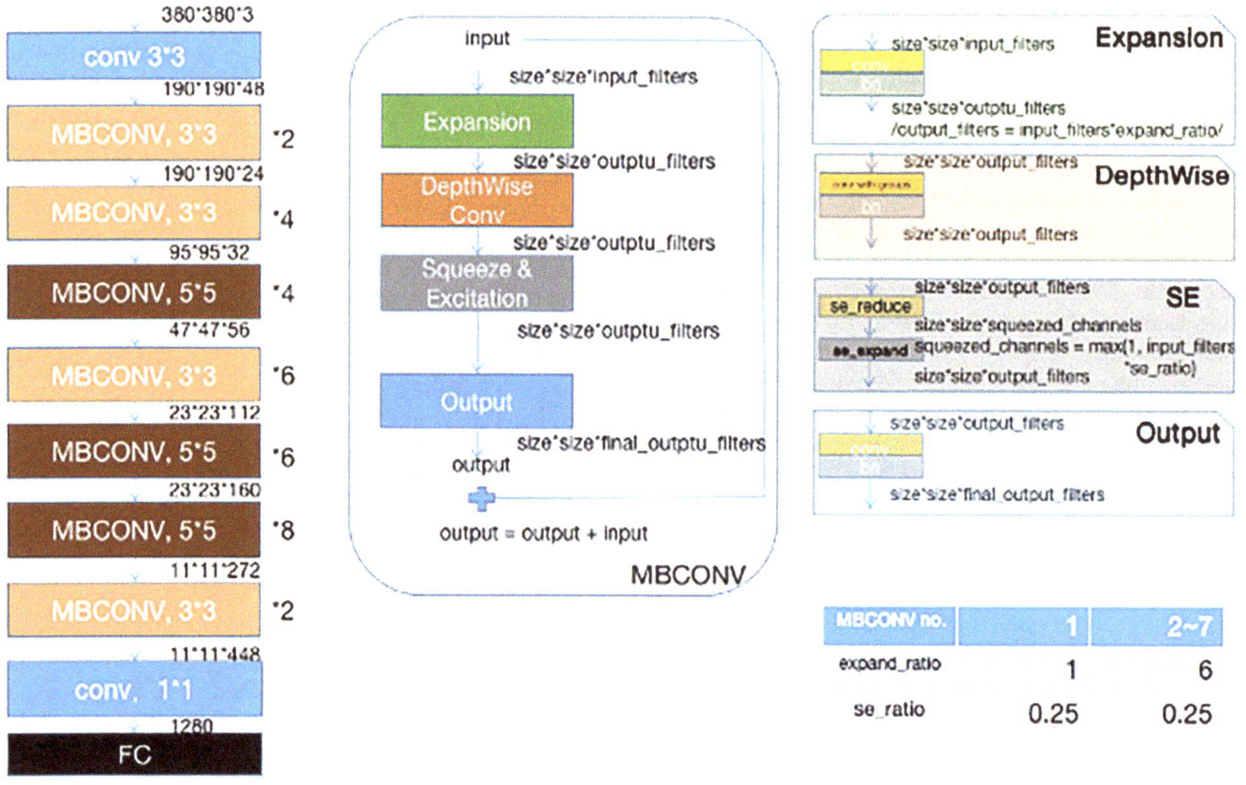


**FIGURE 1** | Original efficientnet-b4 architecture.

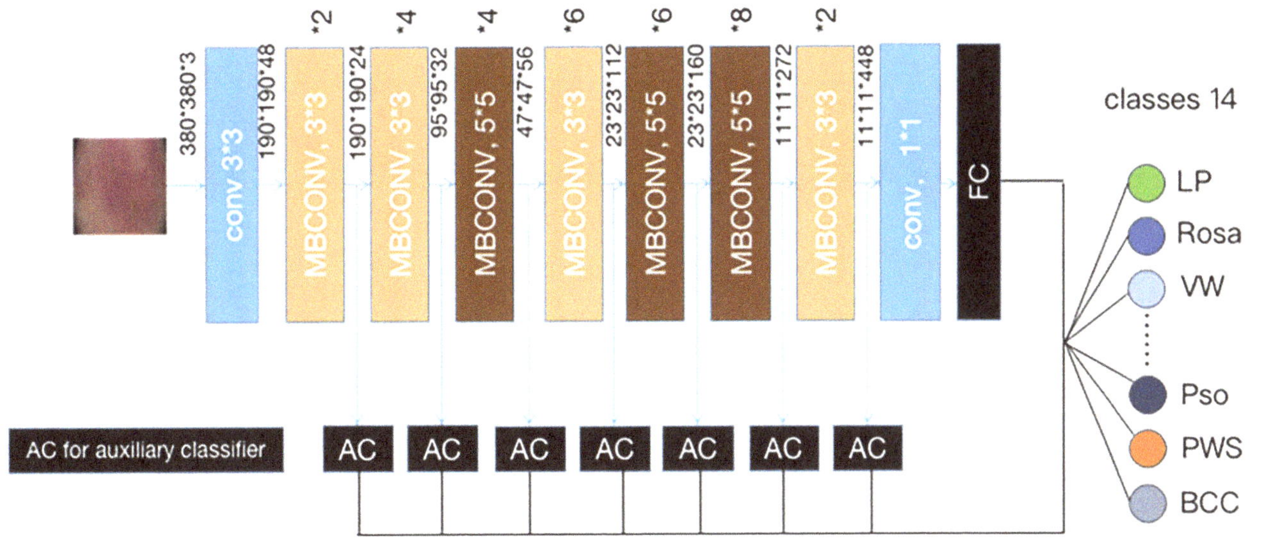


**FIGURE 2 |** Our modified (19) EFFICIENTNET-b4 architecture. Data flow is from left to right: a dermoscopic image is put into the network and finally transformed into a probability distribution over clinical classes of skin disease using our modified EfficientNet-b4 architecture pretrained on the ImageNet dataset and fine-tuned on our own dataset of 13,603 dermoscopic images in 14 categories.

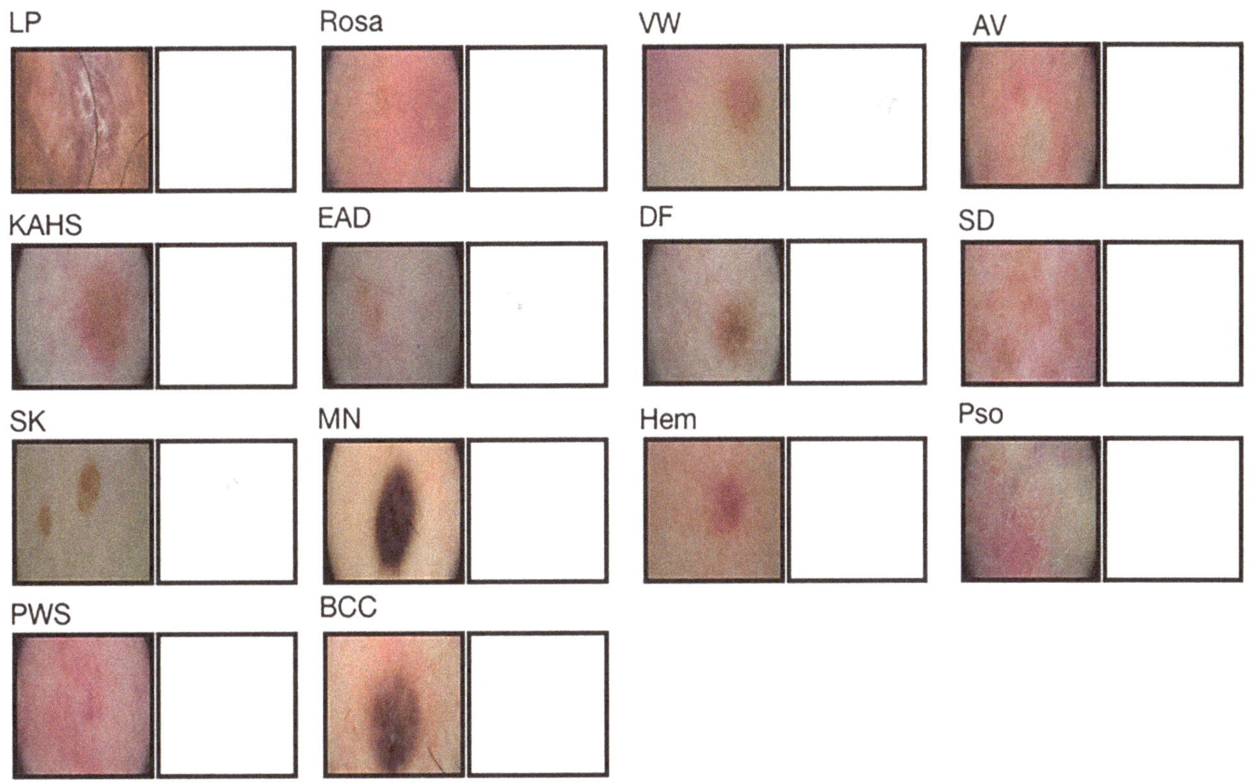


**FIGURE 3 |** Saliency maps for 14 example images from validation set. Saliency maps for example images from each of the 14 disease classes of the validation set reveal the pixels that most influence a CNN's prediction. Saliency maps show the pixel gradients with respect to the CNN's loss function.

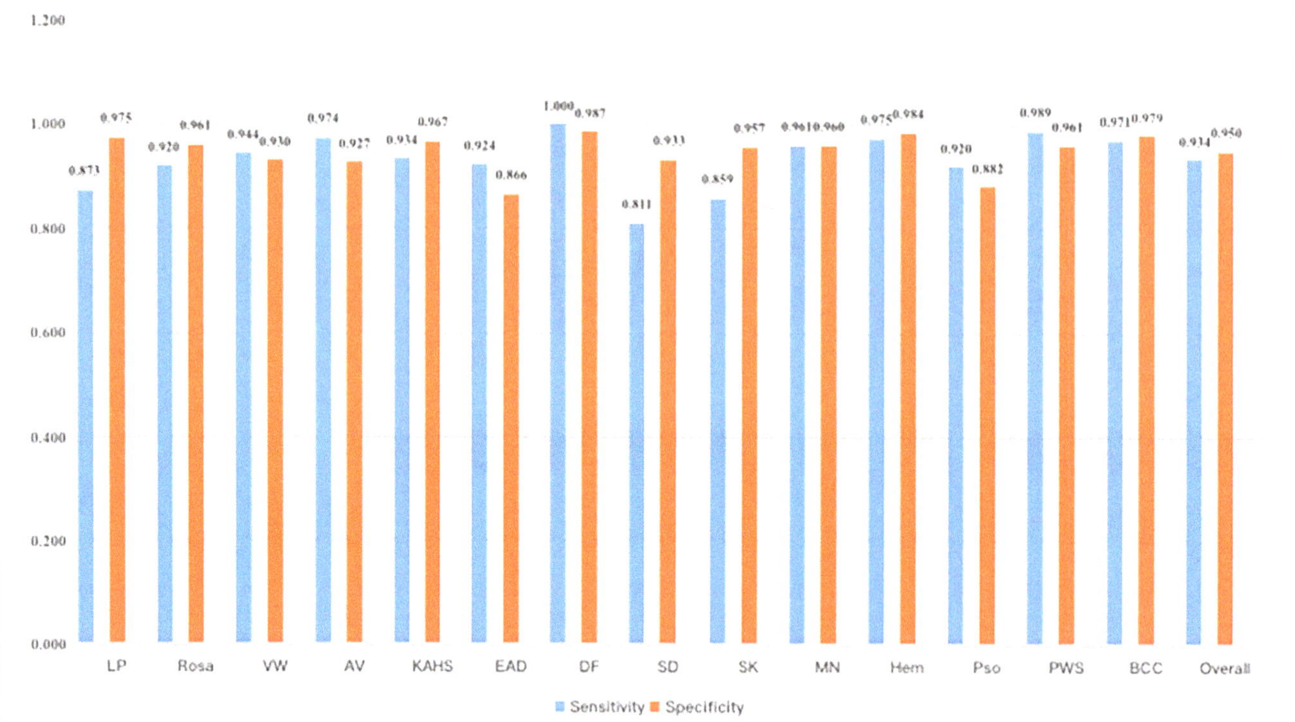


**FIGURE 4** | Sensitivity and specificity of our model. As a result, our model had an overall sensitivity of 93.38 ± 0.08% and specificity 94.85 ± 0.05%.

# RESULTS

## Performance Evaluation

To evaluate the performance of the proposed framework, we applied our method on a dataset of 13,603 dermatologist-labeled images with 14 categories of skin diseases. Sensitivity and specificity defined below are applied as the performance evaluation metrics:

$$\text{Sensitivity} = \frac{\text{true positive}}{\text{positive}}$$

$$\text{Specificity} = \frac{\text{true negative}}{\text{negative}}$$

**Figure 4** demonstrated that the proposed framework achieved a rather high overall accuracy of 0.948 ± 0.001 (mean ± SD), with a sensitivity of 0.934 ± 0.001 (mean ± SD), a specificity of 0.950 ± 0.001 (mean ± SD). The specific diagnostic values according to disease categories were summarized in **Table 2**. Receiver operating characteristic (ROC) curve in **Figure 5** also showed that the proposed model achieved 0.985 of area under curve (AUC) value in 14-way classification. **Figure 6** illustrated the corresponding confusion matrices for the 14 predefined diseases. The diagonal of the matrix showed the overlap of true positives and ground truth for each label, while the other cells of the matrix were misclassification of images with their true labels.

**TABLE 2** | The classification accuracy, sensitivity and specificity of the proposed CNN model according to disease category.

| Disease category | Accuracy | Sensitivity | Specificity |
|---|---|---|---|
| Overall | 0.948 | 0.934 | 0.950 |
| Lichen planus | 0.969 | 0.873 | 0.975 |
| Rosacea | 0.959 | 0.920 | 0.961 |
| Viral warts | 0.932 | 0.944 | 0.930 |
| Acne vulgaris | 0.935 | 0.974 | 0.927 |
| Keloid and hypertrophic scar | 0.969 | 0.934 | 0.970 |
| Eczema/dermatitis | 0.877 | 0.924 | 0.866 |
| Dermatofibroma | 0.987 | 1.000 | 0.987 |
| Seborrheic dermatitis | 0.926 | 0.811 | 0.933 |
| Seborrheic keratosis | 0.953 | 0.858 | 0.957 |
| Melanocytic nevus | 0.960 | 0.961 | 0.960 |
| Hemangioma | 0.984 | 0.975 | 0.984 |
| Psoriasis | 0.886 | 0.920 | 0.882 |
| Port wine stain | 0.963 | 0.989 | 0.961 |
| Basal cell carcinoma | 0.979 | 0.971 | 0.979 |

## Comparative Outcomes Between the Proposed CNN Model and Previous Reported Methods

**Figure 7** demonstrated the comparative results among our model, Inception-v3, ResNet-101 and the original EfficientNet-b4 with respect to the ROC curves and the AUC value. The AUC

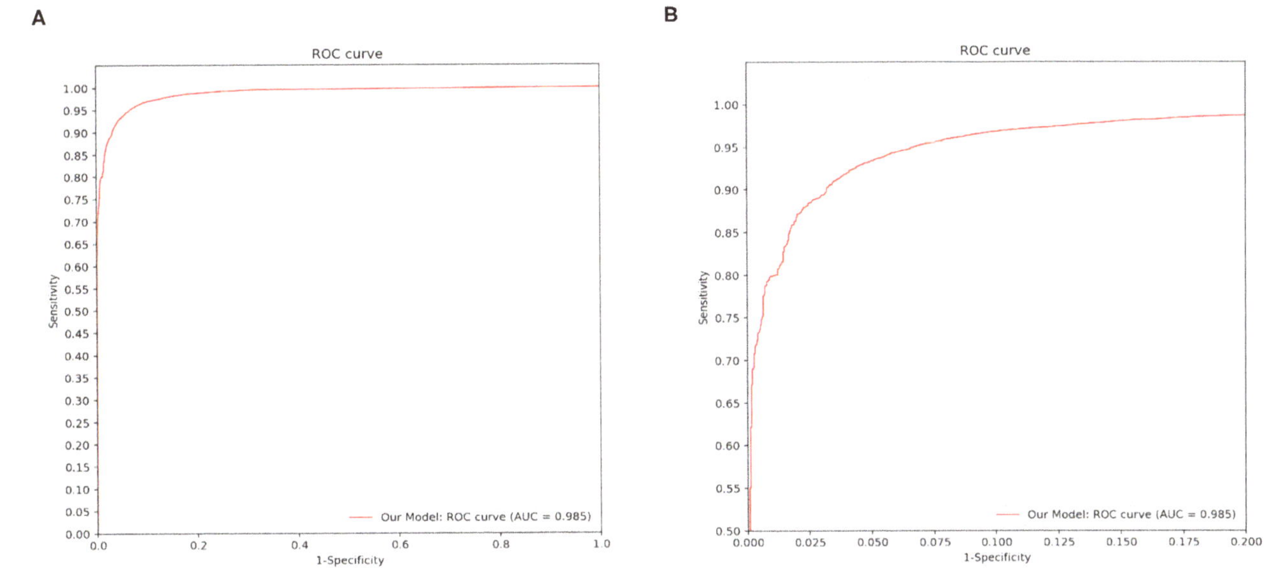


**FIGURE 5 |** Disease classification performance of the proposed model. We fix a threshold probability t such that the prediction y for any image is $y = P \geq t$, and the curve is drawn by sweeping t in the interval 0–1. The AUC is the CNN's measure of performance, with a maximum value of 1. Our model achieves 0.985 AUC in 14-way classification. **(A)** The full view of the ROC curve of the proposed model. **(B)** The local enlarged image of the ROC curve between abscissa 0~0.2.

value can reflect the overall accuracy of each model. As shown in **Figure 7**, our model has the best diagnosis performance over all other models. To be specific, our model outperformed existing models with the highest AUC of 0.985 whereas the Inception-v3 had an AUC of 0.953; the ResNet-101 had an AUC of 0.976; and the original EfficientNet-b4 had an AUC of 0.948, respectively, and the ROC curve of our CNN model was always situated higher than the ROC curves of other 3 models. **Table 3** revealed the detailed overall sensitivity, specificity and accuracy of our and other 3 CNN models.

## Comparative Outcomes Between our CNN Model and Dermatologists

The general information of patients included in an independent dataset is also shown **Table 1**. The performance of our CNN model and that of the dermatologists using the reader study test set is revealed in **Table 4**. The proposed CNN model achieved 92.75% average accuracy for all 200 cases, with a sensitivity of 83.50% and a specificity of 94.07%. While the average accuracy of board-certificated dermatologists is 92.13%, with an average sensitivity of 68.51% and an average specificity of 95.50%. Furthermore, according to the Kappa coefficients and adjusted Z test (summarized in **Table 5**), except for EAD and SD, the CNN model reached better consistency (moderate to good) with the reference standard than the average level of 280 dermatologists, and the difference is statistically significant. It needs to be mentioned that the CNNs is extremely fast, yielding its ranked diagnosis selections within 0.04 s. We also analyzed the diagnostic consistency of dermatologists (as standard) and 4 included CNN models on the 8-class task. Results showed that when taking dermatologists' performance as standard, statistical significance of differences between our model and dermatologists lay merely in psoriasis, and the Kappa coefficient of our model was higher than dermatologists (0.795 vs. 0.675). Furthermore, dermatologists' performance was significantly better than Origin EfficientNet in diagnosing Rosa (0.683 vs. 0.304) and worse in VW (0.533 vs. 0.759). Differences of other classifications between dermatologists and CNNs did not show statistical significance.

## Visualization of Internal Features

To explore the visual characteristics of different clinical classes, we examined the internal features learned by the proposed framework using t-SNE (t-distributed Stochastic Neighbor Embedding) (22). As demonstrated in **Figure 8**, each point represents a skin image projected from the 1792-dimensional output of the last hidden layer of the proposed network into 2-dimensions. We can notice clusters of points from same clinical classes. This visualization represents that our method is capable of separating various skin diseases objectively for referral.

# DISCUSSION

In China, the board-certificated dermatologists are sparse, with the dermatologist to patient ratio as low as 1:60,000. Furthermore, the majority of well-trained dermatologists are practicing in large cities which worsens the reality that the demand for dermatological consultant is increasingly difficult to satisfy in remote and rural areas of China (23). Moreover, the capacity of giving correct diagnosis and management plans of Chinese dermatologists vary tremendously due to the imbalanced training and learning opportunities of

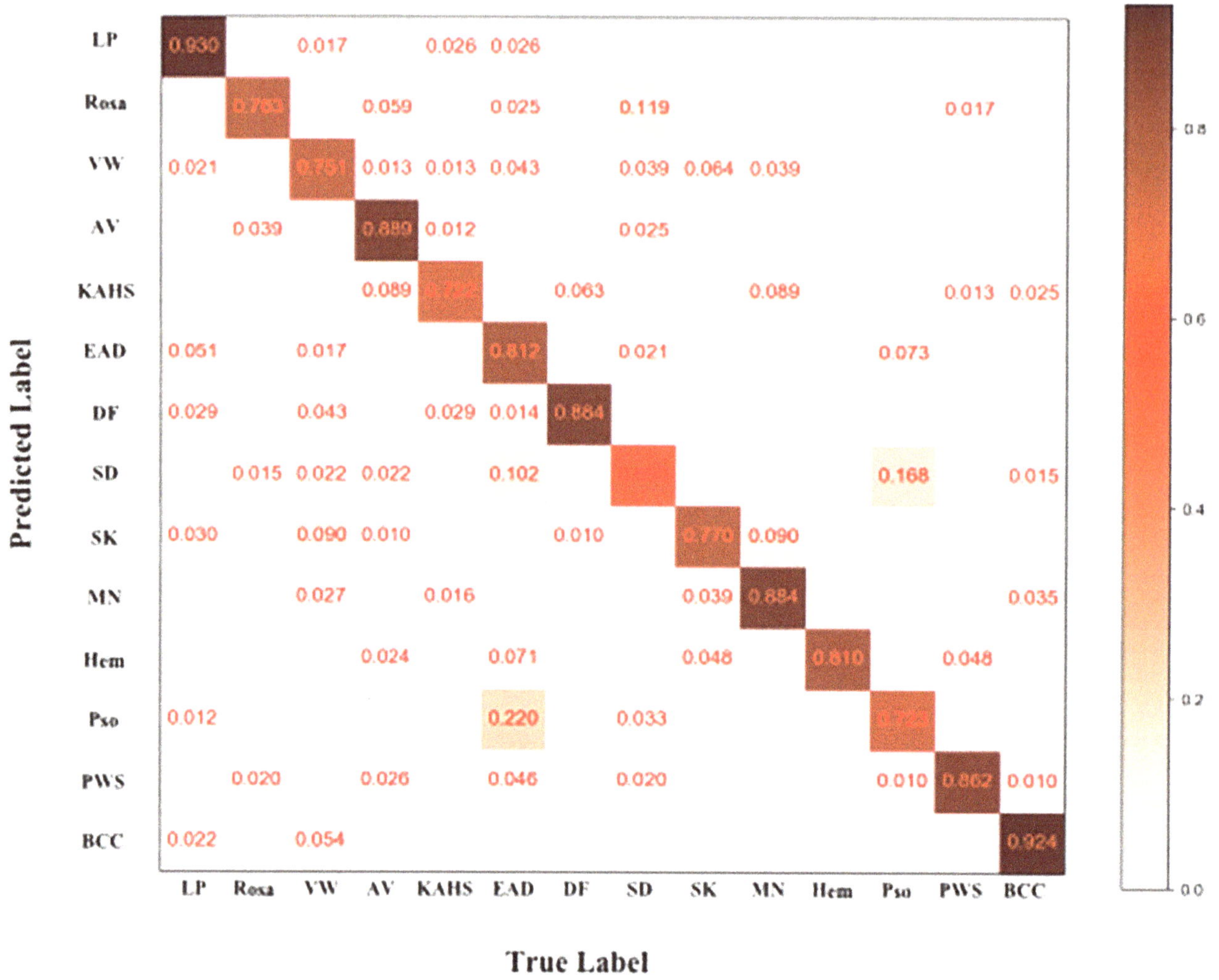


**FIGURE 6 |** Confusion matrix of the classification result. Element (i, j) of each confusion matrix represents the empirical probability of predicting class i given that the ground truth was class j, with i and j referencing classes from **Table 1**. Light red means low percentage and deep red represents high percentage.

medical education system in China. Although the growing application of multiple non-invasive skin imaging techniques such as dermoscopy, high-frequency ultrasonography and reflectance confocal microscopy has to some extent improved the diagnostic accuracy of Chinese dermatologists, the reality is still not optimistic according to a recent study shown that the imaging diagnostic ability for cutaneous tumors of Chinese dermatologists is relatively poor, and the results of dermatologists in different regions are uneven (24). The insufficiency of well-trained dermatologists and the high incidence of misdiagnosis are calling for a more efficient and accurate way of screening and triaging the Chinese patients suffered from cutaneous diseases.

Ever since Esteva et al. (3) reported that their CNN model, utilizing a GoogleNet Inception v3 CNN architecture trained by a large datasets (>120,000 dermoscopic images), could outperform board-certified dermatologists in classification of skin cancer, the number of researches on AI application in dermatology is constantly increasing and many of them could achieve a dermatologist-level accuracy, giving the hope of improving the primary screening process of patients because it is impossible for all the patients to be referred to the skin cancer professionals before a suspicious diagnosis of malignancy. However, the majority of these researches are based on different imaging datasets that mainly include Caucasian patients with cutaneous tumors, especially malignant melanoma because of its relatively high incidences and risks in Western countries. But in Asia, the prevalence of cutaneous diseases is very distinct from that of Western countries, for example, the average annual age-adjusted incidence rate of melanoma in Asian population was reported as <1/100,000 (25, 26). Therefore, the existing CNN models constructed using a large portion of Caucasian patients' images with a preference of those specific skin diseases can hardly meet the real-world clinical needs in Asian countries like China. In fact, recently, Minagawa et al. (27) confirmed that the diagnostic performance of CNN model in diagnosing skin

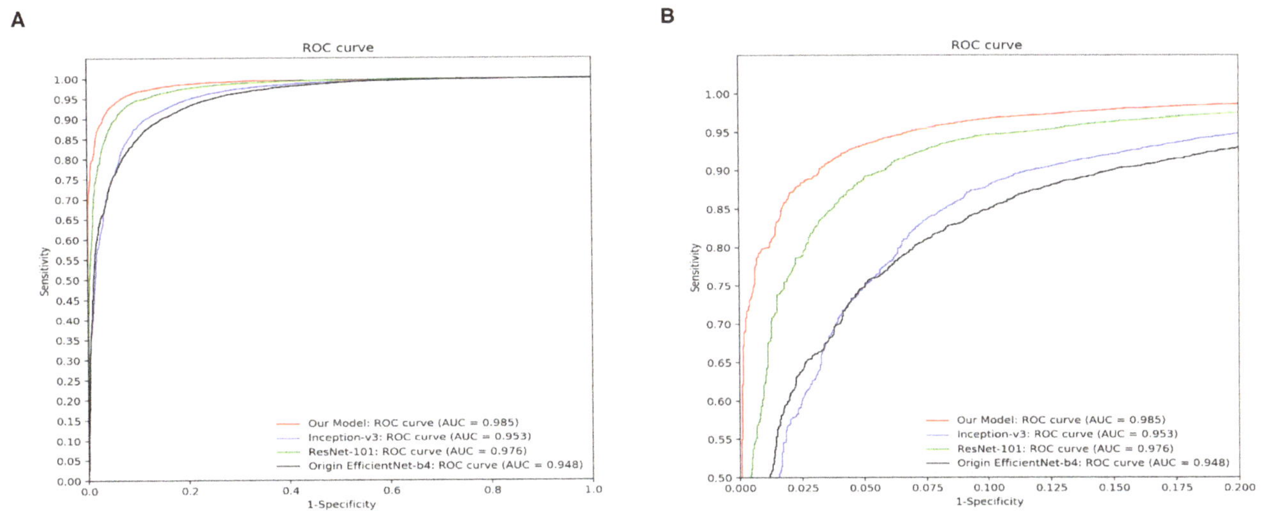


**FIGURE 7** | The ROC curves and the AUC value of our model, Inception-v3, ResNet-101 and the original EfficientNet-b4. Our model outperforms other reported methods for this skin disease diagnosis problem. **(A)** The full view of the ROC curve of the proposed model. **(B)** The local enlarged image of the ROC curve between abscissa 0~0.2.

tumors in Japanese patients would be improved if retrained by a dataset composed of cases with darker skin type.

We developed this CNN model based on pre-trained Google's EfficinetNet-b4 using a unique dataset that consisted of 14 most common skin diseases encountered and examined with dermoscopy in Chinese hospital dermatological clinics, including benign cutaneous neoplasms (MN, SK, DF, and KAHS), cutaneous malignancy (BCC), vascular neoplasm and malformation (Hem and PWS), inflammatory diseases with predilection sites of trunk and extremities (EAD, Pso, and LP) and with predilection sites of facial areas (SD, AV, and Rosa) and infectious diseases (VW). To the best of our knowledge, the construction of this dataset, including 14 categories of diseases, 2,538 cases and 13,603 dermoscopic images, is innovative, with many of the diseases firstly involved in a CNN model training, such as PWS, KAHS, and VW, aiming to propose a CNN model with better adaption of the real, complicated clinical environment in China. We initially chose dermoscopic images to construct the dataset because dermoscopic images usually reveal more valuable information of the lesion morphology than clinical images, and the process of taking a dermoscopic image is easier to standardize, and furthermore the background noises are much more prominent in clinical images which can affect the accuracy of the CNN model. Besides, since each skin diseases included in our research had unique and valuable dermoscopic features for differential diagnosis in clinical practice, we speculated our model would also benefit more from dermoscopic images than clinical images. However, we still tried to perform the 14-classification task using clinical images in the preliminary experiment as well. Results showed that the overall accuracies of clinical-image based CNN was 0.883, while the result our model based on dermoscopic images was 0.948. We thought the modest performance of clinical-image based CNN was relevant to the limited clinical dataset (for each patient, only 1 or 2

**TABLE 3** | The detailed overall sensitivity, specificity and accuracy of our and other 3 CNN models.

| Model / Performance | Our model | Original EfficientNet | ResNet-101 | Inception-v3 |
|---|---|---|---|---|
| Sensitivity | 0.934 | 0.882 | 0.919 | 0.890 |
| Specificity | 0.950 | 0.875 | 0.935 | 0.895 |
| Accuracy | 0.948 | 0.875 | 0.934 | 0.895 |

clinical images were recorded in our imaging database) and the relatively poor standardization of the clinical images (e.g., complex background interferes, different luminous intensity and camera angles). Therefore, we persisted in presenting our research based on the dermoscopy-based CNN. Yet, we would also attempt to construct CNN models based on the combination of clinical and dermoscopic image data since the former would certainly complement the information such as lesion distributions, skin textures and sites of involvement, potentially contributing to an even more satisfying diagnostic accuracy. The detailed performance results of the clinical-image based CNN in our preliminary experiment on the 14-classification task is also provided within the **Supplementary Material**.

In a recent article, Liu et al. (28) developed and validated a deep learning system for differential diagnosis of 26 types of skin diseases using clinical-only images from telemedicine, of which the top-1 diagnostic accuracy was non-inferior to dermatologists and higher than primary care physicians and nurse practitioners. Dermoscopy has been increasingly promoted and used in both dermatologists in the metropolises and general practitioners in the rural areas for its convenience and low costs, while the pace of the qualified telemedicine center construction is relatively

**TABLE 4** | Comparison between doctors and our CNN model in an 8-class task, the better outcomes of our CNN model are colored orange.

| Dermatologists | Rosa (%) | VW (%) | EAD (%) | SD(%) | SK (%) | MN(%) | Pso (%) | BCC(%) |
|---|---|---|---|---|---|---|---|---|
| Sensitivity | 79.70 | 62.04 | 74.96 | 46.53 | 59.43 | 77.23 | 67.66 | 80.54 |
| Specificity | 96.39 | 98.48 | 92.42 | 93.70 | 94.28 | 94.68 | 97.32 | 96.73 |
| Accuracy | 94.31 | 93.93 | 90.24 | 87.81 | 89.92 | 92.50 | 93.61 | 94.71 |
| **OUR MODEL** | | | | | | | | |
| Sensitivity | 92.00 | 92.00 | 84.00 | 48.00 | 76.00 | 96.00 | 92.00 | 88.00 |
| Specificity | 92.57 | 95.43 | 88.57 | 91.43 | 96.00 | 94.86 | 94.29 | 99.43 |
| Accuracy | 92.50 | 95.00 | 88.00 | 86.00 | 93.50 | 95.00 | 94.00 | 98.00 |

**TABLE 5** | Kappa coefficients (95% confidence interval) of the included four CNN models and dermatologists (as standard) on the eight-class task.

| Disease category | Dermatologists | Our model | Original EFFICIENTNET | ResNet101 | Inception-v3 |
|---|---|---|---|---|---|
| Rosacea | 0.683 (0.609~0.757) | 0.712 (0.640~0.783)<br>*P*-value: 0.080 | 0.304 (0.194~0.414)<br>*P*-value: 0.010 | 0.646 (0.567~0.726)<br>*P*-value: 0.358 | 0.691 (0.616~0.765)<br>*P*-value: 0.349 |
| Viral warts | 0.533 (0.445~0.621) | 0.793 (0.731~0.854)<br>*P*-value: 0.057 | 0.759 (0.693~0.825)<br>*P*-value: 0.017 | 0.684 (0.609~0.759)<br>*P*-value: 0.065 | 0.761 (0.695~0.827)<br>*P*-value: 0.095 |
| Eczema/dermatitis | 0.757 (0.694~0.820) | 0.570 (0.484~0.655)<br>*P*-value: 0.104 | 0.507 (0.416~0.598)<br>*P*-value: 0.310 | 0.558 (0.471~0.645)<br>*P*-value: 0.313 | 0.585 (0.500~0.670)<br>*P*-value: 0.347 |
| Seborrheic dermatitis | 0.607 (0.526~0.689) | 0.381 (0.280~0.483)<br>*P*-value: 0.379 | 0.337 (0.233~0.440)<br>*P*-value: 0.137 | 0.352 (0.247~0.457)<br>*P*-value: 0.198 | 0.380 (0.277~0.484)<br>*P*-value: 0.227 |
| Seborrheic keratosis | 0.410 (0.311~0.509) | 0.708 (0.635~0.780)<br>*P*-value: 0.249 | 0.576 (0.489~0.663)<br>*P*-value: 0.239 | 0.576 (0.489~0.663)<br>*P*-value: 0.237 | 0.682 (0.606~0.758)<br>*P*-value: 0.350 |
| Melanocytic nevus | 0.683 (0.609~0.758) | 0.799 (0.738~0.860)<br>*P*-value: 0.224 | 0.786 (0.723~0.849)<br>*P*-value: 0.263 | 0.759 (0.693~0.825)<br>*P*-value: 0.234 | 0.719 (0.648~0.790)<br>*P*-value: 0.237 |
| Psoriasis | 0.675 (0.600~0.749) | 0.759 (0.693~0.825)<br>*P*-value: 0.043 | 0.744 (0.676~0.813)<br>*P*-value: 0.357 | 0.621 (0.539~0.703)<br>*P*-value: 0.387 | 0.701 (0.627~0.774)<br>*P*-value:0.194 |
| Basal cell carcinoma | 0.738 (0.671~0.805) | 0.905 (0.863~0.948)<br>*P*-value: 0.220 | 0.875 (0.826~0.924)<br>*P*-value: 0.204 | 0.725 (0.654~0.796)<br>*P*-value: 0.235 | 0.853 (0.800~0.905)<br>*P*-value: 0.229 |

slower. Therefore, the accessibility of dermoscopy could be better than teledermatology consult in many countries. Furthermore, for inflammatory dermatoses included in our research, each of them has meaningful dermoscopic features for differential diagnosis in clinical practice, well-established and summarized in dermoscopy textbooks, reviews and expert consensuses (29, 30). For example, although clinically similar, Rosa typically appears as multiple polygonal vessels while SD appears as erythema, scattered linear vessels and yellowish scales. According to our experience, CNN might capture those subtle features and make classification more accurate based on dermoscopy images. Moreover, a recent research proposed by Brinker et al. (31) revealed that CNN trained by dermoscopic images could also accurately classify clinical melanoma images, showing that training CNN using images with higher resolution and more details might be able to differentiate images with lower resolution and less information.

Fujisawa et al. (12) previously proposed a CNN model trained by a small dataset of 4,867 clinical images but harvested a satisfactory diagnostic accuracy in classifying 14 skin tumors with an overall accuracy in differentiating benign and malignant conditions of 93.4%. Wang et al. (13) used pre-trained GoogLeNet Inception v3 CNN network trained by 7,192 dermoscopic images also achieved an overall classification accuracy of 81.49% in multiclass model and 77.02% in two-class model. Similarly, considering the classifications are up to 14 categories, the number of images in our dataset is relatively modest, but our CNN model achieved even better results, with an overall sensitivity of 93.38 ± 0.08% and specificity of 94.85 ± 0.05% in this 14-class task, emphasizing that utilizing specific training methods, the CNN model trained by relatively limited imaging data can reach a satisfying performance level as well.

As mentioned above, the proposed CNN model achieved rather high overall classification accuracy, sensitivity and specificity, and was considered capable of aiding the patient screening in real dermatological clinics of China, especially for the remote and rural areas where the medical resources were extremely limited. We also compared our CNN model with previous reported methods including Inception-v3, ResNet-101, and the original EfficientNet-b4. Results showed that our model outperformed all of them in ROC curve and AUC value evaluation using our test set images.

For further verifying the effectiveness of this proposed CNN model, we compared it with 280 board-certificated

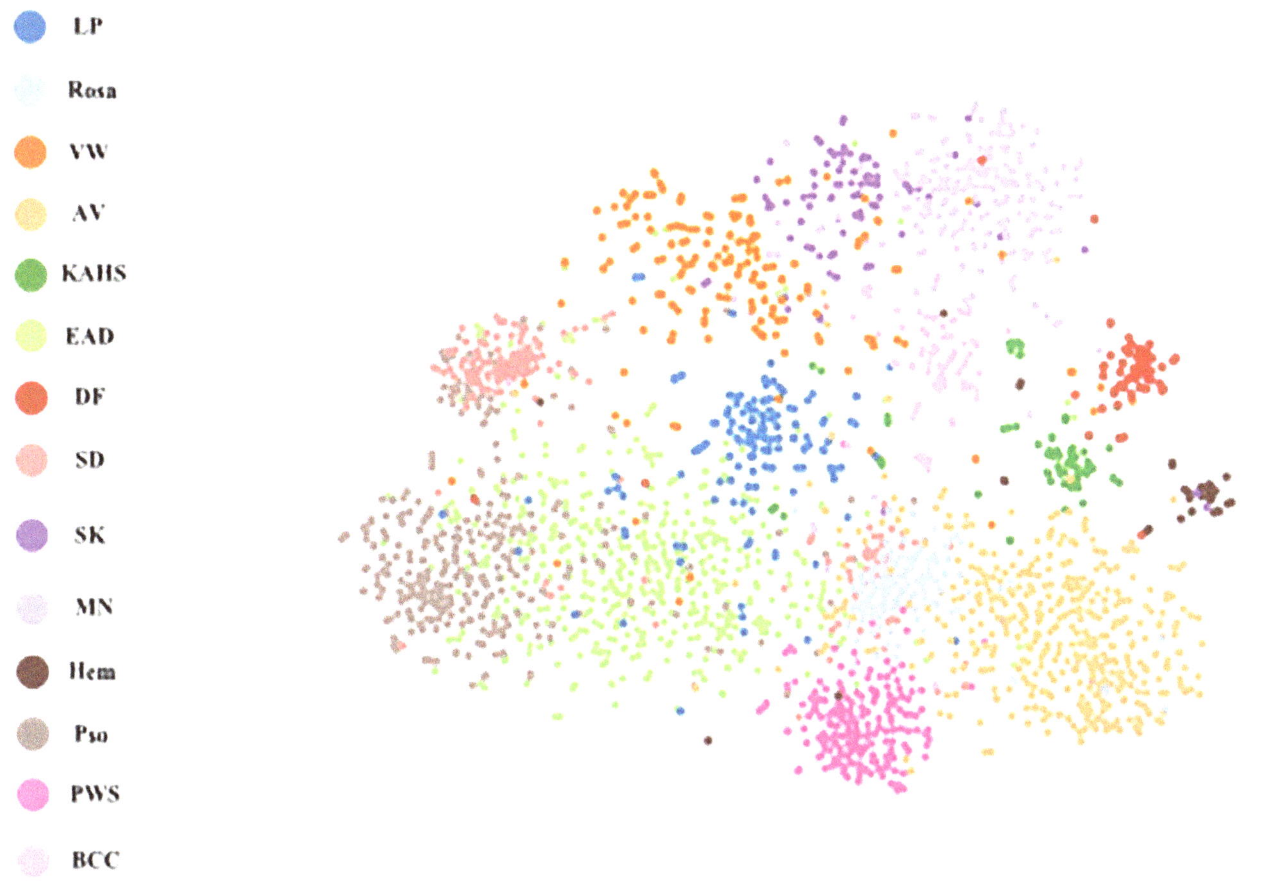


**FIGURE 8** | t-SNE visualization of the last hidden layer representations in the CNN for four disease classes. Here we show the CNN's internal representation of eight disease classes by applying t-SNE, a method for visualizing high-dimensional data, to the last hidden layer representation (1792-D vector) in the CNN. Colored point clouds represent the different disease categories, showing how the algorithm clusters the diseases.

dermatologists who undergone at least 72-h systemic dermoscopic training, using an independent test dataset different from that for the routine performance evaluation process. To the best of our knowledge, this was the largest group of dermatologists included to compare with AI performance (10, 12, 13, 32–34). Results demonstrate that our CNN model has higher sensitivity in all the tested eight categories of skin diseases compared with dermatologists, and higher accuracy in five of them (namely VW, SK, MN, Pso, and BCC), higher specificity in 3 of them (namely, SK, MN and BCC). And statistical analysis revealed that the proposed CNN model reached better consistency (moderate to good) with the reference standard than the average level of 280 dermatologists in 6 of the 8 categories (namely Rosa, VW, SK, MN, Pso, and BCC), and the difference is statistically significant. However, the dermatologists had better outcomes in EAD and SD. According to the confusion matrix of the classification result (**Figure 6**), the proposed CNN model misclassified EAD mostly into Pso and SD, and misclassified SD mostly into Rosa. In our training set, the numbers of Pso images (1707) and EAD images (2440) are much larger than SD images (767) and Rosa images (597), which could lead to an imbalance of data and brought a risk of this inconsistency. Furthermore, in real clinical practice, the diagnosis of EAD is quite straightforward, based on the clinical lesion morphology and symptoms like pruritus in China, including the cases of our dataset, so the morphological diagnosis might include various EAD subtypes (e.g., dyshidrotic, disseminated and nummular) and disease durations (acute, subacute, and chronic), which would at last largely affect the feature extraction of EAD for the CNN. Moreover, it is often quite difficult to differentiate these inflammatory dermatoses in real clinical practice and the conditions of coexistence are not rare. Of note, the dermatologists were even provided with extra clinical images because this process would be more like the real clinical environment. This is critical because for inflammatory dermatoses like EAD, Pso, SD, and Rosa, the lesion distribution and sites of involvement that only shown in clinical images are of vital importance for differential diagnosis, which could also contribute for the relatively worse performance of our CNN in classifying EAD and SD. The outcomes reveal that our CNN model is dependable in classifying theses common cutaneous conditions, and might have a fewer chance to miss the correct diagnosis compared with dermatologists.

However, our study has several limitations. First, our dataset completely came from the imaging database of the Department of Dermatology, Peking Union Medical College Hospital, using the same dermoscopy system. Therefore, it is possible that the accuracy of our CNN model might be lower when the dataset involves cases and images from other hospital or devices because the standardization would be affected. Second, as for the real clinical practice, the diagnosis of cutaneous diseases is not only based on the morphology of the skin lesions but also impacted by the general information and complicated medical history of the present patients, but we still do not know whether the accuracy would increase or decrease if such additional information is provided to the CNN model. Third, the disease spectrum in dermatology is rather wide. Although our dataset could to the best extent mimic the overall clinical conditions in our daily practice, there still lack a vast range of cutaneous diseases, such as skin cancers (e.g., squamous cell carcinoma and melanoma) uncommon in China. For further study, a CNN model should be refined by utilizing data from multiple centers or devices to improve the universality, and including more constantly encountered disease types in clinical practice, and possibly adding the information other than dermoscopic images such as sex, age, disease duration and clinical or high-frequency ultrasonic images. Finally, as forwarded by Tschandl et al. (35), CNN-support diagnosis gains are relative to the clinicians' experience, confidence in diagnosis and specific tasks. Human–computer collaboration will make full use of CNN assistance. The future studies ought to emphasize the cooperation instead of competence between clinicians and CNN. However, our study lacked the validation of the influences of CNN assistance on dermatologists as mentioned above.

In conclusion, we proposed a CNN model based on Google's EfficientNet-b4 with pre-trained weights on ImageNet trained by a novel dermoscopic dataset represented the real dermatological clinics environment of a tertiary class hospital in China with 14 categories of common cutaneous diseases. Our CNN model achieved a rather high level of performance, with an overall accuracy of 0.948 $\pm$ 0.001 (mean $\pm$ SD), a sensitivity of 0.934 $\pm$ 0.001 (mean $\pm$ SD), and a specificity of 0.950 $\pm$ 0.001 (mean $\pm$ SD). Furthermore, we compared this framework with previously reported methods and it outperformed all of them. Also, the performance of this CNN model was comparable to 280 board-certified dermatologists in an eight-class diagnostic task, with higher sensitivity in all of the included diseases.

## ETHICS STATEMENT

The studies involving human participants were reviewed and approved by the Medical Ethics Committee of Peking Union Medical College Hospital. Written informed consent to participate in this study was provided by the participants' legal guardian/next of kin.

## AUTHOR CONTRIBUTIONS

C-YZ, Y-KW, H-PC, K-LG, and JL made the concept and design of this study. C-YZ, Y-KW, and JL were responsible for the literature search, patient enrolment, dermoscopic evaluation, and dataset formation. H-PC, L-FY, and K-LG developed, refined, and validated the proposed CNN model using the dataset mentioned above. C-YZ, Y-KW, CS, J-CW, and JL organized the comparative reader study of 280 board-certificated dermatologists in a formal dermoscopy conference in China. Y-GY and F-YX collected and analysed the classification results of dermatologists. H-PC and Y-GY made the statistical analysis. The manuscript was prepared by Y-KW and H-PC, edited and reviewed by L-FY, JL, and F-YX. All authors contributed to the article and approved the submitted version.

## REFERENCES


1. Litjens G, Kooi T, Bejnordi BE, Setio AAA, Ciompi F, Ghafoorian M, et al. A survey on deep learning in medical image analysis. *Med Image Anal.* (2017) 42:60–88. doi: 10.1016/j.media.2017.07.005
2. Kermany DS, Goldbaum M, Cai W, Valentim CCS, Liang H, Baxter SL, et al. Identifying medical diagnoses and treatable diseases by image-based deep learning. *Cell.* (2018) 172:1122–31.e9. doi: 10.1016/j.cell.2018.02.010
3. Esteva A, Kuprel B, Novoa RA, Ko J, Swetter SM, Blau HM, et al. Dermatologist-level classification of skin cancer with deep neural networks. *Nature.* (2017) 542:115–8. doi: 10.1038/nature21056
4. Menegola A, Fornaciali M, Pires R, Avila S, Valle E. *Towards automated melanoma screening: exploring transfer learning schemes. arXiv [Preprint].* (2016).
5. Huang ML, Hung YH, Lee WM, Li RK, Jiang BR. SVM-RFE based feature selection and Taguchi parameters optimization for multiclass SVM classifier. *Scient World J.* (2014) 2014:795624. doi: 10.1155/2014/795624
6. Jafari MH, Nasr-Esfahani E, Karimi N, Soroushmehr SMR, Samavi S, Najarian K. Extraction of skin lesions from non-dermoscopic images for surgical excision of melanoma. *Int J Comput Assist Radiol Surg.* (2017) 12:1021–30. doi: 10.1007/s11548-017-1567-8
7. Spyridonos P, Gaitanis G, Likas A, Bassukas ID. Automatic discrimination of actinic keratoses from clinical photographs. *Comput Biol Med.* (2017) 88:50–9. doi: 10.1016/j.compbiomed.2017.07.001
8. Xie F, Fan H, Li Y, Jiang Z, Meng R, Bovik A. Melanoma classification on dermoscopy images using a neural network ensemble model. *IEEE Trans Med Imaging.* (2017) 36:849–58. doi: 10.1109/TMI.2016.2633551
9. Garcia-Zapirain B, Elmogy M, El-Baz A, Elmaghraby AS. Classification of pressure ulcer tissues with 3D convolutional neural network. *Med Biol Eng Comput.* (2018) 56:2245–58. doi: 10.1007/s11517-018-1835-y
10. Han SS, Kim MS, Lim W, Park GH, Park I, Chang SE. Classification of the clinical images for benign and malignant cutaneous tumors using a deep learning algorithm. *J Invest Dermatol.* (2018) 138:1529–38. doi: 10.1016/j.jid.2018.01.028
11. Emam S, Du AX, Surmanowicz P, Thomsen SF, Greiner R, Gniadecki R. Predicting the long-term outcomes of biologics in patients with psoriasis using machine learning. *Br J Dermatol.* (2020) 182:1305–7. doi: 10.1111/bjd.18741
12. Fujisawa Y, Otomo Y, Ogata Y, Nakamura Y, Fujita R, Ishitsuka Y, et al. Deep-learning-based, computer-aided classifier developed with a small dataset

of clinical images surpasses board-certified dermatologists in skin tumour diagnosis. *Br J Dermatol.* (2019) 180:373–81. doi: 10.1111/bjd.16924
13. Wang S-Q, Zhang X-Y, Liu J, Tao C, Zhu C-Y, Shu C, et al. Deep learning-based, computer-aided classifier developed with dermoscopic images shows comparable performance to 164 dermatologists in cutaneous disease diagnosis in the Chinese population. *Chin Med J.* (2020) 133:2027–36. doi: 10.1097/CM9.0000000000001023
14. Dreiseitl S, Binder M, Vinterbo S, Kittler H. Applying a decision support system in clinical practice: results from melanoma diagnosis. *AMIA Annu Symp Proc.* (2007) 2007:191–5.
15. Dreiseitl S, Binder M, Hable K, Kittler H. Computer versus human diagnosis of melanoma: evaluation of the feasibility of an automated diagnostic system in a prospective clinical trial. *Melanoma Res.* (2009) 19:180–4. doi: 10.1097/CMR.0b013e32832a1e41
16. Tan M, Le QV. *EfficientNet: rethinking model scaling for convolutional neural networks. arXiv:1905.11946* (2019).
17. Russakovsky O, Deng J, Su H, Krause J, Satheesh S, Ma S, et al. ImageNet large scale visual recognition challenge. *Int J Comp Vision.* (2015) 115:211–52. doi: 10.1007/s11263-015-0816-y
18. Hu J, Shen L, Albanie S, Sun G, Wu E. Squeeze-and-Excitation Networks. *IEEE Trans Pattern Anal Mach Intell.* (2020) 42:2011–23. doi: 10.1109/TPAMI.2019.2913372
19. Szegedy C, Vanhoucke V, Ioffe S, Shlens J, Wojna Z. *Rethinking the inception architecture for computer vision.* In: *2016 IEEE Conference on Computer Vision and Pattern Recognition (CVPR).* Las Vegas, NV: IEEE (2015). p. 2818–26. doi: 10.1109/CVPR.2016.308
20. Selvaraju RR, Cogswell M, Das A, Vedantam R, Batra D. Grad-CAM: visual explanations from deep networks via gradient-based localization. *Int J Comp Vision.* (2019) 128:336–59. doi: 10.1007/s11263-019-01228-7
21. He K, Zhang X, Ren S, Sun J, editors. Deep residual learning for image recognition. In: *2016 IEEE Conference on Computer Vision and Pattern Recognition (CVPR).* p. 27–30. doi: 10.1109/CVPR.2016.90
22. Hinton GE. Visualizing high-dimensional data using t-SNE. *J Mach Learn Res.* (2008) 9:2579–605.
23. Zhao S, Xie B, Li Y, Zhao X, Kuang Y, Su J, et al. Smart identification of psoriasis by images using convolutional neural networks: a case study in China. *J Eur Acad Dermatol Venereol.* (2020) 34:518–24. doi: 10.1111/jdv.15965
24. Shen CB, Shen X, Li CX, Meng RS, Cui Y. Assessment of imaging diagnosis ability of skin tumors in Chinese dermatologists. *Chin Med J (Engl).* (2019) 132:2119–20. doi: 10.1097/CM9.0000000000000389
25. Cress RD, Holly EA. Incidence of cutaneous melanoma among non-Hispanic whites, Hispanics, Asians, and blacks: an analysis of california cancer registry data, 1988-93. *Cancer Causes Control.* (1997) 8:246–52.
26. MacKie RM, Hauschild A, Eggermont AMM. Epidemiology of invasive cutaneous melanoma. *Ann Oncol.* (2009) 20 (Suppl 6):vi1-vi7. doi: 10.1093/annonc/mdp252
27. Minagawa A, Koga H, Sano T, Matsunaga K, Teshima Y, Hamada A, et al. Dermoscopic diagnostic performance of Japanese dermatologists for skin tumors differs by patient origin: a deep learning convolutional neural network closes the gap. *J Dermatol.* (2020) 48:232–6. doi: 10.1111/1346-8138.15640
28. Liu Y, Jain A, Eng C, Way DH, Lee K, Bui P, et al. A deep learning system for differential diagnosis of skin diseases. *Nat Med.* (2020) 26:900–8. doi: 10.1038/s41591-020-0842-3
29. Errichetti E. Dermoscopy of inflammatory dermatoses (Inflammoscopy): an up-to-date overview. *Dermatol Pract Concept.* (2019) 9:169–80. doi: 10.5826/dpc.0903a01
30. Errichetti E, Zalaudek I, Kittler H, Apalla Z, Argenziano G, Bakos R, et al. Standardization of dermoscopic terminology and basic dermoscopic parameters to evaluate in general dermatology (non-neoplastic dermatoses): an expert consensus on behalf of the International Dermoscopy Society. *Br J Dermatol.* (2020) 182:454—67. doi: 10.1111/bjd.18125
31. Brinker TJ, Hekler A, Enk AH, Klode J, Hauschild A, Berking C, et al. A convolutional neural network trained with dermoscopic images performed on par with 145 dermatologists in a clinical melanoma image classification task. *Eur J Cancer.* (2019) 111:148–54. doi: 10.1016/j.ejca.2019.02.005
32. Haenssle HA, Fink C, Schneiderbauer R, Toberer F, Buhl T, Blum A, et al. Man against machine: diagnostic performance of a deep learning convolutional neural network for dermoscopic melanoma recognition in comparison to 58 dermatologists. *Ann Oncol.* (2018) 29:1836–42. doi: 10.1093/annonc/mdy520
33. Brinker TJ, Hekler A, Enk AH, Klode J, Hauschild A, Berking C, et al. Deep learning outperformed 136 of 157 dermatologists in a head-to-head dermoscopic melanoma image classification task. *Eur J Cancer.* (2019) 113:47–54. doi: 10.1016/j.ejca.2019.04.001
34. Maron RC, Weichenthal M, Utikal JS, Hekler A, Berking C, Hauschild A, et al. Systematic outperformance of 112 dermatologists in multiclass skin cancer image classification by convolutional neural networks. *Eur J Cancer.* (2019) 119:57–65. doi: 10.1016/j.ejca.2019.06.013
35. Tschandl P, Rinner C, Apalla Z, Argenziano G, Codella N, Halpern A, et al. Human-computer collaboration for skin cancer recognition. *Nat Med.* (2020) 26:1229–34. doi: 10.1038/s41591-020-0942-0

# 21

# Accuracy of Teledermatology in Skin Neoplasms

*Mara Giavina-Bianchi*, Maria Fernanda Dias Azevedo, Raquel Machado Sousa and Eduardo Cordioli*

*Department of Telemedicine, Hospital Israelita Albert Einstein, São Paulo, Brazil*

***Correspondence:**
*Mara Giavina-Bianchi*
*marahgbianchi@gmail.com*

Teledermatology has been proving to be of great help for delivering healthcare, especially now, during the SARS-CoV-2 pandemic. It is crucial to assess how accurate this method can be for evaluating different dermatoses. Such knowledge can contribute to the dermatologists' decision of whether to adhere to teledermatology or not. Our objective was to determine the accuracy of teledermatology in the 10 most frequent skin neoplasms in our population, comparing telediagnosis to histopathological report and in-person dermatologists' diagnosis. A retrospective cohort study was conducted in São Paulo, Brazil, where a store-and-forward teledermatology project was implemented under primary-care attention to triage surgical, more complex, or severe dermatoses. A total of 30,976 patients presenting 55,012 lesions took part in the project. Thirteen teledermatologists who participated in the project had three options to refer the patients: send them directly to biopsy, to the in-person dermatologist, or back to the general physician with the most probable diagnosis and management. In the groups referred to the in-person dermatologist and biopsy, we looked for the 10 most frequent International Statistical Classification of Diseases and Related Health Problems-10 (ICD-10) of skin neoplasms, which resulted in 289 histopathologic reports and 803 in-person dermatologists' diagnosis. We were able to compare the ICD-10 codes filled by teledermatologists, in-person dermatologists, and from histopathological reports. The proportion of complete, partial, and no agreement rates between the in-person dermatologist's, histopathologic report, and the teledermatologist's diagnosis was assessed. We also calculated Cohen's kappa, for complete and complete plus partial agreement. The mean complete agreement rate comparing telediagnosis to histopathological report was 54% (157/289; kappa = 0.087), being the highest for malign lesions; to in-person dermatologists was 61% (487/803; kappa = 0.213), highest for benign lesions. When accuracy of telediagnosis for either malign or benign lesions was evaluated, the agreement rate with histopathology was 70% (kappa = 0.529) and with in-person dermatologist, 81% (kappa = 0.582). This study supports that teledermatology for skin neoplasms has moderate accuracy. This result reassures that it can be a proper option for patient care, especially when the goal is to differentiate benign from malign lesions.

**Keywords: teledermatology, telemedicine, accuracy: skin neoplasms, skin cancer, benign skin lesions, malign skin lesions, tele-health**

## INTRODUCTION

As we face this pandemic time around the world, telemedicine has been proving to be of great help for delivering healthcare. Any medical specialty that is based on image analysis, such as dermatology, is especially suitable for this method of care. Teledermatology has the potential to improve access to subspecialty expertise, reduce healthcare costs, and improve the overall quality of care. The three main teledermatology delivery platforms are: synchronous (RT: real-time teledermatology), asynchronous (SF-TD: store-and-forward teledermatology), and hybrid (both synchronous and asynchronous forms). Synchronous teledermatology uses live video conferencing between the patient and the dermatologist. Asynchronous teledermatology is a method whereby clinical or dermoscopy dermatologic images are obtained and sent to the responding dermatologist who can review them at a later time. Although it provides high-resolution dermatologic images and promotes an efficient practice, this modality is limited by the ability of the teledermatologist to obtain additional clinical history while evaluating the case (1). Teledermoscopy involves the use of dermoscopic images for remote consultation and decision-making in skin cancer screening. Its addition significantly improved the results of an internet-based skin cancer screening system, compared with clinical images alone (2).

The majority of studies in teledermatology have found rates of accuracy to be in the range of 75–80%, comparable to those with in-person care (1). Many of the articles were focused on skin neoplasms, especially skin cancer and pigmented lesions (3–6), or on general dermatology (7–11). A recent systematic review concluded that robust implementation studies of teledermatology are needed, with attention to reducing the risk of bias when assessing diagnostic accuracy (3). For this purpose, we performed research with the primary goal of determining the accuracy of teledermatology for skin neoplasms in a robust number of cases, assessing the agreement rate between the histopathological report, in-person dermatologists', and the teledermatologists' diagnoses. The secondary aim was to analyze the differential diagnosis of the lesions.

## MATERIALS AND METHODS

This was a retrospective cohort study designed to assess concordance between diagnoses made by in-person dermatologists and teledermatologists, and by histopathological reports and teledermatologists, approved by the Ethics Committee of Hospital Israelita Albert Einstein (CAAE: 97126618.6.0000.0071). We analyzed the reports of 30,976 patients included in a teledermatology triage project conducted in the city of São Paulo, Brazil, from July 2017 to July 2018.

**Abbreviations:** TD, teledermatology; RT, real time; SF-TD, store and forward; IPD, in-person dermatologist; GP, general physician; ICD-10 code, international code of diseases 10; BCC, basal cell carcinoma; SCC, squamous cell carcinoma; AK, actinic keratosis; SK, seborrheic keratosis; Acro/other benign, acrochordon/other benign neoplasms.

### Teledermatology Triage Project

A Teledermatology project implemented from July 2017 to July 2018, in São Paulo. There were 57,832 individuals waiting for a consultation with a dermatologist in the public health system in July 2017. To reduce the waiting list and accelerate the flow of patients with the most severe, complex or surgical dermatoses to in-person dermatologists, the municipal health government requested Hospital Israelita Albert Einstein, a large private hospital in the city with expertise in Telemedicine, to develop a project using Telemedicine to reach these goals. Therefore, an online platform and a mobile app were designed to take photographs with phone cameras and directly upload them to the app and a short clinical history and data of the patient, which were meant to be used by for health technicians or nurses. The photographs and collected information were uploaded to a platform using a secure online process and were accessed only by the 13 Brazilian Board Certified dermatologists associated with this project, for whom the patients were randomly assigned. These 13 dermatologists will be called teledermatologists in this study. All the patients waiting for dermatologist consultations were called consecutively, via phone, by the municipal health care service and scheduled for an appointment in one of the three public city hospitals enabled to carry out the project, depending on the location of the individual's residence. Once there, a short history of the complaint (history of bleeding, pruritus, time from the onset, and location) and demographic data (sex and age) as well as three photographs in different angles and distances from each lesion were taken by a trained health technician: first one at medium distance (50 cm away), second one in close-up (15 cm away) and last one of a lateral view, aiming to evaluate the volume of the lesion. After accessing the patients' pictures and clinical history of the patients, the dermatologists first decided whether the photographs of the lesions were satisfactory for diagnostic purposes. If not, they categorized it under "bad photo," and the patient was referred to a dermatologist for an in-person appointment. If the photo quality was good enough, they formulated the most probable diagnostic hypothesis. They chose one of three options for each lesion assessed: (1) a direct referral for a biopsy (after which the patient would return for an in-person dermatologist appointment), (2) a referral for an in-person dermatologist (IPD) visit, or (3) a referral to go back to the primary care physician (GP) with the most probable diagnosis, treatment and/or recommendation on how to proceed with the investigation and/or management of the lesion. A schematic for this process is shown in **Figure 1**. If the same patient had more than one lesion but different referrals, they were referred to the most specialized one and that would be his/her last referral in terms of statistical accounting. For instance, a biopsy would prevail over a dermatologist visit, which would in turn prevail over general physician referral. This teledermatology project followed the American Medical Association telemedicine policy, adapted for the needs of the Brazilian public health care system (12).

### Study Design

We selected the groups referred to IPD (12,874 patients/16,777 lesions) and biopsy (1,292 patients/1,912 lesions). Then, we assessed the reports that had the International Statistical

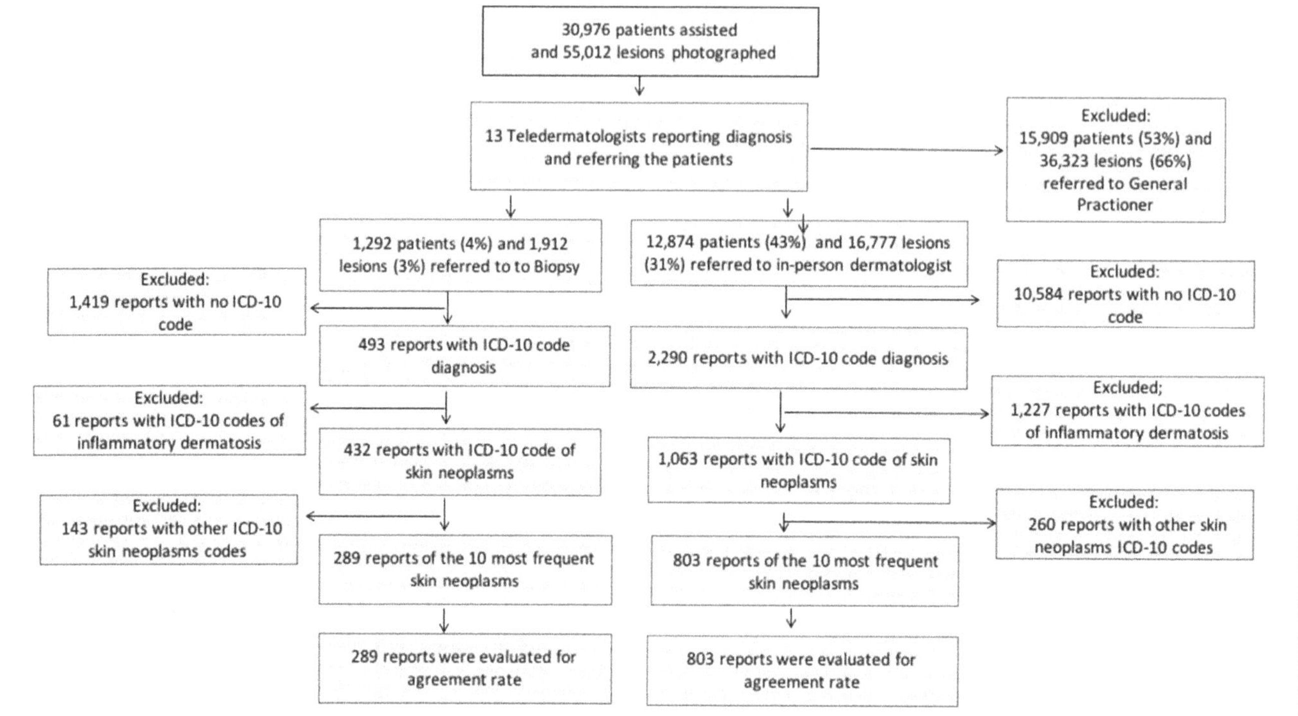


**FIGURE 1 |** Frequency of patients included, photographed lesions and referrals made by the teledermatologists, along with the flow used to assess the diagnosis accuracy for the 10 most frequent skin neoplasms.

Classification of Diseases and Related Health Problems 10th version (ICD-10 code) (13) diagnoses filled by IPD (2,290) and histopathological reports (HP: 493). Next, we separated the reports filled with ICD-10 codes of skin neoplasms sent to IPD (1,063) and from histopathological reports (432). Afterward, we looked for the 10 most frequent dermatoses in each group, 803 in IPD and 289 to include in our study (803 for IPD and 289 in HP **Figure 1**).

We classified the rate of agreement as follows: (1) complete agreement when the ICD-10 code used in both reports were the same, (2) partial agreement when the ICD-10 code used in both reports were different, but in the same group of disease (malign or benign neoplasms), posing as a probable differential diagnosis, and (3) no agreement when both reports did not fill the previous two conditions. Basal cell carcinoma (BCC), squamous cell carcinoma (SCC), melanoma, and actinic keratosis (AK) were considered the malign group. Nevus, seborrheic keratosis (SK), acrochrodon/other benign neoplasms, cyst, lipoma, and wart were the benign group. If the cases did not belong to one of those 10 classes, it was classified as "other." As the gold standard diagnosis is the histopathological diagnosis, the agreement was stated in this research as accurate.

## Statistical Analysis

Rates of concordance were expressed using percentages and Cohen's kappa coefficient, which was used to compare between groups of inter-rater observers (Graph Pad Prism 6.0). The guidelines used to characterize kappa values were created by Landis and Koch (14), as follows: kappa $< 0$: no agreement, 0.00–0.20: slight agreement, 0.21–0.40: fair agreement, 0.41–0.60: moderate agreement, 0.61–0.8: substantial agreement, and 0.81–1.00: almost perfect agreement.

# RESULTS

**Table 1** shows the 10 most frequent skin neoplasms diagnosed by teledermatology according to the frequency of lesions, sex, age, and referral distribution. The total amount represents 31% (17,233/55,012) of the lesions diagnosed in the entire teledermatology project. The female and male proportion was 72 and 28%, respectively, although the female population accounts for 52.6% in the city of São Paulo (2010) (15). Lesions diagnosed as benign were 90% (15,496/17,233) and as malign, 10% (1,727/17,233). Among benign neoplasms, 63% (9,849/15,496) were sent to GP for follow-up, 34% (5,242/15,496) were sent to IPD and only 3% (405/15,496) were sent to biopsy. For malign lesions, 3% (4/1,727) was referred to GP, 51% (880/1,727) to IPD and 46% (803/1,727) to biopsy.

**Figures 2**, **3** demonstrate the comparison between teledermatologists' diagnosis to the histopathological reports and to in-person dermatologists, respectively.

For instance, in **Figure 2**, among the 65 histopathological reports of BCC in this study, the teledermatologists had diagnosed 49 correctly (complete agreement in yellow), 6 as SCC, 2 as melanoma, 3 as AK (all considered partial agreement, in green), 2 as nevus, 2 as SK, and 1 as other (all considered no agreement, in red).

**TABLE 1** | Patient's demographics and referrals for the 10 most frequent skin neoplasms diagnosed in the Teledermatology Project in São Paulo from July 2017–2018.

| | Sex | | Age (years) | | | Referral | | | |
|---|---|---|---|---|---|---|---|---|---|
| **Skin neoplasm** | **M** | **F** | **0–19** | **20–59** | **60+** | **Biopsy** | **IPD** | **GP** | **Total** |
| BCC | 144 | 274 | 0 | 154 | 264 | 341 | 73 | 4 | 418 |
| SCC | 120 | 188 | 5 | 101 | 202 | 267 | 39 | 2 | 308 |
| Melanoma | 45 | 118 | 7 | 68 | 88 | 117 | 46 | 0 | 163 |
| AK | 280 | 558 | 2 | 190 | 646 | 78 | 722 | 38 | 838 |
| Nevus | 917 | 3,434 | 399 | 2,985 | 967 | 166 | 1,491 | 2,694 | 4,351 |
| SK | 784 | 2,251 | 4 | 1,124 | 1,907 | 75 | 507 | 2,453 | 3,035 |
| Acro/other | 889 | 2,872 | 275 | 2,483 | 1,003 | 76 | 539 | 3,146 | 3,761 |
| Cyst | 738 | 1,176 | 119 | 1,172 | 623 | 41 | 1,059 | 814 | 1,914 |
| Lipoma | 394 | 510 | 26 | 590 | 288 | 3 | 362 | 539 | 904 |
| Wart | 592 | 939 | 489 | 722 | 320 | 44 | 1,284 | 203 | 1,531 |
| Total | 4,903 | 12,320 | 1,326 | 9,589 | 6,308 | 1,208 | 6,122 | 9,893 | 17,233 |

| | TELEDIAGNOSIS | | | | | | | | | | |
|---|---|---|---|---|---|---|---|---|---|---|---|
| **HISTOPATHOLOGY REPORT** | BCC | SCC | MELANOMA | AK | NEVUS | SK | ACRO/OTHER | CYST | LIPOMA | WART | OTHER | TOTAL |
| BCC | 49 | 6 | 2 | 3 | 2 | 2 | 0 | 0 | 0 | 0 | 1 | 65 |
| SCC | 5 | 22 | 2 | 2 | 0 | 0 | 0 | 0 | 0 | 0 | 0 | 31 |
| MELANOMA | 1 | 0 | 7 | 0 | 0 | 0 | 0 | 0 | 0 | 0 | 0 | 8 |
| AK | 10 | 8 | 0 | 9 | 0 | 0 | 0 | 0 | 0 | 0 | 3 | 30 |
| NEVUS | 7 | 2 | 7 | 0 | 33 | 0 | 2 | 0 | 0 | 1 | 3 | 55 |
| SK | 1 | 2 | 7 | 2 | 7 | 16 | 1 | 0 | 0 | 2 | 0 | 38 |
| ACRO/OTHER | 8 | 9 | 3 | 1 | 3 | 2 | 6 | 2 | 0 | 0 | 1 | 35 |
| CYST | 2 | 1 | 0 | 0 | 1 | 0 | 0 | 7 | 0 | 0 | 0 | 11 |
| LIPOMA | 0 | 0 | 0 | 0 | 0 | 0 | 0 | 1 | 1 | 0 | 0 | 2 |
| WART | 1 | 2 | 1 | 0 | 1 | 2 | 0 | 0 | 0 | 7 | 0 | 14 |
| TOTAL | 84 | 52 | 29 | 17 | 47 | 22 | 9 | 10 | 1 | 10 | 8 | 289 |

complete agreement
no agreement
partial agreement

**FIGURE 2** | Confusion matrix comparing telediagnosis to histopathology report.

| | TELEDIAGNOSIS | | | | | | | | | | |
|---|---|---|---|---|---|---|---|---|---|---|---|
| **IPD DIAGNOSIS** | BCC | SCC | MELANOMA | AK | NEVUS | SK | ACRO/OTHER | CYST | LIPOMA | WART | OTHER | TOTAL |
| BCC | 26 | 5 | 0 | 3 | 1 | 2 | 1 | 0 | 0 | 1 | 1 | 40 |
| SCC | 2 | 23 | 1 | 5 | 3 | 0 | 2 | 0 | 0 | 1 | 2 | 39 |
| MELANOMA | 0 | 1 | 8 | 0 | 2 | 1 | 1 | 1 | 0 | 0 | 0 | 14 |
| AK | 1 | 5 | 1 | 43 | 1 | 11 | 1 | 1 | 0 | 4 | 9 | 77 |
| NEVUS | 6 | 0 | 13 | 0 | 160 | 7 | 19 | 3 | 0 | 5 | 17 | 230 |
| SK | 2 | 5 | 8 | 9 | 23 | 50 | 8 | 3 | 0 | 6 | 8 | 122 |
| ACRO/OTHER | 6 | 3 | 2 | 4 | 12 | 1 | 32 | 1 | 0 | 6 | 6 | 73 |
| CYST | 2 | 2 | 1 | 0 | 6 | 0 | 3 | 55 | 6 | 0 | 8 | 83 |
| LIPOMA | 0 | 0 | 0 | 0 | 0 | 0 | 0 | 1 | 7 | 0 | 0 | 8 |
| WART | 1 | 4 | 1 | 1 | 5 | 3 | 5 | 1 | 0 | 83 | 13 | 117 |
| TOTAL | 46 | 48 | 35 | 65 | 213 | 75 | 72 | 66 | 13 | 106 | 64 | 803 |

complete agreement
no agreement
partial agreement

**FIGURE 3** | Confusion matrix comparing telediagnosis to in-person dermatologists' diagnosis.

Following the same path, in **Figure 3**, among 40 telediagnosis of BCC, 26 were in agreement with IPD (complete agreement, in yellow), 5 were SCC, 3 were AK (partial agreement, in green) and 1 nevus, 2 SK, 1 acro/other, 1 wart, and 1 other (no agreement, in red).

**Table 2** reveals the percentage of accuracy for complete, partial, and no agreement and Cohen's kappa calculations for complete and complete plus partial agreement, comparing the telediagnosis to histopathological reports (upper part) and in-person dermatologists' diagnosis (bottom part). In the upper part, the mean frequency of complete agreement was 54% for all 10 dermatoses tested (157/289) and its kappa coefficient was 0.087), which is considered a slight agreement. Three malign skin tumors had the highest rates of accuracy: melanoma (7/8), BCC (49/65), and SCC (22/31), respectively with 88, 75, and 71% and kappas = 0.060, 0.326, and 0,117. Among benign neoplasms, cyst, and nevus were the most accurate diagnoses, respectively with 64 and 60% and kappas = 0.335 and 0.298 (fair agreement).

**TABLE 2 |** Agreement between teledermatologists' diagnosis and histopathological reports (upper part) and in-person dermatologists (bottom part).

| | Teledermatologists' diagnosis | | | | |
|---|---|---|---|---|---|
| **Histopathology report** | **Complete agreement (%)** | **Cohen's Kappa complete agreement** | **Partial agreement (%)** | **Cohen's Kappa complete + partial agreement** | **No agreement (%)** |
| BCC | 75 | 0.326 | 17 | 0.680 | 8 |
| SCC | 71 | 0.117 | 29 | 0.627 | 0 |
| Melanoma | 88 | 0.060 | 12 | 0.209 | 0 |
| AK | 30 | −0.146 | 60 | 0.724 | 10 |
| Nevus | 60 | 0.298 | 5 | 0.596 | 35 |
| SK | 42 | 0.129 | 26 | 0.513 | 32 |
| Acro/other benign | 17 | −0.078 | 20 | 0.195 | 63 |
| Cyst | 64 | 0.335 | 9 | 0.717 | 27 |
| Lipoma | 50 | 0.400 | 50 | 1.00 | 0 |
| Wart | 50 | 0.189 | 21 | 0.676 | 29 |
| Total | 54 | 0.087 | 16 | 0.529 | 30 |
| **In-person dermatologists' diagnosis** | | | | | |
| BCC | 65 | 0.213 | 20 | 0.472 | 15 |
| SCC | 59 | 0.067 | 20.5 | 0.496 | 20.5 |
| Melanoma | 57 | −0.138 | 7 | −0.050 | 36 |
| AK | 56 | 0.217 | 9 | 0.427 | 35 |
| Nevus | 70 | 0.446 | 15 | 0.807 | 15 |
| SK | 41 | 0.068 | 34 | 0.527 | 25 |
| Acro/other benign | 44 | −0.117 | 27 | 0.642 | 29 |
| Cyst | 66 | 0.483 | 22 | 0.799 | 12 |
| Lipoma | 87.5 | 0.369 | 12.5 | 1.00 | 0 |
| Wart | 71 | 0.490 | 12 | 0.768 | 17 |
| Total | 61 | 0.213 | 20 | 0.582 | 19 |

Warts, SK and lipomas showed an intermediate rate, around 50%, and acrochordon and other benign neoplasms had the lowest rate (17%; kappa = −0.078). AK had only 30% of agreement, being the least accurate in the malign group (kappa = −0.146). Partial agreement was verified in 22% of all cases (64/289), ranging from 5% in nevus up to 60% in AK. No agreement was found in 24% (68/289); CBC, SCC, and lipoma had zero no agreements while nevus, SK, warts, and cysts had around 30% of no agreement.

Comparing teledermatologists' to in-person dermatologists' diagnosis accuracy, we found a mean frequency of complete agreement in 61% of all 10 skin neoplasms (487/803) and its kappa coefficient was 0.213, which is considered a fair agreement. Benign skin tumors had the highest rates of accuracy: lipoma (7/8), warts (83/116), and nevus (160/230), with 87.5, 72, and 70% and kappas = 0.369, 0.490, and 0.446, respectively. Among malign neoplasms, all four of them were between 56% (AK) and 65% (CBC). The lowest rate was achieved by SK (41%; kappa = 0.068) and acro/other benign (44%; kappa = −0.117). Partial agreement was verified in 20% of all cases (159/803), ranging from 7% in melanoma up to 34% in SK. No agreement was found in 19% (156/803); lipoma had zero no agreements while melanoma, AK, and acro/other benign had around 36, 35, and 29%, respectively.

## DISCUSSION

Analyzing **Table 1**, we can see that most of the benign cases of skin neoplasms in this cohort were not sent to biopsy and in-person dermatologists; they were sent back to the GP to follow-up and, therefore, could not be compared with the teledermatologists' diagnosis. This fact is very relevant when discussing accuracy in this study. As the teledermatology triage project prioritized the severe, more complex, or surgical cases for biopsy and in-person dermatologists, trying to manage the mild cases under the primary-care attention along with the GP, skin neoplasms diagnosed by histopathological analysis or in-person dermatologists have a bias of being the most challenging/difficult cases. Typical or "regular" skin neoplasms were most probably diagnosed and referred back to the GP. In this manner, our results in the rate of agreement would be probably much higher if more typical cases were analyzed.

In terms of health delivery, choosing the proper management of the skin neoplasms is even more important than elaborating the right diagnosis itself. In this way, what is more important than complete agreement (ICD-10 code) is to analyze rates of complete plus partial agreement (benign vs. malign). If the diagnosis fits within the benign neoplasms, an expectant conduct is acceptable, while within the malign neoplasms, a biopsy, or surgery ought to be expected.

Analyzing teledermatogists' diagnosis and histopathological reports' agreement, we showed a mean agreement rate of 70% (54% total + 16% partial agreement rates) and kappa = 0.529 (moderate). Considering studies that compared TD diagnosis and histopathological reports, Silveira et al. (16) included 364 suspected cases of skin malignancy by TD to be confirmed by the biopsy. The majority of the lesions were BCCs with 286 cases, followed by 59 SCCs and 5 melanomas. Two oncologists showed an overall accuracy of 85.3% for the first and 87.3% for the other in categorizing benign x malign lesions. Our results for malign and benign lesions showed 94% (126/134) and 61% (95/155) of agreement, respectively. In another study, 144 pigmented lesions diagnosed via TD were examined histologically, and 63 (43%) showed complete agreement between the clinical and histological diagnoses (17). Comparatively, our study showed 60 and 88% complete agreement for nevus and melanoma respectively. In another article, 201 biopsies were requested to rule out malignancy via TD, which was confirmed in 45.3% (18). A survey among the teledermatologists participating in the project, after its conclusion, showed that the use of dermoscopy would significantly improve the decision to refer nevus and SK to in-person dermatologists, GP or biopsy and, most probably, the agreement rate too. They felt that many cases referred to biopsy or IPD could have been referred to GP if dermoscopic images were available (19). Melanoma had a fair agreement rate. We believe that happened because, when in doubt, one would rather excise it and send it to histopathological than wait to see how it develops. In this project, with no access to dermoscopic images, there were 112 lesions suspected of melanoma and 8 melanomas confirmed (14 benign lesions:1 melanoma). Other studies show that the number of nevus needed to diagnose one melanoma can vary from 4.5 to 22 (20). Acrochordon/other benign neoplasms had slight agreement rate kappa, probably because of the reasons explained before. Only "weird looking" acrochordons would be sent to biopsy, confirming that they were, in fact, not acrochordons.

The results of our study showed a slightly better agreement rate between diagnoses made by teledermatologists and in-person dermatologists in general. If we summed up complete (61%) and partial (20%) agreement rates, we have reached 81% (kappa = 0.582-moderate), but there was an inversion in the accuracy for benign and malign lesions. The agreement rate for benign lesions was 82% and for malign, 73%. Nevus and acrochordons/other benign neoplasms in this referral were probably more typical than the ones sent to biopsy, and that could explain why the agreement rate for benign skin neoplasms had an improvement compared to the previous one. On the other hand, BCC, SCC, and AK showed lower agreement rate to IPD than histopathological reports. The worst agreement rate was for melanoma. Cohen's kappa coefficient showed no agreement (−0.050). This may reflect the same reasons stated before, the absence of dermoscopy images and also the teledermatologists' fear of letting a melanoma diagnosis go undetected. When compared to the previous studies, Kroemer et al. (21) included 104 pigmented lesions and found a kappa = 0.84. Moreno-Ramirez et al. (22) showed a kappa = 0.81 in 890 cases of skin cancer triage.

According to the latest Cochrane review (2018) about teledermatology in skin cancers, using a more widely defined threshold to identify "possibly" malignant cases or lesions that should be considered for excision is likely to appropriately triage those lesions requeiring face-to-face assessment by a specialist. Despite the increasing use of teledermatology on an international level, the evidence base to support its ability to accurately diagnose lesions and to triage lesions from primary to secondary care is lacking and further prospective and pragmatic evaluation is needed (5).

Although this was a retrospective study and much data was missing, we believe this was one of the studies with the largest number of skin neoplasms included in the literature, comparing teledermatologists' diagnosis both to IPD and histopathological reports. Pathologists were responsible for histopathological reports. The study was performed in two centers and different dermatologists performed the tele and in-person examinations. This is a limitation because there is interoperator variability and the technical skills in the groups may be different. Moreover, teledermatologists could diagnose the lesions differently if they were face-to-face. The profile of 12 out of the 13 teledermatologists involved in the project was shown in a previously study (19). Ten had either subspecialty in dermoscopy or skin cancer, which we thought was very suitable for this study. Six had more than 10 years as Board Certified Dermatologists. Five of them integrated the Skin Oncology outpatient unity at University of São Paulo Dermatology Department. Unfortunately, we do not have the profile of the IPD. The risk of false negative cases, which we could not assess, exists and it is another limitation of this research. Nonetheless, during the project, there was always a physician, either a GP or an IPD, responsible for monitoring the patients.

Our study, performed in a large number of patients presenting the 10 most common skin neoplasms, showed moderate accuracy between teledermatology and histopathological reports, and moderate agreement rate between teledermatologists and in-person dermatologists' diagnosis. Accuracy may differ among skin neoplasms. This reassures that store-and-forward teledermatology can be an option for triage skin neoplasms in primary-care attention.

## ETHICS STATEMENT

The studies involving human participants were reviewed and approved by Ethics Committee of Hospital Israelita Albert Einstein (CAAE: 97126618.6.0000.0071). Written informed consent from the participants' legal guardian/next of kin was not required to participate in this study in accordance with the national legislation and the institutional requirements.

## AUTHOR CONTRIBUTIONS

MG-B and EC: study design. MG-B, RS, MA, and EC: data collection and review of the article. MG-B and MA: data analysis. MG-B and RS: writing. All authors contributed to the article and approved the submitted version.

## REFERENCES


1. Lee JJ, English JC. Teledermatology: a review and update. *Am J Clin Dermatol.* (2018) 19:253–60. doi: 10.1007/s40257-017-0317-6
2. Ferrándiz L, Ojeda-Vila T, Corrales A, Martín-Gutiérrez FJ, Ruíz-de-Casas A, Galdeano R, et al. Internet-based skin cancer screening using clinical images alone or in conjunction with dermoscopic images: a randomized teledermoscopy trial. *J Am Acad Dermatol.* (2017) 76:676–82. doi: 10.1016/j.jaad.2016.10.041
3. Finnane A, Dallest K, Janda M, Soyer HP. Teledermatology for the diagnosis and management of skin cancer: a systematic review. *JAMA Dermatol.* (2017) 153:319–27. doi: 10.1001/jamadermatol.2016.4361
4. Warshaw EM, Lederle FA, Grill JP, Gravely AA, Bangerter AK, Frontier LA, et al. Accuracy of teledermatology for pigmented neoplasms. *J Am Acad Dermatol.* (2009) 61:753–65. doi: 10.1016/j.jaad.2009.04.032
5. Chuchu N, Dinnes J, Takwoingi Y, Martin RN, Bayliss SE, Davenport C, et al. Teledermatology for diagnosing skin cancer in adults. *Cochrane Database Syst Rev.* (2018) 12:CD013193. doi: 10.1002/14651858.CD013193
6. Markun S, Scherz N, Rosemann T, Tandjung R, Braun RP. Mobile teledermatology for skin cancer screening: a diagnostic accuracy study. *Medicine (Baltimore).* (2017) 96:e6278. doi: 10.1097/MD.0000000000006278
7. Warshaw EM, Hillman YJ, Greer NL, Hagel EM, MacDonald R, Rutks IR, et al. Teledermatology for diagnosis and management of skin conditions: a systematic review. *J Am Acad Dermatol.* (2011) 64:759–72. doi: 10.1016/j.jaad.2010.08.026
8. Lasierra N, Alesanco A, Gilaberte Y, Magallón R, García J. Lessons learned after a three-year store and forward teledermatology experience using internet: strengths and limitations. *Int J Med Inform.* (2012) 81:332–43. doi: 10.1016/j.ijmedinf.2012.02.008
9. Lim AC, Egerton IB, See A, Shumack SP. Accuracy and reliability of store-and-forward teledermatology: preliminary results from the St. George Teledermatology Project. *Australas J Dermatol.* (2001) 42:247–51. doi: 10.1046/j.1440-0960.2001.00529.x
10. Weingast J, Scheibböck C, Wurm EM, Ranharter E, Porkert S, Dreiseitl S, et al. A prospective study of mobile phones for dermatology in a clinical setting. *J Telemed Telecare.* (2013) 19:213–8. doi: 10.1177/1357633x134 90890
11. O'Connor DM, Jew OS, Perman MJ, Castelo-Soccio LA, Winston FK, McMahon PJ. Diagnostic accuracy of pediatric teledermatology using parent-submitted photographs: a randomized clinical trial. *JAMA Dermatol.* (2017) 153:1243–8. doi: 10.1001/jamadermatol.2017.4280
12. American Medical Association. *AMA Telemedicine Policy.* (2016). Available online at: www.ama-assn.org (accessed october 10, 2020).
13. DATASUS. *CID-10.* (2008). Available online at: http://www.datasus.gov.br/cid10/v2008/webhelp/cid10.htm (accessed May 11, 2017).
14. Landis J, Koch G. The measurement of observer agreement for categorical categorical data. *Biometrics.* (1977) 33:159–74. doi: 10.2307/2529310
15. IBGE. *Censo 2010*, São Paulo: IBGE. (2013). Available online at: https://cidades.ibge.gov.br/brasil/sp/sao-paulo/pesquisa/23/27652 (accessed June 12, 2020).
16. Silveira CE, Silva TB, Fregnani JH, da Costa Vieria RA, Haikel RL Jr., Syrjanen K, et al. Digital photography in skin cancer screening by mobile units in remote areas of Brazil. *BMC Dermatol.* (2014) 14:19. doi: 10.1186/s12895-014-0019-1
17. Jolliffe VM, Harris DW, Whittaker SJ. Can we safely diagnose pigmented lesions from stored video images? A diagnostic comparison between clinical examination and stored video images of pigmented lesions removed for histology. *Clin Exp Dermatol.* (2001) 26:84–7. doi: 10.1046/j.1365-2230.2001.00767.x
18. Tandjung R, Badertscher N, Kleiner N, Wensing M, Rosemann T, Braun RP, et al. Feasibility and diagnostic accuracy of teledermatology in Swiss primary care: process analysis of a randomized controlled trial. *J Eval Clin Pract.* (2015) 21:326–31. doi: 10.1111/jep.12323
19. Giavina Bianchi M, Santos A, Cordioli E. Dermatologists' perceptions on the utility and limitations of teledermatology after examining 55,000 lesions. *J Telemed Telecare.* (2019):1357633X19864829. doi: 10.1177/1357633X19864829
20. Elliott TM, Whiteman DC, Olsen CM, Gordon LG. Estimated healthcare costs of melanoma in Australia over 3 years post-diagnosis. *Appl Health Econ Health Policy.* (2017) 15:805–16. doi: 10.1007/s40258-017-0341-y
21. Kroemer S, Frühauf J, Campbell TM, Massone C, Schwantzer G, Soyer HP, et al. Mobile teledermatology for skin tumour screening: diagnostic accuracy of clinical and dermoscopic image tele-evaluation using cellular phones. *Br J Dermatol.* (2011) 164:973–9. doi: 10.1111/j.1365-2133.2011.10208.x
22. Moreno-Ramirez D, Ferrandiz L, Nieto-Garcia A, Carrasco R, Moreno-Alvarez P, Galdeano R, et al. Store-and-forward teledermatology in skin cancer triage: experience and evaluation of 2009 teleconsultations. *Arch Dermatol.* (2007) 143:479–84. doi: 10.1001/archderm.143.4.479

# Effects of Label Noise on Deep Learning-Based Skin Cancer Classification

*Achim Hekler[1], Jakob N. Kather[1,2], Eva Krieghoff-Henning[1], Jochen S. Utikal[3,4], Friedegund Meier[5,6], Frank F. Gellrich[5,6], Julius Upmeier zu Belzen[7], Lars French[8], Justin G. Schlager[8], Kamran Ghoreschi[9], Tabea Wilhelm[9], Heinz Kutzner[10], Carola Berking[11], Markus V. Heppt[11], Sebastian Haferkamp[12], Wiebke Sondermann[13], Dirk Schadendorf[13], Bastian Schilling[14], Benjamin Izar[15], Roman Maron[1], Max Schmitt[1], Stefan Fröhling[1,16], Daniel B. Lipka[1,16,17] and Titus J. Brinker[1*]*

*[1] National Center for Tumor Diseases, German Cancer Research Center, Heidelberg, Germany, [2] Department of Medicine III, RWTH University Hospital Aachen, Aachen, Germany, [3] Department of Dermatology, Heidelberg University, Mannheim, Germany, [4] Skin Cancer Unit, German Cancer Research Center, Heidelberg, Germany, [5] Skin Cancer Center at the University Cancer Centre and National Center for Tumor Diseases Dresden, Dresden, Germany, [6] Department of Dermatology, University Hospital Carl Gustav Carus, Technische Universität Dresden, Dresden, Germany, [7] Berlin Institute of Health (BIH), Charité, Berlin, Germany, [8] Department of Dermatology and Allergology, Ludwig Maximilian University of Munich, Munich, Germany, [9] Department of Dermatology, Venereology and Allergology, Charité–Universitätsmedizin Berlin, Berlin, Germany, [10] Dermatopathology Laboratory, Friedrichshafen, Germany, [11] Department of Dermatology, University Hospital Erlangen, Erlangen, Germany, [12] Department of Dermatology, University Hospital Regensburg, Regensburg, Germany, [13] Department of Dermatology, University Hospital Essen, Essen, Germany, [14] Department of Dermatology, University Hospital Würzburg, Würzburg, Germany, [15] Department of Medical Oncology, Dana-Farber Cancer Institute, Boston, MA, United States, [16] Translational Cancer Epigenomics, Division of Translational Medical Oncology, German Cancer Research Center (DKFZ), Heidelberg, Germany, [17] Faculty of Medicine, Medical Center, Otto-von-Guericke-University, Magdeburg, Germany*

***Correspondence:**
*Titus J. Brinker*
*titus.brinker@dkfz.de*

Recent studies have shown that deep learning is capable of classifying dermatoscopic images at least as well as dermatologists. However, many studies in skin cancer classification utilize non-biopsy-verified training images. This imperfect ground truth introduces a systematic error, but the effects on classifier performance are currently unknown. Here, we systematically examine the effects of label noise by training and evaluating convolutional neural networks (CNN) with 804 images of melanoma and nevi labeled either by dermatologists or by biopsy. The CNNs are evaluated on a test set of 384 images by means of 4-fold cross validation comparing the outputs with either the corresponding dermatological or the biopsy-verified diagnosis. With identical ground truths of training and test labels, high accuracies with 75.03% (95% CI: 74.39–75.66%) for dermatological and 73.80% (95% CI: 73.10–74.51%) for biopsy-verified labels can be achieved. However, if the CNN is trained and tested with different ground truths, accuracy drops significantly to 64.53% (95% CI: 63.12–65.94%, $p < 0.01$) on a non-biopsy-verified and to 64.24% (95% CI: 62.66–65.83%, $p < 0.01$) on a biopsy-verified test set. In conclusion, deep learning methods for skin cancer classification are highly sensitive to label noise and future work should use biopsy-verified training images to mitigate this problem.

**Keywords: dermatology, artificial intelligence, label noise, skin cancer, melanoma, nevi**

## INTRODUCTION

Deep learning (DL) has revolutionized non-medical image analysis and is starting to change clinical workflows. DL can detect cancer in radiological images (1), can predict molecular changes from histology of cancer (2) and can be used to classify dermatoscopic images (3–6). Based on a large amount of input data and the corresponding class labels, the parameters of a neural network are optimized during the training phase in such a way that for an unknown input the predicted output ideally corresponds to the true class label. Both the input and the class labels are generally noisy, whereby the so-called feature noise has less dramatic effects on the classification quality than the label noise (7).

This is particularly the case in medical applications, since the available medical data sets are normally small and cost-intensive knowledge of experts is required for labeling to be as noise free as possible. Furthermore, there are high inter- and intra-rater variabilities in many medical classification tasks, which additionally increase label noise.

For example in dermatology, the visual inspection of a skin lesion show a significant error rate with respect to the gold standard pathology. In the binary classification task melanoma vs. nevi an average sensitivity and specificity of 82 and 59% is reported in Marchetti et al. (8). The same classification task is also investigated in Haenssle et al. (4), where the dermatologists achieved an average sensitivity and specificity of 86.6 and 71.3%, respectively.

In this paper, the effect of label noise on the performance of convolutional neural networks (CNNs) is to be investigated using the binary classification task between melanoma and nevus. In contrast to many existing studies, label noise is not generated artificially by random noise processes (9, 10), but rather by real-world labels that are either from: (a) several dermatologists or (b) the histopathological diagnosis of a biopsy. The latter diagnostic method has a statistically lower error rate and, therefore, most existing work in digital skin diagnosis attaches great importance to a biopsy-verified test set. However, due to the low availability and the high costs of acquiring biopsy-verified images a large amount of non-biopsy-verified images are often included in the training set whose diagnosis are based solely on a consensus decision of several dermatologists or on the lack of temporal lesion changes over several skin examinations (3, 8, 11–13). In doing so, high label noise is introduced in the modeling process. The hypothesis of this paper is that although the CNN learns the diagnostic performance of dermatologists through such a procedure, the performance for skin cancer classification with respect to the gold standard biopsy is severely limited.

This paper utilizes results of a previous reader study (6) where a total of 804 biopsy-verified images (402 melanoma and 402 nevi) were classified by several German dermatologists. For training and evaluating the CNN model two different ground truths are applied. As a first ground truth, the majority decision (MD) of the dermatologists involved in the reader study is considered for each image without taking the biopsy result into account. This means that both biopsy-verified melanoma can be labeled as nevi as well as biopsy-verified nevi can be labeled as melanoma. Furthermore, the result of a histopathological examination of a biopsy (BIO) is used as a second ground truth, which is the gold standard for skin cancer. In order to investigate the influence of label noise on the skin classification task, all combinations of these two different ground truths are applied for training and test set, so that a total of four scenarios can be distinguished: [1] training with MD and testing with MD, [2] training with MD and testing with BIO, [3] training with BIO and testing with MD, and [4] training with BIO and testing with BIO. For each scenario in this setting, we can evaluate the influence of label noise independent of the image selection for training and test set, since for each image both ground truths are available.

## RESULTS

To obtain the labels based on the majority decision of several dermatologists, we sent six electronic questionnaires each containing 134 images of nevi and melanoma to nine German university hospitals. In total, the six questionnaires were completed 144 times (19,296 images were evaluated); 52 questionnaires were filled out by board-certified dermatologists (evaluation of 6,968 images), and 92 by junior dermatologists (evaluation of 12,328 images). Each of the 804 individual images was evaluated by an average of 21.3 dermatologists (median = 21; standard deviation = 4.8; range = 4–31).

The majority decision of dermatologists correctly classified 261 melanomas, 141 melanomas were wrongly classified as nevus. Among the biopsy-verified nevi, 266 were correctly identified by the majority decision, 136 nevi were misclassified as malignant. This results in an overall sensitivity and specificity of 64.9 and 66.2%, respectively. In the subset of 384 images representing the test set, the dermatologists correctly recognize 135 of 188 melanomas, which corresponds to a sensitivity with respect to the gold standard of 71.8%. Considering only the biopsy-verified nevi in the test set, 115 of 196 nevi are correctly classified by dermatologists resulting in an overall specificity of 58.7%.

Training and evaluating a CNN with identical ground truth labels, high accuracies with 75.03% (95% CI: 74.39–75.66%) for dermatological and 73.80% (95% CI: 73.10–74.51%) for biopsy-verified labels can be achieved. However, if the CNN is trained and tested with different ground truths, the accuracy drops significantly. If the CNN is trained with biopsy-verified labels and tested with dermatological labels, accuracy drops significantly to 64.53% (95% CI: 63.12–65.94%, $p < 0.01$). In the contrary case, an accuracy of 64.24% (95% CI: 62.66–65.83%, $p < 0.01$) is achieved on a biopsy-verified test set. **Table 1** summarizes the results for the primary and secondary study endpoints for all four scenarios.

In **Figure 1**, the boxplots for the primary endpoint accuracy as well as the secondary endpoints sensitivity and specificity are depicted for all four scenarios. The receiver operating characteristic (ROC) curves illustrating the relationship between sensitivity and specificity for different cut-off values are shown in **Figure 2**.

Furthermore, **Figure 3** shows on the left side the four test images for which the outputs of the CNN trained with dermatological labels and those trained with biopsy-verified

**TABLE 1 |** Statistical evaluation of the primary study endpoint (accuracy) and the secondary study endpoints (sensitivity and specificity) for the four different scenarios (training with ground truth majority decision (MD)/testing with ground truth biopsy (BIO), training with MD/testing with BIO, training with BIO/testing with MD, and training with BIO/testing with BIO).

| **Ground truth for training** | **MD** | | **BIO** | |
|---|---|---|---|---|
| **Ground truth for testing** | **MD** | **BIO** | **MD** | **BIO** |
| Mean accuracy | 75.03% | 64.24% | 64.53% | 73.80% |
| 95% CI accuracy | 74.39–75.66% | 62.66–65.83% | 63.12–65.94% | 73.10–74.51% |
| Mean sensitivity | 76.76% | 69.65% | 64.31% | 75.98% |
| 95% CI sensitivity | 75.36–78.15% | 67.92–71.37% | 62.74–65.88% | 74.69–77.26% |
| Mean specificity | 73.00% | 59.05% | 64.79% | 71.85% |
| 95% CI specificity | 71.10–74.90% | 56.56–61.54% | 63.20–66.38% | 71.08–72.61% |

labels differ the most. In the upper part of each image the majority decision of the dermatologists (MD) and the result of the biopsy (BIO) is given. On the right side, the boxplots of the corresponding outputs over the 10 conducted simulation runs are presented.

## DISCUSSION

If a CNN is trained with the diagnosis of several dermatologists, it achieves high-quality results on a test set whose labels have also been created by dermatologists. Convolutional neural networks are therefore able to identify the features in an image that dermatologists are looking for and use them as basis for decision-making. However, with this combination of ground truths it also learns the sources of errors in the dermatological decision. Comparing the achieved sensitivity and specificity with 76.76 and 73.0% with the performance of the dermatologists on the test set (71.8 and 58.7%), the two metrics are substantially higher. This difference may be caused by learning a systematic error of the dermatological diagnosis.

If, however, a CNN trained with majority decisions is tested on a test set with biopsy-verified ground truths, the statistical metrics decrease significantly. In detail, the average accuracy drops from 75.03 to 64.24%. Here it is particularly interesting that the average sensitivity and specificity with 69.65 and 59.05% are in similar orders of magnitude as the statistical metrics of the dermatological diagnoses on the 384 test images regarding the gold standard, i.e., the included.

If a CNN is trained with biopsy-verified images, the accuracy of 73.80% in a test with biopsy-verified images is a little bit lower than the results of a CNN trained and evaluated with dermatological labels. Therefore, learning the relationship between image and corresponding biopsy-verified

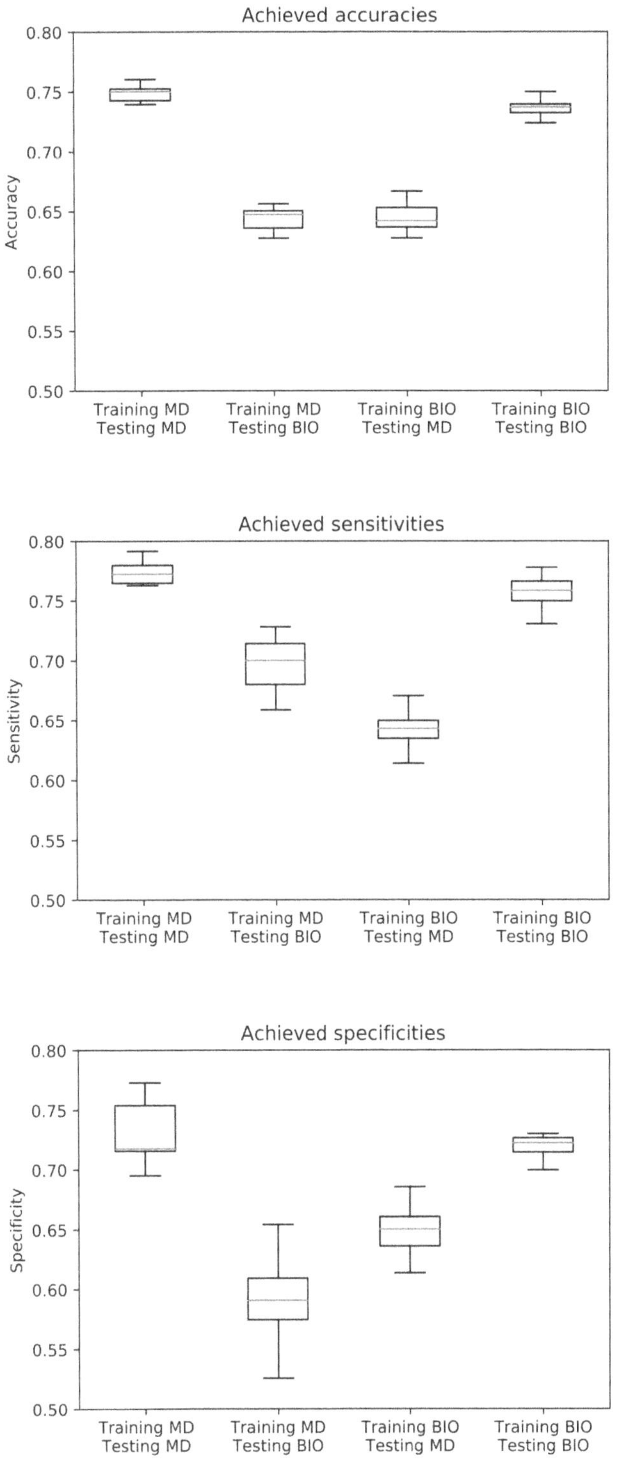


**FIGURE 1 |** Boxplot of the achieved accuracies, sensitivities, and specificities over 10 simulation runs. 804 biopsy-verified images of nevi and melanoma are labeled by both the majority decision of several dermatologists (MD) and by a biopsy-verified ground truth (BIO). All combinations of these two different ground truths are applied for training and test set, so that a total of four scenarios can be distinguished (MD/MD, BIO/MD, BIO/BIO, MD/BIO). 4-fold cross-validation is applied on a test set of 384 images to evaluate the performance of the algorithm.

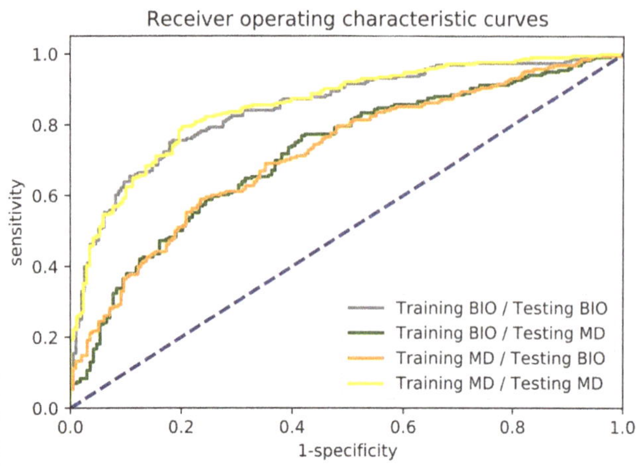


**FIGURE 2 |** Receiver operating characteristic (ROC) curves of all four scenarios. For calculating the ROC curves, the outputs of each image are averaged over the conducted 10 simulation runs.

class labels seems to be a bit harder than learning to mimic the dermatological diagnosis. However, in a test with images whose labels were created by majority decisions of dermatologists, the accuracy also drops to 64.53%. This is also within the range of the label noise.

In all considered scenarios, the accuracies achieved by dermatologists are lower than the reported performance from clinical routine. This is probably due to the selection bias. As all lesions in the study were biopsied, they represent edge cases in general and are naturally difficult to classify. It can be assumed that the accuracy will increase if simpler cases are added to the test set.

There are some limitations of the study. While claiming that deep learning models for skin cancer classification are strongly affected by label noise, only one specific CNN architecture, namely ResNet50, is investigated, thus questioning whether this is truly representative of deep learning models in general. However, the performance of the most common architectures (ResNet, AlexNet, VGGNet, Inception) have been shown to be comparable for most classification tasks.

Furthermore, the overall number of 804 test and training images is very small and as a result the achieved accuracy, sensitivity, and specificity on a biopsy-verified test set are marginally lower than in our previous studies. However, it can be reasonably expected that the relations between the results of the individual scenarios will be comparable for a larger number of images.

## MATERIALS AND METHODS

The reader study (6) included 804 images with biopsy-verified labels (402 melanoma and 402 nevi), all of which randomly selected from the publicly available database HAM10000 and the ISIC archive (14). These images were sent to dermatologists from nine German university hospitals via six randomly assigned electronic questionnaires, each containing 134 images of either melanoma or nevi. In addition to the classification, the dermatologists were also asked to assess the quality of the images. Only images with at least "sufficient" image quality ("excellent," "good," "sufficient"), as rated by the participating dermatologists were included in this study.

To train a CNN with the small number of 804 available images we apply cross-validation which partitions a sample of data into complementary subsets. Since some of the databases in the ISIC archive contain multiple images of the same lesion and the identification of these duplicates is not generally reliably possible with the metadata provided, we restrict the test set to images of HAM10000, where duplicates can be identified by the provided attribute "lesion_id." This results in 384 images remaining for the evaluation of the algorithm, which are splitted into 4 folds for cross-validation. When testing with one of these splits, all images from the ISIC archive as well as all images with different lesions IDs from HAM10000 from the reader study are used for training.

We conducted 10 simulation runs with a pre-defined training procedure and fixed hyperparameter, in each of which a random process generates a mutually disjoint training and test set according to the above-mentioned rules.

### Training of the CNNs

A ResNet-50 pre-trained on the ImageNet database was selected for the classification of melanoma and nevi. A complete training run consisted of 14 epochs.

During training, the network was first trained in a frozen state, where only fully-connected layers were trained at a high learning rate. This was followed by a step where the complete network was trained using differential learning rates. Earlier layers, which were already pre-trained and fine-tuned to detect general features, such as basic shapes and color gradients, were trained on low values. The further the layer is from the input, the larger the learning rate becomes until a pre-set maximum is reached. Differential learning rates allow for a stronger modification of the later layers, which represent application-specific features, and therefore need more adjustment than pre-trained earlier layers.

All work was carried out in Python 3.7.3 and fastai 1.0 for model.

### Statistical Evaluation

The results of the 10 simulation runs are statistically evaluated by the python modules scikit-learn (version 0.21) and scipy (version 1.3). Throughout the paper, the cut-off value is set to 0.5, i.e., if the output of the CNN is higher than 0.5 or equal, the corresponding input image is classified as melanoma, otherwise as nevi. Since the test set is nearly balanced with respect to the two considered classes, accuracy as a scalar measure of classification quality is a suitable choice and therefore represents the primary endpoint of this study. In order to evaluate the influence of the label noise as a function of the two considered classes, sensitivity and specificity are additionally calculated as the secondary study

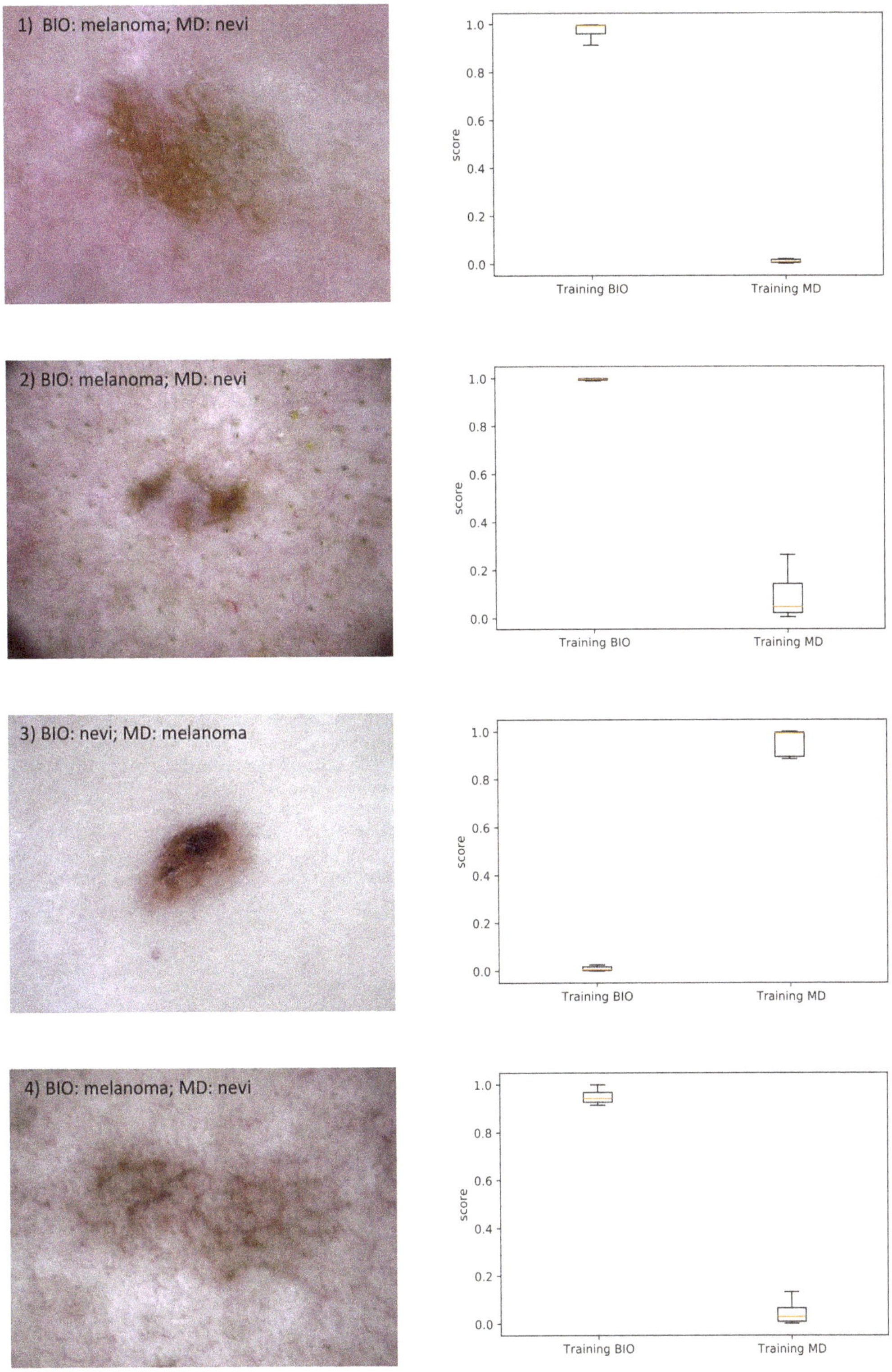


**FIGURE 3 |** On the left side, the 4 test images are shown for which the outputs of the CNN trained with dermatological labels and those trained with biopsy-verified labels differ the most. In the upper part of each image the majority decision of the dermatologists (MD) and the result of the biopsy (BIO) is given. On the right side, the boxplots of the corresponding outputs of the two CNNs over the 10 conducted simulation runs are presented.

endpoints. The primary and secondary endpoints are reported by means and confidence intervals calculated based on the corresponding metrics over the four splits of cross validation. In order to illustrate the relationship between sensitivity and specificity the receiver operating characteristic (ROC) curve is calculated for each CNN based on the averaged outputs of each image over the conducted 10 simulation runs. For statistical testing, we use the Wilcoxon test, which is a non-parametric statistical hypothesis test and compares two related samples. Throughout the paper, the significance level is set to 0.05.

## ETHICS STATEMENT

Ethics approval for the online survey was waived by the ethics committee of the University of Heidelberg due to the fact that all of the participants remained anonymous. Ethical approval for this study was not required in accordance with local legislation and national guidelines.

## AUTHOR CONTRIBUTIONS

AH, JK, EK-H, RM, MS, and TB contributed to the study concept and design. AH carried out the study implementation, data collection and statistical analysis with contributions from RM, EK-H, and JU. JSU, CB, SH, DS, and BS co-organized the reader study and have therefore contributed relevant data to this study. FM, FG, JU, LF, JS, KG, TW, HK, CB, MH, WS, BI, SF, and DL provided data analysis and/or interpretation of data for this study. TB oversaw the study, critically reviewed and edited the manuscript and gave final approval. All authors provided critical review and commentary on the draft manuscript and approved the final version. All authors guarantee the integrity and accuracy of this study.

## REFERENCES


1. McKinney SM, Sieniek M, Godbole V, Godwin J, Antropova N, Ashrafian H, et al. International evaluation of an AI system for breast cancer screening. *Nature.* (2020) 57789–94. doi: 10.1038/s41586-019-1799-6
2. Kather JN, Pearson AT, Halama N, Jäger D, Krause J, Loosen SH, et al. Deep learning can predict microsatellite instability directly from histology in gastrointestinal cancer. *Nature Med.* (2019) 1:12–6. doi: 10.1038/s41591-019-0462-y
3. Esteva A, Kuprel B, Novoa RA, Ko J, Swetter SM, Blau HM, et al. Dermatologist-level classification of skin cancer with deep neural networks. *Nature.* (2017) 542:115–8. doi: 10.1038/nature21056
4. Haenssle HA, Fink C, Schneiderbauer R, Toberer F, Buhl T, Blum A, et al. Man against machine: diagnostic performance of a deep learning convolutional neural network for dermoscopic melanoma recognition in comparison to 58 dermatologists. *Annals Oncol.* (2018) 29:1836–42. doi: 10.1093/annonc/mdy166
5. Tschandl P, Rosendahl C, Akay BN, Argenziano G, Blum A, Braun RP, et al. Expert-level diagnosis of nonpigmented skin cancer by combined convolutional neural networks. *JAMA Dermatol.* (2019) 155:58–65. doi: 10.1001/jamadermatol.2018.4378
6. Brinker TJ, Hekler A, Enk AH, Berking C, Haferkamp S, Hauschild A, et al. Deep neural networks are superior to dermatologists in melanoma image classification. *Eur J Cancer.* (2019) 119:11–7. doi: 10.1016/j.ejca.2019.05.023
7. Zhu X, Wu X. Class noise vs. attribute noise: a quantitative study. *Artific Intelligence Rev.* (2004) 22:177–210. doi: 10.1007/s10462-004-0751-8
8. Marchetti MA, Codella NC, Dusza SW, Gutman DA, Helba B, Kalloo A, et al. Results of the 2016 International Skin Imaging Collaboration International Symposium on Biomedical Imaging challenge: comparison of the accuracy of computer algorithms to dermatologists for the diagnosis of melanoma from dermoscopic images. *J Am Acad Dermatol.* (2018) 78:270–7.e1. doi: 10.1016/j.jaad.2017.08.016
9. Han B, Yao Q, Yu X, Niu G, Xu M, Hu W, et al. Co-teaching: Robust training of deep neural networks with extremely noisy labels. *Adv Neural Inform Proces Syst.* (2018) 2:7–9.
10. Patrini G, Rozza A, Krishna Menon A, Nock R, Qu L (editors). Making deep neural networks robust to label noise: A loss correction approach. In: Proceedings of the IEEE Conference on Computer Vision and Pattern Recognition (2017). doi: 10.1109/CVPR.2017.240
11. Brinker TJ, Hekler A, Hauschild A, Berking C, Schilling B, Enk AH, et al. Comparing artificial intelligence algorithms to 157 German dermatologists: the melanoma classification benchmark. *Eur J Cancer.* (2019) 111:30–7. doi: 10.1016/j.ejca.2018.12.016
12. Codella NC, Gutman D, Celebi ME, Helba B, Marchetti MA, Dusza SW, et al. (editors). Skin lesion analysis toward melanoma detection: A challenge at the 2017 international symposium on biomedical imaging (isbi), hosted by the international skin imaging collaboration (isic). In: *2018 IEEE 15th International Symposium on Biomedical Imaging (ISBI 2018) (2018)* IEEE. doi: 10.1109/ISBI.2018.8363547
13. Haenssle HA, Fink C, Toberer F, Winkler J, Stolz W, Deinlein T, et al. Man against machine reloaded: performance of a market-approved convolutional neural network in classifying a broad spectrum of skin lesions in comparison with 96 dermatologists working under less artificial conditions. *Annals Oncol.* (2020) 31:137–43. doi: 10.1016/j.annonc.2019.10.013
14. Tschandl P, Rosendahl C, Kittler H. The HAM10000 dataset, a large collection of multi-source dermatoscopic images of common pigmented skin lesions. *Sci Data.* (2018) 5:180161. doi: 10.1038/sdata.2018.161

# 23

# High-Frequency Ultrasonography—Possibilities and Perspectives of the Use of 20 MHz in Teledermatology

*Adriana Polańska [1]*, Dorota Jenerowicz [2], Elżbieta Paszyńska [3], Ryszard Żaba [1], Zygmunt Adamski [2] and Aleksandra Dańczak-Pazdrowska [2]*

*[1] Department of Dermatology and Venereology, Poznań University of Medical Sciences, Poznań, Poland, [2] Department of Dermatology, Poznań University of Medical Sciences, Poznań, Poland, [3] Department of Integrated Dentistry, Poznań University of Medical Sciences, Poznań, Poland*

***Correspondence:**
*Adriana Polańska*
*adriana-polanska@wp.pl*

High-frequency ultrasonography (HF-USG) is a non-invasive and *in vivo* method of visualization of the skin and upper part of subcutaneous tissue based on ultrasounds above 20 MHz. Although initially HF-USG was introduced to measure skin thickness, it currently gained widespread acceptance in dermato-oncology, primarily when used to determine skin tumor margins. Moreover, its application in different dermatology fields is known, particularly as a rapidly evolving method in the objective evaluation of the severity of various chronic skin diseases. Among different specialties, teledermatology belongs to leading and continually developing areas of successful telemedicine applications. Various skin conditions are visible to the human eye, which makes them particularly suitable for telemedicine. However, HF-USG enables specialists to look into deeper skin layers, thus extending diagnostic options. On the other hand, teledermatology creates the possibility of sending images for consultation and facilitates the therapeutic decision as HF-USG can be used in an asynchronous store and forward manner. It seems that HF-USG and teledermatology may be regarded as a truly matched pair. The aim of this work is to present current applications of 20-MHz ultrasonography in dermatology, including skin neoplasms and chronic skin diseases. Moreover, the authors aimed to analyze the possibilities of HF-USG use as a valuable tool in teledermatology, especially in diagnosing and monitoring patients suffering from long-lasting skin conditions.

**Keywords: teledermatology, melanoma, atopic dermatitis, mycosis fungoides, high-frequency ultrasonography**

## INTRODUCTION

According to the World Health Organization (WHO), telemedicine utilizes communication technologies in healthcare to exchange medical information for the diagnosis, treatment, prevention, research, evaluation, and education over a distance (1). Therefore, it can be considered a merge of expertise and communication technology, giving patients the possibility of being examined, monitored, and managed by a medical expert in a distant location. Electronic transfer of information may be accomplished in various ways. Still, two basic types currently in practice are "real-time" or "live interactive" (LI) (enables direct communication sender–recipient with an immediate result) and "store-and-forward" (SAF) telemedicine (digital images and patient data are captured, transferred, and stored) (2–4). Teledermatology belongs to the earliest and leading areas of the successful use of telemedicine solutions. Nowadays, it is applied among all kinds of medical facilities, including hospitals, primary care, or nursing homes (5, 6).

The principle aim of teledermatology seems to be to consult and to educate. Digital communication brings possibilities for the exchange of medical information between the patient and the specialist. What is more, a recent modality—"patient-assisted teledermatology," or "home-based teledermatology"—has been vigorously developing (7). After the first visit and face-to-face diagnosis by the dermatologist, a patient is then supposed to send pictures documenting the skin's condition. This form combines SAF teledermatology and mobile technology tools. It is particularly useful for patients with chronic diseases, such as psoriasis, atopic dermatitis, vitiligo, or leg ulcers.

One of the emerging technologies that may find application in teledermatology and implement WHO assumptions seems to be high-frequency ultrasonography (HF-USG). Although initially HF-USG was introduced to measure skin thickness, currently it has gained widespread acceptance in dermato-oncology, particularly to determine margins of skin tumors (8–10). Moreover, its application in different dermatology fields is known, particularly as a rapidly evolving method in the objective evaluation of the severity of the various chronic skin diseases (11–13). The possibility of sending images for consultation may facilitate therapeutic decisions as HF-USG can be used in a SAF manner.

We present the actual applications of 20-MHz ultrasonography in dermatology and analyze the possibility of its use as a valuable tool in teledermatology, especially in managing patients suffering from chronic skin diseases.

## BASIC PRINCIPLES OF HF-USG

The pioneering use of the ultrasound beam in dermatology was carried out in the 1980s by Alexander and Miller with a 15-MHz probe (8). As is known, routine imaging of the abdominal organs is possible with the use of ultrasound waves in the 3–5-MHz range, while for the assessment of more superficial structures (such as lymph nodes, testes, or the thyroid gland), frequencies in the range 7.5–15 MHz are needed. The imaging of the skin became possible with the invention of transducers emitting waves with higher vibration ranges, and now ultrasound scanners of 20 MHz (High Frequency Ultrasonography, HF-USG) and higher (Ultra High Frequency Ultrasonography, UHF-USG) are used for skin examination (14). According to the Guidelines for Performing Dermatologic Ultrasound Examinations, the minimum frequency for dermatological analysis should be 15 MHz (15). However, considering the multifrequency property of available probes, the use of the range from 15 to 22 MHz for better visualization of deeper lesions is suggested (15).

The use of 20-MHz heads allows for images of structures at a depth of 8–10 mm and, according to some manufacturers, even up to 15 mm (14, 16). The higher the frequency, the better the picture resolution. The axial resolution is defined as the minimum distance that can be differentiated between two reflectors located parallel to the ultrasound beam's direction. In comparison, the lateral one is the minimum distance that can be distinguished between two reflectors situated perpendicular to the ultrasound beam's path. Fifty MHz can achieve 20 and 100 μm resolution, respectively, while 20 MHz can achieve 80 and 200 μm (17). The emission of an ultrasound beam by a piezoelectric transducer and its reception enables the analysis of echoes in various presentations. The oldest presentation is of the A-type—it analyzes the echo amplitude as a function of time and allows measurements to be made. However, most often, the B-type presentation is used to analyze the ultrasound image, which is an overlay of many A-type presentations in real time, in which echoes have been converted into glowing spots and mapped on the screen using a grayscale (256-degree grayscale) (18, 19). Thanks to the B-type presentation, it is possible to analyze the echogenicity. The echogenic structures appear bright on ultrasound images (the higher the amplitude of the reflected wave, the brighter the pixel) (14, 16, 18).

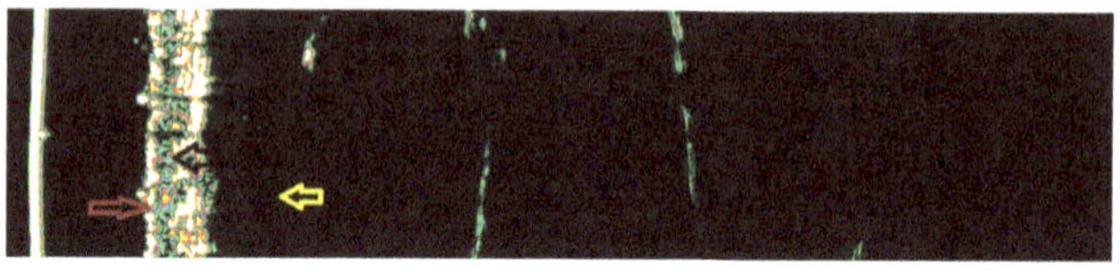

**FIGURE 1** | The HF-USG image of healthy skin of the forearm. Red arrow—the echo from the surface of the epidermis; black arrow—dermis; yellow arrow—subcutaneous tissue.

The ultrasound image of healthy skin corresponds to the skin layers visible on histological examination. We can distinguish three layers that differ in echogenicity (14, 18, 19) (**Figure 1**). The first layer, usually called entrance echo, is hyperechoic and reflects the upper (mainly dead) parts of the epidermis. Below, there is a layer of less echogenicity—which corresponds to the lower layers of the epidermis, the dermoepidermal border, and, above all, the dermis, within which echoes of varying intensity are visible. The lowest layer can be easily distinguishable because it is hypoechogenic in nature and corresponds to the subcutaneous tissue, which (depending on the anatomical location and sex) can be visualized to various depths (14, 18, 19).

## DIAGNOSTIC PROPERTIES OF HF-USG IN TELEDERMATOLOGY

According to an interesting report by Warshaw et al. (20), performed for The American Veterans Health Services Research, in-person dermatology diagnostic accuracy is of a higher quality than teledermatology. While overall management accuracy rates seem to be equivalent, in the case of malignant and premalignant lesions, rates for teledermatology and teledermatoscopy are inferior to the usual care. It is then recommended to be cautious when using teledermatology in such cases. These observations have to be considered in regard to implementing HF-USG in

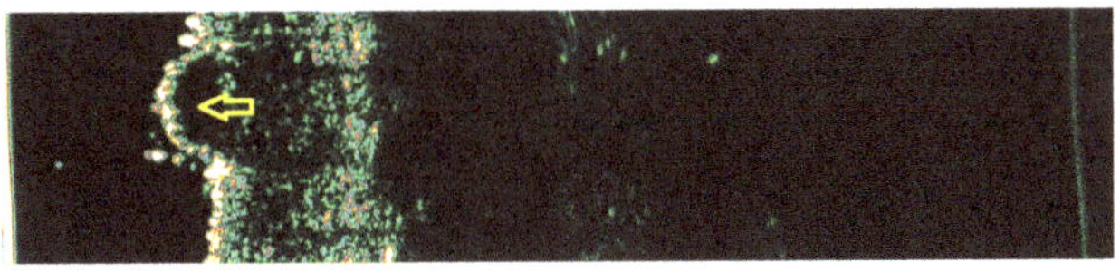

**FIGURE 2 |** Cellular nevus. Yellow arrow—hypoechogenic mass corresponding to the nevus.

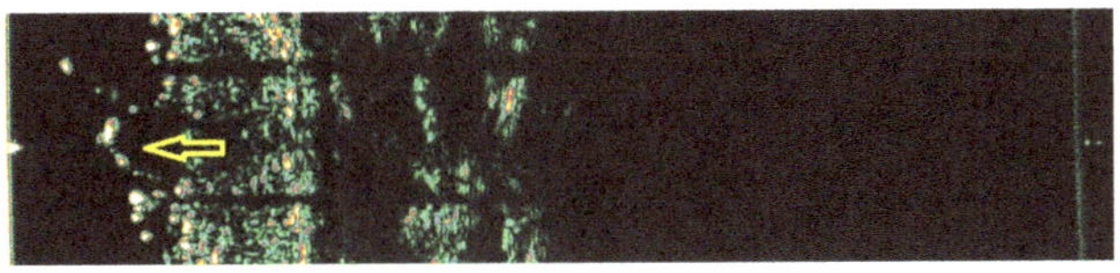

**FIGURE 3 |** Melanoma. Yellow arrow—hypoechogenic mass corresponding to the melanoma.

teledermatology modalities, particularly concerning pigmented lesions and tumors.

Various skin pathologies change the echogenicity of its individual layers, which can be used to analyze the ultrasound image. However, the lack of sufficient resolution does not allow a full interpretation of the image with microscopic examination accuracy. Hypoechoic structures can be both of neoplastic and inflammatory origin (14, 21, 22). Moreover, an identical ultrasound image is observed in melanoma and a benign melanocytic nevus. Due to the insufficient resolution of HF-USG, the process cannot be distinguished at the cell level (**Figures 2, 3**). Although literature has tried to identify more specific features for various skin neoplasms, the final diagnosis should still be supported by histological examination. In melanoma, echolucent areas can be observed, with a shape depending on the subtype. The nodular form may have a spherical arrangement, while superficial spreading melanoma presents as an echolucent area parallel to the entry echo. However, there are no ultrasonographic features pathognomonic for melanoma (14).

What is more, the accuracy of ultrasound analysis may be increased with a Color Doppler ultrasound. This modality is recommended, especially for discriminating between vascular or non-vascular lesions and recognizing the benign or malignant nature of skin tumors (15, 23, 24). In previous studies, vascular signal use in assessing melanoma correlated with the Breslow index and metastatic potential (23). The addition of Color-Doppler in pigmented lesion analysis may have a significant prognostic value (25, 26).

In basal cell carcinoma (BCC), the HF-USG can detect the presence of hyperechoic spots, the so-called cotton flowers; however, in the authors' opinion, this is not a phenomenon that occurs in all tumors and therefore cannot be defining for BCC (14, 21, 27) (**Figure 4**). In squamous cell carcinoma (SCC) and actinic keratosis, scaling may disturb the image's interpretation. This seems to be a crucial limitation of HF-USG in evaluating hyperkeratotic tumors (10, 18, 19).

**FIGURE 4 |** Basal cell carcinoma. Yellow arrow—hypoechogenic mass corresponding to the basal cell carcinoma.

It is worth noting that the usefulness of HF-USG for assessing the thickness of BCC and melanoma infiltration has been well-documented and is now considered a recognized indication for HF-USG (14, 28–32). The preoperative determination of the surgical margins determines the future management and patients' prognosis (particularly in the case of melanoma). Previous studies confirm the agreement between a histological and ultrasonographic measurement with a high compliance rate (28–33). Therefore, the HF-USG assessment of tumor size may be then transferred to a dermato-oncologist or surgeon during teleconsultation to plan the future procedure. This way, teledermatology may globally contribute to better outcomes and radical treatment. However, it should be considered that the thickness of the tumor determined by ultrasound is slightly greater than the thickness determined histologically, due to shrinkage of the material during histological preparation and accumulation of inflammatory cells underneath the tumor (10, 24, 28). Another limitation of the proper margin assessment is the tumor size, mainly when it crosses the dermis border and penetrates the subcutaneous tissue, which is also hypoechogenic. However, the use of a multifrequency probe may reduce this limitation. The preoperative evaluation of the tumor margins may also be difficult in patients with evident photoaging, where elastosis decreases the skin echogenicity, similarly to the neoplasmatic cells (14).

Due to the low diagnostic properties of HF-USG in oncodermatology, the combination of this method with a preliminary dermoscopic evaluation may be extremely useful. Therefore, an initial diagnosis of probable pathology should be performed using a dermoscope, followed by an evaluation of disease extent using HF-USG. Acquired data, provided in the form of telecommunication, may significantly improve the diagnostic and therapeutic process. These observations remain consistent with teledermatology's role in the process of triaging (particularly the SAF method), which influences the cost-effectiveness of therapies and may limit waiting time in the case of urgent patients (34). Moreover, the inclusion of dermatoscopic images improves triaging decisions, including a need for an excision for both melanomas and other skin cancers (35).

## THE MONITORING PROPERTIES OF HF-USG IN TELEDERMATOLOGY

Due to the limited diagnostic value of ultrasonography, the monitoring properties of HF-USG are noteworthy. They allow for observing changes dynamically—occurring in the skin over

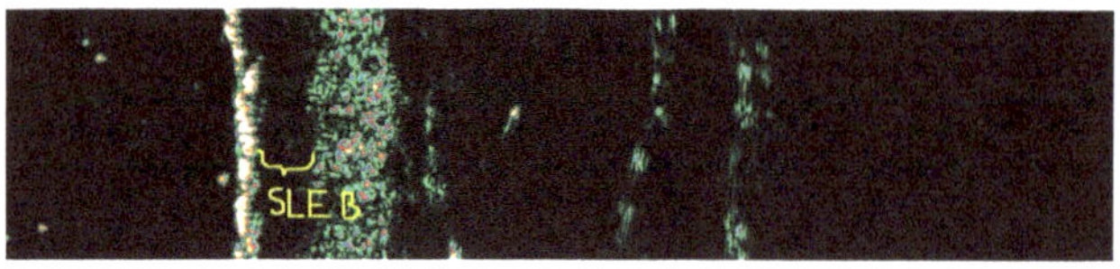

**FIGURE 5 |** Subepidermal low echogenic band (SLEB) within the plaque of mycosis fungoides before treatment (the hypoechogenic band corresponding to the SLEB was marked).

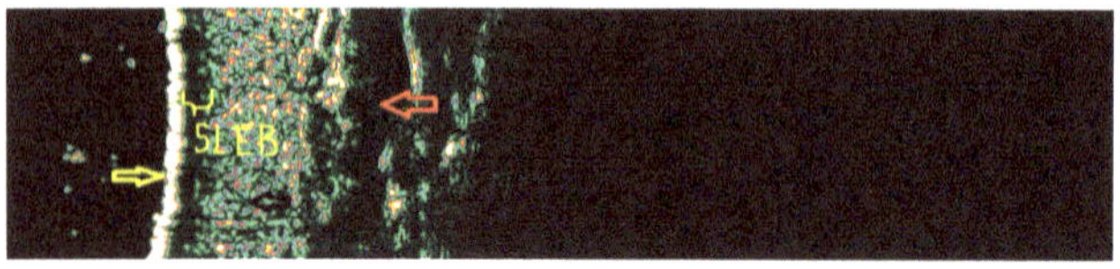

**FIGURE 6 |** The thinning of the SLEB after treatment. Lack of complete disappearance of SLEB still shows the presence of neoplastic T cell infiltrations (the hypoechogenic band corresponding to the SLEB was marked).

time, mainly due to the introduced treatment (**Figures 5**, **6**). Inflammatory and neoplastic cells cause a reduction of skin echogenicity and may result in the formation of a linear band underneath the entry echo, known as the subepidermal low echogenic band (SLEB) (11, 12, 14). Originally, SLEB was observed in photodamaged skin due to glycosaminoglycan accumulation, which possesses an increased water-binding capacity (14, 18). The SLEB formation was well-documented in inflammatory diseases, including psoriasis and atopic dermatitis (11–13, 36, 37). It is not a parameter specific for any skin disease, but its changes over time are of prognostic significance, especially in patients with chronic skin diseases. The areas of reduced echogenicity are mainly related to swelling of the skin and inflammatory cell infiltration. The SLEB thickness in atopic dermatitis correlated with the degree of several histopathologic findings like epidermal hyperplasia, epidermal hyperkeratosis, the degree of parakeratosis, and the degree of spongiosis as well as the intensity of inflammatory infiltrates (38). However, in psoriatic plaque, SLEB's uniformity can be disturbed by streaky shadows perpendicular to the entry echo (most likely caused by air bubbles trapped between the scales). It is observed that SLEB thickness corresponds to the severity of skin lesions and can be used to monitor patients, also potentially as a teledermatology consultation (14, 39).

In one of our first studies, monitoring properties of HF-USG were assessed for atopic dermatitis and so-called proactive therapy, using tacrolimus ointment (40). Six-month ultrasound monitoring was performed in a group of 39 patients with atopic dermatitis (mean age 26 years). It revealed the significant decrease of SLEB value during the undergone therapy, which correlated with the disease severity assessed by measuring scales (40). We found that HF-USG allowed clinicians to visualize pathologic changes of all skin *in vivo*. As a non-invasive and independent of subjective judgment method, HF-USG should be added to the overall patient evaluation, especially in the era of evidence-based medicine (41). We presented that SLEB was detected within lesional skin and in non-affected skin regions, revealing the presence of subclinical inflammation (42, 43). Such patients may significantly benefit most from proactive treatment (40, 42). Information on the decrease of SLEB or lack of its change could be provided in the form of a teleconference to the attending physician with information about the need to intensify the treatment process. It could also be combined with an emerging teledermatology branch—patient-assisted teledermatology (also called home-based teledermatology)—which involves the SAF method and mobile technology tools. It is regarded as especially useful for patients with chronic dermatoses (psoriasis, atopic dermatitis, vitiligo, leg ulcers) and allows the specialist to monitor the phase and the degree of skin lesions. The above method is relatively new (started in 2009) and is used for both diagnosis and follow-up (20, 35).

SLEB thickness objective measurement as a useful, accurate parameter for skin assessment was also performed in psoriasis (14, 36). Queille-Roussel et al. (36) evaluated an innovative aerosol foam formulation's anti-psoriatic effect and analyzed this parameter's thickness. They found a reduction of SLEB in week 4. We also assessed monitoring properties of HF-USG in a prospective, observational study, which included 58 patients diagnosed with recurrent chronic small plaque psoriasis treated with a two-compound ointment containing calcipotriol and betamethasone dipropionate or NB-UVB (311 nm) (11). The SLEB was significantly decreased in both treated groups. The lack of its decrease, similarly to atopic dermatitis, indicated no improvement in the dermatological condition or the need to change/intensify therapy (11, 14). Such information could be consulted with a dermatologist without the need to travel and access the specialist advice more easily, especially in rural areas. What is essential, a high correlation between SLEB and PASI index indicates that HF-USG quickly complements the measurement of the severity of skin lesions in psoriasis in an objective way (11).

Monitoring properties of HF-USG seem to be particularly useful in assessing the therapeutical outcomes in patients with mycosis fungoides. They can be used in teleconsultations also with a non-dermatologist (i.e., hematologist). Neoplastic cells are responsible for decreasing echogenicity, which in mycosis fungoides also manifests in the form of SLEB, similarly to inflammatory diseases (12, 14, 44–46). We have found strong correlations between SLEB thickness and the thickness of subepidermal infiltration in histopathological examination (47). As it is known, in mycosis fungoides, the proper staging is essential in planning the therapy. It should include a detailed evaluation of the skin lesion types and an assessment of the pathological process' extent (45, 47). For 5 years, we followed up patients based on HF-USG, where SLEB was the assessed parameter (48). We evaluated well-known forms of therapies in mycosis fungoides (the effectiveness of UVA1 and PUVA). We monitored these patients' clinical responses compared to the modified Severity Weighted Assessment Tool (mSWAT) (12). Complete response in examined patients correlated with the entire disappearance of SLEB (12, 48). SLEB thickness was associated with disease severity and was wider in stage IIA patients than in stage IA and IB patients (48). For the first time, we revealed that HF-USG is a tool for evaluating the patient's response and can be applied in routine clinical practice.

What is more, using HF-USG, there is a possibility to distinguish a lesion of the type of post-inflammatory hyper/hypopigmentation from a non-specific infiltrative lesion (12, 47, 48). Performing ultrasound measurements enables the patient to be consulted with a dermatologist/hematologist without a face-to-face visit and can significantly improve the therapeutic process. In the case of irradiated patients, a routine practice in our clinic is the ultrasound supervision of patients and making decisions about additional radiation if a visible SLEB is still observed. Again, collected data can be then sent to a photodermatology center.

The practical application of HF-USG is its use in hidradenitis suppurativa (49). Recent studies proposed this method to optimize staging, treatment planning, and monitoring patients suffering from this chronic disease (49). Wortsman et al. (50) proposed a three-point sonographic scoring system for hidradenitis suppurativa, based on the number and distribution of fluid collections, fistulous tracts, and pseudocystic nodules, widening of the hair follicles, and alterations in the dermal thickness/echogenicity. According to the authors, the proper staging of these patients resulted in a management modification in 82% of cases (51). It seems that HF-USG in relation to hidradenitis suppurativa may also be conducted in the form of teleconsultation with other specialists (diagnostic and radiological center, dermatological surgeons). The possibility of an ultrasound consultation can improve diagnosis and help choose an appropriate therapeutic option (depending on the severity of skin lesions).

## THE ADVANTAGES AND LIMITATIONS OF HF-USG

The most significant advantages of HF-USG in a monitoring examination are non-invasiveness, safety, and the possibility of multiple scans without the need to prepare the patient in advance. It seems that in the era of scrupulously determined scales determining the extent and severity of skin lesions during various treatments of skin diseases, especially to qualify patients for biological therapies and research programs, HF-USG can find an application. In the case of teledermatology, the possibility of transmitting images in between clinicians and of archiving images and analyzing them over time contributes an extremely useful visual *in vivo* method. Teleconsultation with the use of HF-USG may improve the treatment process of chronic dermatological diseases requiring long-term care. The possibility of simultaneous dermoscopy and ultrasound of the skin may have a prognostic significance in skin tumors.

Among the main limitations of HF-USG, its high price should be mentioned, as well as restricted availability of the apparatus in a doctor's office. As in the case of dermoscopy, acquiring the ability to interpret an ultrasonographic image requires appropriate training. Lately, also other techniques of non-invasive skin visualization are gaining interest in regard to associations with teledermatology—for example, reflectance confocal microscopy (RCM). RCM allows an *in vivo* evaluation of various skin lesions on the cellular level—nearly to histologic resolution. In comparison to this technique, it has to be emphasized that HF-USG does not possess sufficient resolution and its diagnostic properties are much lower (52).

## AUTHOR CONTRIBUTIONS

All authors listed have made a substantial, direct and intellectual contribution to the work, and approved it for publication.

## ACKNOWLEDGMENTS

The authors are entirely grateful to Dr. Tomasz Maksymiuk (MD, Ph.D.), who provided English grammar editing and really improved the quality and understanding of the whole manuscript.

## REFERENCES

1. *Telemedicine: Opportunities and Developments in Member States: Report on the Second Global Survey on eHealth 2009.* World Health Organization (2010).
2. Waller M, Stotler C. Telemedicine: a primer. *Curr Allergy Asthma Rep.* (2018) 25:54. doi: 10.1007/s11882-018-0808-4
3. Bischoff A. Benefits and risks from telemedicine. *MMW Fortschr Med.* (2016) 158:18–9. doi: 10.1007/s15006-016-8250-9
4. Zaba R. Telemedycyna w dermatologii. *Medicus Mundi Polonia.* (2009) 28:7–8.
5. Coates SJ, Kvedar J, Granstein RD. Teledermatology: from historical perspective to emerging techniques of the modern era: part I: history, rationale, and current practice. *J Am Acad Dermatol.* (2015) 72:563–74. doi: 10.1016/j.jaad.2014.07.061
6. Jankowski M, Klimczak-Wieczorek A, Kloc M, Matuszewski M, Rozum J. *Telemedycyna w Polsce – mozliwości i szanse rozwoju.* Fundacja im. Lesława A. Pagi, Warszawa (2016).
7. Kanthraj GR. Patient-assisted teledermatology practice: what is it? When, where, and how it is applied? *Indian J Dermatol Venereol Leprol.* (2015) 17:136–43. doi: 10.4103/0378-6323.152172
8. Alexander H, Miller DL. Determining skin thickness with pulsed ultrasound. *J Invest Dermatol.* (1979) 72:17–9. doi: 10.1111/1523-1747.ep12530104
9. Pellacani G, Seidenari S. Preoperative melanoma thickness determination by 20-MHz sonography and digital videomicroscopy in combination. *Arch Dermatol.* (2003) 139:293–8. doi: 10.1001/archderm.139.3.293
10. Hoffmann K, el-Gammal S, Winkler K, Jung J, Pistorius K, Altmayer P. Skin tumours in high-frequency ultrasound. In: Altmeyer P, el-Gammal S, Hoffmann K, editors. *Ultrasound in Dermatology.* Berlin; New York, NY: Springer- Verlag (1992). p. 181–202.
11. Polańska A, Gaura T, Bowszyc-Dmochowska M, Osmola-Mańkowska A, Olek-Hrab K, Adamski Z, et al. Calcipotriol/betamethasone ointment compared to narrow-band UVB in plaque psoriasis: first clinical and ultrasonographic study. *Int J Dermatol.* (2019) 58:108–13. doi: 10.1111/ijd.14150
12. Polańska A, Osmola-Mańkowska A, Olek-Hrab K, Molińska-Glura M, Adamski Z, Zaba R, et al. High-frequency ultrasonography in objective evaluation of the efficacy of PUVA and UVA 1 phototherapy in mycosis fungoides. *Arch Dermatol Res.* (2017) 309:645–51. doi: 10.1007/s00403-017-1767-7

13. Wortsman X, Moreno C, Soto R, Arellano J, Pezo C, Wortsmanet J. Ultrasound in-depth characterization and staging of hidradenitis suppurativa. *Dermatol Surg.* (2013) 39:1835–42. doi: 10.1111/dsu.12329
14. Polańska A, Dańczak-Pazdrowska A, Jałowska M, Adamski Z, Zaba R. Current applications of high-frequency ultrasonography in dermatology. *Adv Dermatol Allergol.* (2017) 6:535–42. doi: 10.5114/ada.2017.72457
15. Wortsman X, Alfageme F, Roustan G, Arias-Santiago S, Martorell A, Catalano O, et al. Guidelines for performing dermatologic ultrasound examinations by the DERMUS group. *J Ultrasound Med.* (2016) 35:577–80. doi: 10.7863/ultra.15.06046
16. Dill-Müller D, Maschke J. Ultrasonography in dermatology. *J Dtsch Dermatol Ges.* (2007) 5:689–707. doi: 10.1111/j.1610-0387.2007.06453.x
17. Ng A, Swanevelder J. Resolution in ultrasound imaging. *Continuing Educ. Anaesthesia Crit Care Pain.* (2011) 11:186–92. doi: 10.1093/bjaceaccp/mkr030
18. Jasaitiene D, Valiukeviciene S, Linkeviciute G, Raisutis R, Jasiuniene E, Kazyset R. Principles of high-frequency ultrasonography for investigation of skin pathology. *J Eur Acad Dermatol Venereol.* (2011) 25:375–82. doi: 10.1111/j.1468-3083.2010.03837.x
19. Jemec GB, Gniadecka M, Ulrich J. Ultrasound in dermatology. Part I: high frequency ultrasound. *Eur J Dermatol.* (2000) 10:492–7.
20. Warshaw E, Greer N, Hillman Y, Hagel E, MacDonald R, Rutks I, et al. *Teledermatology for Diagnosis and Management of Skin Conditions: A Systematic Review of the Evidence.* VA-ESP Project #09-009 (2009).
21. Wortsman X, Jemec GBE. High resolution ultrasound applications in dermatology. *Rev Chilena Dermatol.* (2006) 22:37–45.
22. Harland CC, Kale SG, Jackson P, Mortimer PS, Bamberet JC. Differentiation of common benign pigmented skin lesions from melanoma by high-resolution ultrasound. *Br J Dermatol.* (2000) 143:281–9. doi: 10.1046/j.1365-2133.2000.03652.x
23. Scotto di Santolo M, Sagnelli M, Mancini M, Scalvenzi M, Delfino M, Schonauer F, et al. High-resolution Color-Doppler ultrasound for the study of skin growths. *Arch Dermatol Res.* (2015) 307:559–66. doi: 10.1007/s00403-015-1538-2
24. Catalano O, Roldán FA, Varelli C, Bard R, Corvino A, Wortsman X. Skin cancer: findings and role of high-resolution ultrasound. *J Ultrasound.* (2019) 22:423–31. doi: 10.1007/s40477-019-00379-0
25. Catalano O, Voit C, Sandomenico F, Mandato Y, Petrillo M, Franco R, et al. Previously reported sonographic appearances of regional melanoma metastases are not likely due to necrosis. *J Ultrasound Med.* (2011) 30:1041–9. doi: 10.7863/jum.2011.30.8.1041
26. Lassau N, Lamuraglia M. Prognostic value of angiogenesis evaluated with high frequency and Color-Doppler sonography for preoperative assessment of primary cutaneous melanomas: correlation with recurrence after a 5 year follow-up period. *Cancer Imaging.* (2006) 25:24–9. doi: 10.1102/1470-7330.2006.0009
27. Wang SQ, Liu J, Zhu QL, Zhao CY, Qu T, Li F, et al. High-frequency ultrasound features of basal cell carcinoma and its association with histological recurrence risk. *Chin Med J.* (2019) 132:2021–6. doi: 10.1097/CM9.0000000000000369
28. Tacke J, Haagen G, Hornstein OP, Tacke J, Haagen G, Hornstein P, et al. Clinical relevance of sonometry-derived tumour thickness in malignant melanoma: a statistical analysis. *Br J Dermatol.* (1995) 132:209–14. doi: 10.1111/j.1365-2133.1995.tb05015.x
29. Lassau N, Koscielny S, Avril MF, Margulis A, Duvillard P, De Baere T, et al. Prognostic value of angiogenesis evaluated with high-frequency and color Doppler sonography for preoperative assessment of melanomas. *Am J Roentgenol.* (2002) 178:1547–51. doi: 10.2214/ajr.178.6.1781547
30. Serrone L, Solivetti FM, Thorel MF, Eibenschutz L, Donati P, Catricalàet C. High frequency ultrasound in the preoperative staging of primary melanoma: a statistical analysis. *Melanoma Res.* (2002) 12:287–90. doi: 10.1097/00008390-200206000-00013
31. Guitera P, Li LX, Crotty K, Fitzgerald P, Mellenbergh R, Pellacani G, et al. Melanoma histological Breslow thickness predicted by 75-MHz ultrasonography. *Br J Dermatol.* (2008) 159:364–9. doi: 10.1111/j.1365-2133.2008.08681.x
32. Bobadilla F, Wortsman X, Muñoz C, Segovia L, Espinoza M, Jemec G. Pre-surgical high resolution ultrasound of facial basal cell carcinoma: correlation with histology. *Cancer Imaging.* (2008) 22:63–72. doi: 10.1102/1470-7330.2008.0026
33. Seidenari S. High-frequency sonography combined with image analysis: a non-invasive objective method for skin evaluation and desription. *Clin Dermatol.* (1995) 13:349–59. doi: 10.1016/0738-081X(95)00074-P
34. Congalton AT, Oakley AM, Rademaker M, Bramley D, Martin R. Successful melanoma triage by a virtual lesion clinic (teledermoscopy). *J Eur Acad Dermatol Venereol.* (2015) 29:2423–8. doi: 10.1111/jdv.13309
35. Kanthraj GR. Classification and design of teledermatology practice: what dermatoses? Which technology to apply? *J Eur Acad Dermatol Venereol.* (2009) 23:865–75. doi: 10.1111/j.1468-3083.2009.03136.x
36. Queille-Roussel C, Olesen M, Villumsen J, Lacour J. Efficacy of an innovative aerosol foam formulation of fixed combination calcipotriol plus betamethasone dipropionate in patients with psoriasis vulgaris. *Clin Drug Investig.* (2015) 35:239–45. doi: 10.1007/s40261-015-0269-7
37. Yazdanparast T, Yazdani K, Humbert P, Khatami A, Nasrollahi SA, Firouzabadi LI, et al. Biophysical measurements and ultrasonographic findings in chronic dermatitis in comparison with uninvolved skin. *Indian J Dermatol.* (2019) 64:90–6. doi: 10.4103/ijd.IJD_464_17
38. Polańska A, Dańczak-Pazdrowska A, Silny W, Wozniak A, Maksin K, Jenerowicz D. Comparison between high-frequency ultrasonography (Dermascan C, version 3) and histopathology in atopic dermatitis. *Skin Res Technol.* (2013) 19:432–7. doi: 10.1111/srt.12064
39. Gupta AK, Turnbull DH, Harasiewicz KA, Shum DT, Watteel GN, Foster FS, et al. The use of high-frequency ultrasound as a method of assessing the severity of a plaque of psoriasis. *Arch Dermatol.* (1996) 132:658–62. doi: 10.1001/archderm.1996.03890300076011
40. Polańska A, Silny W, Jenerowicz D, Knioła K, Molińska-Glura M, Dańczak-Pazdrowska A. Monitoring of therapy in atopic dermatitis- observations with the use of high-frequency ultrasonography. *Skin Res Technol.* (2015) 21:35–40. doi: 10.1111/srt.12153
41. Osmola-Mańkowska A, Polańska A, Silny W, Zaba R, Adamski A, Dańczak-Pazdrowska A. Topical tacrolimus vs medium-dose ultraviolet al phototherapy in the treatment of atopic dermatitis—a preliminary study in relation to parameters of the epidermal barrier function and high-frequency ultrasonography. *Eur Rev Med Pharmacol Sci.* (2014) 18:3927–34.
42. Dańczak-Pazdrowska A, Polańska A, Silny W, Sadowska A, Osmola-Mańkowska A, Czarnecka-Operacz M, et al. Seemingly healthy skin in atopic dermatitis: observations with the use of high-frequency ultrasonography, preliminary study. *Skin Res Technol.* (2012) 18:162–7. doi: 10.1111/j.1600-0846.2011.00548.x
43. Polańska A, Dańczak-Pazdrowska A, Silny W, Jenerowicz D, Olek-Hrab K, Osmaola-Mańkowska A. Nonlesional skin in atopic dermatitis is seemingly healthy skin - observations using noninvasive methods. *Wideochir Inne Tech Maloinwazyjne.* (2013) 8:192–9. doi: 10.5114/wiitm.2011.33633
44. Polańska A, Osmola-Mańkowska A, Olek-Hrab K. Do we need high-frequency ultrasonography in mycosis fungoides? *Abstract Book* P1065, EADV 2016 Vienna.
45. Mandava A, Koppula V, Wortsman X, Catalano O, Alfageme F. The clinical value of imaging in primary cutaneous lymphomas: role of high resolution ultrasound and PET-CT. *Br J Radiol.* (2019) 92:20180904. doi: 10.1259/bjr.20180904
46. Olek-Hrab K, Silny W, Dańczak-Pazdrowska A, Osmola-Mańkowska A, Sadowska A, Polańska A, et al. Ultraviolet A1 phototherapy for mycosis fungoides. *Clin Exp Dermatol.* (2013) 38:126–30. doi: 10.1111/ced.12001
47. Polańska A, Bowszyc-Dmochowska M, Olek-Hrab K, Adamski Z, Zaba R, Dańczak-Pazdrowska A. High-frequency ultrasonography a new quantitative method in evaluation of skin lymphomas-first comparative study in relation to histopathology. *Skin Res Technol.* (2019) 25:720–4. doi: 10.1111/srt.12708
48. Polańska A, Dańczak-Pazdrowska A, Olek-Hrab K, Osmola-Mańkowska A, Bowszyc-Dmochowska M, Zaba R, et al. High-frequency ultrasonography-new non-invasive method in assessment of skin lymphomas. *Skin Res Technol.* (2018) 24:517–21. doi: 10.1111/srt.12450
49. Lacarrubba F, Dini V, Napolitano M, Venturini M, Caposiena Caro DR, Molinelli E, et al. Ultrasonography in the pathway to an optimal standard of care of hidradenitis suppurativa: the Italian Ultrasound Working Group experience. *J Eur Acad Dermatol Venereol.* (2019) 33:10–4. doi: 10.1111/jdv.15847

50. Wortsman X. Imaging of hidradenitis suppurativa. *Dermatol Clin.* (2016) 34:59–68. doi: 10.1016/j.det.2015.08.003
51. Nazzaro G, Passoni E, Guanziroli E, Casazza G, Muratori S, Barbareschiet M, et al. Comparison of clinical and sonographic scores in a cohort of 140 patients with hidradenitis suppurativa from an Italian referral centre: a retrospective observational study. *Eur J Dermatol.* (2018) 28:845–7.
52. Witkowski A, Łudzik J, Soyer P. Telediagnosis with confocal microscopy: a reality or a Dream? *Dermatol Clin.* (2016) 4:505–12. doi: 10.1016/j.det.2016.05.013

# 24

# Diagnosis of Onychomycosis: From Conventional Techniques and Dermoscopy to Artificial Intelligence

*Sophie Soyeon Lim [1], Jungyoon Ohn [2,3] and Je-Ho Mun [2,3]**

[1] Alfred Health, Melbourne, VIC, Australia, [2] Department of Dermatology, Seoul National University College of Medicine, Seoul, South Korea, [3] Institute of Human-Environment Interface Biology, Seoul National University, Seoul, South Korea

***Correspondence:**
*Je-Ho Mun*
*jehomun@gmail.com*

Onychomycosis is a common fungal nail infection. Accurate diagnosis is critical as onychomycosis is transmissible between humans and impacts patients' quality of life. Combining clinical examination with mycological testing ensures accurate diagnosis. Conventional diagnostic techniques, including potassium hydroxide testing, fungal culture and histopathology of nail clippings, detect fungal species within nails. New diagnostic tools have been developed recently which either improve detection of onychomycosis clinically, including dermoscopy, reflectance confocal microscopy and artificial intelligence, or mycologically, such as molecular assays. Dermoscopy is cost-effective and non-invasive, allowing clinicians to discern microscopic features of onychomycosis and fungal melanonychia. Reflectance confocal microscopy enables clinicians to observe bright filamentous septate hyphae at near histologic resolution by the bedside. Artificial intelligence may prompt patients to seek further assessment for nails that are suspicious for onychomycosis. This review evaluates the current landscape of diagnostic techniques for onychomycosis.

**Keywords: diagnosis, diagnostic imaging, onychomycosis, fungi, pathology, dermoscopy, reflectance confocal microscopy, artificial intelligence**

## INTRODUCTION

Onychomycosis is a fungal nail infection caused by dermatophytes (60–70%), non-dermatophyte molds (NDMs) (20%) and yeast (10–20%) (1–3). It is the most common nail disorder encountered in clinical practice worldwide (4–6). It is a significant public health issue, as human to human transmission occurs *via* direct or indirect contact of surfaces contaminated with scales or keratin from infected patients. Risk of developing onychomycosis increases with advancing age. Thus, onychomycosis is likely to become an even more pertinent issue given the aging population (7, 8). Its other risk factors include diabetes, obesity, trauma, history of tinea pedis, and immunosuppression (9, 10). Onychomycosis is detrimental to patients' quality of life, as its physical appearance can cause significant psychological distress, and the localized pain in severely dystrophic nails can impede everyday living (11).

Onychomycosis is important to diagnose as it is curable with antifungal agents such as oral terbinafine, itraconazole, albaconazole, posaconazole, and fluconazole (12, 13). Topical antifungal solutions including ciclopirox 8%, amorolfine 5%, efinaconazole 10%, and tavaborole 5%, are used as adjuncts to oral agents in severe cases or as alternatives when oral agents are contraindicated or in mild cases (12). Due to costs and long treatment course lasting at least 3 months, patients often find difficulty adhering to therapy (12, 14–16). Ensuring that patients who do not have onychomycosis do not receive antifungal treatment is also important because oral antifungals have adverse systemic effects, including gastrointestinal disturbance and hepatotoxicity (13).

To diagnose onychomycosis, clinical suspicion needs to be confirmed with mycologic testing. This review highlights key characteristics of conventional diagnostic tools, including potassium hydroxide (KOH) testing, fungal culture and histopathology of nail clippings, and newly developed techniques, including dermoscopy, reflectance confocal microscopy, molecular assays and artificial intelligence.

## CLINICAL FEATURES AND DIFFERENTIAL DIAGNOSES

Onychomycosis is typically characterized by a yellow or brown, brittle nail plate with subungual hyperkeratosis causing onycholysis (17–19). It is classified according to the site and involvement of disease: distal and lateral subungual, superficial, endonyx, proximal subungual, and total dystrophic onychomycosis (20). Distal and lateral subungual onychomycosis is the most common, thus the commonly described features of onychomycosis are those observed in this subtype (19, 20). Superficial onychomycosis presents with nail plate discoloration, superficial patches and transverse striae, and endonyx onychomycosis presents with lamellar splitting, discoloration and indentations (19, 20). Proximal subungual onychomycosis predominantly presents with a whitish area in the proximal nail plate (19, 20). This subtype is often seen in immunosuppressed patients, such as those with the human immunodeficiency virus, systemic lupus erythematosus or on immunosuppressants (**Figure 1A**) (10).

According to a prospective cross-sectional diagnosis study in seven dermatology outpatient clinics, features that increase the likelihood of clinically diagnosing onychomycosis are previous diagnosis of fungal disease in feet [likelihood ratio (LR+) for a positive result = 1.84], abnormal plantar desquamation involving > 25% of the sole (LR+ = 3.61), interdigital tinea pedis (LR+ = 1.46) and onychomycosis being considered the most probable diagnosis by dermatologists (LR+ = 1.46) (9). When abnormal plantar desquamation is coupled with onychomycosis being considered the most likely diagnosis, probability of diagnosing onychomycosis is 81% (**Figure 1B**). Onychomycosis can present alongside green nail syndrome. A retrospective analysis of green nail syndrome patients at referral centers revealed fungal co-infection in 65.2% of patients (21). Onychomycosis can present with a dermatophytoma, a compact ball of fungal filaments and large spores which appears as a white/yellow or orange/brown longitudinal streak in the nail plate (22, 23). Features of severe or long-standing disease include dermatophytoma, worsening subungual hyperkeratosis, expanding area of disease involvement and closer proximity of disease to the nail matrix (24). Severe disease can cause pain secondary to onychocryptosis (ingrown nail), nail bed infection and partial or complete nail plate loss (18).

### Differential Diagnoses

#### Trachyonychia

Trachyonychia is an inflammatory nail disease which is commonly idiopathic but can be secondary to systemic inflammatory conditions such as alopecia areata and nail psoriasis (25, 26). It is characterized by a rough and brittle nail plate (opaque trachyonychia) or, less frequently, an opalescent nail plate lined with small geometric pits (shiny trachyonychia) (27). Trachyonychia is diagnosed clinically and dermoscopy is a useful diagnostic aid. Key dermoscopic features of trachyonychia that differentiate it from onychomycosis include red coloration, longitudinal ridging, involvement of the proximal nail plate (at >50% of the nail plate width), splinter hemorrhages, pitting, and onychoschizia (nail plate splitting) (28).

#### Onycholysis

Onycholysis involves separation of the nail plate from the nail bed due to repetitive trauma, phototoxicity, contact dermatitis, underlying tumor or infection, nail psoriasis, or nail lichen planus (29). Onycholysis secondary to trauma can be differentiated from that resulting from onychomycosis on dermoscopic examination. The proximal border of onycholysis is linear with trauma, but jagged with spiked edges in onychomycosis (30).

#### Onychomadesis

Onychomadesis is characterized by complete separation and shedding of the nail plate from the proximal nail bed due to temporary nail matrix arrest (31, 32). Conditions that cause nail matrix arrest include infections such as hand-foot-and-mouth disease and varicella, trauma, chemotherapy, anticonvulsants, lichen planus, and Kawasaki disease (32). Nails affected by onychomadesis are at risk of developing onychomycosis (33).

#### Onychocryptosis

Onychocryptosis (ingrowing nail) involves the nail plate burying within the periungual skin, causing painful inflammation, infection and granulation (34). Although it is observed secondary to severe onychomycosis, it is primarily associated with genetic disposition, trauma, poorly-fitted shoes, and incorrect nail trimming (31, 34).

#### Nail Squamous Cell Carcinoma

Nail SCC is the most common malignant nail disorder and can clinically resemble onychomycosis (35, 36). Like onychomycosis, immunosuppression increases the risk of developing nail SCC. Other risk factors include chronic sun exposure, human papillomavirus infection and trauma (37). Diagnosis delays occur frequently as nail SCC presents with non-specific clinical features, including subungual tumor, lateral onycholysis, subungual hyperkeratosis, painless nail bed erosion, ulceration, purulent discharge, serous ooze, bleeding and nail loss (37, 38).

**Abbreviations:** AI, artificial intelligence; AUC, area under curve; GMS, Grocott-Gomori methanamine silver; KOH, potassium hydroxide; LR+, likelihood ratio for a positive result; NDM, non-dermatophyte mold; PAS, periodic acid-Schiff; PCR, polymerase chain reaction; RCM, reflectance confocal microscopy; R-CNN, region-based convolutional neural network; SCC, squamous cell carcinoma; SDA, Sabouraoud dextrose agar.

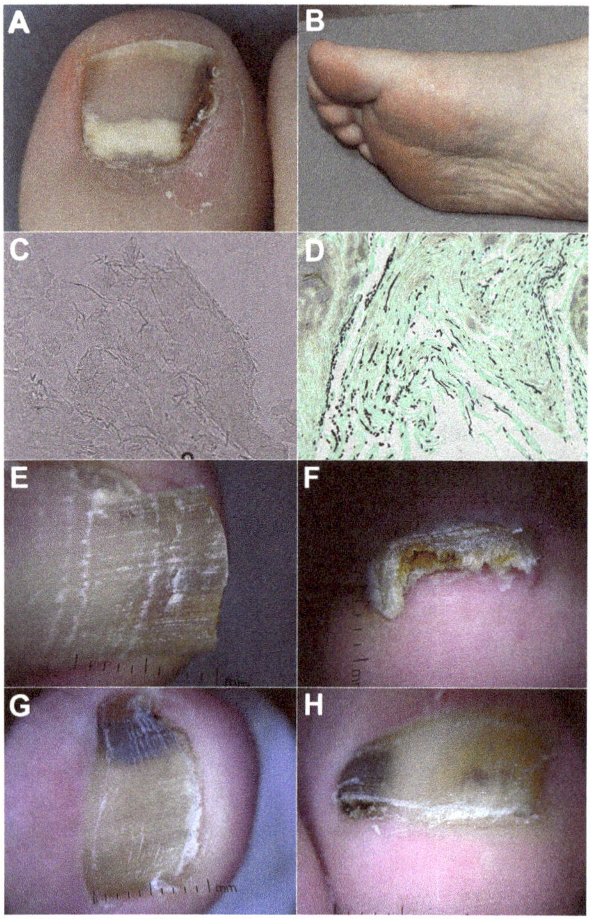

**FIGURE 1 | (A)** Proximal subungual onychomycosis in a patient with systemic lupus erythematosus. **(B)** Abnormal plantar desquamation increases the likelihood of clinically diagnosing onychomycosis. Thus, the sole should also be examined while assessing onychomycosis. **(C)** KOH-test highlighting presence of fungal hyphae (×200 magnification). **(D)** Histopathology (nail clipping) with GMS staining showing numerous fungal hyphae in the nail plate (×400). The fungi are highlighted in black with GMS staining. **(E,F)** Dermoscopic examination of onychomycosis showing yellowish discoloration with spikes pattern and surface scales. Distal edge dermoscopy demonstrating subungual hyperkeratosis. **(G,H)** Dermoscopic examination of fungal melanonychia showing reverse triangular pattern, yellow streaks, black and yellow coloration, scales, and subungual hyperkeratosis.

Therefore, nail dystrophies refractory to treatment need to be carefully investigated.

### Nail Apparatus Melanoma

Nail apparatus melanoma is another malignant nail disorder that warrants prompt diagnosis (39). Its prognosis is poorer than other melanomas due to diagnosis delays resulting from non-specific clinical features and high incidence of amelanosis (40, 41). Nail apparatus melanoma commonly presents with a ≥3 mm-thick brown or black band with variegated borders, nail dystrophy and Hutchinson's sign, where the proximal and/or lateral nail fold is pigmented (41–44). Nail apparatus melanoma can be mistaken for onychomycosis and they may be co-exist with onychomycosis, thus detailed investigation is warranted in onychomycosis with malignant features (45, 46).

## CONVENTIONAL DIAGNOSTIC TOOLS

To diagnose onychomycosis, confirmatory mycologic testing is essential. The potential harm caused by misdiagnosis and inappropriate use of empiric antifungal therapy outweigh the cost benefit of bypassing mycologic testing (18, 47, 48).

### Potassium Hydroxide Testing

Direct potassium hydroxide (KOH) testing is a simple, quick and inexpensive technique integral to dermatological practice for identifying fungal organisms (**Figure 1C**) (49, 50). It involves retrieving the specimen from the nail bed and underneath the nail plate then dissolving it in KOH (51). KOH dissolves the keratin, allowing microscopic visualization of the fungal septate hyphae (51). Specimens can be further treated with stains such as Calcofluor White, Evans Blue, Gram, Giemsa, and India ink (52, 53).

KOH testing has 61% sensitivity and 95% specificity (51). It is cost-effective and can determine the presence of fungal organisms within an hour. However, it cannot specify the exact type of pathogenic organism (19). Retrieving adequate amount of specimen is critical in ensuring the success of KOH testing. To optimize accuracy, specimens should not be interpreted immediately after applying KOH, as it takes at least 15–30 min for the KOH to adequately dissolve the keratin (19). Overall, KOH testing is a quick and inexpensive diagnostic tool for confirming presence of fungi in nails, enabling clinicians to commence treatment for onychomycosis (**Table 1**).

### Fungal Culture

Fungal culture can identify the specific pathogen subtype (53, 64). After removing debris from the nail plate, the subungual specimen is cultured in Sabouraoud dextrose agar (SDA) at 26–30°C for up to a month (18, 52). The media is treated with chloramphenicol and gentamicin to prevent bacteria from interfering with fungal growth (52). Laboratories often culture the subungual specimen in SDA with and without cycloheximide which prevents growth of NDMs. Repeat cultures are required to diagnose NDM onychomycosis, as NDMs are common contaminants of skin surfaces (18).

Fungal culture has 99% specificity, its pooled sensitivity is 56% (range 29–82%) according to a recent meta-analysis (51, 53). Sensitivity of fungal culture is largely dependent on the expertise of the testing center (65). Although specialized mycology centers may report fewer false negatives, most tertiary centers and general clinics observe low sensitivity rates. Clinical utility of fungal culture is further limited by delays in retrieving results (several weeks to months). Therefore, fungal culture is recommended when identifying the fungal organism is necessary (53).

### Histopathology (Nail Clipping)

Histopathological assessment involves examining the microscopic features of nail clipping specimens embedded

**TABLE 1** | Summary of diagnostic techniques for onychomycosis.

| | Sensitivity | Specificity | Advantages | Disadvantages |
|---|---|---|---|---|
| KOH testing (51) | 61% (44–100%) | 95% (75–100%) | Easy to conduct | Diagnostic accuracy dependent on examiner's expertise |
| | | | Inexpensive | Cannot identify pathogen subtype |
| | | | Quick results (15–60 min) | |
| Fungal culture (51) | 56% (29–82%) | 99% (83–100%) | Can identify pathogen subtype | Low sensitivity |
| | | | | Delay in results (up to 1 month) |
| Histopathology (51) | 84% (61–93%) | 89% (44–100%) | Most sensitive conventional mycological test | Expensive |
| | | | | Cannot specify pathogen subtypes |
| Nail dermoscopy | Jagged onycholytic edge with spikes: 86.4% (54), 100% (30) | Jagged onycholytic edge with spikes: 58.3% (54), 100% (30) | Bedside tool, non-invasive | Cannot demonstrate presence of fungi |
| | Longitudinal striae: 25% (54), 86.5% (30) | Longitudinal striae: 83.3% (54), 100% (30) | Quick results | |
| | Ruins aspect: 59.1% (54) | Ruins aspect: 91.7% (54) | Inexpensive | |
| | Homogenous opacity: 34.1% (54) | Homogenous opacity: 83.3% (54) | | |
| Reflectance confocal microscopy | 52.9% (55), 79.5% (56), 91.67% (57) | 57.58% (57), 81% (56), 90.2% (55) | Bedside tool, non-invasive | Moderate sensitivity and specificity |
| | | | | Cannot assess thick nails |
| Polymerase chain reaction | 85% (58) | 94% (58) | Can identify pathogen subtype | Assays still under development |
| | 87.3% (59) | 94.3% (59) | High sensitivity | Risk of false positives |
| | 100% (60) | 100% (60) | Can deliver results with small amount of sample | |
| | Pandermatophyte assay: 90% (61) | Pandermatophyte and panfungal assays: NR | | |
| | Panfungal assay: 47% (61) | | | |
| Flow cytometry and mass spectrometry | NR | NR | Can theoretically identify pathogen subtype | Experimental |
| Artificial intelligence | 70.2% (62) | 72.7% (62) | Inexpensive | Still under development: require improving dataset and considering method of distribution to clinicians |
| | 82.7–96% (63) | 69.3–96.7% (63) | Can be used by patients to screen for highly suspicious nails | Not confirmatory technique |

*NR, not reported.*

in paraffin blocks (18, 52). To acquire an adequate nail sample for examination, at least 4 mm of the free edge of the nail plate should be retrieved using a dual-action or heavy-duty nail nipper (66). Samples can be transported to the laboratory in a dry container or in formaldehyde (67). Softening nail samples before routine processing with solutions such as chitin-softening agent, 4% phenol or 10% Tween 40, facilitates sectioning and thus optimizes the quality of sections (66, 67). After paraffin embedding and sectioning, stains highlight presence of fungi (**Figure 1D**). Using the periodic acid-Schiff (PAS) staining method, periodic acid oxidizes hydroxyl groups of the cell wall in spores, hyphae, pseudohyphae and yeasts into aldehydes (52, 53). These then react with Schiff to produce a red color (52, 53). Using the Grocott-Gomori methanamine silver (GMS) staining method, the chromic acid oxidizes the cell wall then reduces the methanamine silver nitrate into metallic silver to produce a dark brown color (53).

Histopathology of nail clippings is highly sensitive (84%) and specific (89%) (51). It can also be stored and retrospectively reviewed in refractory cases, as the paraffin embedding allows for long-term storage. Histopathology is however rather costly than KOH testing and unable to specify the exact subtype or viability of the causative organism (18, 19, 53, 68).

## NEW DIAGNOSTIC TOOLS

### Nail Dermoscopy (Onychoscopy)

Nail dermoscopy (onychoscopy) is a non-invasive bedside tool that allows clinicians to visualize microscopic features of abnormal nails. Key dermoscopic features of distal and lateral subungual onychomycosis include a jagged proximal edge of the onycholytic area with spikes and longitudinal striae (**Figures 1E,F**) (30, 54). These features and a ruins aspect are associated with total dystrophic onychomycosis (54). Homogenous opacity is found in superficial onychomycosis (54).

Onychomycosis can also present with longitudinal melanonychia (fungal melanonychia). In such cases, white or yellow streaks, non-longitudinal homogenous pattern, yellow coloration, reverse triangular pattern, subungual hyperkeratosis, multicolor pattern and nail scaling are positive predictors of fungal melanonychia (**Figures 1G,H**) compared to nail matrix naevi or subungual melanomas (69). As nail dermoscopy is quick, non-invasive and inexpensive, it has the potential to help physicians identify onychomycosis by the bedside and decide whether to proceed to mycological assessment (70).

## Reflectance Confocal Microscopy

Reflectance confocal microscopy (RCM) is a real-time imaging tool that allows clinicians to observe features of abnormal nails at near-histologic resolution by the bedside. It uses a 830 nm laser in reflectance mode which divides the nail unit into thin horizontal sections for examination (56). Reflectance confocal microscopy of onychomycosis reveals networks of bright filamentous septate hyphae (56, 71, 72). It has 52.9–91.67% sensitivity and 57.58–90.2% specificity for detecting onychomycosis (55–57). Reflectance confocal microscopy is expensive and not subsidized in many countries, and further studies are needed to support its utility in the clinical setting (72). Therefore, it is yet to be integrated into clinical practice in many countries. In addition, it is difficult to assess thick nails with RCM as its depth of imaging is limited to ~200 μm.

## Molecular Assays

Molecular assays including polymerase chain reactions (PCR), flow cytometry and mass spectrometry are advanced diagnostic tools that involve analysis of the fungal DNA causing onychomycosis.

Polymerase chain reactions involves amplifying the fungal DNA then detecting this with specialized fluorescent primers (73). Therefore, it can detect small amounts of pathogenic organisms within nails (74). Real-time PCR is the most frequently used form of PCR as it is relatively simple to conduct, can detect multiple organisms and has a low risk of contamination (73, 74). Various assays have been developed to facilitate commercial use of PCR technology when detecting dermatophytes, but these are not widely available (74). They report sensitivity of 85–100% and specificity of 94–100% (58–60).

Hafirassou et al. investigated usefulness of panfungal and pandermatophyte assays for real-time PCR compared to fungal culture in detecting onychomycosis (61). The pandermatophyte assay was 90% sensitive relative to culture. The panfungal assay showed a low sensitivity of 47% relative to culture due to multiple fungal species residing within diseased and healthy nails, as demonstrated by the candida and aspergillus assays. Further studies are warranted to examine PCR use in a real-world setting and reduce the risk of false positives.

Other molecular assay techniques include flow cytometry and mass spectrometry. Flow cytometry separates cells according to size, granulosity and presence of DNA and protein markers (18). Mass spectrometry involves charging chemical species and separating ions according to their mass-to-charge ratio (18, 53, 75). These techniques are experimental, requiring further research and development prior to integration into clinical practice.

## Artificial Intelligence

Artificial intelligence (AI) has caused a recent paradigm shift in clinical medicine (76, 77). Its diagnostic performance has been shown to be comparable to that of specialist clinicians in identifying diabetic retinopathy and skin cancer (78, 79). Many dermatologists recognize that AI has great potential to improve dermatologic care (80, 81). Currently, it is mainly explored in the setting of skin cancer, ulcers, psoriasis and other inflammatory skin diseases, predicting skin-sensitizing substances, histopathological assessment, and gene expression profiling (82).

Developing a large database of photographs capturing a wide range of disease presentations is critical in AI training (82). Onychomycosis is an ideal candidate for AI as it is a common condition with minimal racial differences (63). Clinics worldwide can contribute to the database, and the AI technology would not be limited to specific populations.

In 2018, Han et al. developed AI for diagnosing onychomycosis (63). Two datasets, A1 ($n$ = 49,567) and A2 ($n$ = 3,741), were generated. A2 consisted of images of clinically diagnosed onychomycosis (63). For A1, standardized clinical images were generated by a hand and foot image selecting convolutional neural network (CNN), followed by a nail part extracting regional CNN (R-CNN) then a fine image CNN. Two CNN algorithms, ResNet-152 and VGG-19, were then trained to classify nails as onychomycosis or one their differential diagnoses using the two datasets. These algorithms were then validated against datasets (B1, B2, C, and D) of mycologically confirmed onychomycosis cases.

Algorithms trained with A1 were more accurate in diagnosing onychomycosis than those trained with A2. Moreover, the AI (two-layered feedforward neural networks computing the combined output of ResNet-152 and VGG-19) achieved test sensitivity/specificity/area under the curve values of (96.0/94.7/0.98), (82.7/96.7/0.95), (92.3/79.3/0.93), and (87.7/69.3/0.82) for the B1, B2, C, and D datasets, respectively. AI performed better than most of the 42 dermatologists. The Youden index (sensitivity + specificity−1) of AI which reflects its diagnostic accuracy was significantly higher than that of the dermatologists ($p$ = 0.01) when evaluating the B1 and C datasets.

More recently, the group reported that the deep neural network at operating point achieved 70.2% sensitivity, 72.7% specificity and AUC of 0.75 in diagnosing onychomycosis in a prospective cohort of 90 patients (62). This was comparable to the performance of dermoscopy (sensitivity 72.7%, specificity 72.9%,

AUC 0.755; $p = 0.952$) and experienced dermatologists (mean Youden index $0.230 \pm 0.176$; $p = 0.667$).

Although there is limited literature on this topic, these results showed that AI has the potential to assist clinicians decide whether they should test nails for onychomycosis. AI can also help improve telemedicine, as it can act as an accessible resource for patients to evaluate their own nails and, if needed, promptly initiate a formal clinician review. To further develop AI, the database should be optimized to include rigorously confirmed onychomycosis and various non-onychomycosis onychopathies that are evaluated with relevant mycological examinations. Finding a suitable means of distributing this technology to the public is also necessary. Finally, whilst integrating AI into clinical practice is important, dermatologists should use their clinical judgment to prevent overdiagnosis and excessive testing which would increase the burden on health care costs.

## CONCLUSION

A wide range of conventional and newly developed tools help diagnose onychomycosis. Each tool has its advantages and disadvantages, and combining these tools improves the sensitivity and specificity of testing (51). KOH testing is best for prompt initial diagnosis. In ambiguous cases, histopathologic assessment of affected nail plates can identify presence of fungi. Fungal culture can be used when the pathogen subtype needs to be specified. Dermoscopy can assist clinicians identify nails that are highly suspicious for onychomycosis. Reflectance confocal microscopy allows visualization of hyphae by the bedside but is not widely

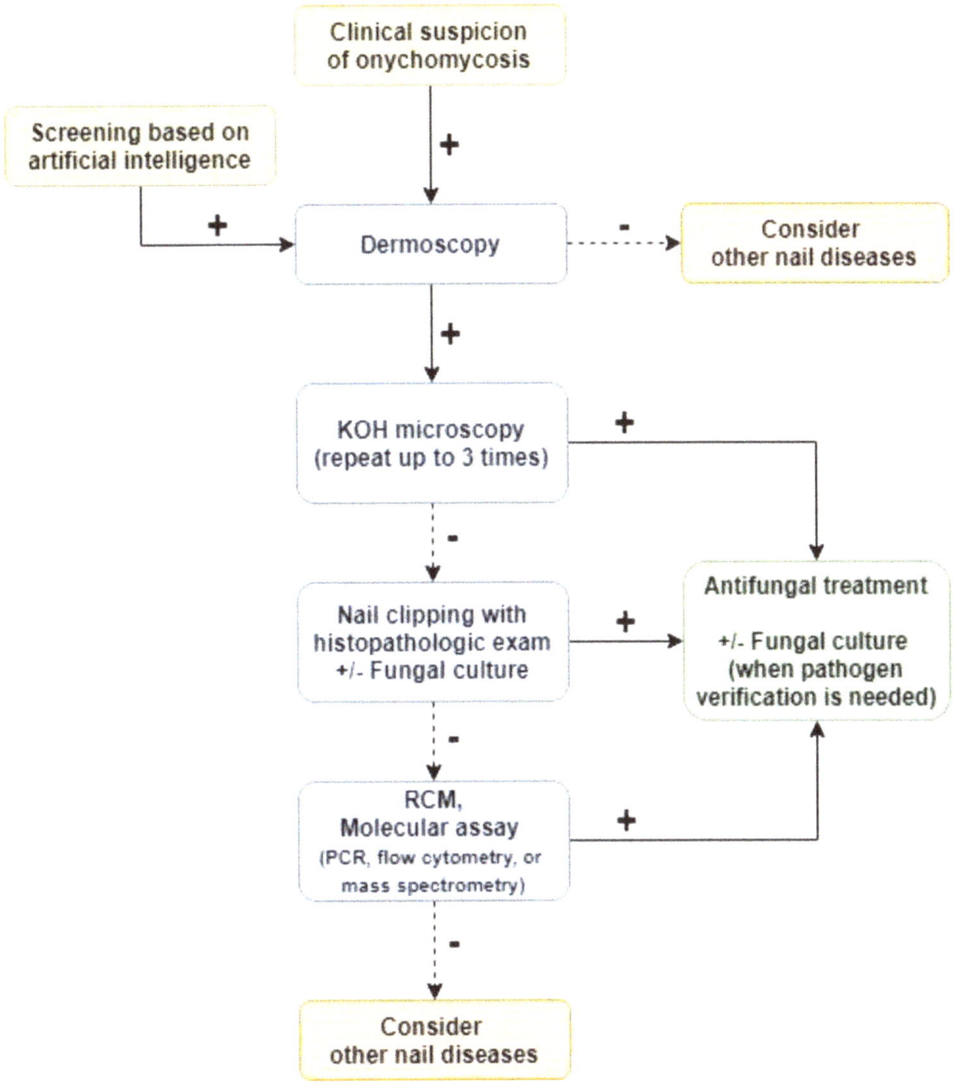


**FIGURE 2** | A flowchart for diagnosing onychomycosis.

available, and molecular assays may act as supplementary diagnostic tests but require more research. AI has the potential to help patients identify affected nails and seek further medical assessment. A diagnostic algorithm integrating these tools can help maximize clinicians' accuracy of diagnosing onychomycosis (**Figure 2**).

## AUTHOR CONTRIBUTIONS

SL: data acquisition, analysis, and manuscript drafting. JO: manuscript critical revision. J-HM: conception of work, manuscript critical revision, and final approval. All authors: contributed to the article and approved the submitted version.

## REFERENCES


1. Ghannoum MA, Hajjeh RA, Scher R, Konnikov N, Gupta AK, Summerbell R, et al. A large-scale North American study of fungal isolates from nails: the frequency of onychomycosis, fungal distribution, and antifungal susceptibility patterns. *J Am Acad Dermatol.* (2000) 43:641–8. doi: 10.1067/mjd.2000.107754
2. Gupta AK, Gupta G, Jain HC, Lynde CW, Foley KA, Daigle D, et al. The prevalence of unsuspected onychomycosis and its causative organisms in a multicentre Canadian sample of 30 000 patients visiting physicians' offices. *J Eur Acad Dermatol Venereol.* (2016) 30:1567–72. doi: 10.1111/jdv.13677
3. Svejgaard EL, Nilsson J. Onychomycosis in Denmark: prevalence of fungal nail infection in general practice. *Mycoses.* (2004) 47:131–5. doi: 10.1111/j.1439-0507.2004.00968.x
4. Faergemann J, Baran R. Epidemiology, clinical presentation and diagnosis of onychomycosis. *Br J Dermatol.* (2003) 149(Suppl. 65):1–4. doi: 10.1046/j.1365-2133.149.s65.4.x
5. Gupta AK, Mays RR, Versteeg SG, Piraccini BM, Takwale A, Shemer A, et al. Global perspectives for the management of onychomycosis. *Int J Dermatol.* (2019) 58:1118–29. doi: 10.1111/ijd.14346
6. Sigurgeirsson B, Baran R. The prevalence of onychomycosis in the global population: a literature study. *J Eur Acad Dermatol Venereol.* (2014) 28:1480–91. doi: 10.1111/jdv.12323
7. Papini M, Piraccini BM, Difonzo E, Brunoro A. Epidemiology of onychomycosis in Italy: prevalence data and risk factor identification. *Mycoses.* (2015) 58:659–64. doi: 10.1111/myc.12396
8. Hwang S, Kim D, Suh M, Kwon K, Kim H, Ro B, et al. Epidemiologic survey of onychomycosis in Koreas: multicenter study. *Korean J Med Mycol.* (2011) 16:35–43. doi: 10.17966/kjmm.2011.16.2.35
9. Garcia-Doval I, Cabo F, Monteagudo B, Alvarez J, Ginarte M, Rodríguez-Alvarez MX, et al. Clinical diagnosis of toenail onychomycosis is possible in some patients: cross-sectional diagnostic study and development of a diagnostic rule. *Br J Dermatol.* (2010) 163:743–51. doi: 10.1111/j.1365-2133.2010.09930.x
10. Tlacuilo-Parra A, Guevara-Gutierrez E, Mayorga J, Garcia-De La Torre I, Salazar-Paramo M. Onychomycosis in systemic lupus erythematosus: a case control study. *J Rheumatol.* (2003) 30:1491–4. Available online at: https://www.jrheum.org/content/30/7/1491
11. Stewart CR, Algu L, Kamran R, Leveille CF, Abid K, Rae C, et al. Effect of onychomycosis and treatment on patient reported quality of life outcomes: a systematic review. *J Am Acad Dermatol.* (2020). doi: 10.1016/j.jaad.2020.05.143
12. Lipner SR, Scher RK. Onychomycosis: treatment and prevention of recurrence. *J Am Acad Dermatol.* (2019) 80:853–67. doi: 10.1016/j.jaad.2018.05.1260
13. Fávero MLD, Bonetti AF, Domingos EL, Tonin FS, Pontarolo R. Oral antifungal therapies for toenail onychomycosis: a systematic review with network meta-analysis toenail mycosis: network meta-analysis. *J Dermatolog Treat.* (2020) 1–10. doi: 10.1080/09546634.2020.1729336. [Epub ahead of print].
14. Singh S, Shukla P. End of the road for terbinafine? Results of a pragmatic prospective cohort study of 500 patients. *Indian J Dermatol Venereol Leprol.* (2018) 84:554–7. doi: 10.4103/ijdvl.IJDVL_526_17
15. Roh D, Kim H, Nam J, Mun J, Park J, Park J, et al. Public awareness of onychosis in Korea: a survey of 621 participants. *J Mycol Infect.* (2018) 23:15–23. doi: 10.17966/jmi.2018.23.1.15
16. Wu AG, Geizhals S, Lipner SR. Retrospective study of factors affecting medication adherence in patients prescribed efinaconazole 10% solution for onychomycosis. *J Am Acad Dermatol.* (2020) 84:208–10. doi: 10.1016/j.jaad.2020.04.126
17. Zaias N. Onychomycosis. *Arch Dermatol.* (1972) 105:263–74. doi: 10.1001/archderm.1972.01620050069017
18. Gupta AK, Mays RR, Versteeg SG, Shear NH, Piguet V. Update on current approaches to diagnosis and treatment of onychomycosis. *Expert Rev Anti Infect Ther.* (2018) 16:929–38. doi: 10.1080/14787210.2018.1544891
19. Leung AKC, Lam JM, Leong KF, Hon KL, Barankin B, Leung AAM, et al. Onychomycosis: an updated review. *Recent Pat Inflamm Allergy Drug Discov.* (2020) 14:32–45. doi: 10.2174/1872213X13666191026090713
20. Hay RJ, Baran R. Onychomycosis: a proposed revision of the clinical classification. *J Am Acad Dermatol.* (2011) 65:1219–27. doi: 10.1016/j.jaad.2010.09.730
21. Ohn J, Yu DA, Park H, Cho S, Mun JH. Green nail syndrome: analysis of the association with onychomycosis. *J Am Acad Dermatol.* (2020) 83:940–2. doi: 10.1016/j.jaad.2020.01.040
22. Lipner SR, Scher RK. Evaluation of nail lines: color and shape hold clues. *Cleve Clin J Med.* (2016) 83:385–91. doi: 10.3949/ccjm.83a.14187
23. Martinez-Herrera E, Moreno-Coutiño G, Fernández-Martínez RF, Finch J, Arenas R. Dermatophytoma: description of 7 cases. *J Am Acad Dermatol.* (2012) 66:1014–6. doi: 10.1016/j.jaad.2010.06.034
24. Carney C, Tosti A, Daniel R, Scher R, Rich P, DeCoster J, et al. A new classification system for grading the severity of onychomycosis: onychomycosis severity index. *Arch Dermatol.* (2011) 147:1277–82. doi: 10.1001/archdermatol.2011.267
25. Jacobsen AA, Tosti A. Trachyonychia and twenty-nail dystrophy: a comprehensive review and discussion of diagnostic accuracy. *Skin Appendage Disord.* (2016) 2:7–13. doi: 10.1159/000445544
26. Starace M, Alessandrini A, Bruni F, Piraccini BM. Trachyonychia: a retrospective study of 122 patients in a period of 30 years. *J Eur Acad Dermatol Venereol.* (2020) 34:880–4. doi: 10.1111/jdv.16186
27. Haber JS, Chairatchaneeboon M, Rubin AI. Trachyonychia: review and update on clinical aspects, histology, and therapy. *Skin Appendage Disord.* (2017) 2:109–15. doi: 10.1159/000449063
28. Jo G, Park JS, Yu DA, Ohn J, Sheu SL, Mun JH. Onychoscopy of trachyonychia: an analysis of 30 patients and comparison with onychomycosis. *Br J Dermatol.* (2018) 179:491–3. doi: 10.1111/bjd.16431
29. Zaias N, Escovar SX, Zaiac MN. Finger and toenail onycholysis. *J Eur Acad Dermatol Venereol.* (2015) 29:848–53. doi: 10.1111/jdv.12862
30. Piraccini BM, Balestri R, Starace M, Rech G. Nail digital dermoscopy (onychoscopy) in the diagnosis of onychomycosis. *J Eur Acad Dermatol Venereol.* (2013) 27:509–13. doi: 10.1111/j.1468-3083.2011.04323.x
31. Smith RJ, Rubin AI. Pediatric nail disorders: a review. *Curr Opin Pediatr.* (2020) 32:506–15. doi: 10.1097/MOP.0000000000000921
32. Salgado F, Handler MZ, Schwartz RA. Shedding light on onychomadesis. *Cutis.* (2017) 99:33–6. Available online at: https://www.mdedge.com/dermatology/article/128565/pediatrics/shedding-light-onychomadesis?sso=true
33. Li M, Chen Z, Yin S, Xue R, Chen Z, Huang H, et al. Onychomycosis secondary to onychomadesis: an underdiagnosed manifestation. *Mycoses.* (2017) 60:161–5. doi: 10.1111/myc.12555
34. Gera SK, PG Zaini DKH, Wang S, Abdul Rahaman SHB, Chia RF, Lim KBL. Ingrowing toenails in children and adolescents: is nail avulsion

superior to nonoperative treatment? *Singapore Med J.* (2019) 60:94–6. doi: 10.11622/smedj.2018106
35. Lecerf P, Richert B, Theunis A, André J. A retrospective study of squamous cell carcinoma of the nail unit diagnosed in a Belgian general hospital over a 15-year period. *J Am Acad Dermatol.* (2013) 69:253–61. doi: 10.1016/j.jaad.2013.02.008
36. Park JH, Lee DY, Kim N. Nail neoplasms. *J Dermatol.* (2017) 44:279–87. doi: 10.1111/1346-8138.13702
37. Starace M, Alessandrini A, Dika E, Piraccini BM. Squamous cell carcinoma of the nail unit. *Dermatol Pract Concept.* (2018) 8:238–44. doi: 10.5826/dpc.0803a017
38. Lee TM, Jo G, Kim M, Lee SH, Cho SI, Jo SJ, et al. Squamous cell carcinoma of the nail unit: a retrospective review of 19 cases in Asia and comparative review of Western literature. *Int J Dermatol.* (2019) 58:428–32. doi: 10.1111/ijd.14306
39. Durbec F, Martin L, Derancourt C, Grange F. Melanoma of the hand and foot: epidemiological, prognostic and genetic features. A systematic review. *Br J Dermatol.* (2012) 166:727–39. doi: 10.1111/j.1365-2133.2011.10772.x
40. Csányi I, Houshmand N, Szucs M, Ócsai H, Kemény L, Oláh J, et al. Acral lentiginous melanoma: a single-centre retrospective review of four decades in East-Central Europe. *J Eur Acad Dermatol Venereol.* (2020) 34:2004–10. doi: 10.1111/jdv.16227
41. Levit EK, Kagen MH, Scher RK, Grossman M, Altman E. The ABC rule for clinical detection of subungual melanoma. *J Am Acad Dermatol.* (2000) 42:269–74. doi: 10.1016/S0190-9622(00)90137-3
42. Sohng C, Han MH, Park D, Park KD, Jang YH, Lee WJ, et al. Clinical features of subungual melanoma according to the extent of Hutchinson's nail sign: a retrospective single-centre study. *J Eur Acad Dermatol Venereol.* (2020) 35:380–6. doi: 10.1111/jdv.16762
43. Phan A, Dalle S, Touzet S, Ronger-Savlé S, Balme B, Thomas L. Dermoscopic features of acral lentiginous melanoma in a large series of 110 cases in a white population. *Br J Dermatol.* (2010) 162:765–71. doi: 10.1111/j.1365-2133.2009.09594.x
44. Ohn J, Jo G, Cho Y, Sheu SL, Cho KH, Mun JH. Assessment of a predictive scoring model for dermoscopy of subungual melanoma *in situ*. *JAMA Dermatol.* (2018) 154:890–6. doi: 10.1001/jamadermatol.2018.1372
45. Riahi RR, Cohen PR, Goldberg LH. Subungual nail bed melanoma masquerading as tinea ungium. *Dermatol Online J.* (2018) 24. Retrieved from: https://escholarship.org/uc/item/4z5191rj
46. Gatica-Torres M, Nelson CA, Lipoff JB, Miller CJ, Rubin AI. Nail clipping with onychomycosis and surprise clue to the diagnosis of nail unit melanoma. *J Cutan Pathol.* (2018) 45:803–6. doi: 10.1111/cup.13333
47. Lipner SR, Scher RK. Onychomycosis—a small step for quality of care. *Curr Med Res Opin.* (2016) 32:865–7. doi: 10.1185/03007995.2016.1147026
48. Lipner SR, Scher RK. Confirmatory testing for onychomycosis. *JAMA Dermatol.* (2016) 152:847. doi: 10.1001/jamadermatol.2016.0785
49. Dasgupta T, Sahu J. Origins of the KOH technique. *Clin Dermatol.* (2012) 30:238–41; discussion 41-2. doi: 10.1016/j.clindermatol.2011.11.020
50. Weinberg JM, Koestenblatt EK, Tutrone WD, Tishler HR, Najarian L. Comparison of diagnostic methods in the evaluation of onychomycosis. *J Am Acad Dermatol.* (2003) 49:193–7. doi: 10.1067/S0190-9622(03)01480-4
51. Velasquez-Agudelo V, Cardona-Arias JA. Meta-analysis of the utility of culture, biopsy, and direct KOH examination for the diagnosis of onychomycosis. *BMC Infect Dis.* (2017) 17:166. doi: 10.1186/s12879-017-2258-3
52. Gupta AK, Simpson FC. Diagnosing onychomycosis. *Clin Dermatol.* (2013) 31:540–3. doi: 10.1016/j.clindermatol.2013.06.009
53. Ghannoum M, Mukherjee P, Isham N, Markinson B, Rosso JD, Leal L. Examining the importance of laboratory and diagnostic testing when treating and diagnosing onychomycosis. *Int J Dermatol.* (2018) 57:131–8. doi: 10.1111/ijd.13690
54. Kayarkatte MN, Singal A, Pandhi D, Das S, Sharma S. Nail dermoscopy (onychoscopy) findings in the diagnosis of primary onychomycosis: a cross-sectional study. *Indian J Dermatol Venereol Leprol.* (2020) 86:341–9. doi: 10.4103/ijdvl.IJDVL_100_19
55. Pharaon M, Gari-Toussaint M, Khemis A, Zorzi K, Petit L, Martel P, et al. Diagnosis and treatment monitoring of toenail onychomycosis by reflectance confocal microscopy: prospective cohort study in 58 patients. *J Am Acad Dermatol.* (2014) 71:56–61. doi: 10.1016/j.jaad.2014.02.020
56. Rothmund G, Sattler EC, Kaestle R, Fischer C, Haas CJ, Starz H, et al. Confocal laser scanning microscopy as a new valuable tool in the diagnosis of onychomycosis—comparison of six diagnostic methods. *Mycoses.* (2013) 56:47–55. doi: 10.1111/j.1439-0507.2012.02198.x
57. Krammer S, Krammer C, Vladimirova G, Salzer S, Ruini C, Sattler E, et al. *Ex vivo* confocal laser scanning microscopy: a potential new diagnostic imaging tool in onychomycosis comparable with gold standard techniques. *Front Med (Lausanne).* (2020) 7:586648. doi: 10.3389/fmed.2020.586648
58. Kondori N, Abrahamsson AL, Ataollahy N, Wennerås C. Comparison of a new commercial test, Dermatophyte-PCR kit, with conventional methods for rapid detection and identification of *Trichophyton rubrum* in nail specimens. *Med Mycol.* (2010) 48:1005–8. doi: 10.3109/13693781003743130
59. Mehlig L, Garve C, Ritschel A, Zeiler A, Brabetz W, Weber C, et al. Clinical evaluation of a novel commercial multiplex-based PCR diagnostic test for differential diagnosis of dermatomycoses. *Mycoses.* (2014) 57:27–34. doi: 10.1111/myc.12097
60. Petinataud D, Berger S, Ferdynus C, Debourgogne A, Contet-Audonneau N, Machouart M. Optimising the diagnostic strategy for onychomycosis from sample collection to FUNGAL identification evaluation of a diagnostic kit for real-time PCR. *Mycoses.* (2016) 59:304–11. doi: 10.1111/myc.12471
61. Hafirassou AZ, Valero C, Gassem N, Mihoubi I, Buitrago MJ. Usefulness of techniques based on real time PCR for the identification of onychomycosis-causing species. *Mycoses.* (2017) 60:638–44. doi: 10.1111/myc.12629
62. Kim YJ, Han SS, Yang HJ, Chang SE. Prospective, comparative evaluation of a deep neural network and dermoscopy in the diagnosis of onychomycosis. *PLoS ONE.* (2020) 15:e0234334. doi: 10.1371/journal.pone.0234334
63. Han SS, Park GH, Lim W, Kim MS, Na JI, Park I, et al. Deep neural networks show an equivalent and often superior performance to dermatologists in onychomycosis diagnosis: automatic construction of onychomycosis datasets by region-based convolutional deep neural network. *PLoS ONE.* (2018) 13:e0191493. doi: 10.1371/journal.pone.0191493
64. Jeelani S, Ahmed QM, Lanker AM, Hassan I, Jeelani N, Fazili T. Histopathological examination of nail clippings using PAS staining (HPE-PAS): gold standard in diagnosis of Onychomycosis. *Mycoses.* (2015) 58:27–32. doi: 10.1111/myc.12251
65. Feuilhade de Chauvin M. New diagnostic techniques. *J Eur Acad Dermatol Venereol.* (2005) 19(Suppl. 1):20–4. doi: 10.1111/j.1468-3083.2005.01287.x
66. Stephen S, Tosti A, Rubin AI. Diagnostic applications of nail clippings. *Dermatol Clin.* (2015) 33:289–301. doi: 10.1016/j.det.2014.12.011
67. Bertanha L, Chiacchio ND. Nail clipping in onychomycosis. *An Bras Dermatol.* (2016) 91:688–90. doi: 10.1590/abd1806-4841.20164968
68. Lilly KK, Koshnick RL, Grill JP, Khalil ZM, Nelson DB, Warshaw EM. Cost-effectiveness of diagnostic tests for toenail onychomycosis: a repeated-measure, single-blinded, cross-sectional evaluation of 7 diagnostic tests. *J Am Acad Dermatol.* (2006) 55:620–6. doi: 10.1016/j.jaad.2006.03.033
69. Ohn J, Choe YS, Park J, Mun JH. Dermoscopic patterns of fungal melanonychia: a comparative study with other causes of melanonychia. *J Am Acad Dermatol.* (2017) 76:488–93.e2. doi: 10.1016/j.jaad.2016.08.013
70. Jo G, Mun J. Dermoscopic findings in onychomycosis. *Korean J Med Mycol.* (2017) 22:50–1. doi: 10.17966/kjmm.2017.22.1.50
71. Hongcharu W, Dwyer P, Gonzalez S, Anderson RR. Confirmation of onychomycosis by *in vivo* confocal microscopy. *J Am Acad Dermatol.* (2000) 42:214–6. doi: 10.1016/S0190-9622(00)90128-2
72. Cinotti E, Fouilloux B, Perrot JL, Labeille B, Douchet C, Cambazard F. Confocal microscopy for healthy and pathological nail. *J Eur Acad Dermatol Venereol.* (2014) 28:853–8. doi: 10.1111/jdv.12330
73. Jensen RH, Arendrup MC. Molecular diagnosis of dermatophyte infections. *Curr Opin Infect Dis.* (2012) 25:126–34. doi: 10.1097/QCO.0b013e32834f5f6e
74. Watanabe S, Ishida K. Molecular diagnostic techniques for onychomycosis: validity and potential application. *Am J Clin Dermatol.* (2017) 18:281–6. doi: 10.1007/s40257-016-0248-7
75. Erhard M, Hipler UC, Burmester A, Brakhage AA, Wöstemeyer J. Identification of dermatophyte species causing onychomycosis and tinea pedis by MALDI-TOF mass spectrometry. *Exp Dermatol.* (2008) 17:356–61. doi: 10.1111/j.1600-0625.2007.00649.x
76. Briganti G, Le Moine O. Artificial intelligence in medicine: today and tomorrow. *Front Med (Lausanne).* (2020) 7:27. doi: 10.3389/fmed.2020.00027

77. Cho SI, Han B, Hur K, Mun JH. Perceptions and attitudes of medical students regarding artificial intelligence in dermatology. *J Eur Acad Dermatol Venereol.* (2020) 35:e72–3. doi: 10.1111/jdv.16812
78. Esteva A, Kuprel B, Novoa RA, Ko J, Swetter SM, Blau HM, et al. Dermatologist-level classification of skin cancer with deep neural networks. *Nature.* (2017) 542:115–8. doi: 10.1038/nature21056
79. Gulshan V, Peng L, Coram M, Stumpe MC, Wu D, Narayanaswamy A, et al. Development and validation of a deep learning algorithm for detection of diabetic retinopathy in retinal fundus photographs. *JAMA.* (2016) 316:2402–10. doi: 10.1001/jama.2016.17216
80. Polesie S, Gillstedt M, Kittler H, Lallas A, Tschandl P, Zalaudek I, et al. Attitudes towards artificial intelligence within dermatology: an international online survey. *Br J Dermatol.* (2020) 183:159–61. doi: 10.1111/bjd.18875
81. Tschandl P, Rinner C, Apalla Z, Argenziano G, Codella N, Halpern A, et al. Human-computer collaboration for skin cancer recognition. *Nat Med.* (2020) 26:1229–34. doi: 10.1038/s41591-020-0942-0
82. Gomolin A, Netchiporouk E, Gniadecki R, Litvinov IV. Artificial intelligence applications in dermatology: where do we stand? *Front Med (Lausanne).* (2020) 7:100. doi: 10.3389/fmed.2020.00100

# 25

# Diagnosis of Primary Cutaneous Amyloidosis Using Dermoscopy and Reflectance Confocal Microscopy

*Xiuli Wang*[1,2,3], *Hui Wang*[1,2,3], *Zhenyu Zhong*[1,2,3], *Liyun Zheng*[1,2,3], *Yifan Wang*[1,2,3], *Ze Guo*[1,2,3], *Hui Li*[1,2,3] *and Min Gao*[1,2,3*]

[1] *Department of Dermatology, The First Affiliated Hospital of Anhui Medical University, Hefei, China,* [2] *Key Laboratory of Dermatology (Anhui Medical University), Ministry of Education, Hefei, China,* [3] *Inflammation and Immune Mediated Diseases Laboratory of Anhui Province, Hefei, China*

***Correspondence:***
*Min Gao*
*ahhngm@126.com*

The dermoscopy and reflectance confocal microscopy (RCM) can provide new insights for diagnosis disease as non-invasive and easy-to-use tool. We described the dermoscopy and RCM characteristics of two patients with primary cutaneous amyloidosis (PCA) respectively. The dermoscopy characteristics were as follows: brownish macules with brown or white centers surrounded by hyperpigmented blotches, and a whitish scar-like center encircled by irregular brownish hyperpigmented spots or patches. The RCM features were increased melanin deposition in the basal layer, highly refractive structures with various shapes in the enlarged papillary dermis, and the increased pleomorphic structure of the dermal papillary ring. This is the first report the dermoscopy and RCM characteristics of PCA. We hope the characteristic dermoscopy and RCM appearances would provide a basis for doctors to diagnose and intervene earlier.

**Keywords: primary cutaneous amyloidosis, dermoscopy, reflectance confocal microscopy, non-invasive technique, diagnosis**

## INTRODUCTION

Primary cutaneous amyloidosis (PCA) is a relatively common disease, but it can cause physical and psychological distress due to itch and potentially disfiguring disorder. There are different subtypes of PCA, including macular amyloidosis, lichen amyloidosis, nodular amyloidosis, or a mixed appearance of macular amyloidosis and lichen amyloidosis, which is described as biphasic amyloidosis (1, 2). We observed two patients with PCA through dermoscopy and reflectance confocal microscopy (RCM). One of them was confirmed by histopathological examination, and the lesions presented as biphasic amyloidosis. Another patient was clinically diagnosed as macular amyloidosis.

Dermoscopy has been proved to be an important noninvasive technique to diagnose cutaneous pigmented diseases, which can magnify the pigmented structures of the epidermis, the dermo-epidermal junction, and the dermis (3, 4). RCM is a valuable, widely used tool for its noninvasive, dynamic real-time and high cellular resolution characteristic (5). These two tools are particularly suitable for disease screening before the histopathological examination, which may avoid some surgical operation.

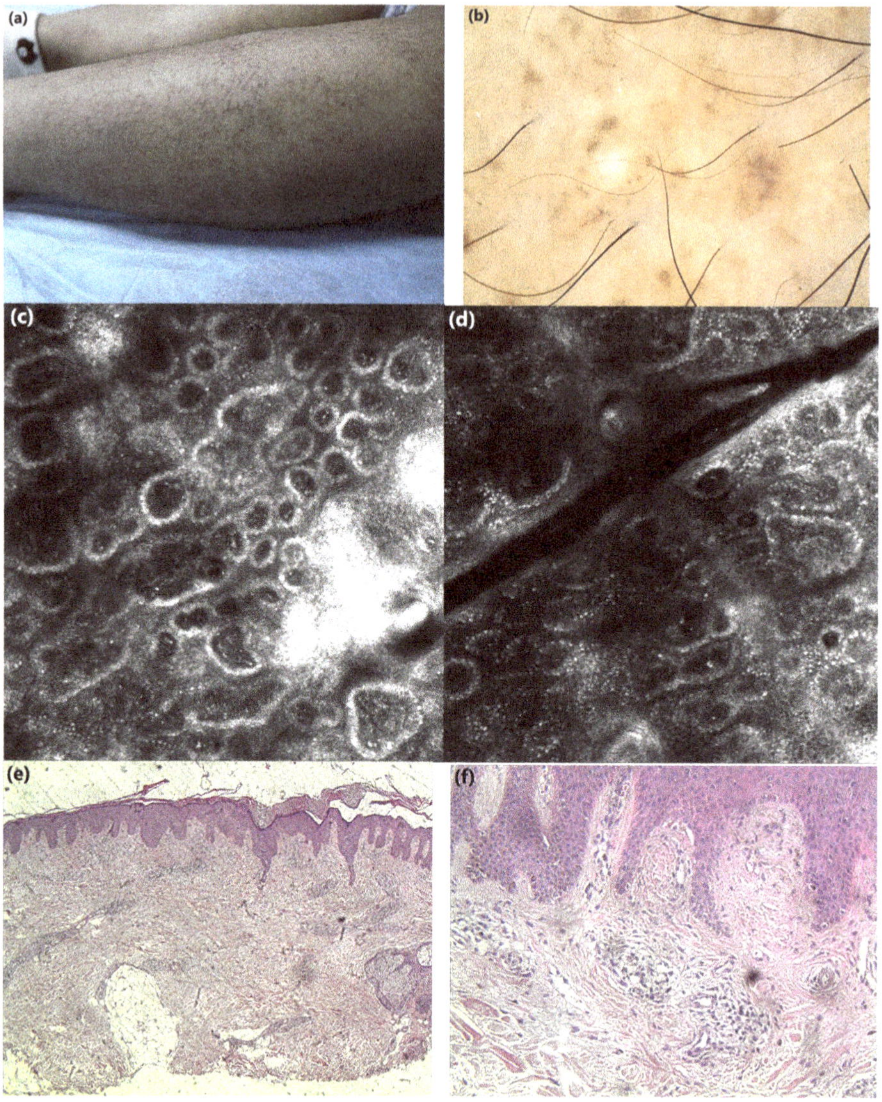


**FIGURE 1 | (a)** Clinical features: macular hyperpigmentation in a rippling pattern and hyperkeratotic brownish papules. **(b)** Under dermoscopic: irregular brownish macules with brown centers surrounded by hyperpigmented blotches, whitish scar-like center encircled by brownish hyperpigmented patches. **(c,d)** Under RCM: hyperkeratosis, melanin deposition in the basal layer, highly refractive structures inside the enlarged papillary dermis in cloud-like agglomerate shape, some round moderately-highly bright round cells in dermis. **(e, f)** Histopathology: hyperkeratosis in the epidermis, increased melanin deposition in the basal layer, focal deposition of homogeneous acidophilic substance in dermal papilla (H&E stain).

## CASE REPORT

Case 1: A 25-years-old woman presented with hyperpigmented macules and maculopapular rash on her lower limbs for 4 years. The lesions were located mainly in the lower legs, which progressed slowly to the thighs and arms, with moderate pruritus. On physical examination, macular hyperpigmentation in a rippling pattern were observed over her limbs, and hyperkeratotic brownish papules in some areas. The patient was otherwise well, with no other skin symptoms or extracutaneous discomfort. The initial clinical diagnosis was consistent with PCA changes, which was more in line with biphasic amyloidosis (because the lesions had both the characteristics of macular amyloidosis and lichen amyloidosus) (**Figure 1a**). Case 2: A 65-years-old woman presented with a 10-year history of tan macules and papules on her back, with a medical history of cardiac disease. The lesions were persistent itching, without other skin discomfort. Physical examination revealed brownish macules fused in a grid pattern. We diagnosed it as macular amyloidosis (**Figure 2a**).

Case 1: Under dermoscopy, the appearance of some smaller brownish macules presented as irregular brown centers

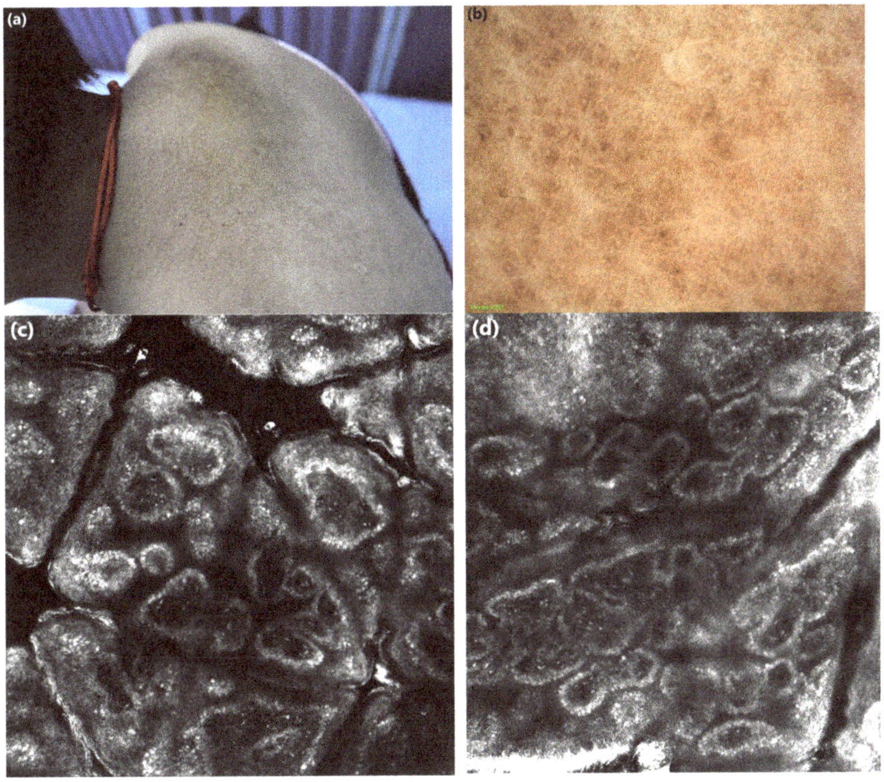


**FIGURE 2 | (a)** Clinical features: brownish macules fused in a grid pattern. **(b)** Under dermoscopic: white center encircled by hyperpigmented blotches, other pigmented patches were partially fused. **(c,d)** Under RCM: highly refractive structures with various shapes (cloud-like agglomerate, dotted substance, coliform substance) gathered in the enlarged papillary dermis, the increased pleomorphic structure of the dermal papillary ring.

with small brown stripes, surrounded by hyperpigmented blotches, while other macules showed irregular inhomogeneous hyperpigmented blotches. The dermoscopic features of hyperkeratotic brownish papules displayed a whitish scar-like center encircled by irregular brownish hyperpigmented spots or patches (**Figure 1b**). Case 2: On dermoscopic examination, the macula lesions showed white center encircled by hyperpigmented blotches, while other pigmented patches were partially fused (**Figure 2b**).

Case 1: Upon RCM, the examination displayed the hyperkeratosis in the epidermis, the increased melanin deposition in the basal layer, the highly refractive structures with cloud-like agglomerate, and dotted substance inside papillary dermis. Part of the dermal papillary rims were obscured, surrounded by some round, moderately-highly bright round cells (**Figures 1c,d**). Case 2: Under RCM, the appearance of PCA were the highly refractive structures with various shapes (cloud-like agglomerate, dotted substance, coliform substance, and so on) gathered in the enlarged papillary dermis, and the increased pleomorphic structure of the dermal papilla ring (**Figures 2c,d**).

Histopathological examination of case 1 showed hyperkeratosis in the epidermis, epidermal hyperplasia, downward extended of part of the epidermis, increased melanin deposition in the basal layer, and focal deposition of homogeneous acidophilic substance in the enlarged dermal papilla (**Figures 1e,f**).

## CONCLUSION

We presented two patient with PCA, and to our knowledge, this is the first report the dermoscopy and RCM characteristics of PCA. The dermoscopic findings of macular amyloidosis often showed a common feature, that is a white or brown central hub surrounded by brownish pigmentation (6). Besides, a white central hub or whitish scar-like center surrounded by pigmentation were often presented in the lichen amyloidosis (6). The RCM features of PCA have not been adequately described in the literature. Only two articles have been published to report the RCM features of PCA (7, 8). Upon RCM, the characteristics of increased melanin in the basal cell layer, cloud-like agglomerate in the dermal papilla, and melanophage infiltrating in the layer of superficial dermis, which were corresponding to histopathological findings: basal hyper pigmentation, amyloid deposition, pigment incontinence (8).

PCA is usually diagnosed clinically. But for cases with atypical presentation, the noninvasive technique, dermoscopy combined with RCM, can be used as a reference for clinicians to diagnose PCA. On our observation, the dermoscopy features were brownish macules with brown or white centers surrounded by hyperpigmented blotches, and a whitish scar-like center encircled by irregular brownish hyperpigmented spots or patches. The RCM features were increased melanin deposition in the basal layer, highly refractive structures with various shapes (cloud-like agglomerate, dotted substance, coliform substance and so on) in the enlarged papillary dermis, and the increased pleomorphic structure of the dermal papilla. We hope the characteristic dermoscopy and RCM appearances would provide a basis for doctors to diagnose and intervene earlier.

## ETHICS STATEMENT

The studies involving human participants were reviewed and approved by Ethical Review Committee of Anhui Medical University. The patients/participants provided their written informed consent to participate in this study. Written informed consent was obtained from the individual(s) for the publication of any potentially identifiable images or data included in this article.

## AUTHOR CONTRIBUTIONS

All authors listed have made a substantial, direct and intellectual contribution to the work, and approved it for publication.

## REFERENCES

1. Fernandez-Flores A. Cutaneous amyloidosis: a concept review. *Am J Dermatopathol.* (2012) 34:1–14. doi: 10.1097/DAD.0b013e31823465c7
2. Brownstein MH, Hashimoto K, Greenwald G. Biphasic amyloidosis: link between macular and lichenoid forms. *Br J Dermatol.* (1973) 88:25–9. doi: 10.1111/j.1365-2133.1973.tb06667.x
3. Bakos RM, Blumetti TP, Roldan-Marin R, Slareni G. Non-invasive imaging tools in the diagnosis and treatment of skin cancers. *Am J Clin Dermatol.* (2018) 19(Suppl.1):3–14. doi: 10.1007/s40257-018-0367-4
4. Argenziano G, Soyer HP. Dermoscopy of pigmented skin lesions – a valuable tool for early. *Lancet Oncol.* (2001) 2:443–9. doi: 10.1016/S1470-2045(00)00422-8
5. Scope A, Benvenuto-Andrade C, Agero AL, Malvehy J, Puig S, Rajadhyaksha M, et al. *In vivo* reflectance confocal microscopy imaging of melanocytic skin lesions: consensus terminology glossary and illustrative images. *J Am Acad Dermatol.* (2007) 57:644–58. doi: 10.1016/j.jaad.2007.05.044
6. Chuang YY, Lee DD, Lin CS, Chang YJ, Tanaka M, Chang YT, et al. Characteristic dermoscopic features of primary cutaneous amyloidosis: a study of 35 cases. *Br J Dermatol.* (2012) 167:548–54. doi: 10.1111/j.1365-2133.2012.11066.x
7. Ionescu A-M, Ilie M-A, Chitu V, Razvan A, Lixandru D, Tanase C, et al. *In vivo* diagnosis of primary cutaneous amyloidosis -the role of reflectance confocal microscopy. *Diagnostics.* (2019) 9:66. doi: 10.3390/diagnostics9030066
8. Lei W, Ai EX. Reflectance confocal microscopy for the characterization of primary cutaneous amyloidosis: a pilot study. *Skin Res Technol.* (2017) 23:441–3. doi: 10.1111/srt.12343

# 26

# Female Pattern Hair Loss in Female and Male: A Quantitative Trichoscopic Analysis in Chinese Han Patients

*Xi Chen [1,2], Xiangqian Li [1], Baifu Chen [1], Yue Yin [2], Jianzhong Zhang [1] and Cheng Zhou [1*]*

*[1] Department of Dermatology, Peking University People's Hospital, Beijing, China, [2] Department of Dermatology, Beijing Tongren Hospital, Capital Medical University, Beijing, China*

***Correspondence:**
*Cheng Zhou*
*chengzhou@live.cn*

**Objectives:** To investigate the trichoscopic features of female pattern hair loss (FPHL) in Chinese Han patients and analyze the difference between male and female patients with FPHL.

**Materials and Methods:** Trichoscopic images were taken in four different scalp areas, including right frontal hairline, vertex, right parietal and occipital areas. Hair density, hair shaft diameter, vellus hair ratio and single hair follicle unit ratio were counted manually and analyzed.

**Results:** Seventy-three subjects were enrolled in this study, including 38 patients with FPHL (28 females and 10 males) and 35 normal controls without hair loss. The hair density and hair shaft diameter of FPHL patients reduced in the whole scalp. Vellus hair ratio and single hair follicle unit ratio were both increased in FPHL compared to normal controls. The vertex was the most affected area and the hair shaft diameter showed the most significant difference. Parietal and occipital area were also affected in FPHL. The reduction or increase was correlated with the severity of Ludwig staging. Very few gender differences were detected in male and female FPHL patients.

**Conclusion:** FPHL patients showed decreased hair density and hair shaft diameter, accompanied by increased vellus hair ratio and single hair follicle unit ratio. Parietal and occipital area can be also affected in FPHL, though not as severe as in vertex area. FPHL in male basically has the same characteristic as those in female patients.

**Limitation:** The main limitation of the study is the small sample size which only enrolled 10 male FPHL patients, in comparison to the female cases. The findings could not be representative of the normal population with the limited sample size.

**Keywords: hair, trichoscopy, female pattern hair loss, Chinese, gender**

## INTRODUCTION

Hair is one of the essential skin appendages in human. Thinning, damaging, or abnormal shedding of hair can not only impair the physical protection of scalp, but also affects mental health, and can even lead to severe social dysfunction. Androgenic alopecia (AGA) is the most common hair loss disease in the world, affecting both male and female. Rather than hair shedding, the process of hair loss in AGA is related to the gradual miniaturization of hair follicles, and eventually, lead to progressive, symmetric baldness (1). Two major hair loss patterns have been widely described in AGA. Male pattern hair loss (MPHL) or named male pattern baldness (MPB) usually manifests as a recession of the frontal hairline, with or without baldness of the vertex area (2). In contrast, female pattern hair loss (FPHL) presents with diffuse hair loss over the middle scalp and show no recession of frontal hairline, mainly affecting women (3).

The nomenclature of male and female pattern hair loss still cause confusion nowadays. Since the pathological changes of hair follicles are similar, most researchers regarded MPHL and FPHL as two variants of the same entity with different clinical presentation and treatment response (3, 4). It is hypothesized that FPHL and MPHL share common susceptibility genes, but genetic studies have not identified any susceptibility locus/gene for FPHL and suggested the etiology differs substantially from that of MPHL (5, 6).

Dermoscopy can magnify the skin lesions while eliminating the reflected light on the skin surface, helping clinicians to fully grasp the characteristics of disease skin lesions. As a branch of dermatoscopy, trichoscopy is cost-efficient, quick, and non-invasive, now is of great significance to evaluate hair and scalp disorders (7). When using a digital dermoscope (trichoscope), dermatologists can easily collect images with higher magnification, then use computer software to analyze the image data, such as hair density and hair shaft diameter. Previous studies have shown that one of the main trichoscopic features of AGA is the increased heterogeneity of hair shaft diameter, which can be quantified by hair shaft diameter and the ratio of vellus hair (8). The increase of single hair follicle units is also a manifestation of hair follicle microminiaturization in AGA patients (9). Besides, yellow dots, brown/white peripilar sign, honeycomb pigmentation, and pinpoint white dots are other important trichoscopic features of AGA, which are potentially related to the severity of the disease (10–12).

In quantitative trichoscpic evaluation, previous studies have analyzed several hair parameters of FPHL in female patients and have come to the consistent conclusion that miniaturization of hair follicles is the characteristics of FPHL in female, which is shown as reduced hair density and hair shaft diameter under trichoscopy (7, 13–15). Hair density and hair shaft diameter are the most used indicators in quantitation evaluation, and the percentage of vellus hair ($< 30\,\mu$m) has also been involved in the studies mentioned above. However, few researches have evaluated the percentage of single-hair follicle units, which is also of significance in FPHL diagnoses (7). In contrast to MPHL, in which occipital and parietal (side of the head) areas are usually not involved, parietal and occipital sites can also be affected in FPHL (14). At present, there still lacks a comprehensive evaluation of all four main hair parameters involving multiple scalp areas (frontal, vertex, parietal, and occipital areas) in FPHL.

Although FPHL is usually used to describe AGA in women, it can also be observed in a proportion of men (16, 17). With an overall AGA prevalence of 21.3% in Chinese male, 3.7% of the male patients showed FPHL type of hair loss (18). However, the trichoscopic feature of FPHL in male patients have not been well-studied yet (4). It is unclear whether the trichoscopic features of FPHL in male and female are the same or not.

In this study, we investigated the quantitative features of FPHL with digital trichoscope, and compared to the normal controls without hair loss. The differences between male and female FPHL patients were also analyzed.

## MATERIALS AND METHODS

### Subjects

Both male and female Chinese Han subjects aged 18–59 years old who visited the dermatology department of Peking University People's hospital from January to August in 2020 were recruited into the study. The participants were screened by two experienced trichologists and categorized in two groups. The FPHL cases were diagnosed according to the Ludwig classification, with diffuse balding process and retention of the frontal hairline (3). The group of normal scalp subjects comprised volunteers who visited the dermatology clinic with complaints except for hair and scalp related diseases. The exclusion criteria included (1) presence of male pattern hair loss, alopecia areata, telogen effluvium, or other hair/scalp disorders; (2) positive results of hair-pull test; (3) history of anemia, thyroid disease, nutritional deficiency, autoimmune disease, or other systemic disease; (4) history of hair-loss treatment within 6 months; (5) hair coloring or perming within 3 months prior to the study; and (6) history of hair restoration surgery or scalp micropigmentation. All participants are agreed to participate in the study and provided written informed consent. The study was approved by the ethics committee of Peking University People's Hospital.

### Trichoscopy and Analysis

Due to the symmetrical hair loss feature of FPHL, trichoscopy was performed in four regions, i.e., right frontal hairline, vertex, right parietal and occipital area, using a polarized contact dermoscope (Fotofinder body studio ATBM, FotoFinder Systems GmbH, Bad Birnbach, Germany). The measurement point of each area is shown in **Figures 1a–d**: (1) the top of right frontotemporal angle (marked as "frontal"); (2) the mid-point of the connection of the left and right external auditory ear canals ("vertex"); (3) 6 cm from the external ear canal on the right side of the participants ("parietal"); (4) the occipital carina ("occipital"). The lateral scalp is divided into three parts by hair transplant surgeons: temporal (anterior one-third), parietal (middle one-third), and occipital (posterior one-third). The measurement area of the lateral scalp used in this study may be called "temporal" or "temporoparietal" in some other previous researches; however, we named this point as "parietal" due to its anatomical location above the parietal bone.

In each area, one 20-fold and four 50-fold figures were taken. All the parameters were all manually measured in Trichoscale 3.0 software Smart Count (Fotofinder Universe 2019, Bad Birnbach, Germany). Hairs and hair follicle units in each 50-fold trichoscopic figure were noted and counted by clicking the mouse, which was conducted by two experienced trichologists. Hair shaft diameter was measured by mouse pointing and

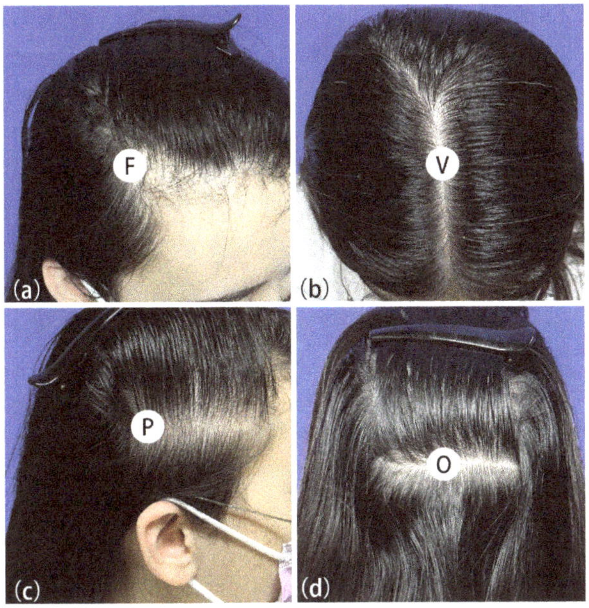


**FIGURE 1** | Measuring points of trichoscopy in frontal **(a)**, vertex **(b)**, parietal **(c)** and occipital **(d)** area.

dragging vertically from one edge of the hair shaft to the other edge, and the average value was calculated.

## Statistical Analysis

Statistical analysis was done using SPSS software (IBM, 25.0, CA, USA). Narrative statistics described the basic characteristics of the population. Independent-sample *t*-tests and Chi-square tests were performed to test the significance between the FPHL patients and the normal subjects. Kruskal-Wallis *H*-tests, Mann-Whitney *U*-tests and Fisher's exact tests were performed to compare results between groups whose data did not subject to normal distribution. The results of the analysis were presented as mean ± standard deviation (SD), and a $p < 0.05$ was considered significant.

PASS 2019 software (NCSS LLC., Kaysville, U.T., USA) was used to calculate the sample size. The primary outcomes of this study are vertex hair density, hair-shaft diameter, vellus hair ratio and single hair follicle unit ratio of normal and FPHL patients. To detect the lowest mean difference of 15 with standard deviations of 19.0 and 11.0 between the two groups with a two-sided 0.0125% significance level (adjusted for multiple comparisons using Bonferroni method) and a power of 90%, a sample size of 33 for each group is needed, at last, 35 normal people and 38 FPHL people were enrolled in this study.

# RESULTS

The participants were subdivided into two groups of 35 normal subjects and 38 FPHL patients based on the clinical diagnosis. The FPHL patients are graded following the Ludwig classification, from L1 to L3. The particular distribution of participants is shown in **Table 1**. The mean age of normal subjects and FPHL patients were 31.40 ± 10.38 and 31.08 ± 8.82 years old, respectively. No significant difference has been detected between normal and FPHL subjects. The typical clinical images of FPHL patients and trichoscopic images in vertex area of both FPHL and normal subjects are shown in **Figure 2**. The values of mean hair density, hair shaft diameter, vellus hair ratio and single hair follicle unit ratio at different scalp sites of FPHL patients are summarized in **Tables 2**, **3**, and the parameters of normal male and female are shown in **Table 4**.

## Hair Density

The mean hair density at different scalp areas of our participants is shown in the first part of **Tables 2–4**. The hair density in parietal area was the lowest in both FPHL and normal participants, and in vertex area, all groups show the highest hair density (**Tables 2, 3**). When compared to the normal subjects, the hair density in FPHL patients tended to reduce and statistically significant differences were detected in all scalp areas, especially in vertex area ($p < 0.0001$). However, no gender difference of hair density was detected in FPHL patients (**Table 3**), though the hair density in parietal area of male normal subjects was significantly lower than female (**Table 4**).

## Hair Shaft Diameter

The second part of **Tables 2–4** has shown the mean hair shaft diameter of male and female participants. In normal participants, the hair of the frontal area was the thinnest, while in the FPHL patients the vertex area showed the lowest hair shaft diameter (**Table 2**). The hair shaft diameter of FPHL patients decreased in the whole scalp with statistically significant differences compared to normal. The highest reduction of hair shaft diameter of FPHL patients was detected in the vertex area ($p < 0.0001$). No gender difference was detected whether in patients or normal (**Tables 3, 4**).

## Vellus Hair Ratio

The vellus hair ratio is shown in the third part of **Tables 2–4**. The frontal area had the highest vellus hair ratio and the lowest ratio was found in occipital area in both FPHL and normal participants. The vellus hair ratio showed a tendency of increase in FPHL patients when compared to normal, and significant differences were detected in all scalp areas (**Table 2**). In vertex area, the vellus hair ratio also showed the highest increase ($p < 0.0001$). In FPHL patients, minor gender difference in vellus hair ratio were detected in parietal area, though no difference was shown between normal male and female participants (**Tables 3, 4**).

## Single Hair Follicle Unit Ratio

The single hair follicle ratio is shown in the last part of **Tables 2–4**. Similar to the vellus hair ratio, the frontal area had the highest single hair follicle ratio and the lowest ratio was found in occipital area in both FPHL and normal participants (**Table 2**). All four areas in FPHL patients showed statistical significance compared to the normal subjects, and the vertex area still had the top decrease among other scalp areas ($p < 0.0001$). There

TABLE 1 | Distribution of participants by hair loss status.

| Classification | | Male | | Female | | Total | |
|---|---|---|---|---|---|---|---|
| | | *n* | Age (year) | *n* | Age (year) | *n* | Age (year) |
| FPHL | Ludwig L1 | 4 | 24.75 (± 3.43) | 15 | 30.13 (± 7.96) | 19 | 29.00 (± 7.51) |
| | Ludwig L2 | 4 | 29.75 (± 7.14) | 9 | 35.78 (± 12.81) | 13 | 33.92 (± 11.43) |
| | Ludwig L3 | 2 | 34.00 (± 1.41) | 4 | 30.25 (± 5.44) | 6 | 31.50 (± 4.68) |
| | Total | 10 | 28.60 (± 5.89) | 28 | 31.96 (± 9.59) | 38 | 31.08 (± 8.21) |
| Normal | | 17 | 29.76 (± 11.02) | 18 | 32.94 (± 9.79) | 35 | 30.40 (± 10.38) |
| *p*-value | | / | 0.786 | / | 0.752 | / | 0.769 |

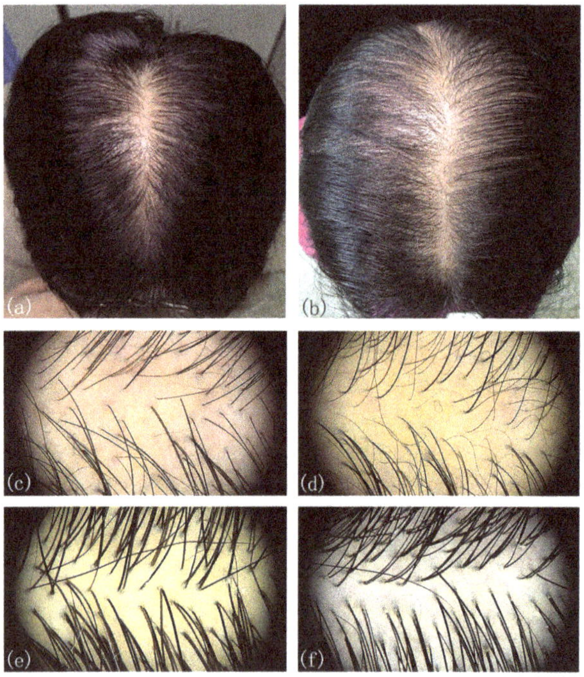

FIGURE 2 | Typical clinical and trichoscopic feature (vertex) of male FPHL **(a,c)** and female FPHL **(b,d)** patients, compared with normal male **(e)**, and female **(f)**.

was no gender difference in both normal and FPHL participants (**Tables 3, 4**).

## Hair Parameters From Grade L1 to L3 in FPHL Patients

We then analyzed the hair parameters of different severity in FPHL patients. According to the FPHL disease severity, patients were stratified into three groups (Ludwig L1-L3). In all scalp areas, the hair density and hair shaft diameter showed a decreasing tendency with the aggravation of the disease, and the ratio of vellus hair in and single hair follicle unit all raised as the disease got worse. Compared with normal group, the significant difference of the parameters was mainly found in vertex area (**Figure 3**) and in L2 and L3 groups. In L1 group, only the hair shaft diameter and vellus hair ratio of vertex area were significantly different with normal subjects.

## DISCUSSION

According to our quantitative trichoscopic analysis, FPHL involved the whole scalp, especially at the vertex area, and primarily manifested as a decrease in hair shaft diameter. All of the four hair parameters including hair density, hair shaft diameter and the ratio of vellus hair and single hair follicle unit, have changed in our FPHL patients when compared to normal, confirmed that the miniaturization of hair follicle is the characteristics of FPHL. Similar to previous research, our study also showed that the involvement of parietal and occipital area is an additional important feature of FPHL (7, 13–15). This pattern of hair involvement is quite different from MPHL. The parietal and occipital parts are usually not involved in MPHL patients, and therefore occipital and even parietal parts are appropriate donor sites for hair transplantation (19). Thus, when consulting hair transplantation with FPHL patients, it should be fully considered that the hair may be abnormal in the whole scalp, and a comprehensive examination should be carried out. Medical treatment of parietal or occipital area is also necessary if the region has been involved. Besides, the frontal area was also involved slightly even though no receding of hairline was observed clinically.

The changes of the hair parameters were correlated with the severity of the disease, from Ludwig grade 1 to 3 (**Figure 3**), and the vertex area was the most severely affected area. In the early stage of disease (L1), significant decreases in hair shaft diameter had been detected and the vellus hair ratio also increased significantly. Although not as severe as the vertex area, all the parameters of parietal and occipital area also showed significant difference in the advanced stages of the disease (L2 and L3).

Though FPHL in male has been described previously (20), studies on the clinical features are extremely limited, especially on trichoscopic features. During a retrospective study of 2,140 male AGA patients, only 84 (3.9%) patients were diagnosed as FPHL (17).

FPHL in male has similar clinical manifestations as FPHL in female, showing diffuse scalp hair loss with no obvious

**TABLE 2** | Hair parameters of FPHL patients and normal subjects.

| Scalp area | Hair density (/cm$^2$) | | | Hair shaft diameter (μm) | | | Vellus hair ratio (%) | | | Single hair follicle unit ratio (%) | | |
|---|---|---|---|---|---|---|---|---|---|---|---|---|
| | FPHL | Normal | *p*-value | FPHL | Normal | *p*-value | FPHL | Normal | *p*-value | FPHL | Normal | *p*-value |
| Frontal | 102.89 (± 20.19) | 117.07 (± 21.49) | 0.010* | 55.71 (± 8.83) | 61.73 (± 6.92) | 0.001* | 22.00 (± 7.88) | 16.89 (± 6.43) | 0.003* | 47.43 (± 16.82 | 35.78 (± 15.53) | 0.005* |
| Vertex | 112.05 (± 25.56) | 140.21 (± 23.91) | <0.001* | 54.23 (± 9.08) | 67.38 (± 7.59) | <0.001* | 20.92 (± 9.74) | 9.26 (± 4.59) | <0.001* | 39.69 (± 18.38 | 18.86 (± 11.37) | <0.001* |
| Parietal | 85.18 (± 27.48) | 96.19 (± 21.63) | 0.028* | 59.91 (± 10.02) | 67.62 (± 8.30) | 0.001* | 16.68 (± 10.71) | 10.72 (± 5.68) | 0.001* | 34.66 (± 18.26 | 17.89 (± 11.60) | <0.004* |
| Occipital | 106.66 (± 22.94) | 127.18 (± 22.7) | <0.001* | 60.78 (± 10.31) | 68.34 (± 7.70) | <0.001* | 15.04 (± 8.2) | 8.88 (± 4.23) | 0.004* | 28.32 (± 16.6) | 13.47 (± 8.74) | <0.001* |

*$p < 0.05$.

**TABLE 3** | Comparisons of hair parameters in FPHL patients between male and female.

| Scalp area | Hair density (/cm$^2$) | | | Hair shaft diameter (μm) | | | Vellus hair ratio (%) | | | Single hair follicle unit ratio (%) | | |
|---|---|---|---|---|---|---|---|---|---|---|---|---|
| | Male | Female | *p*-value | Male | Female | *p*-value | Male | Female | *p*-value | Male | Female | *p*-value |
| Frontal | 92.79 (± 21.29) | 106.5 (± 18.87) | 0.060 | 52.05 (± 8.29) | 57.02 (± 8.79) | 0.088 | 22.49 (± 5.74) | 21.82 (± 8.6) | 0.782 | 49.89 (± 24.29) | 46.54 (± 13.71) | 0.935 |
| Vertex | 113.1 (± 28.84) | 111.68 (± 24.85) | 0.883 | 53.23 (± 9.49) | 54.59 (± 9.08) | 0.636 | 18.15 (± 7.76) | 21.91 (± 10.29) | 0.302 | 38.3 (± 20.87) | 40.18 (± 17.81) | 0.807 |
| Parietal | 77.28 (± 10.14) | 88.00 (± 31.14) | 0.142 | 64.72 (± 9.63) | 58.19 (± 9.74) | 0.194 | 11.89 (± 8.35) | 18.39 (± 11.07) | 0.044* | 34.32 (± 17.36) | 34.78 (± 18.88) | 0.568 |
| Occipital | 95.78 (± 16.38) | 110.55 (± 23.92) | 0.101 | 61.08 (± 11.32) | 60.68 (± 10.14) | 0.732 | 14.32 (± 8.39) | 15.29 (± 8.27) | 0.568 | 33.45 (± 20.65) | 26.48 (± 14.9) | 0.368 |

*$p < 0.05$.

**TABLE 4** | Hair parameter of normal male and female subjects.

| Scalp area | Hair density (/cm$^2$) | | | Hair shaft diameter (μm) | | | Vellus hair ratio (%) | | | Single hair follicle unit ratio (%) | | |
|---|---|---|---|---|---|---|---|---|---|---|---|---|
| | Male | Female | *p*-value | Male | Female | *p*-value | Male | Female | *p*-value | Male | Female | *p*-value |
| Frontal | 114.34 (± 24.12) | 119.63 (± 19.01) | 0.546 | 62.68 (± 5.04) | 60.82 (± 8.37) | 0.318 | 16.75 (± 5.98) | 17.01 (± 6.99) | 0.910 | 39.32 (± 16.40) | 14.31 (± 8.37) | 0.258 |
| Vertex | 137.63 (± 25.44) | 142.63 (± 22.82) | 0.503 | 68.03 (± 8.37) | 66.74 (± 7.30) | 0.590 | 9.00 (± 3.38) | 9.49 (± 5.58) | 0.752 | 18.86 (± 10.90) | 18.87 (± 12.10) | 0.909 |
| Parietal | 85.82 (± 17.23)* | 105.98 (± 21.14) | 0.004* | 69.81 (± 7.51) | 65.54 (± 8.67) | 0.195 | 11.79 (± 5.18) | 9.71 (± 6.09) | 0.286 | 21.02 (± 13.64) | 14.94 (± 8.68) | 0.130 |
| Occipital | 127.51 (± 27.53) | 126.87 (± 17.79) | 0.883 | 68.96 (± 8.61) | 67.75 (± 6.91) | 0.443 | 10.07 (± 4.83) | 7.72 (± 3.30) | 0.105 | 15.83 (± 9.78) | 7.20 (± 6.91) | 0.163 |

*$p < 0.05$.

recession of the frontal hairline (21). Compared with female patients in the present study, we found the hair parameters changed in male FPHL patients are similar to that in female FPHL patients. Importantly, in male FPHL patients, parietal and occipital area can also be involved, which pattern is totally different from MPHL. Therefore, in our experience, diagnosing these male FPHL patients as MPHL or MPB is not appropriate. We suggested that FPHL in male or female should be diagnosed based on different hair loss patterns and trichoscopic alterations, rather than on the basis of gender alone. It is important to establish a classification for assessment and grading of parietal and occipital involvement, which could overcome the limitations in the Ludwig classification, the Sinclair scale and the basic and specific (BASP) classification (3, 22, 23). Oral finasteride 1 mg/day is effective in the majority of male patients with AGA, while in female FPHL patients it could not significantly slow hair thinning, increase hair growth or improve the appearance of the hair unless increasing the dose to 2.5–5 mg/day (24, 25). Whether available treatments for male FPHL patients could be as efficacy as in MPHL is unclear, and further treatment studies on male FPHL patients are needed. This study provides some evidence for clarifying the term of FPHL in male and is of great value for further study on its pathogenesis, treatment, and the similarities and differences with MPHL.

The two parameters, hair density and hair shaft diameter, are trichoscopic features that need precisely quantitative measurement, which might not be practical for daily diagnostics purposes. In our experience, vellus hair ratio and single hair follicle unit ratio are more likely to be perceived and estimated under trichoscopy without quantitative measurements, which are more valuable in clinical practice.

During the progressive and unsynchronized miniaturization of hair follicles in AGA, terminal hairs are gradually replaced by intermediate hair and vellus hairs. Although the relevant quantitative research is relatively limited, researchers have long agreed that hair shaft thickness heterogeneity of more than 20% is a hallmark of AGA, which means that vellus hair percentage for more than 20% of all the hairs in the same view (10, 12). In our study, the vellus hair ratio of FPHL in frontal and vertex areas were both over 20%. In the parietal and occipital area of the FPHL scalp, vellus hair ratio also increased, but not as much as 20%. The present values appear to be similar to the previous study of Caucasian women (9). Mai et al. has also used "terminal/vellus hair ratio" to describe the vellus hair percentage in their study, and we found our results were basically consistent with each other after conversion (15). According to the hair involvement characteristics of FPHL, evaluation of vellus hair ratio should be established on different parts of the scalp.

Hair exists in the form of follicular units on the scalp. The hair follicle unit, also known as the pilosebaceous gland unit, is composed of 1–5 hairs, erect hair muscles, sebaceous glands, and peripheral nerves and blood vessels. Guo et al. indicated that the hair follicle unit types found in healthy Han Chinese are dominated by 2-hair follicle

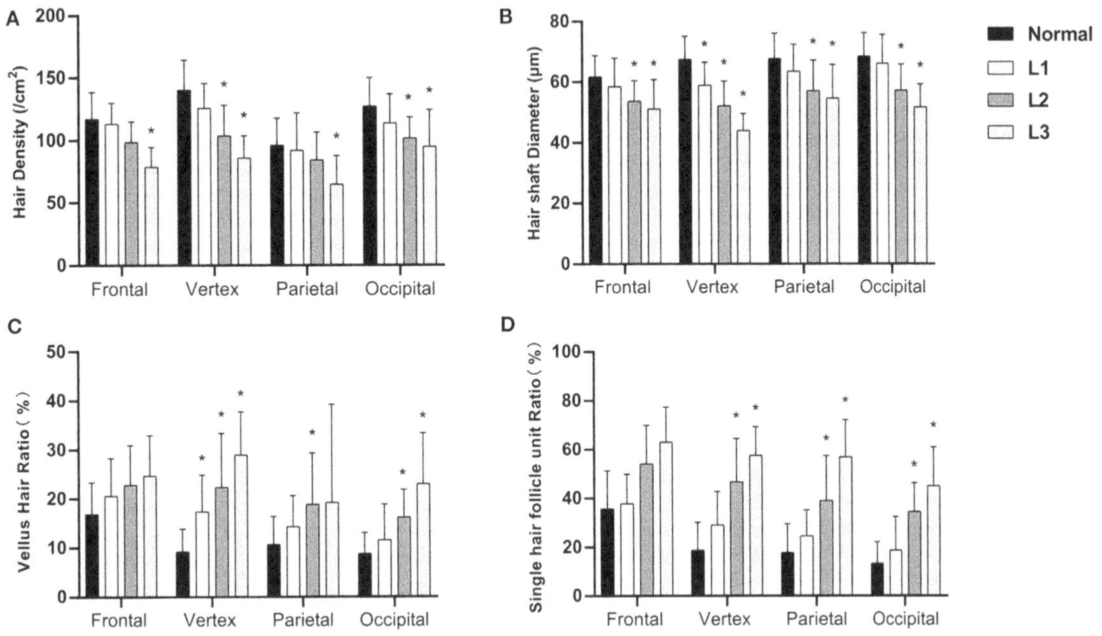


**FIGURE 3 |** Hair density **(A)**, hair shaft diameter **(B)**, vellus hair ratio **(C)**, and single hair follicle unit ratio **(D)** of FPHL patients from Ludwig L1 to L3. *$p < 0.05$ compared with normal subjects.

units, followed by single hair follicle units and 3-hair follicle units (26). The increase of single hair follicle units is also a trichoscopic manifestation of the miniaturization of hair follicles in AGA patients. Rakowska et al. included the increase of single hair follicle units as one of the secondary indicators of the trichoscopy criteria for diagnosing female androgenic alopecia (9). In our study, single hair follicle unit ratio elevated in FPHL patients as expected, however, it was not as high as in Caucasians. Interestingly, the single hair follicle unit ratio in Chinese normal controls was higher than Caucasians (9).

Hair density in this study showed a similar value to the previous study in Southern Chinese women (15). However, when comparing with other studies on Asian women including Korean and Thai women, the hair density of Chinese normal participants was a little bit lower and much lower than Caucasians, Hispanics and Africans (13, 27–29). In terms of hair shaft diameter, our results also seemed to be much "lower" than other similar studies except for the study of Caucasians women conducted by Rakowska et al. (9). The variation of the results in different studies may be caused by different devices and manners for the studies. Most of the previous study included about five randomly selected terminal hairs for hair shaft diameter measurement under 100-fold magnification, using trichoscopy system Folliscope® (LeedM Corporation) (13, 28). While in our study and Rakowska et al. (9) study, vellus hair was also included in the diameter measurement.

Gender factors showed a limited influence on hair parameters. Birnbaum et al. found that the differences in hair density of frontal, vertex and occipital area between men and women were not statistically significant in health Americans (including Hispanic, Caucasian, and African American) (27). A similar study of healthy Thai people also showed the same results (29). The only significant difference we noticed in this study is that the hair density of parietal region of men is lower than that of women, which was blank in the study of American people and not consistent with the data of Thai People. This gender difference in parietal hair density remains to be confirmed by more extensive studies.

## LIMITATION

Compared with other trichoscopic studies on FPHL, the sample size of this study was relatively small. The main limitation of the study cohort is the presence of only 10 male subjects with FPHL, in comparison to the female cases. Though the study could be able to detect the difference of trichoscopic features between FPHL and normal controls, the findings could not be representative of the normal population.

## CONCLUSION

In this study, the hair involvement in FPHL of Chinese Han patients was summarized with quantitative trichoscopic analysis. The miniaturization of hair follicles is the main characteristic of FPHL, which is shown as decreased hair density and hair shaft diameter, accompanied by increased vellus hair ratio and single hair follicle unit ratio. The hair in parietal and occipital area can be also affected, though not as severe as in vertex area. Although the incidence is exceptionally low, FPHL can occur in man, and its characteristics are basically the same as those in female patients.

## ETHICS STATEMENT

The studies involving human participants were reviewed and approved by Ethics Committee of Peking University People's Hospital. The patients/participants provided their written informed consent to participate in this study.

## AUTHOR CONTRIBUTIONS

All authors listed have made a substantial, direct and intellectual contribution to the work, and approved it for publication.

## REFERENCES


1. Drake LA, Dinehart S, Farmer E, Goltz R, Graham G, Hordinsky M, et al. Guidelines of care for androgenetic alopecia. American academy of dermatology. *J Am Acad Dermatol.* (1996) 35:465–9. doi: 10.1016/S0190-9622(96)90627-1
2. Hamilton JB. Patterned loss of hair in man: types and incidence. *Ann N Y Acad Sci.* (1951) 53:708–28. doi: 10.1111/j.1749-6632.1951.tb31971.x
3. Ludwig E. Classification of the types of androgenetic alopecia (common baldness) occurring in the female sex. *Brit J Dermatol.* (1977) 97:247–54. doi: 10.1111/j.1365-2133.1977.tb15179.x
4. Ramos PM, Miot HA. Female pattern hair loss: a clinical and pathophysiological review. *An Bras Dermatol.* (2015) 90:529–43. doi: 10.1590/abd1806-4841.20153370
5. Nuwaihyd R, Redler S, Heilmann S, Drichel D, Wolf S, Birch P, et al. Investigation of four novel male androgenetic alopecia susceptibility loci: no association with female pattern hair loss. *Arch Dermatol Res.* (2014) 306:413–8. doi: 10.1007/s00403-013-1436-4
6. Redler S, Messenger AG, Betz RC. Genetics and other factors in the aetiology of female pattern hair loss. *Exp Dermatol.* (2017) 26:510–7. doi: 10.1111/exd.13373
7. Rudnicka L, Olszewska M, Rakowska A, Kowalska-Oledzka E, Slowinska M. Trichoscopy: a new method for diagnosing hair loss. *J Drugs Dermatol.* (2008) 7:651. doi: 10.1001/archderm.144.8.1007
8. De Lacharrière O, Deloche C, Misciali C, Piraccini BM, Vincenzi C, Bastien P, et al. Hair diameter diversity: a clinical sign reflecting the follicle miniaturization. *Arch Dermatol.* (2001) 137:641–6. doi: 10.1001/pubs.ArchDermatol.-ISSN-0003-987x-137-5-dob10023
9. Rakowska A, Slowinska M, Kowalska-Oledzka E, Olszewska M, Rudnicka L. Dermoscopy in female androgenic alopecia: method standardization and diagnostic criteria. *Int J Trichology.* (2009) 1:123. doi: 10.4103/0974-7753.58555
10. Inui S, Nakajima T, Itami S. Scalp dermoscopy of androgenetic alopecia in Asian people. *J Dermatol.* (2009) 36:82–5. doi: 10.1111/j.1346-8138.2009.00593.x
11. Zhang X, Caulloo S, Zhao Y, Zhang B, Cai Z, Yang J. Female pattern hair loss: clinico-laboratory findings and trichoscopy depending on disease severity. *Int J Trichol.* (2012) 4:23. doi: 10.4103/0974-7753.96082
12. Hu R, Xu F, Han Y, Sheng Y, Qi S, Miao Y, et al. Trichoscopic findings of androgenetic alopecia and their association with disease severity. *J Dermatol.* (2015) 42:602–7. doi: 10.1111/1346-8138.12857
13. Kang H, Kang TW, Lee SD, Park YM, Kim HO, Kim SY. The changing patterns of hair density and thickness in South Korean women with hair loss: clinical office-based phototrichogram analysis. *Int J Dermatol.* (2009) 48:14–21. doi: 10.1111/j.1365-4632.2009.03795.x
14. Rojhirunsakool S, Suchonwanit P. Parietal scalp is another affected area in female pattern hair loss: an analysis of hair density and hair diameter. *Clin Cosmet Investig Dermatol.* (2018) 11:7. doi: 10.2147/CCID.S153768
15. Mai W, Sun Y, Liu X, Lin D, Lu D. Characteristic findings by phototrichogram in southern Chinese women with female pattern hair loss. *Skin Res Technol.* (2019) 25:447–55. doi: 10.1111/srt.12672
16. Norwood OT. Male pattern baldness: classification and incidence. *South Med J.* (1975) 68:1359–65. doi: 10.1097/00007611-197511000-00009
17. Kerkemeyer KL, de Carvalho LT, Jerjen R, John J, Sinclair RD, Pinczewski J, et al. Female pattern hair loss in men: a distinct clinical variant of androgenetic alopecia. *J Am Acad Dermatol.* (in press). doi: 10.1016/j.jaad.2020.09.042. Available online at: https://www.jaad.org/article/S0190-9622(20)32632-3/pdf
18. Wang T, Zhou C, Shen Y, Wang X, Ding X, Tian S, et al. Prevalence of androgenetic alopecia in China: a community-based study in six cities. *Brit J Dermatol.* (2010) 162:843–7. doi: 10.1111/j.1365-2133.2010.09640.x
19. Rousso DE, Kim SW. A review of medical and surgical treatment options for androgenetic alopecia. *JAMA Facial Plast. Surg.* (2014) 16:444–50. doi: 10.1001/jamafacial.2014.316
20. Banihashemi M, Nahidi Y, Meibodi NT, Jarahi L, Dolatkhah M. Serum vitamin D3 level in patients with female pattern hair loss. *Int J Trichol.* (2016) 8:116–20. doi: 10.4103/0974-7753.188965
21. Trüeb RM. Female pattern baldness in men. *J Am Acad Dermatol.* (1993) 29:782–3. doi: 10.1016/S0190-9622(08)81702-1
22. Lee WS, Ro BI, Hong SP, Bak H, Sim Y, Park JK, et al. A new classification of pattern hair loss that is universal for men and women: basic and specific (BASP) classification. *J Am Acad Dermatol.* (2007) 57:37–46. doi: 10.1016/j.jaad.2006.12.029
23. Sinclair R, Torkamani N, Jones L. Androgenetic alopecia: new insights into the pathogenesis and mechanism of hair loss. *F1000Research.* (2015) 4:F1000. doi: 10.12688/f1000research.6401.1
24. Price VH, Roberts JL, Hordinsky M, Olsen EA, Savin R, Bergfeld W, et al. Lack of efficacy of finasteride in postmenopausal women with androgenetic alopecia. *J Am Acad Dermatol.* (2000) 43:768–76. doi: 10.1067/mjd.2000.107953
25. Iamsumang W, Leerunyakul K, Suchonwanit P. Finasteride and its potential for the treatment of female pattern hair loss: evidence to date. *Drug Des Devel Ther.* (2020) 14:951. doi: 10.2147/DDDT.S240615
26. Guo ZH, Wang G, Miao Y, Fan ZX, Liu XM, Qu Q, et al. The distribution of hair in Han Chinese. *Plastic Aesthetic Res.* (2017) 4:150. doi: 10.20517/2347-9264.2017.52
27. Birnbaum MR, McLellan BN, Shapiro J, Ye K, Reid SD. Evaluation of hair density in different ethnicities in a healthy American population using quantitative trichoscopic analysis. *Skin Append Disord.* (2018) 4:304–7. doi: 10.1159/000485522
28. Heo JH, Yeom SD, Byun JW, Shin J, Choi GS. Significant relationship between temporal hair loss and other scalp areas in female pattern hair loss. *J Dermatol.* (2020) 47:334–41. doi: 10.1111/1346-8138.15220
29. Leerunyakul K, Suchonwanit P. Evaluation of hair density and hair diameter in the adult thai population using quantitative trichoscopic analysis. *Biomed Res Int.* (2020) 2020:2476890. doi: 10.1155/2020/2476890

# 27

# Accuracy of Teledermatology in Inflammatory Dermatoses

*Mara Giavina-Bianchi*, Raquel Sousa and Eduardo Cordioli*

*Department of Telemedicine, Hospital Israelita Albert Einstein, São Paulo, Brazil*

***Correspondence:**
*Mara Giavina-Bianchi*
*marahgbianchi@gmail.com*

Teledermatology is assuming a progressively greater role as a healthcare delivery method, especially now, during this pandemic time. It is important to know how accurate this tool is for different skin diseases. Most of the studies have focused on skin neoplasms or general dermatology. Studies based on a large number of inflammatory dermatoses have not yet been performed. Such knowledge can help dermatologists to decide whether endorsing this method or not. Our objective was to determine the accuracy of teledermatology in inflammatory dermatoses in a robust number of cases. A retrospective cohort study was conducted in São Paulo, Brazil, from July 2017–18, where a store-and-forward Teledermatology project was implemented under primary-care attention to triage surgical, more complex, or severe dermatoses. A total of 30,976 patients presenting 55,012 lesions took part in the project. Thirteen participating teledermatologists had three options to refer the patients: directly to biopsy, to the in-person dermatologist or back to the general physician with most probable diagnosis and management. In the group referred to the in-person dermatologist, we looked for the 20 most frequent International Classification of Diseases and Related Health Problems- 10th revision (ICD-10) of inflammatory dermatoses, which resulted in 739 patients and 739 lesions. As patients had been triaged by teledermatology previously, we were able to compare ICD-10 codes filled both by teledermatogists and by in-person dermatologists. The proportion of complete, partial, and no agreement rates between the in-person dermatologist's and the teledermatologist's diagnoses was used for accuracy. We also calculated Cohen's kappa, a statistical measure of inter-rater agreement, for complete agreement. The mean complete agreement rate for all twenty dermatoses was 78% (31–100%) and kappa = 0.743; partial agreement 8%; and no agreement 14%, presenting variability according to the disease. Our study showed that teledermatology for inflammatory dermatoses has a high accuracy. This result reassures that it can be a proper option for patient care.

**Keywords: teledermatology, accuracy, telemedicine, inflammatory dermatoses, telehealth**

## INTRODUCTION

Telemedicine, especially in this pandemic moment, is of great value for delivering healthcare. It has the potential to improve access to subspecialty expertise, reduce healthcare costs, and improve the overall quality of care. Dermatology is particularly suitable for this care system. The three main teledermatology delivery platforms are: synchronous (RT: real-time teledermatology), asynchronous (SF-TD), and hybrid (both synchronous and asynchronous forms). Synchronous teledermatology employs live video conferencing between the patient and the teledermatologist. Asynchronous teledermatology is a method whereby clinical or dermoscopy dermatologic images are obtained, sent to the responding dermatologist, who can review them at later time. Although it provides high-resolution dermatologic images and enables an efficient practice that can be performed across time zones, this modality is limited by the ability of the teledermatologist to obtain additional clinical history while evaluating the case (1).

Rates of diagnostic accuracy by teledermatology vary from study to study; the majority have found rates to be in the range of 75–80%, comparable to those with in-person care (1). Nevertheless, most of the studies were focused on skin neoplasms, especially skin cancer and pigmented lesions (2–5), or on general dermatology (6–10). A recent systematic review concluded that robust implementation studies of teledermatology are needed, with attention to reducing risk of bias when assessing diagnostic accuracy (2). For this reason, we performed a study with the aim of determining the accuracy of teledermatology for inflammatory dermatoses in a robust number of cases, assessing the agreement rate between the in-person dermatologist's and the teledermatologist's diagnoses.

## MATERIALS AND METHODS

This was a retrospective cohort study designed to assess concordance between diagnoses made by in-person dermatologists and teledermatologists, approved by the Ethics Committee of Hospital Israelita Albert Einstein (CAAE: 97126618.6.0000.0071). We analyzed the reports of 30,976 patients included in a teledermatology triage project conducted in the city of São Paulo, Brazil, from July 2017 to July 2018.

### Teledermatology Triage Project

Since there was a long patients' waiting list for an appointment with a dermatologist in the public health service, the aim of the teledermatology project was to triage the patients, in such a way that the severe, more complex, or surgical cases would be prioritized for biopsy procedure and in-person dermatologists, and the mild cases would be managed in the primary care attention along with the general physician (GP). Briefly, there were 57,832 patients under public primary-care attention who were on a waiting list for an appointment with a dermatologist, after being referred by the primary care physician. All of them were consecutively phoned to go to one of the three public municipal hospitals. Once there, their demographic data, a short clinical history and photographs of their skin lesions were taken by a nurse or a health technician, utilizing a cell phone app created for this purpose. Thirty thousand nine hundred seventy-six individuals responded to the call and attended the project. All their data and images were securely uploaded to a platform accessed by thirteen teledermatologists from Hospital Albert Einstein, authorized to do so through login and password at a later time (store-and-forward telemedicine). The thirteen dermatologists were Brazilian Board-certified to decrease the chance of diagnostic error. Once logged, the teledermatologists evaluated the cases, and they had to elaborate the most probable diagnosis and management. Next, they had to decide among three options to refer the patients: (1) directly to biopsy (with subsequent follow-up with an in-person dermatologist), (2) to an in-person dermatologist and (3) back to the general physician who had referred him/her to the dermatologist in the first place. **Figure 1** shows the frequency of patients included, photographed lesions, and referrals made by the teledermatologists, along with the flow used to select the reports to assess the accuracy. Teledermatologists were Hospital Israelita Albert Einstein employees (a private institution), and in-person dermatologists were public health service employees.

### Study Design

We selected only the group referred to in-person dermatologist (12,874). Then, we assessed the reports that had the International Code of Diseases diagnoses filled by the in-person dermatologists (2,290). Next, we separated the reports filled with ICD-10 codes of inflammatory dermatoses (1,227). Afterwards, we looked for the 20 most frequent dermatoses to include in our study (1,143). As the last step, we eliminated duplicity of reports from the same patient, totalizing 739 reports from 739 patients (**Figure 1**).

We classified the rate of agreement as: (1) complete agreement when ICD-10 code used in both reports were the same, (2) partial agreement when ICD-10 used in both reports were different, but in the same group of disease (**Table 1**), posing as a probable differential diagnosis, and (3) no agreement when both reports did not fill the previous two conditions. As many inflammatory diagnoses are based on clinical diagnosis, we considered in-person dermatologist diagnosis as our gold standard diagnosis. For this reason, the rate of agreement between in-person dermatologists and teledermatologists was stated in this research as accuracy.

### Statistical Analysis

Rates of concordance were expressed using percentages and Cohen's kappa coefficient, which was used to compare between groups of inter-rater observers (Graph Pad Prism 6.0). The guidelines first created by Landis and Koch (11) used to characterize kappa values are as follows: kappa $< 0$: no agreement, 0.00–0.20: slight agreement, 0.21–0.40: fair agreement, 0.41–0.60: moderate agreement, 0.61–0.8: substantial agreement, and 0.81–1.00: almost perfect agreement.

## RESULTS

**Table 2** shows the 26 most frequent inflammatory dermatoses diagnosed by teledermatology according to number of patients, lesions, and sex distribution. This constitutes 78% (24,210/30,976) of the total number of patients and 50% (27,519/55,012) of the lesions diagnosed in the overall teledermatology project. The female and male participation was 70 and 30%, respectively, although the female population accounts for 52.6% in the city of São Paulo (12). The mean number of inflammatory dermatosis lesion per patient was 1.1.

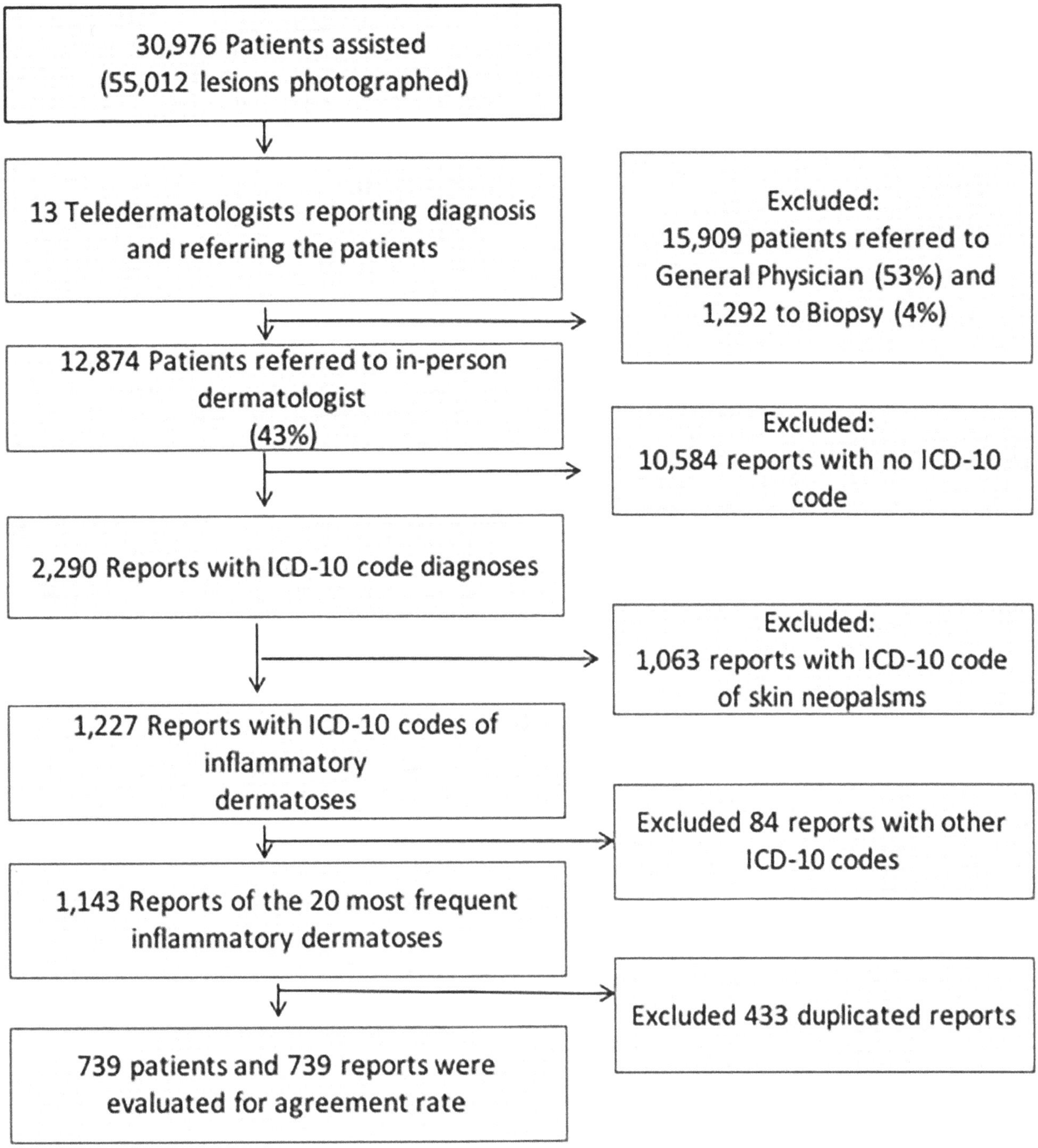


**FIGURE 1** | Frequency of patients included, photographed lesions and referrals made by the teledermatologists, along with the flow used to select the reports to assess the diagnosis accuracy.

**Table 3** assesses the 20 most frequent inflammatory dermatoses diagnosed by in-person dermatologists of which we were able to recover the ICD-10 codes, along with the accuracy of teledermatology found in our study. The mean frequency of complete agreement was 78% for all 20 dermatoses tested (573/739) and its kappa coefficient was 0.743, which is considered a substantial agreement. Xerosis had the lowest rate (31%; kappa = 0.173) and psoriasis and focal hyperhidrosis showed the greatest (100%; kappa = 1.00). A partial agreement was verified in 8% of all cases (60/739), ranging from 0% (dermatophytosis, atopic dermatosis, molluscum, psoriasis, pityriasis versicolor, and focal hyperhidrosis) to 46% (xerosis). No agreement was found in 14% (106/739); psoriasis and focal hyperhidrosis with the lowest rate (0%) and pityriasis versicolor with the highest (44%).

**TABLE 1 |** Group of skin disorders and respective dermatoses present in this study considered as partial agreement between in-person dermatologists' and teledermatologists' diagnosis.

| Group of disorder | Dermatoses |
|---|---|
| Skin adnexal glands (sebaceous, sweat) | Acne, rosacea, hidradenitis |
| Skin Hyperpigmentation | Chloasma, post-inflammatory hyperpigmentation |
| Erythematous-scaly patches | Psoriasis, dermatophytosis, pityriasis versicolor, actinic keratosis, seborrheic dermatitis, lupus erythematosus |
| Skin Hypopigmentation | Vitiligo, leukoderma |
| Eczematous | Atopic dermatitis, contact dermatitis, dyshidrosis, stasis dermatitis, nummular dermatitis, xerosis, lichen simplex chronicus, pityriais alba, urticaria, photoallergy, seborrheic dermatitis |
| Alopecia | Androgenetic alopecia, alopecia areata, telogen effluvium, cicatricial alopecia |

Partial agreement frequency and the description of each inflammatory dermatoses are shown in **Table 4**. Post-inflammatory hyperpigmentation reached the highest number, with 16 cases, all of them with the same diagnosis. On the other hand, seborrheic dermatitis had 13 cases of partial agreement with 11 different diagnoses.

## DISCUSSION

The differences in frequency for the inflammatory dermatoses between **Tables 2** and **3** are due to the fact that although one disease could be very frequently diagnosed by the teledermatologists (**Table 2**), but it could not be referred as frequently to the in-person dermatologists (**Table 3**). That, in fact, was the reason for solar lentigo, leukoderma, pityriasis alba, dyshidrosis, lichen simplex chronicus and stasis dermatitis to be left out of the second table. These dermatoses were mostly referred back to the GP along with the diagnosis/management, and they were present only in few cases for the in-person dermatologist, not included in the 20 most frequent ones as the inclusion criteria.

This fact is also very relevant when discussing accuracy. Since the aim of the teledermatology triage project was to prioritize the severe, more complex, or surgical cases for biopsy and

**TABLE 2 |** Most frequent inflammatory dermatoses diagnosed by teledermatologists according to number of patients, sex distribution, and number of photographed lesions.

| ICD-10 code | Dermatosis | Patients (*n*) | Male (*n*) | Female (*n*) | Photographed lesions (*n*) |
|---|---|---|---|---|---|
| B35 | Dermatophytosis | 3,064 | 843 | 2,221 | 3,496 |
| L70 | Acne | 2,662 | 851 | 1,811 | 3,217 |
| L81.1 | Chloasma | 1,749 | 121 | 1,628 | 1,840 |
| L20.9 | Atopic dermatitis | 1,648 | 603 | 1,045 | 2,058 |
| L85.3 | Xerosis | 1,632 | 478 | 1,154 | 1,815 |
| L57.9 | Solar lentigo | 1,584 | 223 | 1,361 | 1,870 |
| L21.9 | Seborrheic dermatitis | 1,259 | 426 | 833 | 1,421 |
| L23/L24/L25 | Contact dermatitis | 1,203 | 325 | 878 | 1,333 |
| L81.0 | Post-inflammatory hyperpigmentation | 1,139 | 256 | 883 | 1,303 |
| L81.5 | Leukoderma | 1,029 | 829 | 200 | 1,102 |
| L65 | Telogen effluvium | 881 | 20 | 861 | 891 |
| L30.5 | Pityriasis alba | 796 | 282 | 514 | 881 |
| L64.9 | Androgenetic alopecia | 765 | 135 | 630 | 774 |
| B36.0 | Pityriasis versicolor | 727 | 264 | 463 | 862 |
| L60 | Nail disorders | 586 | 94 | 492 | 629 |
| L40.0 | Psoriasis | 551 | 249 | 302 | 760 |
| L80 | Vitiligo | 550 | 228 | 322 | 694 |
| B08.1 | Molluscum contagiosum | 366 | 168 | 198 | 423 |
| L30.1 | Dyshidrosis | 358 | 84 | 274 | 387 |
| L28 | Lichen simplex chronicus | 340 | 157 | 183 | 368 |
| L63 | Alopecia areata | 331 | 135 | 196 | 348 |
| L71 | Rosacea | 248 | 60 | 198 | 257 |
| I83.1 | Stasis dermatitis | 202 | 92 | 110 | 209 |
| L30.0 | Nummular dermatitis | 201 | 59 | 142 | 218 |
| L74.5 | Focal Hyperhidrosis | 200 | 86 | 114 | 209 |
| L50 | Urticaria | 139 | 40 | 99 | 154 |
| Total | | 24,210 | 7,108 | 17,112 | 27,519 |

**TABLE 3 |** Most frequent inflammatory dermatosis diagnosed by in-person dermatologists and agreement with teledermatology diagnoses.

| Diagnoses(*n* =) | Complete agreement *n* (%) | Complete agreement kappa | Partial agreement *n* (%) | No agreement *n* (%) |
|---|---|---|---|---|
| Acne (122) | 113 (93) | 0.924 | 1 (1) | 8 (6) |
| Dermatophytosis (83) | 52 (63) | 0.564 | 0 (0) | 31 (37) |
| Atopic Dermatitis (81) | 75 (93) | 0.923 | 0 (0) | 6 (7) |
| Post-inflammatory hyperpigmentation (59) | 20 (34) | 0.206 | 16 (27) | 23 (39) |
| Contact dermatitis (52) | 40 (77) | 0.743 | 5 (10) | 7 (13) |
| Androgenetic alopecia (49) | 38 (78) | 0.751 | 8 (16) | 3 (6) |
| Chloasma (36) | 32 (89) | 0.883 | 2 (5.5) | 2 (5.5) |
| Molluscum contagiosum (36) | 34 (94) | 0.943 | 0 (0) | 2 (6) |
| Vitiligo (30) | 27 (90) | 0.895 | 1 (3) | 2 (7) |
| Seborrheic dermatitis (29) | 10 (34) | 0.213 | 13 (45) | 6 (21) |
| Psoriasis (26) | 26 (100) | 1.000 | 0 (0) | 0 (0) |
| Telogen effluvium (24) | 23 (96) | 0.957 | 1 (4) | 0 (0) |
| Alopecia areata (21) | 20 (95) | 0.951 | 1 (5) | 0 (0) |
| Rosacea (20) | 17 (85) | 0.839 | 1 (5) | 2 (10) |
| Pityriasis versicolor (16) | 9 (56) | 0.481 | 0 (0) | 7 (44) |
| Nail disorders (14) | 12 (86) | 0.847 | 0 (0) | 2 (14) |
| Focal hyperhidrosis (11) | 11 (100) | 1.000 | 0 (0) | 0 (0) |
| Xerosis (13) | 4 (31) | 0.173 | 6 (46) | 3 (23) |
| Urticaria (9) | 7 (78) | 0.754 | 2 (22) | 0 (0) |
| Nummular dermatitis (8) | 3 (37.5) | 0.247 | 3 (37.5) | 2 (25) |
| Total (739) | 573 (78) | 0.743 | 60 (8) | 106 (14) |

**TABLE 4 |** Differences between teledermatogists' and in-person dermatologists' diagnosis in cases considered partial agreement for inflammatory dermatosis.

| Teledermatologist diagnosis | Partial agreement (*n*) | In-person diagnosis |
|---|---|---|
| Acne | 1 | 1 hidradenitis |
| Rosacea | 1 | 1 acne |
| Contact dermatitis | 5 | 4 atopic dermatitis, 1 lichen simplex chronicus |
| Nummular dermatitis | 3 | 2 pitiryasis alba, 1 dyshidrosis |
| Urticaria | 2 | 1 atopic dermatitis, 1 contact dermatitis |
| Xerosis | 6 | 4 atopic dermatitis, 1 pityriasis alba; 1 photoallergy |
| Seborrheic dermatitis | 13 | 3 androgenic alopecia, 1 contact dermatitis,<br>1 psoriasis, 1 dermatophytosis,<br>1 rosacea, 1 hidradenitis suppurativa,<br>1 pityriasis alba, 1 phototoxic allergy,<br>1 perifolicullitis capitis,<br>1 lupus erythematosus, 1 actinic keratosis |
| Vitiligo | 1 | 1 leukoderma |
| Post-inflammatory hyperpigmentation | 16 | 16 chloasma |
| Chloasma | 2 | 2 post-inflammatory hyperpigmentation |
| Androgenetic alopecia | 8 | 4 alopecia areata, 3 telogen effluvium, 1 cicatricial alopecia |
| Alopecia areata | 1 | 1 androgenetic alopecia |
| Telogen effluvium | 1 | 1 androgenetic alopecia |

in-person dermatologists and to manage the mild cases under the primary-care attention along with the GP, the inflammatory disorders diagnosed by in-person dermatologists in **Table 2** have a potential bias of being the most challenging cases. Typical or "regular" inflammatory dermatoses were most likely diagnosed and referred to the GP. Therefore, the rate of agreement found would be probably even higher if the more typical cases were analyzed. The results of our study showed a high agreement rate between diagnoses made by teledermatologists and in-person dermatologists, corroborating the idea that teledermatology is accurate for inflammatory dermatoses. If we add the total (78%) and partial (8%) agreement rates, we will achieve 86% (kappa = 0.846), which is considered an almost perfect agreement, and only 14% of no agreement. This would be remarkable even if we were not discussing the potential bias above. According to literature, SF-TD had an accuracy in general of 64 and 65% in medium size studies ($n$ = 109 and 163, respectively) and 90 and 95% in small size studies ($n$ = 50 and 10, respectively) (6). Another article found an agreement of 90% in 120 cases of SF-TD consultations (7). Lim et al. reported 88% agreement in 53 cases (8). Weingast et al. evaluated 263 patients and found accuracy of 80% (9). O'Connor et al. assessed 40 patients and encountered accuracy of 83% (10).

There were different accuracies among the 20 most frequent dermatoses diagnosed by in-person dermatologists in our study. Eight diseases reached very high complete agreement rate, 90% or above: acne, atopic dermatitis, molluscum contagiosum, vitiligo, psoriasis, telogen effluvium, alopecia areata, and focal hyperhidrosis. Six disorders showed a good total agreement rate, 70–89%: contact dermatitis, androgenetic alopecia, chloasma, rosacea, nail disorders, and urticaria. Six inflammatory dermatoses were less accurate (<60% of total agreement): dermatophytosis, post-inflammatory hyperpigmentation, seborrheic dermatitis, pityriasis versicolor, xerosis, and nummular dermatitis. What were those diseases mistaken for? In order to verify that, we checked if they could be classified as possible differential diagnosis, which we considered to be a partial agreement.

Examining the six diseases with total agreement ranging from 70–89% and considering the partial agreement rate, three of them would have a considerable change. Contact dermatitis would increase from 77 to 87%, due to five cases that were in fact four atopic dermatitis and one lichen simplex chronicus. Androgenetic alopecia (AGA) would increase from 78 to 94%, due to four alopecia areata, three telogen effluvium and one cicatricial alopecia. Chloasma would also raise from 89 to 94.5% accuracy if we included the two cases of post-inflammatory hyperpigmentation in **Table 4**.

Most interestingly, anyhow, is to look for the diseases showing the least accuracy. Post-inflammatory hyperpigmentation (PIH) should have a separate interpretation once all 16 cases of partial agreement had the same diagnosis: chloasma. One hypothesis is a typing error, because their ICD-10 codes are almost the same (L81.0 and L81.1). Another one is that dermatologists misuse chloasma ICD-10 code for PIH, since chloasma is a very frequent disease and its ICD-10 code may be already known by heart while PIH code would not. Nummular dermatitis and xerosis would at least double the accuracy (37.5–75% and 31–77%, respectively) if we considered the partial agreement diagnosis. Seborrheic dermatitis (SD) was the disease with the highest number of differential diagnosis (13) and considering the partial agreement rate, accuracy would go from 34 to 79%. On the scalp, SD was diagnosed as AGA and perifolicullitis capitis, which could even occur simultaneously, and on the skin, could be confused with many diseases such as psoriasis, eczemas, lupus erythematous, dermatophytosis, rosacea, and actinic keratosis. Dermatophytosis and pityriasis versicolor were the least accurate diagnosis when total and partial agreement were considered, 63 and 56%, respectively. This may be due to some limitation in assessing the lesions through teledermatology or to a great variety of possible differential diagnoses. Again, in our study, the fact that the most typical cases were meant to be treated by teledermatology and not sent to in-person dermatologists could have played an important role in these two dermatoses.

Although this was a retrospective study and much data was missing, we believe this was one of the studies with the largest number of inflammatory diseases included in the literature. The study was performed in two centers and different dermatologists performed the tele and in-person examinations. This is beneficial, in a way that we assessed the agreement between different examiners, but it also may have some bias, since the technical skills in the two groups may be different.

Our study in a large number of patients presenting the most common inflammatory dermatoses showed that the mean accuracy of teledermatology was high, varying according to the disease. This result reassures that store-and-forward teledermatology is as proper option for patient care.

## ETHICS STATEMENT

The studies involving human participants were reviewed and approved by Ethics Committee of Hospital Israelita Albert Einstein (CAAE: 97126618.6.0000.0071). Written informed consent from the participants' legal guardian/next of kin was not required to participate in this study in accordance with the national legislation and the institutional requirements.

## AUTHOR CONTRIBUTIONS

MG-B, RS, and EC were responsible for the study design. MG-B was responsible for writing the article. MG-B and RS were responsible for data analyzes. All authors contributed to the article and approved the submitted version.

## REFERENCES


1. Lee JJ, English JC. Teledermatology: a review and update. *Am J Clin Dermatol.* (2018) 19:253–60. doi: 10.1007/s40257-017-0317-6
2. Finnane A, Dallest K, Janda M, Soyer HP. Teledermatology for the diagnosis and management of skin cancer: a systematic review. *JAMA Dermatol.* (2017) 153:319–27. doi: 10.1001/jamadermatol.2016.4361
3. Warshaw EM, Lederle FA, Grill JP, Gravely AA, Bangerter AK, Fortier LA, et al. Accuracy of teledermatology for pigmented neoplasms. *J Am Acad Dermatol.* (2009) 61:753–65. doi: 10.1016/j.jaad.2009.04.032
4. Chuchu N, Dinnes J, Takwoingi Y, Matin RN, Bayliss SE, Davenport C, et al. Teledermatology for diagnosing skin cancer in adults. *Cochrane Database Syst Rev.* (2018) 12:CD013193. doi: 10.1002/14651858.CD013193
5. Markun S, Scherz N, Rosemann T, Tandjung R, Braun RP. Mobile teledermatology for skin cancer screening: a diagnostic accuracy study. *Medicine.* (2017) 96:e6278. doi: 10.1097/MD.0000000000006278
6. Warshaw EM, Hillman YJ, Greer NL, Hagel EM, MacDonald R, Rutks IR, et al. Teledermatology for diagnosis and management of skin conditions: a systematic review. *J Am Acad Dermatol.* (2011) 64:759–72. doi: 10.1016/j.jaad.2010.08.026
7. Lasierra N, Alesanco A, Gilaberte Y, Magallón R, García J. Lessons learned after a three-year store and forward teledermatology experience using internet: strengths and limitations. *Int J Med Inform.* (2012) 81:332–43. doi: 10.1016/j.ijmedinf.2012.02.008
8. Lim AC, Egerton IB, See A, Shumack SP. Accuracy and reliability of store-and-forward teledermatology: preliminary results from the St George Teledermatology Project. *Aust J Dermatol.* (2001) 42:247–51. doi: 10.1046/j.1440-0960.2001.00529.x
9. Weingast J, Scheibböck C, Wurm EM, Ranharter E, Porkert S, Dreiseitl S, et al. A prospective study of mobile phones for dermatology in a clinical setting. *J Telemed Telecare.* (2013) 19:213–8. doi: 10.1177/1357633x13490890
10. O'Connor DM, Jew OS, Perman MJ, Castelo-Soccio LA, Winston FK, McMahon PJ. Diagnostic accuracy of pediatric teledermatology using parent-submitted photographs: a randomized clinical trial. *JAMA Dermatol.* (2017) 153:1243–8. doi: 10.1001/jamadermatol.2017.4280
11. Landis J, Koch G. The measurement of observer agreement for categorical categorical data. *Biometrics.* (1977) 33:159–74. doi: 10.2307/2529310

# 28

# Imaging of Vulva Syringoma With Reflectance Confocal Microscopy

*Lin Feng*[1], *Yan Lin*[2], *Leilei Wang*[3], *Hongxiao Chen*[4], *Min Gao*[3*], *Huaxu Liu*[2] *and Hongyu Yang*[5]

*[1] Chongqing Hospital of Traditional Chinese Medicine, Chongqing, China, [2] Shandong Provincial Institute of Dermatology and Venereology, Shandong First Medical University & Shandong Academy of Medical Sciences, Jinan, China, [3] Shandong Cancer Hospital and Institute, Shandong First Medical University & Shandong Academy of Medical Sciences, Jinan, China, [4] Linyi People's Hospital, Linyi, China, [5] Department of Pathology, St. Vincent Evansville Medical Center, Evansville, IN, United States*

***Correspondence:**
*Min Gao*
*gmlhx@163.com*

**Objectives:** To investigate the application of reflectance confocal microscopy (RCM) imaging in diagnosis of vulva syringoma.

**Methods:** Patients with lesions suspicious of syringoma on vulva were enrolled in the study. After informed consent was taken, the lesions were photographed and imaged with RCM. The features of the lesion in confocal images were then analyzed and compared with the biopsy findings for histology correlation.

**Results:** Eleven cases in total were included in the study. The typical RCM features observed in syringoma are the presence of round to oval high refractive, and relatively monomorphous mass of varying sizes in the superficial and middle dermis, usually surrounded with 1–2 layers of light-dark line structures, which were further confirmed by histological evaluation. Ten cases showed classic features of syringoma and 1 case exhibited milia in RCM images.

**Conclusions:** Syringoma has distinct features in RCM imaging, which correlates well with histological findings, highlighting the potential role of RCM in the diagnosis and differential diagnosis of vulva syringoma.

**Keywords:** ***in vivo*** **imaging, reflectance confocal microcopy, vulva, syringoma, histology, differential diaenosis**

## INTRODUCTION

Syringoma is a benign sweat gland tumor derived from eccrine ducts and it occurs predominantly in women at puberty or later in life (1). The typical lesions of syringoma present as multiple, small, firm, skin-colored papules, usually 1–3 mm in diameter, and symmetrically distributed on the periorbital region (1, 2). Although the most common site of localized involvement is periorbital, syringoma in other areas have also been reported, including the vulva, penis, palms, scalp, and axillae (2, 3). The classification criterion of syringoma proposed by Friedman and Butler (4) was based on clinical features and consists of 4 variants: localized, familial (5), a form associated with Down Syndrome (DS), and a generalized variant, including multiple and eruptive syringoma (6).

The characteristics of lesions on the eyelids and forehead can be easily identified, while lesions in other areas especially on the vulva were not easily identifiable and the definitive diagnosis was usually made by histological examination. However, the invasive biopsy procedure for histology analysis reduced the compliance of the patients with suspicious vulva lesions, therefore developing a non-invasive skin imaging modality in the diagnosis and differential diagnosis of syringoma seems more appealing to potential patients.

The reflectance confocal microscopy (RCM) is a non-invasive skin imaging modality with high "cellular" resolution (7), which could compare the cellular changes of epidermis and superficial dermis *in vivo* in real time, and its accuracy is comparable with the histological evaluation of syringoma. In this study, we investigated the role of RCM in the diagnosis of vulva syringoma.

## PATIENTS AND METHODS

The study had been approved by Ethics Committee of Shandong Cancer Hospital and Institute and was conducted from 2018 to 2019. Cases with lesions suspicious of syringoma on vulva (**Figures 1a**, **2a**, **3a**, **4a**) were enrolled in the study. After written informed consent was signed, the lesions were photographed and imaged by a commercially available, reflectance mode confocal microscope (Vivascope 1500; Caliber Imaging & Diagnostics, Inc. formerly Lucid, Inc., Rochester, NY, USA). The captured horizontal images in a 500 × 500 μm field, and viva-block image of 3 × 3 mm at different layers were obtained. A detailed description of the technique and the device has been published previously (7, 8). After imaging with RCM, the same lesions were biopsied and fixed in phosphate-buffered neutral formalin, embedded in paraffin, and stained with hematoxylin-eosin (HE), then analyzed using an optical microscope to investigate the accuracy of RCM imaging.

## RESULTS

A total of 11 female adults were enrolled in the study (**Table 1**). The average age of the cases was 30.5 years old, and the average duration of the lesion was 17 months.

On clinical examination, multiple small, light brown papules are scattered in the vulva area (**Figures 1a**, **2a**, **3a**, **4a**), or in a "beaded" distribution along the outer margin of labia Majora. The main characteristics of lesions from the patients observed

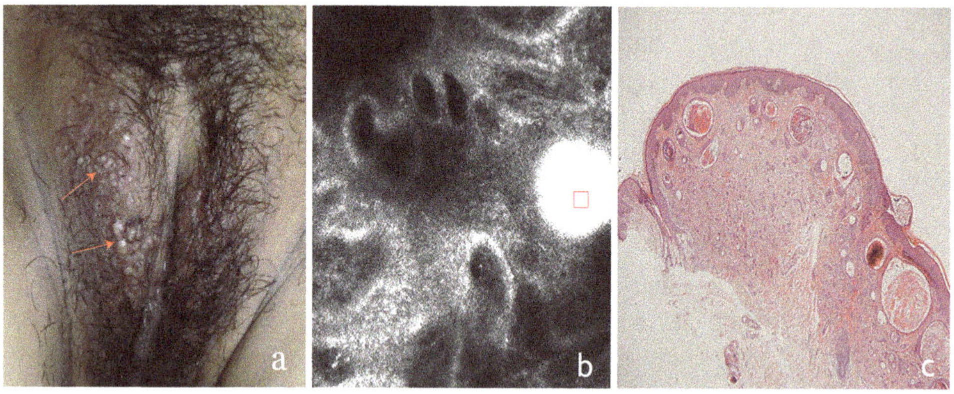


**FIGURE 1 |** The clinical presentation, RCM findings and histology of vulva syringoma (case 1). **(a)**, the clinical image of case 1, **(b)**, the RCM image findings; **(c)**, the histology findings. The presence of round to oval high refractive, and relatively monomorphous mass of varing sizes (the red square)was prensent in the superficial dermis, with 1–2 layers of surrounding light-dark line structure (red arrowhead) in **(b)**.

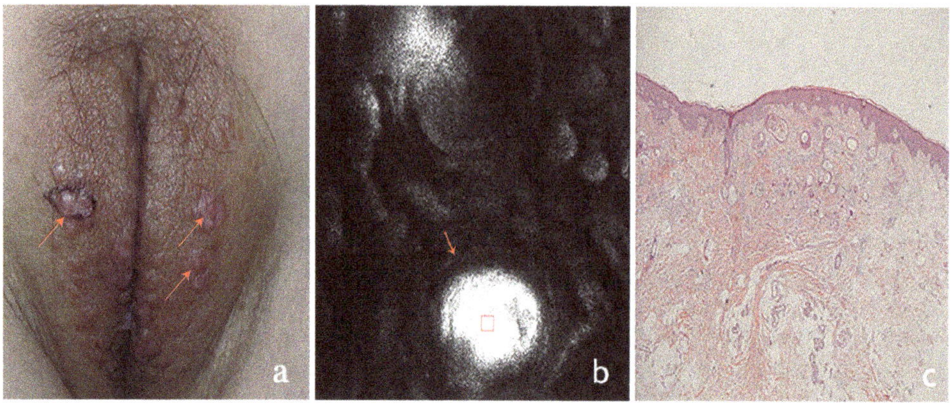


**FIGURE 2 |** The clinical presentation, RCM findings and histology of vulva syringoma (case 2). **(a)**, the clinical image of case 2, **(b)**, the RCM image findings; **(c)**, the histological findings. The presence of round to oval high refractive, and relatively monomorphous mass of varing sizes (the red square) was present in the superficial dermis, with 1–2 layers of surrounding light-dark line structure (red arrowhead) in **(b)**.

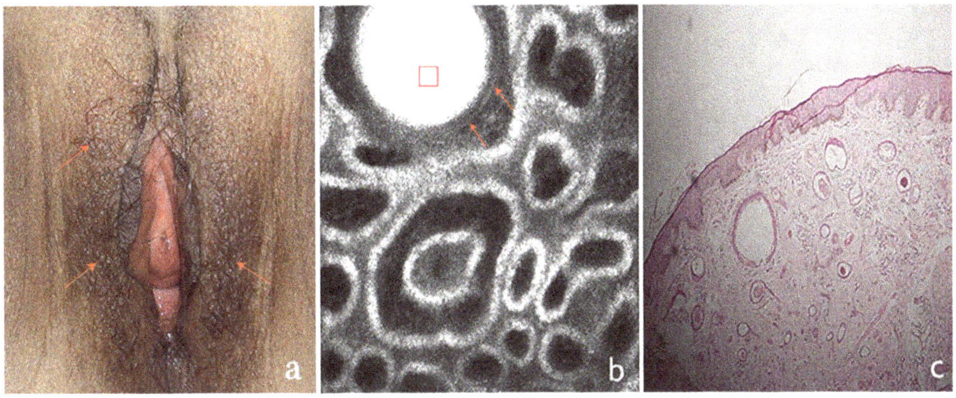


**FIGURE 3 |** The clinical presentation, RCM findings and histology of vulva syringoma (case 3). **(a)**, the clinical image of case 3, **(b)**, the RCM image findings; **(c)**, the histological findings. The presence of round to oval high refractive, and relatively monomorphous mass of varing sizes (the red square)was present in the upper dermis, with 1–2 layers of surrounding light-dark line structures (red arrowhead)in **(b)**.

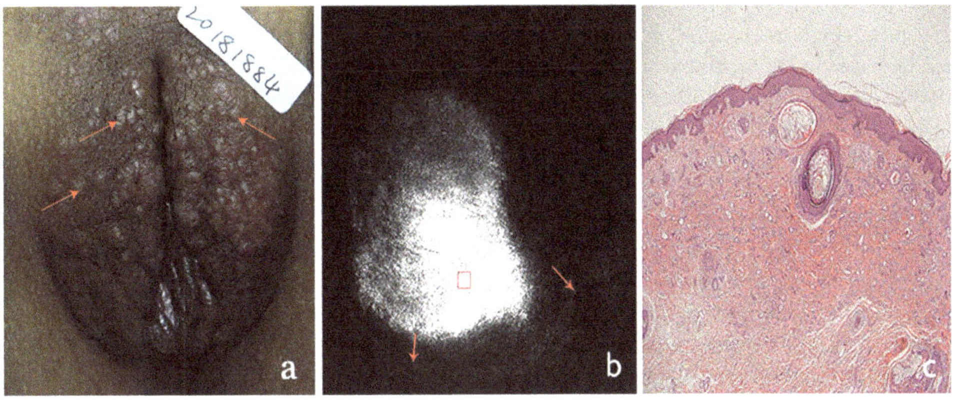


**FIGURE 4 |** The clinical presentation, RCM findings and histology of vulva syringoma (case 4). **(a)**, the clinical image of case 4, **(b)**, the RCM image findings; **(c)**, the histological findings.

**TABLE 1 |** The age and medical history of the patients enrolled in the study.

| Case number | Age | Medical history (month) | RCM imaging (+ or –) | Histology results (+ or –) |
|---|---|---|---|---|
| 1 | 23 | 12 | + | + |
| 2 | 32 | 16 | + | + |
| 3 | 44 | 20 | + | + |
| 4 | 21 | 30 | + | + |
| 5 | 32 | 23 | + | + |
| 5 | 34 | 14 | + | + |
| 7 | 25 | 11 | + | + |
| 8 | 27 | 17 | + | + |
| 9 | 28 | 9 | + | + |
| 10 | 31 | 13 | + | + |
| 11 | 39 | 22 | -(milia) | -(milia) |
| Average | 30.5 | 17 | | |

*+ with significant changes of syringoma in RCM or histology images.*
*– other changes.*

by RCM were very similar. There were no significant cellular changes in superficial epidermis, and the keratinocytes appeared regular and small, and the architectural pattern of the honeycomb was similar with the peri-lesional normal skin. Deeper level imaging showed brighter keratinocytes in the basal cell layer in lesional zone and the melanin contents in the basal cell layer were also increased compared with the adjacent normal skin.

The most characteristic changes were observed in the upper and middle dermis. Evenly distributed varying sizes of round to oval structures show high refractive mass with surrounding light-dark lines (**Figures 1b**, **2b**, **3b**, **4b**). In comparison, there was just mild to moderate refracted collagen in upper and middle dermis in adjacent non-lesional areas.

The definitive histological diagnoses were all confirmed by biopsy finding in all cases studied, which show classic findings of syringoma with superficial to mid-dermal nests of eccrine ducts and tadpole-like structures embedded in fibrous stroma. clear cell changes of epithelial cells were occasional present. The ductal lumina are filled with an amorphous, periodic

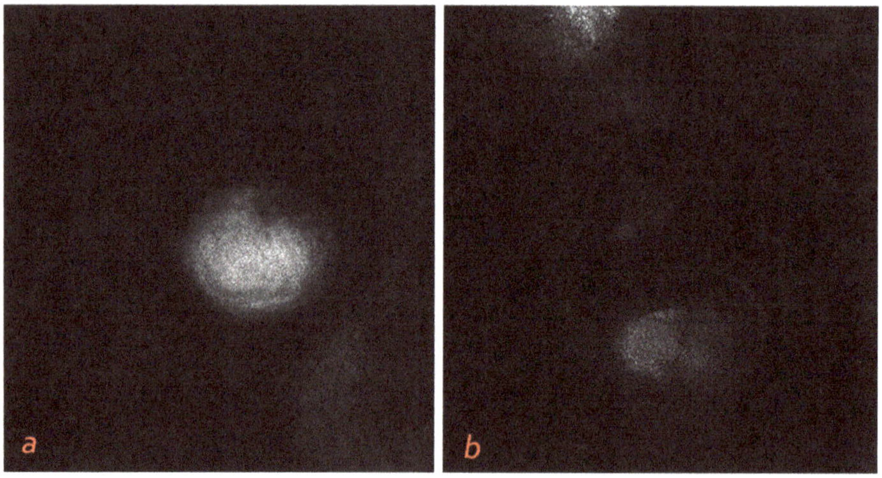


**FIGURE 5 |** Deeper level imaging of syringoma of vulva area **(a,b)** showed that the refraction of the round structures tends to be slightly decreased as they go deep.

acid-Schiff-positive material (**Figures 1c**, **2c**, **3c**, **4c**), Deeper level imaging showed that the refraction of the round structures tends to be slightly decreased as they go deep (**Figures 5a,b**).

## DISCUSSION

Syringoma occurs more frequently in adult female with distinct histopathologic features (1, 2). In cases with characteristic clinical presentation, syringoma can be easily diagnosed clinically. For lesions on unusual sites such as the genital area, the clinical manifestation was usually atypical. They need to be confirmed by biopsy and histological diagnosis. However, the invasive biopsy procedure would reduce the compliance of the patients, and a non-invasive method for the diagnosis and differential diagnosis of syringoma on vulva sites is definitely sought after by various medical professionals.

The application of dermoscopy imaging in diagnosis of syringoma has been reported and dermoscopy may contribute to the imaging diagnosis of syringoma by revealing multiple bright cystic enlargements in dermis (9). While comparing with dermoscopy, RCM provides more details of those lesions studied with more sensitivity and specificity.

The RCM is also non-invasive and dynamically shows the cellular-level morphology in human skin *in vivo* (7, 10). Imaging is based on the detection of single back scattered photons from the optical section and contrast due to the relative variations in refractive indices and sizes of organelles and micro-structures (7). The cellular changes of the lesion in epidermis and superficial dermis could be imaged and compared with that of the adjacent normal skin. The RCM had been widely used in the screening of skin tumors, such as melanoma (10, 11), basal cell carcinoma (12), and actinic keratosis (13). In recent years, the RCM was reported to be useful in the diagnosis, differential diagnosis, and follow-up of pigmented and inflammatory skin disorders (14, 15) with high sensitivity and specificity.

The typical changes of syringoma are in mostly confined to superficial and mid-dermis, which is in the imaging depth of RCM. And we found the presence of round to oval, high refractile, and relatively evenly distributed substances of varying sizes in the superficial and mid-dermis with surrounding light-dark line structures based on RCM imaging to be characteristic for synringomas, which were confirmed by histology results. The well-demarcated high refractile substances noted in confocal image correlate with the amorphous, periodic acid-Schiff-positive material in the ductal lumina in histological findings, while the surrounding 1–2 layers of light-dark line structures seen in confocal images correlate with the lining epithelial cells and myoepithelial cells seen in histological images.

Vulva areas can be affected by many papular skin lesions, which should be differentiated from syringoma, those entities include milia, Fox-Fordyce disease, epidermal cysts, lichen planus, and lichen simplex chronicus (9, 16, 17). The confocal images of milia showed relatively high refractile, but unevenly distributed keratin in superficial dermis (18), which is more superficial compared with syringoma in confocal image findings. The major difference between syringoma and milia in confocal images is the "evenly" refractile substance in dermis and the presence of surrounding 1–2 layers of light and dark lines noted in the former and not present in the latter (18). Our observations are all confirmed with the histological findings. As to other cutaneous adnexal tumors, the RCM could also detect the changes around the follicles and cellular changes in epidermis and superfical dermis, which is useful in the screening and differential diagnosis of those lesions.

A recent case report of syringoma considered the dark areas surrounded by rims of epithelia as the characteristic of syringoma based on RCM findings (19). They interpreted the encircling hollow dark areas as lumina. However, in our study, we identified the round to oval, high refractile, and relatively monomorphous substances of varying sizes in the superficial and middle dermis to represent lumina. And future studies with a larger sample size coupled with histological analysis is needed to confirm our findings.

Our preliminary study showed the novel features of syringoma in RCM imaging, which could be useful as a non-invasive "*in vivo*" tool in the screening and differential diagnosis of suspicious vulva syringomatous lesions. The appropriate clinical application of RCM or other skin imaging methods will potentially reduce the invasive biopsy procedure and related medical cost, and in the end benefit the patients.

## ETHICS STATEMENT

The studies involving human participants were reviewed and approved by The ethic committe of Shandong Provincial Hospital for Skin Diseases. The patients/participants provided their written informed consent to participate in this study.

## AUTHOR CONTRIBUTIONS

LF, YL, and LW collected the cases and che clnical and RCM data. HC collected the histology data. MG and HL designed the study and prepared the manuscript. HY revised the manuscript. All authors contributed to the article and approved the submitted version.

## REFERENCES


1. Ghanadan A, Khosravi M. Cutaneous syringoma: a clinicopathologic study of 34 new cases and review of the literature. *Indian J Dermatol.* (2013) 58:326. doi: 10.4103/0019-5154.113956
2. Williams K, Shinkai K. Evaluation and management of the patient with multiple syringomas: a systematic review of the literature. *J Am Acad Dermatol.* (2016) 74:1234–40. doi: 10.1016/j.jaad.2015.12.006
3. Ciarloni L, Frouin E, Bodin F, Cribier B. Syringoma: a clinicopathological study of 244 cases. *Ann Dermatol Venereol.* (2016) 143:521–8. doi: 10.1016/j.annder.2015.06.025
4. Friedman S, Butler D. Syringoma presenting as milia. *J Am Acad Dermatol.* (1987) 16:310–14. doi: 10.1016/S0190-9622(87)70041-3
5. Lau J, Haber RM. Familial eruptive syringomas: case report and review of the literature. *J Cutan Med Surg.* (2013) 17:84–8. doi: 10.2310/7750.2012.12027
6. Soler-Carrillo J, Estrach T, Mascaró JM. Eruptive syringoma: 27 new cases and review of the literature. *J Eur Acad Dermatol Venereol.* (2001) 15:242–6. doi: 10.1046/j.1468-3083.2001.00235.x
7. Rajadhyaksha M, Marghoob A, Rossi A, Halpern AC, Nehal KS. Reflectance confocal microscopy of skin *in vivo*: from bench to bedside. *Lasers Surg Med.* (2017) 49:7–19. doi: 10.1002/lsm.22600
8. Liu H, Lin Y, Nie X, Chen S, Chen X, Shi B, et al. Histological classification of melasma with reflectance confocal microscopy: a pilot study in Chinese patients. *Skin Res Technol.* (2011) 17:398–403 doi: 10.1111/j.1600-0846.2011.00517.x
9. Corazza M, Borghi A, Minghetti S, Ferron P, Virgili A. Dermoscopy of isolated syringoma of the vulva. *J Am Acad Dermatol.* (2017) 76:S37–S9. doi: 10.1016/j.jaad.2016.06.009
10. Farnetani F, Manfredini M, Longhitano S, Chester J, Shaniko K, Cinotti E, et al. Morphological classification of melanoma metastasis with reflectance confocal microscopy. *J Eur Acad Dermatol Venereol.* (2019) 33:676–85. doi: 10.1111/jdv.15329
11. Uribe P, Collgros H, Scolyer RA, Menzies SW, Guitera P. *In vivo* reflectance confocal microscopy for the diagnosis of melanoma and melanotic macules of the lip. *JAMA Dermatol.* (2017) 153:882–91. doi: 10.1001/jamadermatol.2017.0504
12. Couzan C, Cinotti E, Labeille B, Vercherin P, Rubegni P, Cambazard F, et al. Reflectance confocal microscopy identification of subclinical basal cell carcinomas during and after vismodegib treatment. *J Eur Acad Dermatol Venereol.* (2018) 32:763–7. doi: 10.1111/jdv.14650
13. Peppelman M, Nguyen KP, Hoogedoorn L, van Erp PE, Gerritsen MJ. Reflectance confocal microscopy: non-invasive distinction between actinic keratosis and squamous cell carcinoma. *J Eur Acad Dermatol Venereol.* (2015) 29:1302–9. doi: 10.1111/jdv.12806
14. Ardigo M, Agozzino M, Franceschini C, Lacarrubba F. Reflectance confocalmicroscopy algorithms for inflammatory and hair diseases. *Dermatol Clin.* (2016) 34:487–96. doi: 10.1016/j.det.2016.05.011
15. Cinotti E, Perrot JL, Labeille B, Cambazard F. Reflectance confocal microscopy for cutaneous infections and infestations. *J Eur Acad Dermatol Venereol.* (2016) 30:754–63. doi: 10.1111/jdv.13254
16. Heller DS. Benign tumors and tumor-like lesions of the vulva. *Clin Obstet Gynecol.* (2015) 58:526–35. doi: 10.1097/GRF.0000000000000133
17. Naveen KN, Pai VV, Sori T. Syringoma masquerading as steatocystoma multiplex. *Indian J Dermatol Venereol Leprol.* (2012) 78:365–6. doi: 10.4103/0378-6323.95458
18. Gao M, Lin Y, Wang L, Yu Y, Zhou Y, Chen S, et al. The differential diagnosis of syringoma and milia based on the imaging of reflectance confocal microscopy. *Skin Res Technol.* (2020) 26:951–3. doi: 10.1111/srt.12879
19. Jiménez MR, Rocchetto H, Ferreira PS, Sangueza M, Lourenço SV, Nico MMS. Evaluation of syringomas by *in vivo* reflectance confocal microscopy: a report of two cases. *Am J Dermatopathol.* (2017) 39:845–8. doi: 10.1097/DAD.0000000000000751

# Permissions

All chapters in this book were first published by Frontiers; hereby published with permission under the Creative Commons Attribution License or equivalent. Every chapter published in this book has been scrutinized by our experts. Their significance has been extensively debated. The topics covered herein carry significant findings which will fuel the growth of the discipline. They may even be implemented as practical applications or may be referred to as a beginning point for another development.

The contributors of this book come from diverse backgrounds, making this book a truly international effort. This book will bring forth new frontiers with its revolutionizing research information and detailed analysis of the nascent developments around the world.

We would like to thank all the contributing authors for lending their expertise to make the book truly unique. They have played a crucial role in the development of this book. Without their invaluable contributions this book wouldn't have been possible. They have made vital efforts to compile up to date information on the varied aspects of this subject to make this book a valuable addition to the collection of many professionals and students.

This book was conceptualized with the vision of imparting up-to-date information and advanced data in this field. To ensure the same, a matchless editorial board was set up. Every individual on the board went through rigorous rounds of assessment to prove their worth. After which they invested a large part of their time researching and compiling the most relevant data for our readers.

The editorial board has been involved in producing this book since its inception. They have spent rigorous hours researching and exploring the diverse topics which have resulted in the successful publishing of this book. They have passed on their knowledge of decades through this book. To expedite this challenging task, the publisher supported the team at every step. A small team of assistant editors was also appointed to further simplify the editing procedure and attain best results for the readers.

Apart from the editorial board, the designing team has also invested a significant amount of their time in understanding the subject and creating the most relevant covers. They scrutinized every image to scout for the most suitable representation of the subject and create an appropriate cover for the book.

The publishing team has been an ardent support to the editorial, designing and production team. Their endless efforts to recruit the best for this project, has resulted in the accomplishment of this book. They are a veteran in the field of academics and their pool of knowledge is as vast as their experience in printing. Their expertise and guidance has proved useful at every step. Their uncompromising quality standards have made this book an exceptional effort. Their encouragement from time to time has been an inspiration for everyone.

The publisher and the editorial board hope that this book will prove to be a valuable piece of knowledge for researchers, students, practitioners and scholars across the globe.

# List of Contributors

**Zeinab Schäfer and Andreas Mathisen**
Department of Computer Science, Aarhus University, Aarhus, Denmark

**Katrine Svendsen**
Research Unit for Mental Public Health, Department of Public Health, Aarhus University, Aarhus, Denmark

**Susanne Engberg**
Steno Diabetes Center, Copenhagen, Denmark

**Trine Rolighed Thomsen**
Department of Chemistry and Biosciences, Center for Microbial Communities, Aalborg University, Aalborg, Denmark
Life Science, Danish Technological Institute, Taastrup, Denmark

**Klaus Kirketerp-Møller**
Steno Diabetes Center, Copenhagen, Denmark
Department of Dermatology, Venereology and Wounds, Copenhagen Wound Healing Center, Bispebjerg Hospital, Copenhagen, Denmark

**André P. dos Santos**
Department of Telemedicine, Hospital Israelita Albert Einstein, São Paulo, Brazil

**Hong Gi An and Sejung Yang**
Department of Biomedical Engineering, Yonsei University, Wonju, South Korea

**Byung Ho Oh**
Department of Dermatology and Cutaneous Biology Research Institute, Yonsei University College of Medicine, Seoul, South Korea

**Kumutnart Chanprapaph, Wuttidej Fakprapai, Preeyachat Limtong and Poonkiat Suchonwanit**
Division of Dermatology, Faculty of Medicine, Ramathibodi Hospital, Mahidol University, Bangkok, Thailand

**Abder-Rahman Ali and Jingpeng Li**
Faculty of Natural Sciences, Computing Science and Mathematics, University of Stirling, Stirling, United Kingdom

**Summrina Kanwal**
Department of Computing and Informatics, Saudi Electronic University, Al-Dammam, Saudi Arabia

**Guang Yang**
National Heart and Lung Institute, Imperial College London, London, United Kingdom

**Amir Hussain**
Cognitive Big Data and Cybersecurity Research Lab, Edinburgh Napier University, Edinburgh, United Kingdom

**Sally Jane O'Shea**
Mater Private Hospital, Cork, Ireland

**Jing Gao, Minghui Sun, Qing Li, Tingfang Zhang and Chunjun Yang**
Department of Dermatology, The Second Affiliated Hospital, Anhui Medical University, Hefei, China

**Wenmin Fei and Yong Cui**
Department of Dermatology, China-Japan Friendship Hospital, Beijing, China
Institute of Skin Health, China-Japan Friendship Hospital, Beijing, China
Graduate School, Peking Union Medical College and Chinese Academy of Medical Sciences, Beijing, China

**Changbing Shen, Ning Xu and Cong Huang**
Department of Dermatology, Peking University Shenzhen Hospital, Shenzhen, China
Shenzhen Key Laboratory for Translational Medicine of Dermatology, Shenzhen Peking University–The Hong Kong University of Science and Technology Medical Center, Shenzhen, China

**Xue Shen**
Department of Dermatology, Chengdu Second People's Hospital, Chengdu, China

**Randy Ko**
Division of Molecular Medicine, Department of Internal Medicine, University of New Mexico Health Sciences Center, Albuquerque, NM, United States

**Amy X. Du and Robert Gniadecki**
Division of Dermatology, Faculty of Medicine and Dentistry, University of Alberta, Edmonton, AB, Canada

**Sepideh Emam**
Information Services and Technology, University of Alberta, Edmonton, AB, Canada

**Sarah Beicht, Veronika Baghin, Sebastian P. Stark, Tilo Biedermann and Felix Lauffer**
Department of Dermatology and Allergy, Technical University of Munich, Munich, Germany

**Natalie Garzorz-Stark**
Department of Dermatology and Allergy, Technical University of Munich, Munich, Germany
Division of Dermatology and Venereology, Department of Medicine Solna, Center for Molecular Medicine, Karolinska Institutet, Stockholm, Sweden

**Tanja B. Jutzi, Eva I. Krieghoff-Henning, Stefan Fröhling, Roman C. Maron and Titus J. Brinker**
Division of Translational Oncology, National Center for Tumor Diseases (NCT), German Cancer Research Center (DKFZ), Heidelberg, Germany

**Tim Holland-Letz**
Division of Biostatistics, German Cancer Research Center, Heidelberg, Germany

**Jochen Sven Utikal**
Department of Dermatology, Heidelberg University, Mannheim, Germany
Skin Cancer Unit, German Cancer Research Center, Heidelberg, Germany

**Axel Hauschild**
Department of Dermatology, University Hospital Schleswig-Holstein, Kiel, Germany

**Dirk Schadendorf and Wiebke Sondermann**
Department of Dermatology, University Hospital Essen, Essen, Germany

**Marta Szymoniak-Lipska and Dorota Jenerowicz**
Department of Dermatology, Poznan University of Medical Sciences, Poznan, Poland

**Adriana Polańska and Ryszard Żaba**
Department of Dermatology and Venereology, Poznan University of Medical Sciences, Poznan, Poland

**Adam Lipski**
Department of Urology, Poznań University of Medical Sciences, Poznan, Poland

**Arieh Gomolin, Elena Netchiporouk and Ivan V. Litvinov**
Division of Dermatology, McGill University Health Centre, Montreal, QC, Canada

**Xiaohua Shen**
Princess Alexandra Hospital, Woolloongabba, QLD, Australia

**H. Peter Soyer**
Princess Alexandra Hospital, Woolloongabba, QLD, Australia
Dermatology Research Centre, The University of Queensland Diamantina Institute, The University of Queensland, Brisbane, QLD, Australia
Department of Dermatology, Princess Alexandra Hospital, Brisbane, QLD, Australia

**Harrison A. Edwards**
Princess Alexandra Hospital, Woolloongabba, QLD, Australia
School of Public Health, University of Queensland, Herston, QLD, Australia
Dermatology Research Centre, The University of Queensland Diamantina Institute, The University of Queensland, Brisbane, QLD, Australia

**Rocío del Amor, Sandra Morales, Adrián Colomer and Valery Naranjo**
Instituto de Investigación e Innovación en Bioingeniería, I3B, Universitat Politècnica de València, Valencia, Spain

**Mette Mogensen**
Department of Dermatology, Bispebjerg Hospital, University of Copenhagen, Copenhagen, Denmark

**Mikkel Jensen, Niels M. Israelsen and Ole Bang**
DTU Fotonik, Department of Photonics Engineering, Technical University of Denmark, Kongens Lyngby, Denmark

**Chen-Yu Zhu, Yu-Kun Wang, Chang Shu, Jun-Cheng Wang and Jie Liu**
Department of Dermatology, State Key Laboratory of Complex Severe and Rare Diseases, Peking Union Medical College Hospital, Chinese Academy of Medical Sciences and Peking Union Medical College, Beijing, China

**Hai-Peng Chen, Kun-Lun Gao and Li-Feng Yan**
DeepWise AI Lab, Beijing, China

**Yi-Guang Yang and Feng-Ying Xie**
Image Processing Center, School of Astronautics, Beihang University, Beijing, China

**Achim Hekler, Eva Krieghoff-Henning, Roman Maron and Max Schmitt**
National Center for Tumor Diseases, German Cancer Research Center, Heidelberg, Germany

**Jakob N. Kather**
National Center for Tumor Diseases, German Cancer Research Center, Heidelberg, Germany
Department of Medicine III, RWTH University Hospital Aachen, Aachen, Germany

**Jochen S. Utikal**
Department of Dermatology, Heidelberg University, Mannheim, Germany
Skin Cancer Unit, German Cancer Research Center, Heidelberg, Germany

**Friedegund Meier and Frank F. Gellrich**
Skin Cancer Center at the University Cancer Centre and National Center for Tumor Diseases Dresden, Dresden, Germany
Department of Dermatology, University Hospital Carl Gustav Carus, Technische Universität Dresden, Dresden, Germany

**Julius Upmeier zu Belzen**
Berlin Institute of Health (BIH), Charité, Berlin, Germany

**Lars French and Justin G. Schlager**
Department of Dermatology and Allergology, Ludwig Maximilian University of Munich, Munich, Germany

**Kamran Ghoreschi and Tabea Wilhelm**
Department of Dermatology, Venereology and Allergology, Charité–Universitätsmedizin Berlin, Berlin, Germany

**Heinz Kutzner**
Dermatopathology Laboratory, Friedrichshafen, Germany

**Carola Berking and Markus V. Heppt**
Department of Dermatology, University Hospital Erlangen, Erlangen, Germany

**Sebastian Haferkamp**
Department of Dermatology, University Hospital Regensburg, Regensburg, Germany

**Bastian Schilling**
Department of Dermatology, University Hospital Würzburg, Würzburg, Germany

**Benjamin Izar**
Department of Medical Oncology, Dana-Farber Cancer Institute, Boston, MA, United States

**Stefan Fröhling**
National Center for Tumor Diseases, German Cancer Research Center, Heidelberg, Germany
Translational Cancer Epigenomics, Division of Translational Medical Oncology, German Cancer Research Center (DKFZ), Heidelberg, Germany

**Daniel B. Lipka**
National Center for Tumor Diseases, German Cancer Research Center, Heidelberg, Germany
Translational Cancer Epigenomics, Division of Translational Medical Oncology, German Cancer Research Center (DKFZ), Heidelberg, Germany
Faculty of Medicine, Medical Center, Otto-von-Guericke-University, Magdeburg, Germany

**Sam Polesie, Martin Gillstedt and John Paoli**
Department of Dermatology and Venereology, Institute of Clinical Sciences, Sahlgrenska Academy, University of Gothenburg, Gothenburg, Sweden
Region Västra Götaland, Sahlgrenska University Hospital, Department of Dermatology and Venereology, Gothenburg, Sweden

**Phillip H. McKee**
Retired, Boston, MA, United States

**Jerad M. Gardner**
Department of Laboratory Medicine, Geisinger Medical Center, Danville, PA, United States

**Jan Siarov and Noora Neittaanmäki**
Region Västra Götaland, Sahlgrenska University Hospital, Department of Dermatology and Venereology, Gothenburg, Sweden
Department of Pathology, Institute of Biomedicine, Sahlgrenska Academy, University of Gothenburg, Gothenburg, Sweden

**Raquel Sousa**
Department of Telemedicine, Hospital Israelita Albert Einstein, São Paulo, Brazil

**Mara Giavina-Bianchi, Maria Fernanda Dias Azevedo, Raquel Machado Sousa and Eduardo Cordioli**
Department of Telemedicine, Hospital Israelita Albert Einstein, São Paulo, Brazil

**Huaxu Liu, Yan Lin and Xiaofeng Shan**
Shandong Provincial Institute of Dermatology and Venereology, Shandong First Medical University & Shandong Academy of Medical Sciences, Jinan, China

**Leilei Wang**
Shandong Cancer Hospital and Institute, Shandong First Medical University & Shandong Academy of Medical Sciences, Jinan, China

**Xiuli Wang, Hui Wang, Zhenyu Zhong, Liyun Zheng, Yifan Wang, Ze Guo and Hui Li**
Department of Dermatology, The First Affiliated Hospital of Anhui Medical University, Hefei, China
Key Laboratory of Dermatology (Anhui Medical University), Ministry of Education, Hefei, China
Inflammation and Immune Mediated Diseases Laboratory of Anhui Province, Hefei, China

**Min Gao**
Department of Dermatology, The First Affiliated Hospital of Anhui Medical University, Hefei, China
Key Laboratory of Dermatology (Anhui Medical University), Ministry of Education, Hefei, China
Inflammation and Immune Mediated Diseases Laboratory of Anhui Province, Hefei, China
Shandong Cancer Hospital and Institute, Shandong First Medical University & Shandong Academy of Medical Sciences, Jinan, China

**Liam J. Caffery**
Centre for Online, Centre for Health Services Research, The University of Queensland, Brisbane, QLD, Australia
Dermatology Research Centre, The University of Queensland Diamantina Institute, The University of Queensland, Brisbane, QLD, Australia

**Veronica Rotemberg and Jochen Weber**
Dermatology Service, Department of Medicine, Memorial Sloan Kettering Cancer Center, New York, NY, United States

**Josep Malvehy**
Department of Dermatology, Institut d'Investigacions Biomèdiques August Pi i Sunyer, Hospital Clinic of Barcelona, University of Barcelona, Barcelona, Spain

**David Clunie**
PixelMed Publishing, Bangor, PA, United States

**Zygmunt Adamski and Aleksandra Dańczak-Pazdrowska**
Department of Dermatology, Poznań University of Medical Sciences, Poznań, Poland

**Elżbieta Paszyńska**
Department of Integrated Dentistry, Poznań University of Medical Sciences, Poznań, Poland

**Lin Feng**
Chongqing Hospital of Traditional Chinese Medicine, Chongqing, China

**Hongxiao Chen**
Linyi People's Hospital, Linyi, China

**Hongyu Yang**
Department of Pathology, St. Vincent Evansville Medical Center, Evansville, IN, United States

**Marta Cullell-Dalmau, Sergio Noé and Carlo Manzo**
The QuBI Lab, Facultat de Ciències i Tecnologia, Universitat de Vic - Universitat Central de Catalunya, Vic, Spain

**Marta Otero-Viñas**
Tissue Repair and Regeneration Laboratory, Facultat de Ciències i Tecnologia, Universitat de Vic - Universitat Central de Catalunya, Vic, Spain

**Ivan Meić**
The QuBI Lab, Facultat de Ciències i Tecnologia, Universitat de Vic - Universitat Central de Catalunya, Vic, Spain
University of Zagreb, Zagreb, Croatia

**Xiangqian Li, Baifu Chen, Jianzhong Zhang and Cheng Zhou**
Department of Dermatology, Peking University People's Hospital, Beijing, China

**Xi Chen**
Department of Dermatology, Peking University People's Hospital, Beijing, China
Department of Dermatology, Beijing Tongren Hospital, Capital Medical University, Beijing, China

**Wenju Wang, Lixin Fu, Bei Kan and Yonghong Lu**
Department of Dermatovenereology, Chengdu Second People's Hospital, Chengdu, China

**Yansen Liao and Xiaodong Peng**
Department of Oncology, Chengdu Second People's Hospital, Chengdu, China

**Sophie Soyeon Lim**
Alfred Health, Melbourne, VIC, Australia

**Jungyoon Ohn and Je-Ho Mun**
Department of Dermatology, Seoul National University College of Medicine, Seoul, South Korea
Institute of Human-Environment Interface Biology, Seoul National University, Seoul, South Korea

**Li Li**
Department of Dermatology, Plastic Surgery Hospital, Chinese Academy of Medical Sciences and Peking Union Medical College, Beijing, China

**Jiaosheng Xu**
Department of Dermatology, Beijing Children's Hospital, National Center for Children's Health, Capital Medical University, Beijing, China

**Siwei Wang**
Department of Radiology, Beijing Children's Hospital, National Center for Children's Health, Capital Medical University, Beijing, China

**Jun Yang**
Institute of Biomedical Engineering, Chinese Academy of Medical Sciences, Tianjin, China

# Index

www.ingramcontent.com/pod-product-compliance
Lightning Source LLC
LaVergne TN
LVHW082147200926
848484LV00008B/2118